"Just as *Freedom of the Hills* is the go-to bible of mountaineering, *Conditioning for Outdoor Fitness* could become THE reference manual for health and fitness information geared for an outdoor lifestyle."
—*Adventure Sports Journal*

"Whether you're a hard-core athlete or someone who wants to get back into shape, the second edition of *Conditioning for Outdoor Fitness* . . . has practical information you can use."
—*Star-Gazette* (Elmira, NY)

"America could do well to read this exhaustive guide."
—*Reno Gazette-Journal*

"Thorough explanations of exercise physiology, with solid chapters on balance, stretching, structuring an aerobic workout, functional core and strength training."
—*Arkansas Democrat Gazette* (Little Rock, AR)

"This book addresses the entire scope of outdoor fitness better than perhaps any other publication . . . It's well-written . . . The doctor and trainer [authors] are a near-perfect combination to discuss outdoor conditioning. The cover is a fantastic motivator itself."
—*Deseret Morning News* (Salt Lake City, UT)

"Offers people of all fitness levels something to help them to the next level."
—*Great Falls Tribune*

"The one book . . . where an outdoorsman can turn for all fitness needs."
—*Tennessean* (Nashville, TN)

"Just what every outdoor enthusiast and every trainer of an outdoor enthusiast needs on the bookshelf."
—*Fitness Business Pro*

"Will help keep both the enthusiasm and fitness level on an upward swing all year-round . . . This book is excellent, and a 'must-have' for your library."
—*Ottawa Outdoors*

"If you are serious about conditioning, this is the book for you."
—*The Cascadian*

"Very thorough, covering all aspects of fitness, diet, and conditioning for all parts of the body . . . One of the best aspects of the book is how it goes through each exercise explaining what part of the body is strengthened and how to make it most effective."
—*Dayton Daily News*

"Full of helpful bits of information."
—*Cedar Rapids Gazette*

"As outdoors recreation becomes more specialized, the second edition of *Conditioning for Outdoor Fitness* is likely to become a bible of sorts . . . It is as scientifically thorough as one can imagine . . . This comprehensive guide is all-inclusive."
—*Tucson Citizen*

"Helpful guide to functional exercise and nutrition."
—*St. George Magazine*

"Extremely easy to use . . . Simply pick a sport, and turn to the corresponding page and pictures and details on how to do the exercises."
—*Tacoma News Tribune*

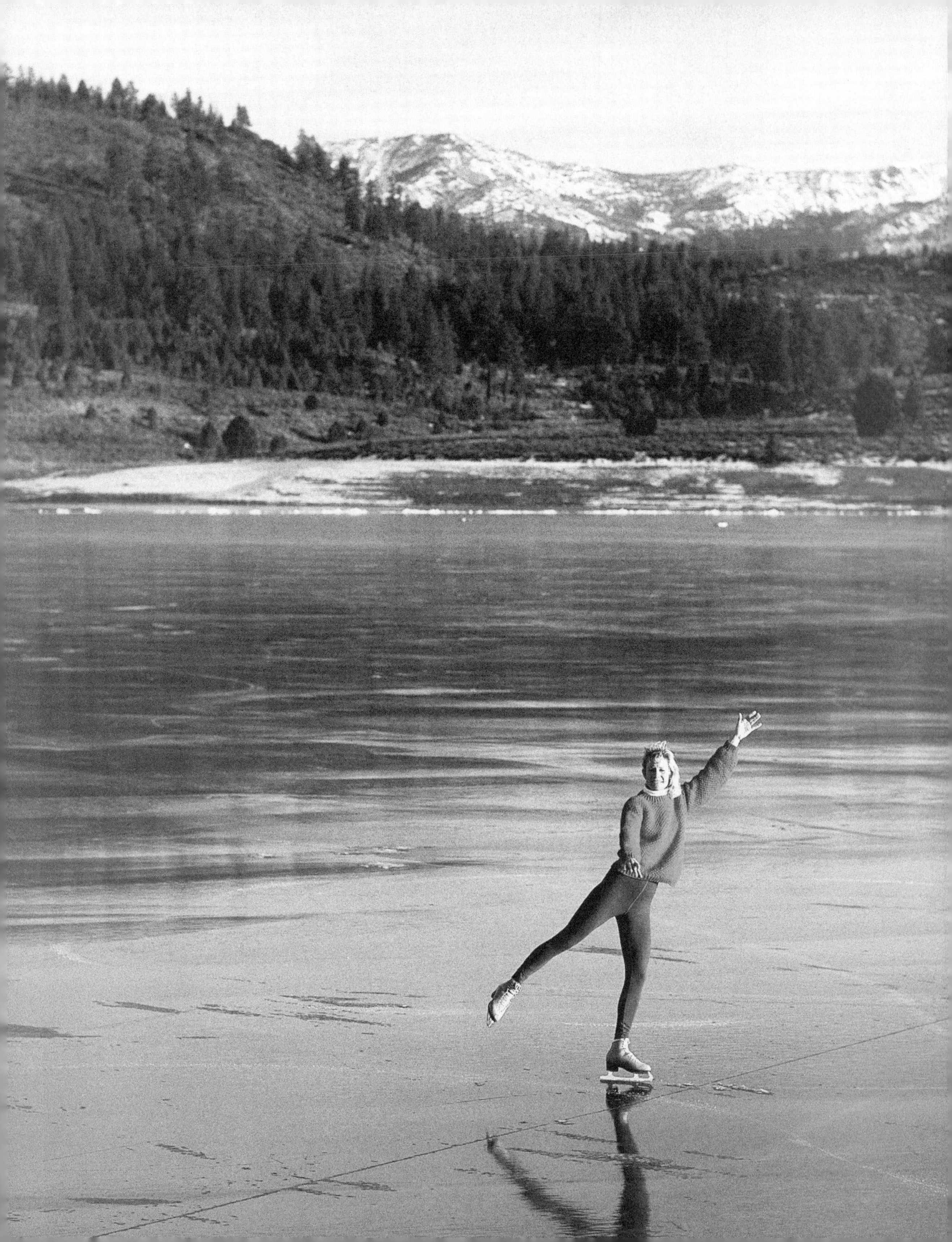

FUNCTIONAL EXERCISE AND NUTRITION FOR EVERY BODY

Conditioning for Outdoor Fitness

SECOND EDITION

David Musnick, M.D.
and Mark Pierce, A.T.C.

THE MOUNTAINEERS BOOKS

To my father, Henry Musnick, M.D., who took me on my first hike when I was in elementary school. My early introduction to aerobic exercise was fast walking with him. He set an example for me that persistence and hard work are important in order to achieve life's important goals.

To my father James P. Pierce: father, husband, scholar, professor, musician, linguist, and gentleman farmer. My fondest memories are those of working with him on the farm, which taught me the life values of hard work, focus, and dedication to one's goals. Sie sind lieb liebten und vermißten.

THE MOUNTAINEERS BOOKS
is the nonprofit publishing arm of The Mountaineers Club, an organization founded in 1906 and dedicated to the exploration, preservation, and enjoyment of outdoor and wilderness areas.

1001 SW Klickitat Way, Suite 201, Seattle, WA 98134

First edition 1999, second edition: first printing 2004, second printing 2005

Published simultaneously in Great Britain by Cordee, 3a DeMontfort Street, Leicester, England, LE1 7HD

Printed in the United States of America

Project Editor: Julie Van Pelt
Copyeditor: Julie Van Pelt
Cover and interior design: The Mountaineers Books
Layout Artist: Ani Rucki
Front cover photograph: *Jumping off rock onto trail* © PatitucciPhoto
Back cover photographs: © Getty Images/EyeWire
Frontispiece: *Woman figure skating on lake* © Getty Images/Photodisc

Library of Congress Cataloging-in-Publication Data
Musnick, David.
Conditioning for outdoor fitness : functional exercise and nutrition for every body / by David Musnick and Mark Pierce.— 2nd ed.
p. cm.
Includes bibliographical references and index.
ISBN 0-89886-756-8 (pbk.)
1. Exercise. 2. Physical fitness. 3. Outdoor recreation. I. Pierce, Mark. II.itle.
GV481.M89 2004
613.7'11—dc22

2004013588

Printed on recycled paper

Seattle Running Company
919 E. Pine St.
Seattle, WA, 98122
(206) 329-1466

Fit Specialist PK

1	9780898867565	25.00
	Conditioning for Outdoor Fitness, 2n	

Sub Total	$25.00
Tax	$2.20
Total	$27.20
Cash:	$40.00
Change	$12.80

Thank You!
Are You A Club Member Yet?
www.seattlerunningcompnay.com

06/18/06 13:07:38
INVOICE: 18 Register 7SU

Seattle Running Company
919 E. Pine St.
Seattle, WA, 98122
(206) 329-1466

Fit Specialist PK

1	9780898867565	25.00
	Conditioning for Outdoor Fitness, 2n	

Sub Total	$25.00
Tax	$2.20
Total	$27.20
Cash:	$40.00
Change	$12.80

Thank You!
Are You A Club Member Yet?
www.seattlerunningcompnay.com

06/18/06 13:07:38
INVOICE: 18 Register 750

Contents

Preface to the Second Edition 7
Introduction 9

PART I. BASIC PRINCIPLES

1. Exercise Physiology 24
   Energy Production; Cardiac, Respiratory, and Muscle System Function; and Training Adaptations
2. Nutritional Considerations for Conditioning 29
3. Aerobic Conditioning and Interval Training 44
4. Warm-Up and Stretching 65
5. Functional Core and Strength Training 83
6. Balance and Agility Training 125
7. Training Concepts, Conditioning Goals, and Program Planning 154
8. Creative Use of the Outdoors in Training 161

PART II. BODY REGIONS

9. Anatomy and Musculoskeletal Injury: Prevention and Treatment 176
10. The Abdominals 185
11. The Knee, Thigh, Hip, and Buttock 206
12. The Ankle and Leg 226
13. The Foot 228
14. The Neck, Mid Back, and Low Back/Core 232
15. The Shoulder, Upper Torso, and Arm 244
16. The Forearm and Hand 273

PART III. CONDITIONING FOR OUTDOOR ACTIVITIES

17. Conditioning for Hiking, Backpacking, and Snowshoeing 280
18. Conditioning for Scrambling and Rock Climbing 285
19. Conditioning for Mountaineering 297
20. Conditioning for Snowboarding and Skiing 301
21. Conditioning for Canoeing, Kayaking, and Rowing 318
22. Conditioning for Road and Mountain Bicycling 327
23. Conditioning for Running 337
24. Conditioning for Windsurfing 347

PART IV. OPTIMAL WELLNESS

25. Body Posture and Movement Patterns 350
An Aston-Patterning™ Approach

26. Exercise, Nutrition, and Lifestyle for Optimal Wellness 360

27. Conditioning for Seniors, Deconditioned Individuals, and People with Neurodegenerative Conditions 369

28. Special Issues for the Conditioning Woman 374

29. Weight Loss: A Functional and Holistic Approach 378

30. Energy, Fatigue, Overtraining, and Exercising with Fibromyalgia 387

31. Arthritis and Nutrient Support for Joint Health 390

Appendix 392
Selected References 393
Index 402
Acknowledgments 410
About the Contributors 411
Photo and Illustration Credits 414

Preface to the Second Edition

This second edition has been extensively updated and revised. Chapter 2 has significantly new material on food quality, protein, and the glycemic index. Chapter 5 has been completely revised and updated to include information on core strengthening and activating the core in all exercises. Strength training for injury prevention, weight management, and for slowing down the aging process is also discussed, and new exercises with Freemotion machines have been added. Chapter 6 about balance is completely new, with a series of balance self-tests and new information on balance equipment. Chapter 9 includes new information on ligament laxity and muscle recruitment issues. All of the body region chapters have been extensively updated with new exercises. Chapter 14 is now a state-of-the-art core and spine chapter with a series of core and spine exercises.

Part III offers revised activity-specific programs, especially in regards to balance and lower-body exercises. Part IV is completely new, with most chapters bringing new material, including nutrition and conditioning for optimal health, as well as chapters for seniors, weight loss, and energy and fatigue issues. The chapter on women's conditioning has been significantly updated.

NOTE ABOUT SAFETY

The exercises in this book vary in difficulty. When you do these exercises you are doing them at your own risk. The authors and the publisher are in no way responsible for your outcomes from doing these exercises or for any injury you may incur. Please consult your health-care professional with any questions about whether a particular exercise is risky for your condition.

David Musnick, M.D., and Mark Pierce, A.T.C.

Safety is an important concern in all conditioning activities. No book can alert you to every hazard or anticipate the limitations of every reader. The descriptions of techniques and procedures in this book are intended to provide general information. This is not a complete text on physical conditioning and nutrition. Nothing substitutes for formal instruction, routine practice, advice from health-care practitioners, and plenty of experience. When you follow any of the procedures described here, you assume responsibility for your own safety and health. Use *Conditioning for Outdoor Fitness* as a general guide to further information.

The Mountaineers Books

Introduction

This is an exercise and nutrition guide for everyone. It is for the average person, the athlete, the outdoor enthusiast, and for health-care professionals, including physical therapists, trainers, and all types of physicians. No matter who you are, what you do, what your sport or activity, whether you prefer indoor or outdoor activities, whether you are an experienced athlete or are just beginning to exercise and would like to develop a program tailored to your needs, this book is for you.

There are many books about exercise, but no one book written for the layperson combines comprehensive information on functional and core strength training, basic exercise concepts, posture, movement patterns, balance, and agility with detailed discussions of exercises that embody state-of-the-art thinking on these subjects. Written by specialists in sports medicine, nutrition, physical therapy, fitness training, and athletic training, and designed to be the one volume you turn to for all your conditioning needs, this book:

- Can be used by people of all ages.
- Teaches basic concepts so that you will be able to better evaluate exercises, programs, and equipment.
- Contains many unique exercises.
- Focuses on functional conditioning so your muscles and your aerobic system are trained in ways that mimic how you actually use them in indoor or outdoor activities.
- Uses a body-region approach designed to increase your knowledge of your musculoskeletal system and how it functions.
- Will help you develop awareness of muscle imbalances in your own body and how to correct them.
- Will help you self-test and improve your balance.
- Emphasizes safety and injury prevention.
- Emphasizes proper movement patterns and posture.
- Places particular emphasis on the important areas of the back/core and neck, both in terms of maintaining their health and strength and in exercising safely.
- Extensively details the health benefits of exercise.
- Will help you set fitness goals and plan your own conditioning program.
- Devotes entire chapters to the specific exercises required to excel in particular activities.
- Gives you state-of-the-art nutrition and wellness information.

The structure and function of the musculoskeletal and cardiorespiratory systems have been extensively studied, but much of the research is unavailable to laypeople, or when it is available is written in language aimed at scientists or medical personnel. Because we feel strongly that knowing these basic concepts will enhance both your understanding of your body and the hows and whys of exercising, this book is packed with the most up-to-date information, translated into terms that you can understand. In the more complex sections, you may find you need to read carefully, so take a deep breath and take it slow, but do take the time to understand this material. Doing so will benefit you far more than any recipe list of generic exercises.

Many people find that they can get by with cars that they take to the shop for maintenance, without learning about the car's parts or how it functions. This approach might work fine for cars, but it does not work well for the human body, especially the musculoskeletal system. You can greatly improve your present and future health just by improving how you sit, stand, move, nourish, and condition the amazing machine that is your body.

Our bodies are physiological and biomechanical structures that change gradually with time. In order to optimize your time and health and to maximally enjoy your outdoor activities, you need to choose wisely from a wide range of options for maintaining and conditioning your musculoskeletal and cardiovascular systems. It can be difficult to get advice on what type of conditioning will best achieve a particular goal or on how to devise an exercise program that is challenging, that is specific to and functionally supportive of your chosen activities, and that keeps you interested. Although you might employ the help of a health-care or fitness professional along the way, ultimately you are in charge of your own conditioning program. The components of any conditioning program should address:

- Basic aerobic fitness and endurance.
- Muscular strength (for tone and function).
- Balance and agility.
- Flexibility.
- Activity-specific coordination and skill.
- Nutrition for wellness, weight management, and optimal performance.

In this book, we emphasize functional and activity-specific training not only because they are extremely important but also because they are overlooked in most fitness-training programs and books. *Functional conditioning* is exercise in which your muscles and joints are deployed in positions similar to those of the particular sport or activity being pursued; in these exercises the muscles and joints have the same relationship to gravity and must meet the same, or similar, balance and coordination challenges as in the activity itself. We have also integrated into the exercises presented the concepts of proper posture, core activization, safe movement patterns, and injury prevention.

HOW TO USE THIS BOOK

This book is organized into four parts: Part I covers the basic principles of conditioning; Part II discusses the anatomy and function of specific body regions and details appropriate exercises for each; Part III focuses on conditioning for specific outdoor activities; and Part IV addresses general fitness, nutrition, and wellness, including chapters on posture and movement patterns, conditioning and nutrition for optimal wellness, exercise plans for seniors, women's conditioning concerns, weight loss, and discussion of fatigue and fibromyalgia. Each chapter begins by highlighting its objectives; you can get an overview of any chapter by reading its objectives as well as its brief introduction and the "practical point" pullouts found throughout.

The main exercise chapters are chapters 3, 4, 5, 6, 8, 10, 11, 14, and 15. The main nutrition and wellness chapters are chapters 2 and 26–30.

The chapters in **Part I, Basic Principles**, cover exercise physiology, sports nutrition, aerobic conditioning, warm-up and stretching, strength training, balance and agility training, planning your conditioning program, and training outdoors. **Chapter 3**, Aerobic Conditioning and Interval Training, **chapter 4**, Warm-Up and Stretching, and **chapter 5**, Functional Core and Strength Training, lay the foundations for building endurance and strength and should be read before moving on to the activity-specific chapters. **Chapter 6**, Balance and Agility Training, will help you test balance and use balance and agility exercises in your program. **Chapter 7**, Training Concepts, Conditioning Goals, and Program Planning, will help you if you have a specific activity goal (climbing a mountain, biking a long ride, running a race, etc.), if you plan on a season of physically demanding activity such as skiing or climbing, or if you want to make progress in your conditioning program. **Chapter 8**, Creative Use of the Outdoors in Training, is an excellent source of exercises as well as ideas on how to improve your agility, add diversity to your training, and how to exercise in outdoor settings.

Part II, Body Regions, educates you about the anatomy, common muscle imbalances, movement faults, and preferred ways to functionally exercise your major body regions. It contains descriptions and pictures of particular exercises as well as recommendations on how to keep a particular body region in shape. Read **chapter 9**, Anatomy and Musculoskeletal Injury: Prevention and Treatment, for an overview before reading about a specific body region. It will give you a lot of basic information about anatomy, medical terms, and how to prevent injuries. Chapters 10–16 present the most current and exciting information from the physical therapy and sports medicine fields. Much of this material is normally available to individuals only after they have been injured. Why wait for an injury?

The exercises in Part II and throughout the book have been designed by physical therapists, athletic trainers, and sports medicine doctors, all of whom are experts in their fields. Safe positioning and movement patterns are emphasized, and for many exercises additional variations are given as well as cross-references to further choices in other chapters. **Chapter 10**, The Abdominals, presents unique abdominal and core exercises and should be read by anyone seeking to improve tone, balance, or back health. **Chapter 11**, The Knee, Thigh, Hip, and Buttock, presents a comprehensive set of functional lower-body exercises; it should be read by anyone doing a general conditioning program or performing any lower-body activity. Everyone should read **chapter 14**, The Neck, Mid Back, and Low Back/Core. Knowing about how to keep your spine safe during exercises is essential for a healthy strength-training program. **Chapter 15**, The Shoulder, Upper Torso, and Arm, discusses common areas of injury. Problems with these parts of your body can keep you away from activities for prolonged periods, and this body region is frequently underemphasized when it comes to safety and muscle balance.

The chapters in **Part III, Conditioning for Outdoor Activities**, provide exercises and training programs to help you prepare for specific activities. The chapters include activity-specific exercises as well as cross-references to exercises found throughout the book that are applicable to the given activity. If you engage in any of the activities discussed, you will benefit from learning about common muscle imbalances and training activity errors. You will learn more about functional exercises and activity-specific training to help you achieve your goals. Some chapters contain conditioning plans that are examples of training programs, with time scales you can use or modify. Before launching into conditioning for your chosen activity, be sure to read Part I's chapter 3, Aerobic Conditioning and Interval Training, and chapter 5, Functional Core and Strength Training. See Part II's chapter 9, Anatomy and Musculoskeletal Injury: Prevention and Treatment, for illustrations of skeletal and muscular anatomy. See the relevant body region chapter(s) in Part II for information on the muscles or joint areas discussed in an activity chapter.

Part IV, Optimal Wellness, contains chapters of special interest to any person interested in staying healthy, slowing the aging process, and learning about healthy nutrition. **Chapter 25**, Body Posture and Movement Patterns, is important for better understanding neutral spine posture and movement patterns. If you are trying to stay healthy and prevent disease, **chapter 26**, Exercise, Nutrition, and Lifestyle for Optimal Wellness, is for you. It will also give you a vast amount of information about healthy lifestyle and nutrition choices. If you are over the age of 60, start with **chapter 27**, Conditioning for Seniors, Deconditioned Individuals, and People with Neurodegenerative Conditions, in order to develop a safe program of exercise. Women will get additional information on exercise and nutrition in **chapter 28**, Special Issues for the Conditioning Woman. **Chapter 29**, Weight Loss: A Functional and Holistic Approach, is for you if you are trying to lose weight. **Chapter 30**, Energy, Fatigue, Overtraining, and Exercising with Fibromyalgia, is appropriate if you are feeling fatigue, have fibromyalgia, or wish to prevent either. Finally, **chapter 31**, Arthritis and Nutrient Support for Joint Health, addresses the special exercise and nutrition needs of people who experience varying levels of joint pain.

In this book, most distances are listed in inches, feet, yards, and miles, and most other units of measurement are also in standard American units. In some chapters, metric measurements are used for chemical and physiological data; in discussions of running, shorter distances and marathon distances are in meters or kilometers (abbreviated as K). The Appendix gives conversions for standard and metric units of measurement.

Where Should You Start?

If you are just beginning an exercise program, read chapters 3, 4, 5, 6, and 14. This will help you develop a basic understanding of aerobic exercises and strength training. Seniors, add chapter 27.

If you are an outdoor enthusiast, start with chapters 3, 5, 6, and 14 and then move to the chapter describing your chosen activity.

If you are a health-care professional, start with chapters 3, 5, 6, 9, and 14 as your base of knowledge for exercise planning. Use chapter 6 to test your patients'/clients' balance and to select appropriate balance exercises. Choose exercises from chapters 5, 6, or any of the body-region chapters (11–16) to help your patients/clients improve their strength and tone. You can use the exercises throughout the book and the nutrition chapters to build comprehensive exercise and nutrition programs for your patients/clients, no matter what their level of fitness.

About the Exercises

To assist you in keeping track of the many exercises described in this book, the following system has been devised. Each exercise, beginning with Exercise 1 in chapter 4, has been assigned a unique number, which is also used to identify any photographs or drawings used to illustrate it. If more than one part of an exercise is shown, each part is labeled, for example, 1a, 1b, and so on. Variations of a particular exercise are labeled 1.1, 1.2, and so on. Illustrations or photographs that are not exercise-specific are identified by captions that include the word "figure" (Figure 1, etc.).

Each exercise description includes equipment, purpose, and technique; some exercises also discuss variations as well as tips and precautions.

In each exercise's "purpose" summary, icons indicate the exercise's appropriateness for specific outdoor activities (see Figure 1a). Figure 1b, Exercises by Activity, generally shows which exercises are appropriate for any given activity; but for detailed activity-specific exercise programs and explanations, please refer to the activity chapters in Part III.

Each of us has only one body, but we all have a wide range of potential in our aerobic and musculoskeletal systems. The conditioning programs you choose can affect your motion and strength capabilities and your tendency to stay healthy or become injured. You can enhance your enjoyment of life and of your activities by choosing the most appropriate conditioning programs. Take charge of your health and maximize your potential by learning as much as possible about your body and how it functions. Become involved—choose the exercise and training that is right for you. We hope that this book will be an excellent resource for you as you move in that direction.

FIGURE 1a. OUTDOOR-ACTIVITY ICONS

- climbing, gym or rock
- mountaineering, rock or glacier or both
- scrambling, nontechnical peak ascents
- hiking
- backpacking
- snowshoeing
- downhill skiing
- telemark skiing
- cross-country and skate skiing
- snowboarding
- cycling, road or mountain bike
- running or jogging
- canoeing
- kayaking
- crew
- windsurfing
- general conditioning

FIGURE 1b. EXERCISES BY ACTIVITY

Exercise	climbing	mountaineering	scrambling	hiking	backpacking	snowshoeing	downhill skiing	telemark skiing	cross-country/ skate skiing	snowboarding	cycling road/ mountain bike	running/jogging	canoeing	kayaking	crew	windsurfing	general conditioning
CHAPTER 4. WARM-UP AND STRETCHING																	
1. Hamstring Stretch, p. 72	●	●	●	●	●	●	●	●	●	●	●	●	●	●	●		●
2. Sitting and Supine Active Hamstring Stretch, p. 73							●				●		●	●	●		●
3. Quadriceps Stretch, p. 73	●	●	●	●	●	●	●	●	●	●	●	●	●	●	●	●	●
4. Active Quadriceps Stretch, p. 74				●	●	●	●	●	●	●		●					●
5. Iliotibial Band (ITB) Stretch, p. 74	●	●	●	●	●	●	●	●	●	●	●	●	●	●	●	●	●
6. Hip Flexor Stretch, p. 75	●	●	●	●	●	●	●	●	●	●	●	●	●	●	●		●
7. Active Hip Stretch, p. 76	●	●	●	●	●	●	●					●				●	●
8. Adductor Stretch, p. 76	●	●	●	●	●	●	●	●	●	●	●	●	●	●	●	●	●
9. Heel Cord (Achilles) Stretch, p. 77	●	●	●	●	●	●	●				●	●	●	●	●		●
10. Active Squat Stretch to the Heel Cord, p. 77							●					●				●	●
11. Chest Stretch, p. 78	●	●	●					●	●	●	●	●	●	●	●	●	●
12. Rhomboid and Posterior Shoulder Stretch, p. 78	●	●	●	●	●	●	●	●	●	●	●		●	●	●	●	●
13. Active Shoulder Stretch, p. 78	●	●	●	●	●	●	●	●	●	●	●		●	●	●	●	●
14. Rotator Cuff and Shoulder Capsule Active Stretch, p. 79	●	●	●	●	●	●	●	●	●	●	●		●	●	●		●
15. Triceps Stretch, p. 80	●	●	●	●	●	●	●	●		●		●	●	●	●	●	●
16. Forearm Stretch, p. 80	●	●	●	●	●		●	●		●	●		●	●	●	●	●
17. Cat/Camel Stretch, p. 81		●		●		●	●		●	●	●	●	●	●	●		●
18. Pelvic Circles, p. 81	●	●	●	●	●	●	●	●	●				●	●	●		●
19. Active Spine Rotations, p. 82	●	●	●	●	●	●					●						●
CHAPTER 5. FUNCTIONAL CORE AND STRENGTH TRAINING																	
20. X-Combo, p. 104	●	●	●										●	●			●
21. Core Cable Flys, p. 105	●	●	●				●	●	●	●	●	●	●	●		●	●
22. Dynamic Core: Chest-Abdominal Exercise, p. 106	●	●	●				●	●		●	●	●					●

Exercise	climbing	mountaineering	scrambling	hiking	backpacking	snowshoeing	downhill skiing	telemark skiing	cross-country/ skate skiing	snowboarding	cycling, road/ mountain bike	running/jogging	canoeing	kayaking	crew	windsurfing	general conditioning
23. Standing and Seated Torso Rotations, p. 107	•	•	•				•	•	•		•	•	•	•	•	•	•
24. Standing Push-Pull Core Rotations, p. 108									•		•			•			•
25. Staggered Stance Overhead Diagonal Arm Crosses, p. 109		•	•								•			•			•
26. Squat with Alternate Forward-Overhead Presses, p. 110		•	•	•	•								•	•	•	•	
27. Single-Leg Balance Alternate Biceps Curl, p. 111						•	•	•	•	•		•					•
28. Forward Lunge with a Biceps Curl, p. 112	•	•	•	•	•	•	•	•	•	•	•	•					•
29. Anterior Lunge with Opposite Knee Reach, p. 113	•	•	•	•	•		•	•	•	•	•	•	•	•			
30. Lunge Matrix/Combos, p. 113	•	•	•			•	•	•	•	•		•	•	•		•	
31. Lawnmower Pulls to a Row or an External Rotation, p. 115	•	•			•	•	•	•		•	•	•			•	•	
32. Double-Arm Combination Row Squat, p. 118	•	•					•	•	•				•	•	•	•	•
33. Single-Arm Pulley Rows, p. 119	•	•						•					•	•	•	•	•
34. Standing Latissimus (Lat) Pull-Down, p. 119	•	•	•		•	•	•	•	•	•						•	•
35. Anterior Step-Up with Overhead Shoulder Press, p. 120	•	•	•			•		•	•								•
36. Anterior Step-Up with Resisted Shoulder Extension, p. 121	•	•	•	•	•	•		•	•		•					•	•
37. Make Your Own Rowing Erg, p. 122													•	•	•		
38. Seated Single-Arm Pulley Pushes, p. 122								•	•				•	•	•		
39. Seated Push-Pull Double-Arm Pulley Rows, p. 123													•	•	•	•	
CHAPTER 6. BALANCE AND AGILITY TRAINING																	
40. (BST). Basic Self-Test, p. 136																	•
41. (BST). Bent-Knee Basic Self-Test, p. 136	•	•	•	•	•		•	•	•	•							•
42. (BST). Sagittal Plane Balance with Arm Swing, p. 137	•	•	•	•	•	•	•	•	•	•	•	•	•	•	•	•	•
43. (BST). Seated Sagittal Plane Balance with Arm Swing, p. 137																	•
44. (BST). Sagittal Plane Balance with Opposite-Leg Swing, p. 138												•					•
45. (BST). Frontal Plane Balance with Arm Swing, p. 138																	•

Exercise	climbing	mountaineering	scrambling	hiking	backpacking	snowshoeing	downhill skiing	telemark skiing	cross-country/ skate skiing	snowboarding	cycling, road/ mountain bike	running/jogging	canoeing	kayaking	crew	windsurfing	general conditioning
46. (BST). Frontal Plane Balance with Opposite-Leg Swing, p. 139	•	•	•	•	•	•	•	•	•	•	•	•				•	•
47. (BST). Transverse Plane Balance with Arm Swing, p. 139	•	•	•	•	•	•	•	•	•	•	•	•				•	•
48. (BST). Transverse Plane Balance with Opposite-Leg/Knee Swing, p. 140	•	•	•	•	•	•	•	•	•	•	•	•				•	•
49. (BST). Single-Leg Balance and Reach with Opposite Foot, p. 140	•	•	•	•	•	•	•	•	•	•	•	•				•	•
50. (BST). Single-Leg Balance and Reach with Both Arms, p. 141	•	•	•	•	•	•	•	•	•	•	•	•				•	•
51. (BST). Frontal Plane Balance and Reach with Opposite Foot, p. 141	•	•	•	•	•	•	•	•	•	•	•	•				•	•
52. (BST). Frontal Plane Balance and Reach with Both Arms, p. 142	•	•	•	•	•	•	•	•	•	•	•	•				•	•
53. (BST). Transverse Plane Balance and Reach with Opposite Foot, p. 142				•	•	•	•	•	•	•	•	•				•	•
54. (BST). Sagittal Plane Lunge, p. 143	•	•	•	•	•	•	•	•	•	•	•	•				•	•
55. (BST). Frontal Plane Lunge, p. 144	•	•	•	•	•	•	•	•	•	•	•	•				•	•
56. (BST). Transverse Plane Lunge, p. 144	•	•	•	•	•	•	•	•	•	•	•	•				•	•
57. Skier/Climber/Cyclist/Windsurfer Position Holds, p. 145	•	•	•				•	•	•	•	•					•	
58. Arm and Leg Balance and Reach, p. 146	•	•	•			•	•	•	•	•		•	•			•	
59. Clock Leg Reach, p. 147	•	•	•	•	•	•	•	•	•	•		•				•	•
60. Single-Leg Stance Upper-Extremity Chopping Pattern, p. 148	•	•	•		•	•	•	•		•	•					•	
61. Single-Leg Ball Toss, p. 149	•	•	•	•	•	•	•	•	•	•		•				•	
62. Sitting Ball Toss, p. 150											•		•	•	•		
63. Rocker Board Sagittal Plane Static Balance, p. 150	•	•			•	•		•	•	•	•	•				•	•
64. Rocker Board Frontal Plane Static Balance, p. 151							•	•	•	•							
65. Wobble Board Static Multiplanar Challenge, p. 151	•	•	•		•	•	•	•	•	•	•	•				•	•
66. Disc Pillow Static Balance, p. 152	•	•	•			•	•	•	•	•	•	•					•
67. Bosu Ball Squat, p. 152	•	•	•		•	•	•	•	•	•	•	•				•	•
68. The Fitter Skiing and Frontal Plane Dynamic Balance, p. 153							•	•	•	•							
69. Body Blade Single-Leg Multiplanar Challenge, p. 153	•	•	•		•	•	•	•	•	•	•	•				•	•

	climbing	mountaineering	scrambling	hiking	backpacking	snowshoeing	downhill skiing	telemark skiing	cross-country/ skate skiing	snowboarding	cycling, road/ mountain bike	running/jogging	canoeing	kayaking	crew	windsurfing	general conditioning
CHAPTER 8. CREATIVE USE OF THE OUTDOORS IN TRAINING																	
70. Outdoor Step-Ups, p. 165	•	•	•	•	•	•		•									
71. Squat Hops and Jumps, p. 166	•	•				•	•	•		•		•					
72. Sitting Ball Rotation, p. 168	•	•	•										•	•	•		
73. Over and Back, p. 168	•	•			•		•	•							•		
74. Dips, p. 169	•	•	•						•				•	•	•		•
75. Pull-Ups, p. 170	•	•	•														•
76. Push-Ups, p. 170	•	•	•								•					•	•
77. Plyometric Push-Ups, p. 171	•	•	•								•					•	
CHAPTER 10. THE ABDOMINALS																	
78. Lower Abdominal Progression, p. 188	•	•	•	•	•	•	•	•	•		•	•	•	•	•	•	•
79. Upper Abdominal Strengthening, p. 191	•	•	•		•	•	•	•	•		•	•	•	•	•		•
80. Torso Rotations: The Twister, p. 193		•	•		•	•	•	•	•	•	•	•	•	•	•	•	•
81. Supine Physioball Alternating Press, p. 194	•	•	•				•	•	•	•	•	•	•	•	•	•	•
82. Squat to Double-Arm Overhead Diagonal Wall Reach, p. 195	•	•	•	•	•	•	•	•	•	•			•	•		•	
83. Staggered Stance Abdominal Crunch with Rotation, p. 196	•	•	•		•	•	•	•	•	•	•		•	•	•	•	•
84. Single-Leg Stance Trunk Side Bend with Medicine Ball, p. 197	•	•	•	•	•	•	•	•	•	•	•	•	•	•	•	•	•
85. Standing Single-Leg Abdominal Challenge with Dynamic Partner Resistance, p. 197	•	•	•		•	•	•	•	•	•	•	•					
86. Single-Leg Balance Overhead Double-Arm Tubing Challenge, p. 198	•	•	•			•	•	•	•	•		•	•	•	•	•	
87. Bosu Ball Core Challenge, p. 199	•	•	•				•	•	•	•	•	•			•	•	•
88. Kneeling Ab Dolly/Roller Core Challenge, p. 201	•	•	•				•	•		•	•		•	•	•		
89. The Prayer, p. 202	•	•	•				•	•	•		•		•	•	•		•
90. The Plank, p. 202							•	•									•
91. The Skier, p. 203							•	•	•								
92. Supine Crunch on Physioball, p. 203	•	•	•	•	•	•							•	•	•	•	•

Exercise	climbing	mountaineering	scrambling	hiking	backpacking	snowshoeing	downhill skiing	telemark skiing	cross-country/ skate skiing	snowboarding	cycling, road/ mountain bike	running/jogging	canoeing	kayaking	crew	windsurfing	general conditioning
93. Supine Ball Toss with Partner, p. 204	•	•					•	•		•	•		•	•	•		
94. Seated Physioball Boaters/Cyclist Reaction Challenge, p. 205											•		•	•	•		
CHAPTER 11. THE KNEE, THIGH, HIP, AND BUTTOCK																	
95. Squat, p. 209	•	•	•	•	•	•	•	•	•	•	•	•	•	•	•	•	•
96. Hamstring Curls, p. 210	•	•	•	•	•	•	•	•	•	•	•	•			•		•
97. Lunges, p. 211	•	•	•	•	•	•	•	•	•	•	•	•	•	•	•	•	•
98. Step-Ups, p. 216	•	•	•	•	•	•	•	•	•	•	•	•					
99. Step-Downs, p. 217	•	•	•	•	•	•	•	•	•	•		•					
100. The Basic Jump, p. 220	•	•			•	•	•	•		•		•			•	•	
101. The Basic Hop, p. 222	•	•	•	•	•	•	•	•	•	•	•	•			•	•	
102. Gluteus Medius Side Lying, p. 223																	•
103. Gluteus Medius Standing Pulley, p. 223																	•
104. Quadruped Gluteus Maximus, p. 224																	•
105. Gluteus Maximus Standing Pulley, p. 224																	•
106. Reverse Lunge, p. 225	•	•	•		•	•	•	•	•	•	•	•				•	•
CHAPTER 14. THE NECK, MID BACK, AND LOW BACK/CORE																	
107. Spine Extension Series, p. 240	•	•	•				•	•		•	•					•	•
108. Suspension Bridge, p. 241																	•
109. T-Pose, p. 242	•	•	•		•	•	•	•	•	•	•	•				•	•
110. Waiter's Bow, p. 243	•	•	•	•	•		•	•	•	•						•	
CHAPTER 15. THE SHOULDER, UPPER TORSO, AND ARM																	
111. Dumbbell Flat Bench Press, p. 248		•	•			•	•	•	•	•	•		•	•	•	•	•
112. Dumbbell Incline Bench Press, p. 249	•	•	•			•	•	•	•				•	•	•		•
113. Dumbbell Decline Bench Press, p. 249	•	•	•			•	•	•	•		•		•	•	•		•
114. Flat, Incline, or Decline Bench Press, p. 250		•	•			•	•	•	•		•		•	•	•		•

	climbing	mountaineering	scrambling	hiking	backpacking	snowshoeing	downhill skiing	telemark skiing	cross-country/ skate skiing	snowboarding	cycling, road/ mountain bike	running/jogging	canoeing	kayaking	crew	windsurfing	general conditioning
115. Push-Up, p. 250	•	•	•								•	•	•	•		•	•
116. Flat Bench Dumbbell Flies, p. 251	•	•	•										•	•	•		•
117. Stomach-Lying Elbow Lift, p. 252	•	•	•			•	•	•	•		•		•	•	•	•	
118. Pulley/Cable Row, p. 254		•	•			•		•	•		•		•	•	•	•	
119. Bent Barbell Row, p. 254		•	•			•	•				•		•	•	•	•	
120. Latissimus (Lat) Pull-Downs to the Front and Rear, p. 255	•	•	•	•	•	•	•	•	•		•		•	•	•	•	•
121. Rotator Cuff Rotations, p. 256	•	•	•		•	•	•	•	•		•		•	•	•	•	•
122. Dumbbell Overhead Press, p. 258	•	•											•	•	•		
123. Lateral Dumbbell Raise, p. 258	•	•	•	•	•	•							•	•	•		•
124. Front Dumbbell Raise, p. 259	•	•	•	•	•	•	•	•	•		•		•	•	•	•	
125. Dumbbell and Barbell Curls, p. 259	•	•	•		•	•	•	•	•		•		•	•	•	•	•
126. Triceps Extensions, p. 261		•	•		•	•	•	•	•		•		•	•	•	•	•
127. Dips, p. 263	•	•	•			•	•	•	•		•		•	•	•	•	•
128. Chin-Ups, p. 264	•	•	•					•			•						•
129. Single-Arm Dumbbell Press, p. 265		•	•		•	•	•	•	•	•	•		•	•	•	•	
130. Variable-Level Push-Ups, p. 266	•	•	•			•	•	•		•	•		•	•			
131. Single-Arm Dumbbell Row, p. 267	•	•	•	•	•	•		•	•	•	•		•	•	•	•	•
132. Single-Leg Hip, Knee Extension/Pull-Down, p. 268	•	•	•	•	•	•	•	•	•		•		•	•	•	•	
133. Staggered Stance Cross-Diagonal Row with Dumbbells, p. 268	•	•	•			•	•	•	•	•	•	•	•	•	•	•	
134. Prone Reach/Row/Kick-Back, p. 269	•						•			•			•	•	•		•
135. Shoulder Butt Burner Combo, p. 270	•	•	•	•	•		•	•	•	•		•				•	•
136. Standing-Weight Shift Triceps Press, p. 272	•	•					•	•	•								
CHAPTER 16. THE FOREARM AND HAND																	
137. Finger Flexor Grip, p. 276	•	•	•										•	•	•	•	
138. Weight Roll-Up, p. 276	•	•	•										•	•	•	•	•

Exercise	climbing	mountaineering	scrambling	hiking	backpacking	snowshoeing	downhill skiing	telemark skiing	cross-country/ skate skiing	snowboarding	cycling, road/ mountain bike	running/jogging	canoeing	kayaking	crew	windsurfing	general conditioning
139. Dumbbell Palms-Up Wrist Curl, p. 277	•	•	•										•	•	•	•	•
140. Dumbbell Palms-Down Wrist Curl, p. 277	•	•	•										•	•	•	•	•
141. Sitting Olympic Plate Hand Squeeze, p. 278	•	•	•										•	•	•	•	
CHAPTER 18. CONDITIONING FOR SCRAMBLING AND ROCK CLIMBING																	
142. Climbing Rest Position for Your Fingers and Body, p. 291	•	•															
143. Traversing, p. 291	•	•	•														
144. Five Moving Parts, p. 292	•	•															
145. Round-the-Clock Weight Shifting, p. 293	•	•															
146. Flagging, p. 294	•	•															
147. Fingerboards, p. 294	•																
148. Endurance Climbing, p. 295	•	•															
149. Redpointing, p. 296	•	•															
CHAPTER 20. CONDITIONING FOR SNOWBOARDING AND SKIING																	
150. Balance Boards, p. 308							•	•	•	•						•	
151. Shuffle Lunge with Reach, p. 309							•	•	•	•						•	
152. The Fitter, p. 309							•	•	•	•						•	
153. Alpine Ski Circuit, p. 310							•										
154. Snowboard Circuit, p. 310									•	•						•	
155. Telemark Circuit, p. 311								•									
156. Pole-Running Agility Circuit, p. 311							•			•							
157. The "Z" Agility Course, p. 311							•	•		•							
158. Dynamic Jumping Warm-Up, p. 312							•	•	•	•							
159. 45-Degree Hopping, p. 312							•	•	•								
160. Simulated Ski Turns, p. 313							•	•	•								
161. Slalom Jumps, p. 313							•			•							

	climbing	mountaineering	scrambling	hiking	backpacking	snowshoeing	downhill skiing	telemark skiing	cross-country/ skate skiing	snowboarding	cycling, road/ mountain bike	running/jogging	canoeing	kayaking	crew	windsurfing	general conditioning
162. Dynamic Jumping Warm-Up 2, p. 313							•	•	•	•							
163. Telemark Jump, p. 314							•	•									
164. Progressive Power Jumps, p. 314							•	•									
165. Single-Leg Lateral Jumps, p. 314							•	•		•							
166. Crossover Bench Jumps, p. 315							•			•							
167. The Hex Circuit, p. 315							•	•	•								
168. Acceleration Sprints, p. 316							•	•	•	•							
169. Slide Boards, p. 316							•	•	•	•							
170. Tuck Drills, p. 317							•		•								
CHAPTER 22. CONDITIONING FOR ROAD AND MOUNTAIN BICYCLING																	
171. Balance-Ready Position, p. 333											•						
172. Maintaining a Straight Line, p. 333											•						
173. Level Slalom, p. 334											•						
174. Downhill Slalom, p. 334											•						
175. Ride the 2x4 Line, p. 335											•						
176. Lifting the Front Wheel, p. 335											•						
177. Lifting the Back Wheel, p. 336											•						
178. Bunny Hop, p. 336											•						
CHAPTER 25. BODY POSTURE AND MOVEMENT PATTERNS																	
179. Ground Reaction Force, p. 355																	•
180. Sitting Arcing Exercise: Finding Neutral in Sitting, p. 355																	•
181. Gravity's Effect on Sitting, p. 357																	•
182. Standing Arcing Exercise: Finding Neutral in Standing, p. 357				•	•	•											•
183. Base of Support, p. 358																	•
184. Weight-Shifting in Standing, p. 359																	•

PART I

Basic Principles

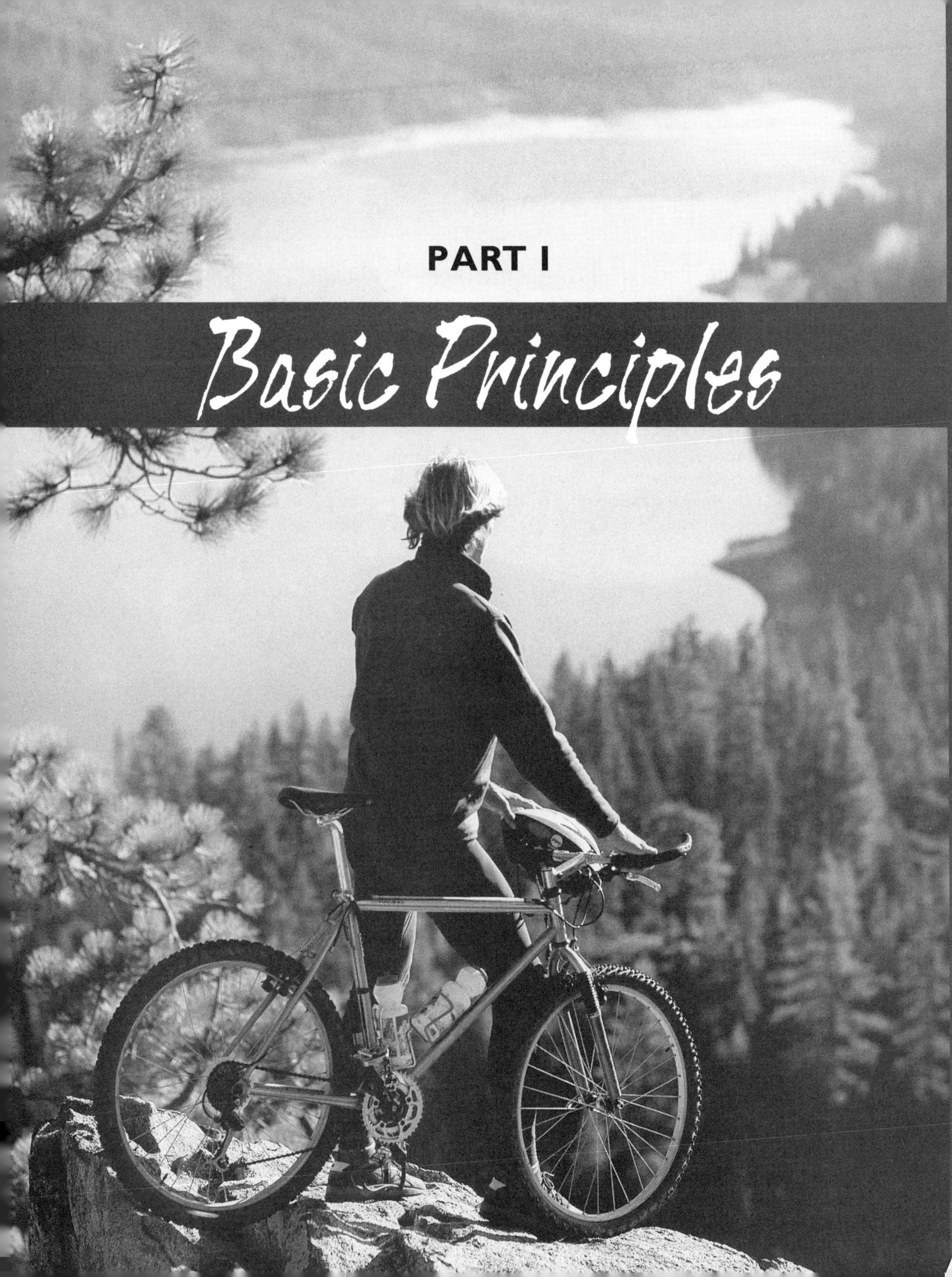

chapter 1 EXERCISE PHYSIOLOGY

Energy Production; Cardiac, Respiratory, and Muscle System Function; and Training Adaptations

By David Musnick, M.D.

THIS CHAPTER WILL HELP YOU:

- Understand your body's energy systems.
- Understand the difference between aerobic and anaerobic exercise.
- Understand how your respiratory and cardiovascular systems respond to exercise.
- Understand the physiological changes that occur when exercising at altitude.

In order to undertake any exercise, your body requires energy to power your muscles. To obtain this energy, your body must convert food into a substance known as adenosineriphosphate (ATP). The molecules of ATP are held together by high-energy bonds, and when these bonds are broken, energy becomes available to do biological work such as muscle contractions. The amount of ATP that can be stored in your cells is very limited. In fact, at any one time, your body contains only about 100 grams of ATP, which is enough to exercise at a maximum level for just a few seconds. Thus, a crucial function of your muscle cells is their ability to quickly recycle and synthesize ATP molecules—a task they do best in the presence of adequate oxygen supplies, that is, under "aerobic" conditions.

AEROBIC VS. ANAEROBIC EXERCISE

The terms aerobic and anaerobic refer to whether oxygen is being used in the chemical reactions—metabolic pathway—that your body uses to create energy. The amount of ATP manufactured by your muscle cells is directly proportional to the amount of oxygen available in relation to the intensity of the exercise. Activities that are performed at low to moderate intensity for prolonged periods (such as hiking, jogging, cross-country skiing, or kayaking) are aerobically fueled. Such activities involve the repetitive use of major muscle groups, which leads to an elevated heart rate. As your heart rate increases, the amount of blood flowing to your muscles also increases, as does the amount of oxygen in your blood. As the available oxygen increases, the production of ATP becomes more efficient, allowing movement to be sustained over time.

Conversely, brief, intense activities (for example, sprinting or a few minutes of very difficult climbing) are usually anaerobically fueled. When you undertake such activities, there is inadequate oxygen available to meet the demand in the oxygen-utilizing pathways.

Anaerobic Exercise

In the absence of adequate oxygen, energy can be created in a variety of ways. These anaerobic reactions include: (1), The small amount of ATP stored in muscle cells can be broken down;

(2) ATP can be recycled from creatine phosphate (CP), a compound present in muscles; (3) glucose (a sugar) can be broken down to a smaller molecule called pyruvate, a process called glycolysis; or (4) glycogen (stored in the muscles and liver) can be broken down into glucose.

Because the amounts of ATP and CP stored in our bodies are quite small, the first two reactions are only sufficient to sustain about 20 seconds of very high-intensity activity. High-intensity activity of any longer duration (up to 90 seconds) is fueled by the third reaction, glycolysis.

One by-product of anaerobic reactions is the accumulation of lactic acid. The enzymes necessary for muscle contraction work less effectively in acidic conditions, so as the amount of lactic acid increases, the efficiency of muscle contraction decreases. Also, in the absence of oxygen, the muscle cells cannot regenerate ATP quickly enough to meet the demands of high-intensity exercise, with the result that the muscles become fatigued and the intensity of the activity must be lessened or stopped altogether. These natural limits on energy production under anaerobic conditions explain why a runner can sprint for only a short distance or why a climber can do very difficult moves for only a short period before needing a rest break.

Our bodies generate lactic acid whenever we exercise, but as the intensity of exercise increases, the level of lactic acid in the blood also increases. Each individual has a "lactate threshold," beyond which the level of lactic acid rises steeply with any further increase in exercise intensity. Less aerobically trained individuals reach their lactate threshold sooner than those who are physically fit.

Furthermore, individuals who train for endurance have a greater ability to metabolize ("clear") lactic acid and may even produce less of it than untrained individuals. Endurance training may also increase the production of enzymes that support anaerobic energy production, making it more efficient (see chapter 3 for information on interval training for endurance).

Aerobic Exercise

Aerobic exercise relies on energy produced via metabolic pathways in which oxygen is delivered from the lungs to the blood, and from the blood to mitochondria within the cells of muscle tissues, where the production and breakdown of ATP occurs. The chemical reactions that produce energy require the assistance of various enzymes (enzymes are catalysts that can speed up chemical reactions without themselves being altered in the process). Enzymes are critical to the transfer of electrons in the mitochondria of your cells, and they function best within a narrow range of acid (pH) and temperature balance. Enzymes become less efficient as acidity in the cell increases, and more efficient with slightly increased temperatures (one reason why warming up before exercise is a good idea).

Aerobic energy production involves a number of other biochemical reactions, including the Krebs—or citric acid—cycle, which is approximately eighteen times more efficient at producing ATP than are anaerobic reactions. You can continue sustained low- to moderate-intensity aerobic activities primarily because of this ongoing production of energy.

FUEL SOURCES FOR ENERGY PRODUCTION

Energy production is fueled by food, which, once it is digested, can enter the series of metabolic reactions described above at a number of biochemical points. Each of the three types of food—carbohydrates (including glycogen), fats (lipids), and proteins—functions a bit differently.

Carbohydrates

Carbohydrates, which are composed of carbon, hydrogen, and oxygen, are the body's primary source of energy. When you consume carbohydrates, they are broken down into glucose (also called dextrose), which is transported directly to your muscle cells and used as fuel. The consumption of carbohydrates is especially important in the production of energy for activities lasting more than 60–90 minutes, such as a long run, hike, climb, bike ride, or kayak trip.

If they are not immediately used for energy production, carbohydrates are stored in the body, mostly in the form of glycogen, but they may also be stored as fat. Your daily intake of carbohydrates must be sufficient to supply the energy needs of your body as well as to maintain its stores of glycogen. Two hours of aerobic activity will almost fully deplete the glycogen stored in your liver and your muscles. If you use up your glycogen stores and don't consume additional carbohydrates, you will likely experience fatigue, decreased efficiency, and possibly even weakness, hunger, and lightheadedness, as glucose is pulled from your bloodstream (causing low blood sugar) for energy production.

Fats (Lipids)

Fats (lipids) are stored in both fat cells and muscle cells, usually in the form of triglycerides. Because a gram of fat has a caloric value of 9 kilocalories (kcals), compared with 4 kcals for a gram of carbohydrate, it has the potential to provide even more energy.

Your body begins to use fat as fuel after about a half hour of light to moderate activity, and fat may contribute 50–80% of energy needs during prolonged exercise. Regular aerobic conditioning increases the body's efficiency in extracting fat from your fat cells and increases the use of fatty acid for fuel in your muscles. It is for this reason that prolonged aerobic activity can result in weight loss. Your body's ability to break down fat for energy does not significantly decrease your need for carbohydrates during a lengthy activity.

PRACTICAL POINT

To burn more fat and lose weight, perform aerobic exercise of low to moderate intensity (50–70% of maximum heart rate; see chapter 3) for prolonged periods of time (greater than 30 minutes). This can be almost any type of activity, including walking and hiking, as long as the intensity does not increase to a high level.

Proteins

Proteins are made from amino acids, which are made from the basic building blocks of carbon, hydrogen, oxygen, and nitrogen. Proteins serve many purposes: they support your body's enzymatic functions and are in all its tissues—muscles, ligaments, intracellular components, and so on. Systematic resistance training increases the protein component of your skeletal muscle, which can lead to increased muscle size and strength. Protein normally plays only a minimal role in energy production. However, if the usual fuel sources (carbohydrates and fats) are lacking, the body can use protein as fuel.

PRACTICAL POINT

In summary, your body uses fuels for exercise in these ways:

At rest: free fatty acids and glucose.

For the first 20 seconds of exercise: reserves of ATP and CP.

As exercise progresses: glycogen, glucose, and fat.

After 2–4 hours of exercise: glycogen, glucose (if carbohydrates have been consumed during the activity), fatty acids, and protein; except during bursts of activity, when anaerobic use of ATP and CP resumes.

YOUR LUNGS AND RESPIRATORY SYSTEM

Aerobic conditioning increases the efficiency of the muscles you use to breathe, with the result that your breathing rate (i.e., number of breaths per minute) is lower than that of less trained individuals. Because aerobically conditioned individuals take fewer, but more efficient, breaths per minute, they are less likely to feel winded at higher exercise intensities. This response is fairly specific to the type of training and activities you regularly do.

YOUR HEART AND VASCULAR SYSTEM

Another benefit of aerobic training is that your cardiac output improves. Cardiac output is calculated by multiplying your heart rate (number of beats per minute) by your stroke volume (the amount of blood pumped per contraction). Regular aerobic training increases stroke volume. As your stroke volume increases, your resting heart rate decreases because your heart does not need to beat as many times per minute as it did in your untrained condition to output the same amount of blood. Your heart thus becomes a more efficient pump, both during exercise and at rest.

As the intensity of your exercise increases, so does your heart rate. Monitoring your heart rate is thus an excellent means of determining the intensity level of your exercise to keep it within the heart-rate target zone that meets your fitness goals (see chapter 3 for a discussion of target zones).

Maximal Oxygen Uptake (VO_2 Max)

VO_2 max is a clinical measurement of the maximal oxygen consumption that a particular individual can achieve at the highest intensity of exercise. VO_2 max is related to the efficiency of numerous body systems, including the respiratory, cardiovascular (particularly hemoglobin concentration and blood volume), and aerobic systems within the muscles.

If you participate in regular aerobic training, you can increase your VO_2 max. Because you won't usually be performing at maximum intensity, you will be able to perform at various levels of exercise intensity with less effort. About half your endurance improvement will come from improved heart pumping ability and half from increased efficiency of your muscles at extracting oxygen and using it to supply energy.

YOUR MUSCULAR SYSTEM

Your muscular system is made up of a series of motor units. A motor unit is a set of motor nerves combined with the group of muscle fibers to which they supply motor impulses. The amount of force you are able to exert in a contracting muscle is correlated to the percentage of motor units recruited (used), the intensity of the effort, and the percentage of faster or slower fiber types that you have in a muscle. Fibers are recruited from slower to faster. An increasing number of motor units are used as exercise intensity increases. For more powerful and rapid strength demands, the faster fibers are activated. You can train for increased recruitment to increase your speed and strength.

The Effects of Aerobic Training on Muscle

Aerobic conditioning can increase the size and volume of your muscles' mitochondria (where ATP is synthesized), the levels of certain enzymes related to energy production, the extent of your capillary plumbing system (very small blood vessels), and the efficiency of your muscles in using fat as fuel. It can also decrease lactic acid production, the muscles you use in aerobic exercise will become much more efficient metabolically, but this training is pretty specific to how you use the muscles, meaning that if you are a jogger you may not have much swimming or kayaking endurance.

Muscular Benefits of Strength Training

Strength training can enhance your performance in any outdoor activity, as well as in many work and home activities. It can improve body tone and shape, and slow the increase in the ratio of fat to lean body mass that typically occurs as you age. There is also evidence that strength training to the point of muscle fatigue can stimulate the release of growth hormone. Growth hormone facilitates protein synthesis and increases mobilization and utilization of fat as a fuel source, thereby increasing your muscle mass and decreasing fatty tissue. The release of growth hormone may occur with very high-intensity exercise, such as interval and anaerobic training, as well as strength training.

Activity-Specific Training

The effects of training on a particular muscle or group of muscles are specific to the fibers and motor units used, the range of motion of the joints, the length of the muscles used, and the speed of use. Activity-specific training means training to simulate the muscular demands of your activities using aerobic, strength, and balance training.

EXERCISE AT ALTITUDE

For the most part, altitude does not affect exercise performance until you reach an elevation of 6,000 feet. Then a number of physiological changes occur, all of which are primarily related to a decrease in total amount of oxygen delivered to the muscles, brain, and other organs. There are other changes, including a decrease in blood volume that can worsen with dehydration, an increase in the effort it takes to breathe, and a decrease in the ability to do activities at submaximal and maximal levels.

> **PRACTICAL POINT**
>
> There are a number of methods to acclimatize to increasing altitude, but in general all involve gradual increases in elevation gain (1,000 feet per day above 9,000 feet, or 2,000 feet every 2 days if base camps are being moved). It is a good idea to spend 2–4 extra days hiking at 7,000–8,000 feet, as well as at 12,000–13,000 feet, before going to higher altitudes. Rest days with lower-intensity activity are a good idea above 10,000 feet. Sleep at lower altitudes if symptoms start to arise. If symptoms of altitude illness are detected, descend at least 2,000–3,000 feet, accompanied by at least one other person.

Other changes can occur at higher elevations, including a decrease in arterial oxygen during sleep and a decrease in your ability to exercise to your maximum capacity. Sleep problems, including headaches, insomnia, and frequent awakening, can impede daytime performance.

At 10,000 feet, about half the amount of oxygen is available in the blood as at sea level. If you gradually move up in altitude, your body can adapt somewhat, but cannot fully compensate for altitude in regard to your ability to exercise and perform other activities.

chapter 2 NUTRITIONAL CONSIDERATIONS FOR CONDITIONING

By David Musnick, M.D., Bobbi Lutack, N.D., and Leslie Moskowitz, M.S., R.D.

THIS CHAPTER WILL HELP YOU:

- Understand your energy needs.
- Understand the importance of carbohydrates, including complex vs. simple carbohydrates and carbohydrate loading.
- Clarify your needs for protein.
- Understand how you can make good fat choices.
- Clarify the issue of vitamin, mineral, and antioxidant needs as they relate to exercise, and free radical risk.
- Understand your fluid needs.
- Understand energy and fluid needs for high-altitude activities.
- Clarify issues regarding food quality.

What you eat supplies the energy you need and affects both your performance and your health. Good training habits and nutrition help you function optimally. Whether you are a competitive athlete, an outdoor enthusiast, or just trying to stay in shape or be healthy, you need to know the latest nutrition information.

ENERGY REQUIREMENTS

Understanding your energy requirements is important if you are trying to lose or gain weight or if you are trying to plan food amounts for a backpacking, kayaking, or climbing trip. Your approximate total daily energy expenditure consists of the kilocalories (kcals) needed for your resting metabolic rate (RMR), plus kcals needed for the light activities of daily living and those related to exercise.

Your RMR is measured in kcals and can be estimated with some equipment that has become more widely available in the past few years. Barring access to such equipment, you can use the Harris and Benedict formula to calculate RMR fairly precisely, but the calculation is not as accurate as direct measurement and may underestimate your RMR.

Harris and Benedict RMR formula for men:

66.5 + (13.75 × weight in kg) + (5 × height in cm) – (6.78 × age in years) = kcals

For a 40-year-old man who is 5 feet, 9 inches tall and weighs 160 pounds, this means:

66.5 + (13.75 × 72.72 kg) + (5 × 175.26 cm) – (6.78 × 40) = 1,671 kcals

Harris and Benedict RMR formula for women:

655 + (9.56 × weight in kg) + (1.85 × height in cm) – (4.68 × age in years) = kcals

For a 36-year-old woman who is 5 feet, 4 inches tall and weighs 135 pounds, this means:

655 + (9.56 × 61.36 kg) + (1.85 × 162.56 cm) – (4.68 × 36) = 1,373 kcals

You can **estimate the kcals needed for**

your RMR using an abbreviated version of this formula (women should use 0.95 kcals/kg):

weight in kg × 1 kcal/kg × 24 hours = kcals

Calculating exercise calories burned during the day depends on what type of activity is being performed, the intensity, the load carried, and the weight of the individual. Exercise and outdoor activities can vary from 5–20 kcals per minute (walking to all-out cross-country skiing), with the average being 7–11 kcals. Most typical 30- to 40-minute aerobic workouts burn 300 kcals, and most rigorous backpacking or mountaineering trips can burn 450–600 kcals per hour. (The lower number would be appropriate for a 120-pound individual with a light pack, and the higher number would be appropriate for a 160-pound person with a heavy pack.) You can calculate your expected kcal output for an activity by estimating the amount of time spent in the activity and using a chart to estimate kcals burned per minute or hour. (Excellent charts are available in Katch and McArdle, *Exercise Physiology* and in Ainsworth et al., "The Compendium of Physical Activities"; see Selected References.)

For example, the RMR for an average 40-year-old, 160-pound male is 1,671 kcals; if he carries a 44-pound pack while mountaineering for 8 hours (taking 2 hours in breaks), this adds 6 hours × 600 kcals per hour (or 3,600 kcals) for exercise, for a total of 5,271 kcals of energy needed for each day. You can see that the largest variable here is the exercise, especially in outdoor activities lasting many hours. It is important to plan for enough calories to meet your energy needs if you are on an outdoor trip.

If you are going to participate in competition or longer-duration outdoor activities, you must plan for and take in a significant amount of food to provide this energy. Hunger is not the best guide to food intake during vigorous outdoor activities, especially if you are at higher altitudes. Inadequate food intake can lead to a feeling of general fatigue and can be dangerous in activities such as mountaineering and sea kayaking.

FOOD QUALITY AND PURITY

It has become apparent since this book's first edition that there are significant issues that influence the purity and quality of the food supply in the United States and likely most other countries. For this reason the first author recommends that athletic individuals who seek the best performance and health choose organic food products (whenever possible) and use a good multivitamin supplement. For more information on this issue, see chapter 26 as well as Vitamins, Minerals, and Free Radicals in this chapter.

FOOD AS FUEL

Carbohydrate, fat, and protein all yield energy, and this energy is measured in kcals. Carbohydrates and protein supply 4 kcals per gram, and fat supplies 9 kcals per gram. Most foods contain a mixture of these three, but usually have a higher percentage of one nutrient. In general your body obtains energy best by breaking down carbohydrates.

Carbohydrates

The main emphasis in nutrition for sports, especially endurance exercise, has been on the role of carbohydrates for energy. Carbohydrates are composed of carbon, hydrogen, and oxygen molecules combined into different biochemical structures. They are classified as monosaccharides such as glucose and fructose. Oligosaccharides such as sucrose form when 2–10 monosaccharides bond together. Polysaccharides are large chains of linked monosaccharides such as starch and glycogen.

Carbohydrates can be classified as complex, which means they are composed of three or more glucose molecules, or as simple, composed of one or two sugar molecules. Examples of complex carbohydrates are breads, pasta, and certain vegetables. Examples of simple carbohydrates are sucrose (table sugar), honey, corn syrup (used in many foods as a sweetener), fruit, and fruit juices. In general, these simple carbohydrates should not be eaten immediately prior to exercise or a race because they can stimulate a rapid rise in insulin and a subsequent drop in blood glucose levels. Certain fruits are more likely to cause this problem, including bananas, watermelon, and papaya. Also, the rise of insulin inhibits fat mobilization and increases the use of muscle glycogen (stored starch). The normal effect of insulin combined with the effects of exercise can cause a significant drop in blood glucose. Simple sugars are appropriate to eat during a race and are usually mixed in with fluids to maintain adequate blood glucose levels during activities prolonged for more than 1 1/2–2 hours.

Both complex and simple carbohydrates can fuel your muscles and brain, but foods containing complex carbohydrates supply you with additional nutrients such as B vitamins, minerals, and fiber. The degree to which these other nutrients are supplied depends on how processed the food is, your choice of carbohydrates, and the health of the soil in which the product was grown. In general, the soils in most countries, including the United States, are markedly depleted in essential minerals. Carbohydrates that are made from organic flours are more likely to have a higher mineral content. They are also less likely to be processed.

FIBER TIP

Fiber does not directly provide energy for exercise, but it confers many important health benefits. By improving the health of the gastrointestinal system it may indirectly contribute to improved metabolic function. Although you can take a fiber supplement, you need to get fiber primarily from your diet. For further details on the health benefits and selection of fiber, see chapter 26. Athletes can get their fiber from wheat-bran cereals, oatmeal, legumes and beans, other grains, and from fruits and vegetables. It is recommended that 25–35 grams of fiber be consumed each day for gastrointestinal and cardiovascular health.

Most of both simple and complex carbohydrates in the diet are converted into glucose during digestion, to be used for fuel or stored for future energy use as glycogen in the muscles and liver. The liver can store about 100 grams of glycogen, and muscles can store 300–500 grams of glycogen. Any carbohydrates consumed in excess are stored as fat.

When we eat carbohydrates, the subsequent rise in blood glucose signals the hormone insulin to circulate in the blood. Insulin promotes utilization of carbohydrates for energy by transporting glucose into your body's cells. When glucose concentration is high, insulin secretion is stimulated and carbohydrates are used for energy. When glucose levels are low, insulin is suppressed and fat is used preferentially for energy.

Carbohydrates are important sources of energy for contracting muscles during prolonged and strenuous exercise. High-carbohydrate diets seem to be more effective than high-fat diets in supplying energy for endurance athletes. Fatigue is often associated with muscle glycogen depletion and/or hypoglycemia (low blood sugar; see below).

During active training periods, especially around competition times, or significant aerobic events like climbing a mountain, the usual carbohydrate recommendation is approximately 60–70% of total energy intake for the day, with 12–20% going to protein, leaving a total of about 20–25% calories from fat. The amount of carbohydrates needed may decrease in long-duration backpacking or mountaineering, in which high-calorie, dense fat is often used to supply adequate energy.

The carbohydrate calories you need depend on your calculated daily energy expenditure and the percent of carbohydrate in your diet. For example, if your total energy requirements are 2,500 kcals per day, 1,500 kcals should come from carbohydrate (60% × 2,500 = 1,500). Since there are 4 kcals per gram of carbohydrate, there are 375 grams of carbohydrate in 1,500 kcals

(1,500/4 = 375). Note that 15 grams equals 1 serving, so that you have to calculate the number of portions of a particular carbohydrate-containing food (see American Dietetics and American Diabetes Associations, *Exchange Lists for Meal Planning*, in Selected References.)

FOOD TIP

At mealtime, have two-thirds of your plate covered with carbohydrate to obtain about 60–65% carbohydrate calories. This is the best percentage if you are an active athlete, training regularly. You may vary and decrease this amount in your off-season depending on your health goals and your metabolic type (see Metabolic-Type and Low-Carb Diets below).

Because the benefits of a high-carbohydrate diet for improving sport performance are so highly touted, many athletes and exercisers believe they can eat all they want of any type of carbohydrate, as long as it is a complex carbohydrate. Not so. Complex carbohydrates such as refined pasta and breads are milled and lose vitamins and minerals during the process. Individuals whose diets are high in these complex carbohydrates may suffer from vitamin and mineral deficiencies. Fatigue, poor recovery, staleness, and aching muscles may reflect a lack of critical nutrients, glycogen depletion, or other medical conditions. It is better to eat relatively unprocessed whole grains such as oats, barley, wheat, millet, amaranth, spelt, and rice, along with a variety of vegetables and fruits, for your carbohydrate sources.

Choosing carbohydrates with a low to moderate glycemic index (see Glycemic Index below) is also a good idea for the majority of your carbohydrates unless you are actively trying to replace glycogen stores (see Glycogen Reserves and Carbohydrate Loading below). Becoming familiar with the nutrient and fiber composition and the glycemic index of various complex carbohydrates will enable you to choose a variety of foods to meet your nutritional needs.

Hypoglycemia

Hypoglycemia occurs when blood sugar levels are less than approximately 65 milligrams per deciliter. The condition can occur in type 1 diabetics as well as in nondiabetics. The symptoms are a fast heart rate at rest, palpitations, anxiety, hunger, and irritability. In people with type 1 diabetes there are specific predictable causes of hypoglycemia and there are specific treatments.

Causes of hypoglycemia in insulin-dependent diabetics:

- Improper timing of meals or snacks
- Excessive insulin, improper timing or dosing of insulin
- Excessive exercise or unplanned exercise with inadequate food intake

HEALTH TIP FOR DIABETICS

Before aerobic exercise: If your glucose level is 100–180 mg/dl, take 15 grams of carbohydrate (60 kcals), for example, a small can of juice. If your glucose level is 180–250 mg/dl, it is not necessary to increase food intake. If your glucose level is more than 250 mg/dl, don't start aerobic exercise.

Hypoglycemia can also occur as "reactive hypoglycemia" in nondiabetics. If you have an exaggerated response to sugar or simple carbohydrates, your insulin level can rise abruptly and cause low blood sugar. You can prevent this by eating every 2 hours, making sure to eat a combination of complex, unrefined carbohydrate with protein or some healthy fat. Adding foods with fiber will slow the rise of insulin and decrease the likelihood of hypoglycemia. Avoid eating simple carbohydrates alone.

FOOD TIP

Good snacks for avoiding hypoglycemia: a protein bar (not low carbohydrate), mixed nuts with rye crisps, apples with almond butter, granola with nuts.

Glycemic Index

The glycemic index is an index of the glucose and insulin responses induced by carbohydrate foods. It refers to the digestion and entry rate of glucose from the digested food into the bloodstream and is related to the rise of insulin. A lower glycemic index indicates a slower and more prolonged increase in blood glucose and less of an insulin increase. A higher glycemic index indicates a rapid rise in blood glucose and insulin and a shorter duration of blood-sugar elevation. In general, it is desirable to have your blood sugar elevated for longer periods of time to prevent hunger and the need for more frequent eating. It is also very important to eat lower glycemic foods if you are diabetic or overweight. In general it is healthy to eat carbohydrates that have a low to moderate glycemic index except during a long-duration aerobic activity/competition, in which case you should eat high-glycemic carbohydrates. High-glycemic carbs are also reasonable to eat after an endurance event to replace glycogen stores.

Glycemic response is affected by the type of simple sugar present (glucose, fructose, galactose) and by the type and the amount of fiber content (soluble or insoluble). Glycemic response is also affected by the percentage of fat and protein in the carbohydrate or present in the rest of the meal. The higher the fiber, fat, or protein content, the lower the glycemic index. The sugars found in grains, pastas, bread, cereal, and sweets are usually absorbed quickly. Dairy products contain galactose, which is next to be absorbed, and fruits contain fructose, which has the lowest glycemic index.

Note that the glycemic index measure is usually based on 50 grams of the isolated carbohydrate food. But most of the time people don't eat a food by itself and often don't eat that quantity of it. Therefore, you should consider the healthful qualities of any one food, the quantity of the food eaten, and where that food falls on the glycemic index, as well as what you might be eating at the same time. Eating carrots alone might be of some concern just in regard to glycemic index, but when eaten with protein foods at a meal the meal's glycemic load is quite different.

FOOD TIP

Dried fruit is an excellent carbohydrate source and has a moderate glycemic index. Mix it with nuts to create a source of long-lasting energy and to increase your carbohydrate calories.

Health-care providers who support eating lower glycemic foods suggest that a steady blood-glucose level is maintained by preventing an overstimulation of insulin and a more prolonged release of glucose. As a result, hypoglycemia is avoided and excessive storage of calories as fat may be reduced. To maintain a reasonable level of blood glucose, eat lower glycemic carbohydrates as well as meals that have some protein and fat. This is especially true for outdoor activi-

FIGURE 2. GLYCEMIC INDEX OF SOME COMMON FOODS

High	Moderate	Low	Lowest
Breakfast cereals	Pastas	Barley	Soybeans
Rice cakes	Candy bars	Apples	Peanuts
Glucose	Whole-grain rye	Oranges/Orange juice	Other nuts
Carrots	Most breads	Milk	Lentils
Potatoes	Raisins	Yogurt	Fructose
Bananas	Brown rice	Protein bars	

ties of low to moderate intensity. Figure 2 gives some examples of various foods' glycemic index (for a more extensive chart, see chapter 29 and the websites listed in Selected References for chapters 2 and 29). Eat lower to moderate glycemic foods during the day and use higher glycemic foods (including sports drinks) for a more rapid supply of energy if you are in an endurance activity or a race and need a quick energy source, especially after 1–2 hours of the activity. Eating high glycemic index carbohydrates for 8–12 hours after an endurance event also appears to be very important for replacing muscle glycogen stores quickly. Replenishing your glycogen stores after such an event is quite important; if not done adequately, you may feel excessive exercise-related fatigue or have poor endurance for the next training session. See Selected References for good sources discussing the glycemic index.

Glycogen Reserves and Carbohydrate Loading

Your glycogen reserves may vary from 300 to 500 grams, depending on the duration and intensity of your exercise. This could provide you with 1,200–2,000 kcals from glycogen alone, and this is combined with energy released from fat, depending on the intensity of the exercise. Your glycogen reserves could be used up within 1 1/2–6 hours of prolonged outdoor activities. People seem to feel less energetic and have less exercise capacity when their glycogen stores have been used up. Low muscle glycogen stores before an event or a workout can be a cause for poor exercise endurance or performance (though there are many other causes of exercise-related fatigue or poor performance; see chapter 30). You can increase your muscles' glycogen storage to aid you in long-duration activities and competitions by consuming higher-than-normal amounts of carbohydrates and by tapering your training activities prior to the event or activity.

An example of a carbohydrate (glycogen)-loading plan is to start 1 week before the long-distance event. Consume a high-carbohydrate diet, starting with about 60% of your total kcals in carbohydrate (or 350–400 grams) and working up to 70% carbohydrate by day 4 (500–550 grams per day). Stay with this level of intake until the night before your event or activity. Perform your current intensity level of aerobic exercise for the first 4 days, but gradually decrease your training sessions from 60–90 minutes the first day to 20 30 minutes on the fourth day. Day 5 would be a very light training day, and day 6 would be a rest day. Only adults who are in excellent aerobic condition and have no health problems such as diabetes should attempt carbohydrate loading. Try to include adequate protein during carbohydrate loading.

Meal Timing Suggestions for Carbohydrates

Ingestion of a meal with a high percentage of carbohydrate 2–3 hours prior to exercise ensures adequate glycogen availability (as long as your glycogen stores were adequate the day prior) and enhances exercise performance. So it is especially important to eat a high-carbohydrate breakfast on an event day. Test out particular meals to make sure that you choose a pre-event meal you will tolerate well. It is OK to eat a mixed meal of carbohydrates, protein, and good fat if you eat it at least 3 hours prior to working out. Most people will need 2 hours between finishing eating a regular meal and doing aerobic exercise. You will need less time if you are going to participate in weight-lifting activities. Try not to eat any simple sugars within 1 1/2 hours of your exercise or event to decrease the possibility of low blood sugar.

Replacement of body glycogen stores is important if you have been involved in intensive exercise lasting more than 1 hour and especially if you are doing endurance activities that last more than a few hours. Glycogen replacement can be achieved most rapidly if extra carbohydrates are consumed as soon as possible after exercise and at repeated 1–2 hour intervals for at least 8 hours after the event. In general, you want to eat a variety of carbohydrates of low, mid, and high glycemic index during this period. One strategy to achieve this is to eat 50–75 grams of moderate to high glycemic carbohydrates every 2 hours after the event until reaching 500 grams or until eating a high-carbohydrate meal. It also makes sense to eat very soon after an endurance event. Carbohydrate replacement should be done within 24 hours after a prolonged, high-intensity event lasting longer than 1 1/2–2 hours. Finally, glycogen is replenished best if you avoid significant exercise for 8 hours after the event. You can continue to replenish glycogen during endurance and outdoor activities by eating snacks and meals with moderate to high glycemic index during your activity.

FOOD TIP

For healthy carb loading before an event or replacement after an endurance event, consider a mix of the following:

- Fruit juices and fruits (especially within the first 4 hours postevent)
- Whole-grain, minimally processed foods, including breads (multigrain and seed breads), cereals, crackers, muffins, pasta
- Potatoes, corn, rice, or boiled whole grains such as wheat, barley, spelt, or quinoa
- Snacks with mixed nuts, granola, and seeds (pumpkin and sunflower)

Metabolic-Type and Low-Carb Diets

Since the first edition of this book there has been an explosion of new diets. The majority of these have been low-carbohydrate diets. Unfortunately, low-carbohydrate diets are not good for endurance athletes, though they might work just fine for individuals trying to lose weight (see chapter 29) or for individuals trying to maintain optimal wellness (see chapter 26). A metabolic-type diet may be OK for an endurance athlete if it allows at least 60% carbohydrate, otherwise such diets are best for weight loss and improving wellness.

Protein

Protein and its amino acids are a major structural material of our bodies. Adequate amounts of protein are necessary for the active individual to repair and build muscle tissue. Protein-containing foods are a good source of B vitamins and iron. Protein (especially the amino acid alanine) is a secondary source of energy during prolonged aerobic activity.

Protein Quality

Protein is composed of amino acids, and nine of the twenty-two amino acids in the human body are essential because they must come from the food we eat and cannot be made by the body. Meat, fish, poultry, eggs, milk, and soy products contain all the essential amino acids and are called complete proteins. There is also protein in grains, legumes, nuts, and seeds. The meat- and milk-based protein sources are the most likely to be compromised in regard to toxins because these sources concentrate toxins. It is best when choosing meat- or milk-based protein sources to choose organic and grass-fed (if beef) items whenever possible. It is also wise to choose organic vegetarian proteins for health reasons.

Protein Requirements

Your need for protein varies depending on your body weight and its percent of fat, and the type, intensity, and duration of activity. The usual recommendations are that adults should have 0.8 gram of protein per kilogram (2.2 lb) of body weight, equivalent to about 0.4 gram per pound. This is likely enough for most individuals. While it was once thought that protein deficiency was mostly the result of being poor (protein generally being more expensive than either grains or vegetables), it is noteworthy that today many people with reasonable incomes don't eat even the minimal amount of protein recommended. This is probably related to the fact that it takes more time to prepare some proteins and that simple carbohydrates are used for breakfast and snacks rather than carbohydrates with protein.

There is some evidence indicating that regular exercise at high volumes does in fact increase protein needs. The range of 0.8 1 gram of protein per kilogram of body weight (gm/kg body weight) should be adequate for the majority of people doing a moderate amount of exercise (i.e., simply trying to stay fit). If you strength-train intensely and are trying to build significant muscle mass, you may need as much as 1.2–1.8 gm/kg body weight. If your activities are primarily aerobic and you are training for an endurance event, you will need about 1.2 gm/kg body weight. If you are trying to heal a muscular related injury (strain), consider increasing your daily protein intake to 1–1.2 gm/kg body weight. A diet with 12–15% of total daily calories from protein can usually meet these extra requirements (unless total caloric intake is insufficient, or the diet is a vegetarian one containing no soy, milk, or egg products and inadequate protein combining).

FOOD TIP

Try to have protein at each meal, especially at breakfast and lunch. Try to start your day with 20–30 grams of protein. You can do this with a protein smoothie. Doing so can improve your likelihood of getting enough protein and can improve your body's ability to regulate blood-sugar levels.

There are many methods to calculate your protein requirements. You can calculate your needs by figuring out your lean weight in kilograms (or in pounds/2.2) and using one of the formulas above. Your lean body weight is your ideal body weight and is mainly important if you are moderately to significantly overweight. Another method is to estimate your total calorie needs per day and multiply by 15%.

For example, if you need 2,500 calories per day, 15% × 2,500 = 375 kcals of protein. Since protein has 4 kcals per gram, you would need 93 grams of protein a day from complete and incomplete sources.

Examples of grams of protein per common serving:

Meat, 1 oz	7 gm
Fish, 1 oz	5–7 gm
Eggs, 1 medium	6 gm
Milk, 8 oz	8 gm
Yogurt, milk, 1 cup	11 gm
Beans, 1/2 cup	12–14 gm
Potatoes, white, medium size	6–8 gm
Peanuts, 1/4 cup	8 gm
Peanut butter, 1tbs	4.5 gm
Almonds, 1/4 cup	6.5 gm
Tofu, 3 oz	10–12 gm

Most protein bars have 10–14 grams of protein (some have up to 30 gm), but have varying ratios of carbohydrate and fat. Protein bars that have more than 15 grams of protein often don't taste good or have quite a bit of additives in them. You need to enjoy the taste of the bar and have no reactions to any of the ingredients to make it a regular source of additional protein.

Most protein supplementation can be done with protein-rich foods low in saturated fats, but you could use protein bars or powders of soy, whey, or rice origin to start your day with protein. When evaluating a protein bar, make sure it has at least 12 grams of protein and that it has no partially hydrogenated oils. For additional benefit, some high-quality protein bars have extra vitamins and minerals. It may be reasonable to make yourself a protein smoothie as part of your breakfast, with at least 20–25 grams of protein. For more on high-quality protein bars and powders, see Selected References for chapter 26.

> **FOOD TIP**
>
> To make a protein smoothie, use a blender to mix 1 1/2–2 scoops of protein powder with 8–10 ounces of liquid (e.g., organic milk or vanilla-flavored almond, oat, rice, or soy milk). Add a banana or organic berries (black- or blueberries); using different fruit combinations can improve taste and variety. If you are not getting omega-3 oils from fish or fish oil, you could add 1 tablespoon of flaxseed oil.

Protein on Outdoor Excursions

On outdoor excursions (unless they are in the winter), you will need to take vegetarian sources of protein because they don't spoil as rapidly in warmer weather. Excellent protein sources to take on long trips are peanuts, almonds, nut butters, soy nuts, and certain protein bars. They can be eaten separately or added to other foods to enhance taste.

Protein Precautions

Excessive protein may be detrimental because (1) it causes frequent urination to eliminate urea, a waste product formed when protein is digested, thus making the kidneys work overtime and possibly lose important electrolytes in the urine; (2) it can be high in fat, particularly saturated fat, and thus is a contributing factor in heart disease and certain types of cancer; and (3) a high-protein diet may cause more calcium to be excreted in your urine. This is particularly problematic for women because of their higher risk of osteoporosis. Remember, unused protein is stored as fat, like any other unused fuel source.

Vegetarian Diets

Vegetarians will usually be able to get enough protein and will not have any difficulty getting enough carbohydrates. Vegetarians can get complete protein from eggs, soy, or dairy products. If you don't eat those foods, you must eat a variety of incomplete proteins to supply the essential amino acids. Most vegetarian proteins don't contain the full complement of essential amino acids, so it is good practice to eat at least two different types of vegetarian food groups at each meal. It has been found that if you eat vegetarian protein sources from two different groups during the same day you will get a reasonable supply of all essential amino acids as long as you ingest an adequate number of overall protein grams per day. You can do this by eating legumes with grains or seeds (e.g., peanut butter with wheat crackers or bread), beans with grains (e.g., with tortillas or rice), or legumes with seeds (e.g., chickpeas with crushed sesame seeds or tahini).

Obtaining enough protein in a vegetarian diet requires more planning but is not difficult, especially if you eat soy products, beans, grains, nuts, and a variety of protein-containing foods.

> **FOOD TIP**
>
> Try increasing your intake of soy (especially organic and fermented soy products such as tempeh, tofu, and miso). It is an excellent protein source, and certain compounds in soy are thought to have many health benefits, including decreased risks of prostate and breast cancer, as well as a decreased chance of prostate hypertrophy. There is also evidence that soy can help decrease cholesterol levels. Soy-based foods include tofu, tempeh, soy powders and milk, soy nuts, and soybean sprouts. The less the soy product is processed, the better it is for your health.

Vegetarians may be at risk for vitamin B_{12} deficiency and should consider taking it as a supplement. This is especially important if you don't drink milk or eat eggs. Other areas of concern if your diet has minimal or no dairy products are vitamin D, calcium, and riboflavin. You can get some of these in fortified food products, but vitamin and mineral supplementation is advised for vegetarians. In a supplement, look for at least 200 micrograms of B_{12} and 400 IUs of vitamin D. If you don't eat dairy, consider a daily calcium supplement with 800–1,000 milligrams of calcium citrate.

> **FOOD TIP**
>
> To get enough vegetarian protein you can use dairy, eggs, and soy as complete (i.e., with all essential amino acids) nonflesh protein sources. If you combine dairy (preferably organic) with grains or legumes, you will be getting all of your essential amino acids. If you are vegan, combine grains (barley, corn, quinoa, rice, rye, spelt, or wheat) with legumes (beans, lentils, chick peas, peanuts, or soy).

Iron levels may also be low in vegetarians, especially in exercising and menstruating women, because iron from nonmeat sources is less well absorbed than iron from meats. Iron-deficiency anemia can develop and lead to decreased exercise performance and fatigue.

> **FOOD TIP**
>
> Vitamin C–containing foods (citrus fruits or certain vegetables) or low-dose supplements (100–250 mg) can be eaten with meals to enhance iron absorption.

Modified Carb-to-Protein-Ratio Diets

A number of popular diets have proposed lowering the carb-to-protein ratio for the purpose of regulating insulin and its subsequent effects. They are being advocated for weight loss as well as other health benefits. They are also interesting because they may have a favorable effect on fat burning and general health. There have been some reports of good endurance being possible on these diets. The science of nutrition is continually evolving, and our biochemical individuality may dictate different percentages of nutrients for different individuals. Although the optimal percentage of carbohydrate intake probably varies from person to person, it is likely that a reasonable range of intake is 50–70% especially if you are athletic or exercise frequently.

The lower carb-to-protein-ratio diets are not recommended for long mountaineering trips at higher altitudes because they have not been adequately studied and because rapid replenishment of glycogen stores each day is needed. The majority of health professionals and nutritionists still recommend the higher carbohydrate diet. Consult a health-care provider trained in nutritional and functional medicine for more information.

Fat

Fat is a stored source of energy, serves as a carrier for the fat-soluble vitamins (A, D, E, and K), protects vital organs, helps make hormones, and is an essential part of all cell membranes. At 9 kcals per gram, it is the most concentrated source of energy you can take on long outdoor excursions. Unfortunately, fat has gotten a bad reputation because of the relationship of saturated and partially hydrogenated fat to heart disease and cancer, and for contributing excess calories toward obesity.

Essential Fatty Acids

We need essential fatty acids (a form of fat) such as linoleic acid (omega-6) and alpha-linolenic acid (omega-3), which we cannot manufacture in our bodies. Eating the correct balance of fats is important to your nutrition and can influence the structure of your cell membranes and your general health. Most peoples' diets are very high in nonessential, saturated, and hydrogenated fat and are low in beneficial fatty acids. Some people, because of their concern over fats in general, eat an extremely low-fat diet that is actually deficient in essential fatty acids as well as the beneficial omega-3 fatty acids. This can lead to skin and other health problems. Follow the fat guidelines below to avoid such problems.

Certain fatty acids, namely, omega-3 fatty

acids found in flaxseed products and certain fish (salmon, sardines, and mackerel) and omega-6 fatty acids found in plant sources (primrose, borage, pumpkin, and walnuts), have been found to be beneficial to your health. The omega-3 oils have been shown to decrease risks of coronary artery disease, improve mood, and decrease some inflammatory disorders, especially of the gastrointestinal tract. They also can have a beneficial and regulatory effect on eicosanoid production in the body and may lead to decreases in inflammation when taken in certain amounts. It is recommended that we have about 1 part omega-3 oil for every 4–10 parts omega-6 oil in our diet. Most people have about a 1:20 ratio in their present diets, which is inadequate.

FOOD TIP

You can increase your intake of omega-3 oil by adding 1 gram of fish oil per day or by eating ocean-based cold-water fish. When purchasing a fish-oil product make sure it is tested for PCBs, pesticides, and heavy metals. For vegetarian sources of omega-3s, use 1–2 tablespoons of flaxseed oil per day. You can add it to smoothies, put it on salads or veggies, or add it to foods such as salsa or hummus. Don't heat flaxseed oil. You can also get a lesser amount of omega-3s from walnuts, pumpkin seeds, and canola oil.

Since the first edition of this book there has been a lot of media attention on the issue of mercury and PCBs in fish. For this reason it is recommended that you limit or eliminate your consumption of any large fish such as tuna and swordfish until the oceans become less polluted. It is also recommended that pregnant women stay away from fish during their pregnancy and probably during breast-feeding. Sources of purified fish oils are available and can be used to supplement your diet without the risk of the toxins.

The current recommendation is to consume less than 30% of total calories from fat and to get most of it from mono- and polyunsaturated fats such as olive, walnut, sesame, and flaxseed oil. To calculate your fat needs, take your total food calorie requirement per day (e.g., 2,500 kcals) and multiply it by a fat percentage of 20–30%. For example, $25\% \times 2{,}500 = 625$ kcals from fat. Fat has 9 kcals per gram, so divide your fat calorie requirement by 9, which in this example comes to 69 grams of fat per day.

Fats are abundant in foods, but you should pay attention to the right type of fat. Try especially to stay away from the hydrogenated and partially hydrogenated fats in processed carbohydrates as well as in nut butters and margarines. Examples of good sources of fat include avocados, artichokes, olives, fish, nuts and seeds, tofu, soy milk, and almonds.

FOOD TIP

It is important to bring adequate and diverse sources of fat on long outdoor trips (especially mountaineering trips), because they are compact, high-energy food sources. Good choices are cheese, olive oil, almonds and peanuts and their butters, other nuts, and sesame seeds. These can also be added to other foods to improve their flavor.

Fat Intake Guideline Summary

Limit your caloric intake of fat per day to 20–30% of total calories.

Increase this amount when you are on a multiday outdoor activity, especially a mountaineering expedition.

Try to limit the majority of your fat intake to poly- and monounsaturated fats, and decrease animal-related fat. Don't worry about this when planning for food during outdoor activities.

Avoid food products with partially hydrogenated oils.

Increase your intake of omega-3 fatty acids by using walnuts and flax oils, and using safe sources of small, cold-water fish or purified fish-oil supplements.

VITAMINS, MINERALS, AND FREE RADICALS

The percentage of daily value (% daily value) is an estimate of a safe and adequate nutrient intake that will prevent deficiency diseases. It is based on estimates for the population at large and not on individual needs. Humans have some biochemical individuality, and so some % daily values are limited in their usefulness. Always try to get as many nutrients from your food as possible. However, supplementation may be required because of poor soil quality where some foods are grown, and because of personal eating habits, the demands of exercise, and to achieve optimal health.

Free Radicals and Antioxidants

Increasing scientific evidence suggests that exercise causes an increase of free radicals in the body, particularly if you exercise outdoors and live in a metropolitan area or other place where the air is polluted. Free radicals are extremely reactive molecules that have an unpaired electron, which may seek to pair up with electrons from other molecules and can lead to cell damage. By stealing electrons, new free radicals are created and chain reactions can occur. Free radicals can harm your body by damaging your cells, impairing enzyme production, and by leading to damaged arteries and cardiovascular disease.

Free radicals are created by the body as a byproduct of oxygen metabolism. When we exercise, we breathe faster and require more oxygen for exercising muscles. Your body has an inherent capacity to rid itself of free radicals with naturally occurring antioxidants, but free radicals can exceed your body's ability to neutralize them, and supplements may be helpful. Antioxidants should not be taken separately in isolated form. It is better to combine them and take a formula that mixes a number of antioxidants or to take individual antioxidants together. Research shows the following antioxidants to be beneficial.

Alpha-lipoic acid is an antioxidant that works in water and fat components of cells. It can help to regenerate vitamins C and E and glutathione. Doses of 50–150 milligrams per day may be used to decrease free-radical damage.

Vitamin E scavenges free radicals produced in the fat (lipid) component of cells. Endurance exercise generates lipid free radicals, and vitamin E supplements can protect against exercise-induced tissue damage. Supplement with 400–600 IUs of mixed natural-source vitamin E per day.

Vitamin C is a water-based antioxidant that your body cannot synthesize. Our recommendation is 250–1,000 milligrams per day of vitamin C, and you might wish to take it in divided doses 2–3 times per day. You can get about 30–60 milligrams of vitamin C per serving in the following foods: cantaloupe, kiwi fruit, broccoli, kale, cabbage, brussels sprouts, green peppers, and citrus fruits.

Selenium is a trace mineral that is required as a component of an important antioxidant enzyme. It may also, on its own, decrease harmful changes to fat and have some role in preventing cancer and premature aging. The typical American diet is marginal or deficient in selenium. (The % daily value is 55–70 micrograms per day, but 200 mcg per day may be more protective.) Good food sources of selenium include seafood, whole grains, nuts, lean meats, and chicken. As our soils are becoming depleted in minerals, selenium is more difficult to get through diet alone.

Zinc, copper, and manganese are among the other trace minerals that are essential for the function of superoxide dismutase, one of the body's natural antioxidants. A good multiple vitamin should contain sufficient amounts of these nutrients. Recommended daily intakes are: zinc (aspartate or citrate form), 15–25 milligrams per day; copper, 1–2 milligrams per day; and manganese, 5–10 milligrams per day. Good food sources of these trace minerals include poultry, meat, fish, beans, eggs, and nuts.

Iron, another trace mineral involved in antioxidant enzyme activation, is paradoxically both a promoter as well as a scavenger of free radicals. Studies have demonstrated an increased relative risk of coronary artery disease as serum iron levels rise. There is no increase in the amount of iron needed for exercising individuals. It is recommended that you avoid food supplemented with a high percentage of iron and avoid vitamins with iron unless you have laboratory tests demonstrating an iron-deficiency anemia. Adolescents and premenopausal women need adequate iron because of increased needs. If you are not sure, have blood drawn by your physician to check for anemia and to see if iron supplementation is appropriate. Good food sources of iron include dark green vegetables, egg yolk, meat, fish, fortified cereals, and blackstrap molasses. If you are deficient in iron, take iron supplements or eat iron-rich foods along with vitamin C or vitamin C–rich foods to increase absorption.

ERGOGENIC AIDS

Ergogenic aids are substances that may enhance performance in aerobic, anaerobic, or weight-lifting activities. They may be appropriate for athletes involved in high-performance activities, races, or body building. Ergogenic aids include food, drugs, vitamins, herbs, hormones, nutritional supplements, and blood products. They range from accepted techniques such as carbohydrate loading to unsafe approaches such as anabolic-androgenic steroid use. To date, many substances have been studied, but few other than caffeine and creatine have shown much benefit. High-performance athletes should look at the reference works available and keep up with the literature before trying an ergogenic aid. It is important to look at the proposed mechanism of action and safety of the approach as well as studies that document improved exercise performance. You should also look at the guidelines for your sport and look into any regulating commissions, as many substances are banned if you enter into competitions. Remember that no ergogenic aid will replace good nutrition, proper rest, and good training habits.

There is evidence that creatine monohydrate can increase your ability to do anaerobic intervals and repeated brief spurts of strength moves. This might be helpful if you are racing or if you are climbing in a rock gym. There has not been adequate research using creatine at higher altitudes to know whether it is safe. The dosing schedule is 20–25 grams per day, in amounts of 5 grams 5 times per day, for 5 days for loading. Take 2 grams per day for maintenance during your training season. The main side effect is water weight gain, and it should not be taken if you have high blood pressure.

WATER AND FLUIDS

Water is essential to sustain the metabolic processes of your cells, your blood pressure, and all vital functions. It is also a key factor in your ability to regulate your temperature by sweating and getting rid of heat. You need to take in fluids to replace your body's losses.

Your body can lose water from waste excretion, moisture in the air you exhale (12 oz per day and up to 0.07–0.17 oz per minute with very strenuous exercise), and sweat (17 oz per day and up to 35 oz per hour of very strenuous exercise in hot weather). Your sweat losses are the most significant variable when you are physically active.

FOOD TIP

Even if you are not exercising, you need 8 glasses of good-quality fluid (filtered or bottled) per day. If possible, store your fluid in glass bottles rather than plastics, because of by-products in plastics. If you are exercising in hot weather, you need to replace your losses from sweating. Your kidneys have the ability to get rid of extra water if you drink more than you need. In this case, your urine will usually be lighter in color. Light or clear urine is desirable during an outdoor activity or after you have rehydrated following an exercise session or endurance event.

If you don't replace fluid losses, you can become dehydrated and lightheaded, have poor exercise performance and stamina, and risk more serious problems such as very low blood pressure or heat-related illnesses. The average daily fluid loss amounts to about 2,500–3,000 milliliters in the average person on an average temperature day without significant physical activity.

Your fluid input consists of the fluid you drink, the fluid in the food you eat, and the fluid generated by your metabolism.

FOOD TIP

Avoid alcohol and caffeinated beverages before long activities in the heat, because they can cause fluid loss. In warm weather, drink cold beverages. In cold weather, drink warm beverages.

Replacing Your Fluid Losses from Sweating

You can lose 32–64 ounces of fluid per hour of exercise. For every 16 ounces of fluid lost, you will lose a pound of body weight. The following are recommendations to prevent dehydration. Before regular and longer-duration exercise, drink 12–16 ounces of fluid 1 1/2–2 hours prior to your event or workout. After a vigorous short workout, drink 16–24 ounces of fluid. If you are in a race or competition, drink 6–8 ounces every 15–20 minutes. Drink enough after the competition is over to get your weight back to what it was before the competition. Drink 16 ounces (2 cups) for every pound of weight lost. If you are on a hike or cross-country ski trip, have your water handy and drink at least every hour, so that you feel good and have relatively clear urine. Carry at least two 32-ounce containers with you, and purify your water. You may need to drink 16–32 ounces per hour, depending on how vigorously you exercise and how hot it is. Your fluid requirements will increase in warmer weather, at higher altitudes, and with higher-intensity exercise.

Sport Drinks

Sport drinks contain a quick-acting carbohydrate as well as some sodium and potassium (electrolytes). They can provide carbohydrate calories and replace electrolytes, especially during a competitive event lasting more than 1 hour. The carbohydrate percentage should be about 6–8%. There is some evidence that drinks containing maltodextrin as the sugar may have the best benefit. Drink carbohydrate beverages during an event at a rate of 30–70 grams per hour. Read the label on a sport drink to determine how much carbohydrate it contains, and drink accordingly; usually 16–32 ounces per hour is equal to 30–70 grams per hour. If you are participating in an outdoor activity away from civilization, or if you are on a more leisurely bicycling event and can eat foods with some salt and potassium in them (such as salted foods and dried fruit), you don't need to carry a sport drink. As sport drinks are constantly changing, refer to Selected References for more information on particular sports drinks.

ALTITUDE, COLD WEATHER, AND MOUNTAINEERING TRIPS

Mountaineering and trekking at altitudes above 8,000 feet present numerous challenges, including getting enough calories and fluids. Fluid losses can increase because of increased breathing rates and fluid lost from expired air. Because everything seems more difficult at high altitude, extra effort and awareness must be given to maintaining adequate fluid balance. Every hour, drink approximately 8–32 ounces, depending on the temperature and how much sweating and rapid breathing you are doing. If your urine is dark yellow, you need to drink more. Your water should be conveniently situated so you don't have to remove your pack to get at it. All water should be filtered or treated. Consider bringing different flavored powders to flavor water if you cannot drink enough plain water. Bring a few packets of oral rehydration powder if you are going to less-developed countries where traveler's diarrhea is a possibility. If you develop diarrhea, make sure you increase your fluid intake to keep up with the water loss.

A large quantity of calories needs to be consumed because of the amount of energy used to hike or climb for long duration on slopes, snow, and rugged terrain. Every 1–2 hours, consume snacks with a combination of fats and carbohydrate. Try to have a variety of nuts and nut butters to provide protein and fat. Pack many different crackers, dried fruits, and cereals, and don't worry about the fat content. Remember, you often need to eat more than you feel like eating, especially at higher altitudes or when you are feeling weak or tired. Try saving some diverse, tasty, easy-to-eat food for high altitudes when you will need maximum calories and may have little appetite. Don't worry about gaining weight on a multiday trip or expedition. The problem is usually one of weight loss, not weight gain.

FOOD TIP

You can usually pack enough food to meet your energy needs on an outdoor excursion if you plan for three meals and at least four snacks per day. Use bars or handfuls of energy-dense snack foods with protein and fat to add extra calories during the day. Eat during at least every other water or rest break. A bar or a handful of gorp usually has 200–250 kcals.

There is no consensus concerning diets for exercise in the cold. The evidence is strong that increased amounts of carbohydrates, and high calorie and fluid intake, are necessary. Foods with a high fat content are reasonable. Remember to drink frequently even though it is cold.

chapter 3 AEROBIC CONDITIONING AND INTERVAL TRAINING

By David Musnick, M.D. and Dorothy Sager Dolan, B.A., L.M.P.

THIS CHAPTER WILL HELP YOU:

- Understand what makes aerobic exercise aerobic.
- Understand the minimum aerobic program needed to achieve health benefits from exercise.
- Be able to modify the minimum aerobic program to meet the specific endurance demands of your planned outdoor activity.
- Be able to evaluate appropriate aerobic activities and equipment you can use to accomplish sport-specific goals.
- Understand the importance of the intensity at which you exercise and how to calculate intensity levels.
- Develop a complete program through goal setting and a heart-zone-intensity approach.

Aerobic exercise is the repetitive use of large muscle groups at submaximal effort for prolonged periods. This type of exercise utilizes oxygen at the cellular level to enable efficient production of energy storage molecules to supply energy for contracting muscles. With regular aerobic exercise, you can increase your stamina (endurance) and be able to exercise at your previous intensity, or a higher intensity, with more ease and less feeling of fatigue. The aerobic component of your conditioning program improves basic endurance and can lead to health benefits.

Health Benefits of Aerobic Exercise

To achieve health benefits from exercise, you must do at least a regular aerobic (cardio) workout program. Aerobic exercise can have significant positive impacts on overall health.

One health benefit is a decreased risk of developing complications from coronary artery disease, including fatal heart attacks. Compared to individuals of comparable age and risk factors, you can reduce your risk of heart attack by 50% and your risk of stroke by 40% by following this chapter's guidelines for a minimum aerobic program.

Aerobic exercise may lower blood pressure and total cholesterol, including low-density cholesterol (LDL), and increase beneficial high-density cholesterol (HDL). The potential for blood clotting is also reduced, which is a presumed factor in decreased cardiovascular risk. The incidence of some types of cancer may decrease, especially colon cancer.

Regular aerobic exercise can improve sensitivity to the hormone insulin, which will decrease the risk of developing type 2 diabetes. If you have type 2 diabetes, you can improve the condition with regular exercise.

Metabolic syndrome, also called Syndrome X, is a set of metabolic problems associated with insulin resistance. These include diabetes, elevated LDL and total cholesterol, low HDL cholesterol, and elevated blood pressure. Aerobic exercise can decrease insulin resistance and thus improve such symptoms. Aerobic exercise is important for Syndrome X even if it is only 10–15 minutes of walking or cycling 1–2 times a day. If you have Syndrome X, it is best to work up to the minimum aerobic program described in this chapter and to exercise at a lower intensity (60–70% of your maximum heart rate; see Intensity below). Your Syndrome X symptoms will improve more rapidly if you exercise for sessions of longer than 30 minutes, especially if you are overweight.

Aerobic exercise is a very important component of any weight-loss program. It helps an overweight person increase calorie usage. For weight loss, it is important to start with some short periods of exercise (10–15 minutes) and to gradually work up to 30-minute sessions (longer exercise sessions as well as occasional interval training can also be helpful for weight loss, if your schedule and body permit; see chapter 29).

You can help to maintain or possibly improve the bone density in your legs, hips, and back by doing moderately impact-loaded exercise (see the Impact of Aerobic Options section later in this chapter). This is especially important for women beginning in their 50s (i.e., for peri- or postmenopausal women), but maintaining bone density is important for men and women of any age.

Regular aerobic exercise can lead to improved sleep, especially if the exercise is done prior to 6 P.M. You can also reduce stress and stress-related muscle pain with regular exercise. A decrease in anxiety and an improved mood often result as well. The risk of developing, and the severity of, depression may also decrease.

Risks of Aerobic Exercise

There are possible risks to starting or increasing the intensity of aerobic exercise, predominantly related to complications of preexisting coronary artery disease, or other heart or lung problems. Consult a doctor familiar with exercise evaluation and testing if:

- You have physical symptoms with exercise.
- You have a known disease condition.
- You are male and over 40 or female and over 50 and would like to begin or significantly increase the intensity of an aerobic exercise program or activity. This is especially important when starting interval training.

Other risks include overuse injuries such as strains and sprains, which are usually related to excessive exercise impact, quantity, or high-intensity interval training. Poor posture, excessive weight-loading (such as a backpack that's too heavy), and inadequate equipment can also play a significant role. See chapter 9, Anatomy and Musculoskeletal Injury: Prevention and Treatment, for more information on injuries.

Free radicals and aerobic exercise. There is evidence that free-radical oxygen molecules are generated during aerobic activity. These are molecules with one or more unpaired electrons that seek out other molecules to complete their unpaired electrons. They may contribute to damage in your tissues if there is an imbalance of free radicals with antioxidant reactions. (For more on this subject, see chapter 2, Nutritional Considerations for Conditioning.) The amount of free-radical load is likely to increase with increasing aerobic exercise, especially with increased intensity and when exercising in areas with poor air quality. It is recommended that you have adequate antioxidants in your diet (see chapter 2) to help prevent such harmful side effects from your exercise.

THE FIVE VARIABLES OF AEROBIC CONDITIONING

Frequency, duration, intensity, specificity, and progression are the five variables of aerobic conditioning. **Frequency:** How often should you train? **Duration:** How long should you train? **Intensity:** How hard should you train? **Specificity:** What specific activity should you do? **Progression:** How should you progress your workout once you have obtained your desired initial level of fitness? Your aerobic conditioning goals and knowledge of the effects and risks of modifying the variables will influence your answers to these questions.

The Minimum Aerobic Program

The American College of Sports Medicine and the Surgeon General's Physical Activity and Health Report recommend a minimum aerobic program, so named because it is the "dose" of exercise that can help you increase your likelihood of experiencing certain health benefits discussed above. It has been found that aerobic exercise of less intensity or duration will still improve stamina, decrease stress, and aid in weight loss. If you are presently sedentary or exercising very irregularly, the minimum aerobic program, outlined below, can enable you to increase your stamina and increase your chances of improved health.

Frequency: 5-6 times per week.

Duration: 30 minutes within your intensity range; may require an addition of 5–10 minutes of warm-up and cooldown time.

Intensity: Within your target zone, 60–85% of your maximum heart rate (70% is ideal).

Calories: the activity should use a minimum of 200–300 kilocalories (kcals).

FREQUENCY

Frequency is the number of aerobic conditioning sessions you do per week. Six sessions a week results in the best physiological response. If you have been sedentary, begin with 2–3 sessions a week. For full cardiovascular risk reduction, increase your exercise frequency gradually.

DURATION

Duration is the amount of time you maintain the proper intensity in your exercise session. Gradually increase your intensity level until you reach your heart-rate training zone, and do 30–50 minutes of continuous activity at this "plateau" intensity. If you are a beginner, start with 10–20 minutes. Optimum duration depends on the intensity you maintain and what your goals are. In order to achieve health and fitness benefits, exercise should be long enough to expend at least 200–300 kcals per session, but stress reduction can occur with exercise of any duration. Thirty minutes of moderate-intensity exercise can usually expend 200–300 kcals. In general, limit your aerobic training sessions on consecutive days to 50 minutes or less so that you don't overtrain.

If you are training for outdoor activities that last longer than a few hours, plan a lower-intensity, longer-duration (LILD) exercise session each week at an exercise intensity and difficulty level that are similar to your outdoor activity (usually 50–65% of your maximum heart rate). You should feel comfortable at this intensity and be able to sustain it for 2–4 hours, so as to achieve approximately three-quarters of the expected duration of your first major outdoor activity. You can increase the duration 10–15% per week; if it is a lower-impact activity such as cross-country skiing, hiking, or paddling, you can increase the duration 20% per week. These longer sessions should usually consist of the outdoor activity that you are training for, or one very similar to it, using similar muscle groups. It is good to start these longer training sessions within 6–8 weeks of your expected activity or sooner if your goal is ascending a high mountain or running a long race. As the weeks go by, you may decide to add both distance and difficulty gradually so your body can adapt to the training stresses without injury.

INTENSITY

The intensity of aerobic activity is related to the level of oxygen consumption and the energy demands of your contracting muscles. Intensity is perhaps the most important variable that can affect your fitness, endurance, and aerobic power. Think of intensity as a percentage of your maximum aerobic ability that responds to increases in variables such as speed, slope, resistance, and so on. As you increase any or all of these variables, and thus increase your exercise intensity, you will feel like you are working harder. Your exercise will stimulate a demand for increased oxygen and blood flow and a corresponding increase in your heart rate. Your heart rate increases in direct correlation with increasing exercise intensity and oxygen consumption.

The intensity at which you exercise is measured in heartbeats per minute (your pulse). The intensity range (target zone) that you choose (and within which you try to stay after you have warmed up) is related to many factors, including:

- Present fitness level.
- Desire to burn fat and lose weight.
- Activity goals and the intensity demands of your desired activity.
- Health-related exercise goals.
- Health status, including your risks for heart disease, presence of any heart rate–lowering drugs, and any musculoskeletal problems.

All of these factors, except the last, are covered in the sections below. Any individual with health problems should seek an evaluation and advice as to safe exercise-intensity zones from a physician trained in stress testing and familiar with exercise prescription.

A threshold of intensity to elicit a training stimulus seems to be an exercise pulse rate of about 50–70% of your maximum heart rate, though this varies among individuals. The percentage and type of fuel used are also directly related to exercise intensity, with a higher percentage of fat burned for fuel at lower-intensity levels (less than 70% of maximum heart rate). Remember that working out at very high-intensity levels (85% of maximum heart rate, or higher) might be associated with higher risks of injury or medical problems. Intensity can be expressed in many ways, including:

1. Calories expended per unit of time.
2. Percentage of maximum oxygen consumption (% VO_2 max).
3. Rating of perceived exertion (RPE).
4. Percentage of maximum heart rate (% max HR).
5. Anaerobic threshold, a level related to the lactate threshold.

Methods 3 and 4 are the most practical for the average exercising individual. These, along with methods 1 and 5, are described below. Method 2 is the most accurate but is expensive and requires the most equipment. It is not practical for most people.

Calories

Calories expended per unit of time is an important factor if you are trying to accurately estimate your calorie needs to maintain your weight or to lose weight. This is especially true for long outdoor trips, to ensure that you have enough food to meet your energy needs. Calorie expenditure in kcals per minute is dependent on your body composition, intensity of the exercise, and the workload, such as whether you are carrying a pack. Although there is a great deal of individual variability, a fit person weighing about 150 pounds burns or metabolizes 7–10 kcals per minute for most moderate activities, including aerobic dance classes, cycling, rowing, backpacking, and mountaineering. Walking, swimming, and kayaking usually burn 5–6 kcals per minute unless they are very vigorous. Running, cross-country skiing, snowshoeing, and mountaineering with a heavy pack can use more than 10 kcals per minute, and up to 20. In general, the calorie values listed on exercise machines, especially stair-climbers, are overestimated.

Rate of Perceived Exertion

Rating your perceived exertion (RPE) is a method that can help you evaluate your exercise intensity by how hard you feel the exercise is on a scale from 0 to 10, with 0 being nothing at all and 10 being very, very heavy. Your RPE can be correlated to your heart rate response to exercise by using a heart rate monitor or by taking your exercise pulse.

An adequate work intensity for achieving aerobic conditioning elicits a response of a value of 3–6. Interval high-intensity training leads to an RPE of 7–10. Most outdoor activities can be sustained at an RPE of 2–5.

FIGURE 3. RATE OF PERCEIVED EXERTION

RPE	Exercise intensity	(% max HR)
0	Resting	
2	Light work	50–60%
4	Somewhat hard	60–70%
5	Heavy (strong), moderately hard	70–80%
7	Very heavy	80–90%
10	Very, very heavy (almost maximum)	90–100%

Heart Rate

Heart rate is a guiding factor for the intensity level of aerobic training. Most heart rate calculations of intensity use your maximum heart rate (max HR), which is the highest heart rate you can attain during hard exercise. The safest way to determine your maximum heart rate is to take a graded exercise stress test on a treadmill. This should be done for people who fall into a higher risk category for coronary artery disease or other diseases due to age, symptoms, family history, and other factors. If you have questions about this, consult a physician trained in exercise testing.

As a rule, any man over 40 or woman over 50 who is thinking about exercising at moderate to high intensities should consider having a stress test. It will screen for electrical changes indicative of decreased heart blood supply and give you a maximum heart rate and a training zone prescription. You can also get an idea of your maximum heart rate from supervised short aerobic testing (2–4 minutes of running or cycling) while wearing a heart rate monitor (see Edwards, *Heart Zone Training*, in Selected References). This is usually safe for people under 40 with no other medical problems or risks for heart disease.

Heart Rate Calculations

There can be a substantial error of up to plus or minus 25 beats per minute when using any formula to predict your maximum heart rate. You can estimate your maximum heart rate by subtracting your age from the number 220. Fit people over 40 may have a maximum heart rate that is underestimated by that formula. Maximum heart rate times a range of percentages, from 60% to 85% max HR, will give you an estimate of your various training zones.

During times of higher-volume training, occasionally take your pulse before getting out of bed in the morning to determine if you are training too hard. If you are, you might find a morning resting pulse that is elevated past (8–10 beats per minute higher than) your normal one. This, along with a feeling of fatigue, may be an indication that you are overtraining.

PRACTICAL POINT

To find your resting heart rate, take your pulse (turn your left forearm palm side up, and place two or three fingers from your right hand on your left wrist below the base of your left thumb) in a standing position for 15 seconds, and multiply it times 4 to get your per minute pulse rate (see Figure 4). You can also take your pulse right above your collarbone's midsection, if you have difficulty finding it at the base of your thumb. In general, it is not good to take your pulse right below your jaw, as putting pressure on this area can stimulate a response that may slow the pulse rate or make you lightheaded.

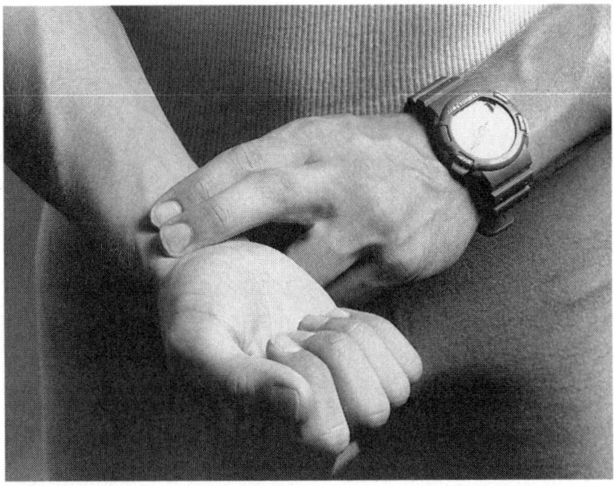

FIGURE 4

Calculate Your Heart-Rate Training Zones

Calculating various heart-rate intensity zones allows you to choose intensity zones appropriate for accomplishing certain goals. If you don't want to be this specific, calculate a 60% max HR and start there. Gradually increase your intensity until you are at 70–85% (closer to 70%) for the majority of your exercise. Try doing these calculations for yourself using an actual tested maximum, or estimate your maximum by subtracting your age from 220. Calculate your heart rate zones by using the formulas below.

Zone 5: 90–100% max HR

(my zone 5 =   ). Zone for intervals and training for speed and power, anaerobic/very, very hard exertion (sprints of less than 1 minute). Improved performance can occur from training in this zone, but there is a higher risk of musculoskeletal injuries and possible cardiovascular problems. Do most of your training below this zone.

Zone 4: 80–90% max HR

(my zone 4 =   ). Zone for intervals and training for aerobic and anaerobic power at or beyond the lactate threshold. Fast HR and breathing rate. Very hard RPE (brief push in a kayak in rough water or tough, steep parts of a climb, hike, etc.).

Zone 3: 70–80% max HR

(my zone 3 =   ). Moderately hard RPE (your average workout after you have achieved a basic aerobic fitness level).

Zone 2: 60–70% max HR

(my zone 2 =   ). Somewhat hard RPE. An average level for longer-duration activities such as hiking, or for when you are gradually building aerobic fitness or working on weight loss.

Zone 1: 50–60% max HR

(my zone 1 =   ). Zone with high percentage of fat metabolized, and for lower-intensity, longer-duration (LILD) workouts. A light work RPE. A common zone for prolonged outdoor activities or when you are starting your fitness training.

Heart Rate Monitors

Using a heart rate monitor is one of the most effective ways to monitor your aerobic intensity. These generally consist of transmitter units mounted in chest straps that pick up electrical signals from your heart and transmit them to a receiver on your wrist or to a readout on your exercise machine. The continuous, accurate feedback allows you to be aware of your heart rate response and adjust the intensity of your exercise to stay within your desired intensity. Heart rate monitors are available at exercise equipment and sporting good stores.

Lactate Threshold

Your breathing response is also a good indicator of exercise intensity. If you are in aerobic training zones 1–3, you should feel relatively comfortable breathing and be able to talk while you exercise.

As you increase the intensity, you will notice a level of breathing that feels difficult and at which it is not easy to carry on a conversation. This will be associated with a feeling that it is very hard work and that you would not like to continue very long at this intensity level. There may also be a feeling of muscle discomfort. This is approximately the level at which you accumulate excessive lactic acid; this is called your lactate threshold. Your lactate threshold is usually some point between 80% and 90% of your maximum heart rate. Interval training helps increase your tolerance for lactic acid as it builds up in your system, and your body learns to use lactate as an alternate fuel source.

Interval Training

Interval training is the performance of an aerobic activity done at high intensities for brief periods of time. The energy systems used by your body may be aerobic or anaerobic, depending on how intense your exercise is. The goal of interval training is to increase your ability to do short spurts of high-intensity aerobic activity and to improve your aerobic fitness. In outdoor activities, very high-intensity aerobic activity may last less than 5 minutes. Moderately high-intensity activity may last for longer periods. Examples are going up a very steep, short trail, snow, or crevasse field; crossing a stream or boulder field; kayaking or paddling through a rough or dangerous area of water; or sprinting at the end of a race. Training for this short, high-intensity output can greatly improve your ability to accomplish these tasks well and without injury when the need arises.

You can use a variety of interval techniques, depending on the activities you are interested in. Try to simulate the conditions in which you do your bursts of activity, such as walking up slopes on trails or snow fields, bicycling up hills, or paddling through rough water. You can also add different types of interval training to more quickly improve your overall aerobic conditioning.

Interval training risks. Many people never do high-intensity activity spurts and may prefer not to do interval training because of the injury risks or because they are content with their fitness level. Because interval training puts a higher demand on your cardiovascular and musculoskeletal systems, it is not recommended for anyone with heart, lung, or musculoskeletal problems. A solid level of aerobic fitness (at least 6 weeks of training and an ability to exercise briefly at close to 80% max HR) is necessary before beginning interval training. Precautions:

- Don't do intervals on consecutive days or when you are recovering from an injury that involves your back, hips, or legs.
- Don't do intervals if you have an infection or are anemic.
- Slow down or stop the interval if you have chest pain or excessive pain elsewhere.

Designing an interval workout. Consider adding intervals to your workout 2 times a week. The goal for each interval is to work out at an intensity of 80–100% max HR, depending on where your lactate threshold is (but usually in the 80–90% range). Interval training can be done as a separate activity or within a regular aerobic workout or outdoor activity, such as Fartlek training (see below). You can do intervals while running, stair climbing, or doing any outdoor activity, as well as while using any indoor aerobic exercise machine (treadmill, stair-climber, etc.).

In interval training, the workout time segments are split into alternating periods of hard efforts, called the exercise interval, and recovery periods, called the recovery interval. The recovery periods usually consist of lower-intensity aerobic activity (50–70% max HR), and they are related to the length of the exercise interval by a ratio of work:rest. Recovery times are indicated in Figure 5, but you may need a longer rest period depending on how you feel. Based on the demands of your sport, you can choose the appropriate work interval that would be most applicable to your athletic goal. The intervals can be done as part of your general training or as a component of your activity-specific conditioning program.

Practical aspects of interval training. Warm up for 10–15 minutes at 60–70% max HR

FIGURE 5. SAMPLE INTERVAL WORKOUT

	Interval Distance Training	Interval Mid-Distance Training	Interval Sprint Training
Work:Rest Ratio	1:1	1:2	1:3+
Heart Rate Zone	Zone 2–3	Zone 4	Zone 4–5
Exercise Load Duration(s)	240 sec–15 min	30 sec–240 sec	10 sec–30 sec
Recovery Time(s)	240 sec–15 min	60 sec–480 sec	30 sec–90 sec
Repetitions	2–5	5–15	5–20
Energy Supply	Aerobic	Anaerobic	Anaerobic

before you begin an interval effort. Increase your heart rate to 80–95% max HR or work until you perceive your effort as very hard (6+ RPE). Hold the intensity there for the amount of time in your exercise interval, then reduce the workload to a recovery level by reducing speed, incline, or resistance until your heart rate has dropped to approximately 50–70% max HR. Hold your intensity at this level for the duration of your rest interval.

Based on how you feel, you can begin the next intense effort and try the sequence again. Initially try intervals of 30–60 seconds and do 2–4 of them. Gradually build up to 4–10 intervals per workout. You can decide on the duration of the intervals based on the demands of your activity. If your activity demands very short bursts of maximum intensity, then do intervals of 20–30 seconds. Your average intermediate intervals should be 30–120 seconds, the most common duration for interval training. Endurance anaerobic intervals are 120–240 seconds. Endurance aerobic intervals are 5–20 minutes.

Fartlek Interval Training

Fartlek interval training is interval training that is randomly dispersed throughout your workout in regard to when you start the interval. The interval duration, the rest period, and so on. When you are training outside, you can use the distance between telephone poles, hill to hill, tree to tree, stone to stone, or any landmarko measure your interval. You can also use time periods.

Fartleks usually involve spurts of increased intensity that last 30 seconds–4 minutes. Try to exercise in a low- to moderate-intensity zone as a baseline (60–75% max HR), and then work out in higher-intensity intervals in various zones (zones 4 and 5), depending on the terrain and how you feel. This can be done on exercise equipment and can also be done outside by hiking, running, biking, or cross-country skiing. In a Fartlek interval, you usually continue some baseline aerobic activity between intervals. You can do the intervals at different intensities, speeds, and slopes. Below are some sample Fartlek programs.

Cycling. Do 2–4 repetitions (reps) of 30-60-90-120-90-60-30 seconds of Fartlek intervals, keeping your heart rate at 80–85% max HR. Each rest interval should be twice as long as the exercise interval.

Hiking. Try this on a training day hike. After hiking for at least 30 minutes at a moderate pace, begin some random fast hiking. Pick a tree, stone, or bend in a switchback to head for, and use varying times of 20 seconds–2 minutes. Start with the 20-second interval and hike as fast as you can to your landmark, then slow down your pace until you feel only a light to moderate RPE. Try these short intervals on relatively level or gradual slopes, then try them on steeper trail sections. Within about a half hour from your major rest stop, try some longer intervals of 1–2 minutes at a slightly lower intensity than the first set of intervals. Rest at least 1–2 times the interval length until you are in your recovery heart rate, and try again 1–3 more times. Avoid doing these on downhill sections. Make sure you drink enough water, and avoid doing this on very hot days or on slippery or exposed terrain.

Aerobic machines. You can do Fartlek intervals on any piece of aerobic exercise equipment if there is a manual setting and you feel very comfortable and well balanced on the equipment. Increase the intensity by putting more effort into self-propelled equipment such as cycles or cross-country ski machines. For machines with intensity buttons, such as stair-climbers and treadmills, you can dial up the speed. Some equipment has programmed interval settings. Look at these beforehand to see if they are appropriate for you.

Slope Intervals

Slope intervals are intervals you could do on short hiking, snowshoe, or climbing trips in which you are on slopes rather than relatively flat terrain. Slope intervals are done like Fartlek intervals. The duration of slope intervals is usually less than that of intervals on level ground. It is best to try these with and without a pack.

SPECIFICITY

The options for aerobic exercise are numerous. Modes of Aerobic Conditioning, later in this chapter, gives details and the pros and cons of equipment, classes, and outdoor activities. As a general rule, choose two or three options to give you a variety and to prevent overuse injuries.

To achieve health benefits, try walking, cycling, or using a treadmill, elliptical trainer, or stair-climber, as well as aerobic classes. Chapter 26 discusses aerobic options for overall health benefits; chapter 29 details aerobic options for weight loss. If you are a senior or have a neurological condition, refer to chapter 29; see chapter 30 if you have a fatigue-related condition.

If you are working on specific training or activity goals, your training should be specific to the demands of your outdoor activity, in regard to the muscles used, patterns of motion, loads (if any), and duration and intensity of your activity. If you usually do lower-body activities, there is not a great deal of transfer of aerobic capacity when you first try a predominantly upper-body activity such as crew, kayaking, or swimming. The optimal way to train for a specific activity is to do it, or something closely resembling it in regard to the muscles used. For suggestions on specificity of activities, refer to Figure 6, Aerobic Cross Training and Specificity.

Cross Training

While repeatedly using the same training machines or doing the same activities may enhance your performance in your chosen activity, over-reliance on the specificity principle can cause problems. Overuse injuries such as tendonitis and bursitis can result from training the same way all the time. If you never train the rest of your body, you may sustain injury from strength imbalances. Cross training means training with various activities or types of exercise equipment. You can choose standing vs. seated positions, for example, to change the stress on your hip, knee, and ankle joints.

Cross training can also mean choosing an alternate training mode that will train muscles not usually used in your primary activity. Many injuries can be avoided if you avoid overuse and incorporate some cross training. Figure 6 suggests some ways you can train specifically for a sport, as well as some options for cross training.

PROGRESSION

As you plan your aerobic program, consider base development, intensity development, and maintenance. This is a way to plan how to use the total training time you have available. If you are training for a specific event, there will be a definite target date for your peak. If you are training for a seasonal activity, there will be a range of

FIGURE 6. AEROBIC CROSS TRAINING AND SPECIFICITY

Activity/Exercise	**Stair climbing**	**Stair-climber**	**Cross-country skiing**	**Cross-robics**	**Treadmill**	**Climbing wall**	**EFX Cross-trainer**	**Cycling**	**Rowing**	**In-line skating**	**Step aerobics**	**Swimming**	**Running**	**Hiking**	**Slideboard**
Windsurfing	S	X	X	X	X	X	X	X	S	X	X	S	X	X	S
Walking	X	X	X	X	S	X	X	X	O	X	X	O	S	S	X
Hiking	S	S	X	X	S	X	S	X	O	X	S	O	S	S	X
Running	X/S	X/S	X	X	S	X	S	X	O	X	X	O	S	X	X
Rock Climbing	S	S	X	X	X	S	X	X	S	X	S	O	X	X	X
Scrambling	S	S	S	X	S	S	X	O	X	X	S	O	S	S	X
Mountaineering	S	S	S	X	S	S	X	O	X	X	S	O	S	S	X
Skiing, Downhill	X	X	X	X	X	X	X	X	X	X	X	O	X	X	X
Snowboarding	X	X	X	X	X	X	X	O	X	X	X	O	X	X	S
Skiing, Telemark	S	S	S	X	X	X	X	X	X	S	S	O	S	S	S
Skiing, Skate	X	X	S	X	X	X	X	X	X	S	X	O	S	X	S
Skiing, Cross-Country	X	X	S	X	X	X	X	X	X	S	X	O	S	X	S
Snowshoeing	S	S	S	X	S	X	S	X	X	X	S	O	S	S	S
Cycling	X	X	X	X	X	X	X	S	X	X	X	O	X	X	X
Rowing	X	X	X	X	O	X	O	X	S	X	X	O	X	X	O
Canoeing	O	O	X	O	O	X	O	O	S	O	O	X	O	O	O
Kayaking	O	O	X	O	O	O	O	O	X	O	O	X	O	O	O

S = Specific: Choose this option to train muscles and joints in ways similar to the demands of your sport.
X = Cross train: Choose this option to train muscles and joints with different demands from those used in your sport.
O = Cross train other: Choose this option to train other muscles than those used in your sport in order to balance your body.

time in which you want to maintain high levels of aerobic conditioning. You can enter this sequence at any stage, depending on your fitness level.

About 6 weeks after beginning a conditioning program, you can restructure your training cycle to include increases in intensity and interval training. Always keep in mind the demands of the actual sport you are pursuing. Use that specific activity to monitor the progress you are making. The closer you get to the event or season, the more sport-specific your training activities should be. For example, if your plan is to climb a mountain, spend more time on stair-climbers and hiking than on bicycles or kayaking.

Rate of Progression

Initial conditioning stage. If you have not been doing regular aerobic conditioning, start at this stage to build your aerobic base and achieve the physiological adaptations required for an event or season. This stage may last 4–6 weeks. Frequency should be 3–4 nonconsecutive days. Duration should be 12–15 minutes initially and gradually increase to 30 minutes. Intensity as measured by heart rate should be 50–70% max HR, starting at the low end. This stage should also include strength training at 2–3 sessions per week of light resistance with a higher number of repetitions (15–20 per set). Try to increase your exercise duration by 10–15% per week, and gradually increase the intensity.

Improvement conditioning stage. This lasts 12–20 weeks. Frequency should be 5–6 days per week. Consider 1–2 aerobic sessions of 40–50 minutes, with your other sessions closer to 30 minutes. Increase duration every 1–3 weeks by 10–15% until you reach 30–50 minutes. Intensity as measured by heart rate should be 70–80% max HR for fitness and health benefits. In addition, there might be a longer period of a lower-intensity, 50–60% max HR, if you are conditioning for an aerobic outdoor activity requiring endurance or if you are trying to lose weight. Consider doing some cross training 1 day a week to avoid injuries, especially if you are exercising more than 30 minutes 3 times a week. You may add intervals after 4–8 weeks in this stage, if you have goals of doing high-intensity spurts of activity or to more quickly increase your aerobic fitness. This stage should also include strength training with increased resistance and lower repetitions (8–12) per set. Specificity can be added if you are training for a specific activity; do activity-specific balance and skill exercises.

Maintenance conditioning stage. When you have reached your desired level of conditioning, your emphasis can be redirected to activity challenges. It is easier to maintain strength and endurance levels than it is to achieve them initially. Maintenance can be sustained with a frequency of 3 sessions per week, but the activities should be of the same duration and intensity used to achieve the improvements. Try to do aerobic conditioning 5–6 days a week if you wish to achieve maximum health benefits.

Making a 1-Week Plan

Begin by looking at a 1-week plan. Include 1 rest day and 1 day of active rest. Active rest is when you are physically active doing something other than your usual training. (Individuals 50 and older may do better with an additional rest day.) This leaves you with 5–6 days of specific training. Alternate between hard days and easy days. (Hard days are those on which you do interval training, or longer time or distance.) Try to use particular HR or RPE targets for every workout.

Heart-Rate Zone Training

A heart-rate zone training approach can be used to progress your aerobic conditioning and achieve an activity goal. Such an approach is based on periods of times in various training zones. See chapter 19 for an example of an aerobic program for mountaineering-based heart-rate zone training.

Building an endurance base. In this period, you are training primarily to improve your cardiovascular and muscular systems' adaptation to aerobic exercise, and to build your general endurance.

Spend 10% of your total training time at 50–60% max HR (zone 1).

Spend 80% of your total training time at 60–70% max HR (zone 2).

Spend 10% of your total training time at 70–80% max HR (zone 3), after you have been working out in zone 2 for at least 3 weeks.

Increasing your endurance. In this period, you are training primarily in your aerobic heart rate zones.

Spend 20% of your total training time at 50–70% max HR (zones 1 and 2).

Spend 70% of your total training time at 70–80% max HR (zone 3).

Spend 10% of your total training time above 80% max HR (zone 4); make sure you have spent 2 weeks at 70–80% max HR before you begin this interval training.

Increasing your speed. In this period, your focus shifts to adding more anaerobic interval training.

Spend 20% of your total training time at 50–70% max HR (zones 1 and 2).

Spend 60% of your total training time at 70–80% max HR (zone 3).

Spend 10% of your total training time above 80% max HR (zone 4).

Spend 10% of your total training time above 90% max HR (zone 5).

Reaching your peak. In this period, you further increase your percentage of time in interval training. This is especially appropriate for racing or competition, for which a very high level of aerobic fitness is critical. This period likely would not be necessary for most recreational activities such as mountaineering, kayaking, noncompetitive cycling, and running, but is included for completeness.

Spend 10% of your total training time below 70% max HR (zones 1 and 2).

Spend 60% of your total training time at 70–80% max HR (zone 3).

Spend 20% of your total training time above 80% max HR (zone 4).

Spend 10% of your total training time above 90% max HR (zone 5).

Developing a plan. If you have 12 weeks to train for your target, spend the first 4 weeks building your endurance base, the second 4 weeks increasing aerobic endurance zones, and the third 4 weeks increasing your speed. Include time in the peak period if you are training for a race or competing. It is good to plan a reduced volume of training 1 week before your event so your body can rest and charge up its fuel stores.

These periods are similar to periods of progression discussed above and the periods discussed in chapter 7, but they are more specific to a zone type of training. Of important note is that some of the zones include a significant amount of high-intensity training (intervals), and you should be very healthy and medically cleared for this type of activity. It is possible to accomplish most goals with very little or no interval training if you cannot do that part of conditioning.

THE AEROBIC EXERCISE SESSION

Warm-up period. For a short period before you achieve your training zone, start at a low intensity of the aerobic activity you will be doing and gradually increase the intensity until you are in your heart-rate training zone. The warm-up period may last 5–10 minutes and can decrease the likelihood of overuse injuries.

Plateau period. Your target training heart rate zone is the range of heartbeats per minute within which you can achieve conditioning benefits. The best method for an individual aerobic session is to warm up (see above) and then stay in a plateau period of intensity for a prescribed time, until the cooldown period.

Cooldown period. After you have completed your aerobic training, gradually decrease your level of intensity for 2–5 minutes (longer after very high-intensity or endurance events, or 10% of your workout time). This has been shown to decrease the likelihood of heart rhythm disturbances and may decrease muscle soreness. Abruptly stopping an aerobic exercise or activity is not a good idea.

Figure 7 shows a typical aerobic training session. This is an example of a 45-minute aerobic period for a 50-year-old training at a 70–80% max HR. Notice the gradual increase of intensity in the warm-up period and the gradual decrease in intensity in the cooldown period. Also notice the heart rate in the training zone.

FIGURE 7

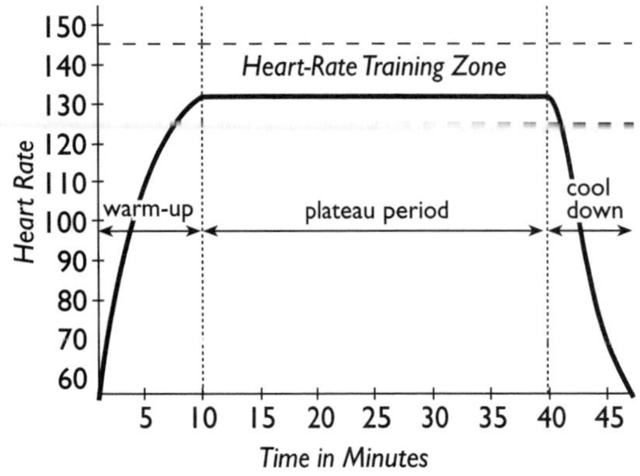

Modes of Aerobic Conditioning

The modality you select for developing cardiorespiratory fitness should use large muscle groups, be rhythmical, and be maintained continuously throughout your workout. Consider the following when choosing your activity:

- If you are training for a specific activity, you should spend a high percentage of time (at least 60%) in activity-specific aerobic sessions that use muscles and motion patterns similar to those you will use in your chosen activity or sport.
- Choose activities that are less likely to exacerbate existing injuries or restricted areas of motion, if you have any.
- Spend some time doing activities that you enjoy, to prevent becoming bored with your exercise program.
- Vary your activities to decrease the amount of impact if you are doing a high volume of aerobic conditioning. This might include lower-impact activities after a day of interval or long-distance training, or after 3 consecutive days of conditioning.

The following evaluation covers joint and muscle demands, sports activities best trained for in each modality, potential concerns, and tips on form.

Using a stair-climber. Stair-climbers target the large muscles of the hip, buttock, and thigh that flex and extend your hip and knee and also engage the calf muscles that lift your heel when you step. The movement challenges each leg individually from a standing position. A stair-climber is excellent for lower-body workouts and provides functional training for activities that require you to carry your own body weight up an incline, including hiking and rock and mountain climbing. Stair-climbers that include a revolving step (a "stepmill") are particularly useful and provide an excellent cardio workout. They use a more natural climbing motion. When you feel like your posture is good on the stepmill, you can try it without holding on, thus using your arms and legs at the same time. For added benefit consider adding a pack when you are within 4 weeks of a significant mountaineering trip (see Figure 8a). It is important to step with your whole foot and keep off your toes to get the most out of your gluteal muscles and to reduce strain on your foot (Figure 8b illustrates good stair-climbing posture). Machines that have revolving full steps usually offer a more intense, full workout, but may be harder on your kneecaps. Try to take deeper steps with a definite force downward if you don't have knee problems. Place a minimum amount of weight on your hands, as this will decrease your energy expenditure (Figure 8c gives an example of poor stair-climbing posture). Maintain an upright posture, otherwise you will get less of a buttock workout. Also stay alert for kneecap pain, back pain, and foot tingling and numbness.

Climbing stairs. This is one of the best aerobic and anaerobic training modes for good cardiovascular fitness as well as for mountaineering, backpacking, snowshoeing, and telemark and cross-country skiing. It is best done outdoors if you can find an area with at least 5 flights of stairs. Bleachers or stairs inside tall buildings can also be used. Warm up with a fast walk or jog for 5–10 minutes before stair climbing. Stair climbing can be done as an aerobic or an interval

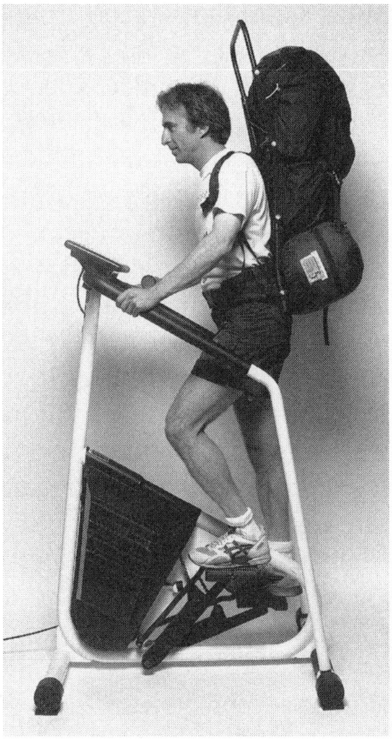

FIGURE 8a. Train with a pack.

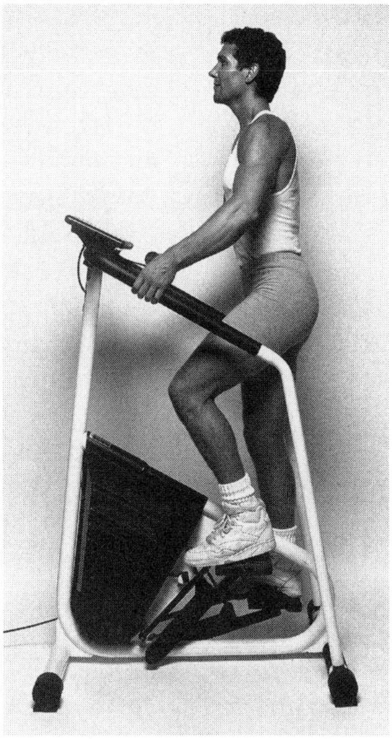

FIGURE 8b. Correct posture.

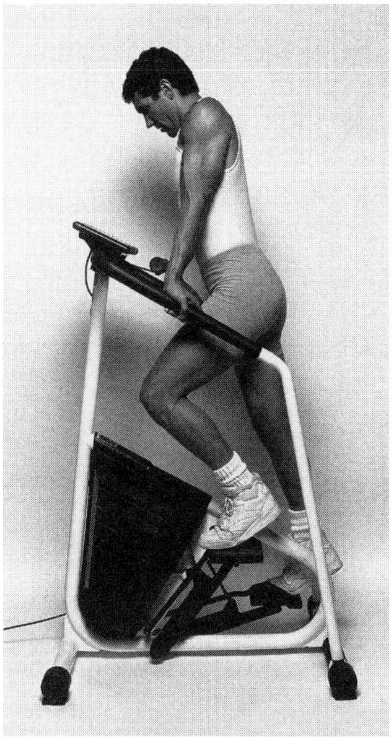

FIGURE 8c. Incorrect posture.

workout. Options include:

1. Run up or down single stairs.
2. Run up double stairs.
3. Fast-walk double or triple stairs.
4. Descend double stairs.

Using a cross-country skiing machine. The motion on cross-country skiing machines is functional and bilateral. Muscles trained include hip flexors and extensors, quadriceps, hamstrings, shoulders, upper back, and triceps. The movement also trains coordination and balance. These machines vary in their design. Some have foot cars and poles connected so that more of your upper-body muscles can be trained. This training is suitable for general conditioning and any hiking or running activity, in-line skating, skiing, and snowshoeing. Some people report discomfort when they first train with this mode, and it should not be used if it aggravates an existing shoulder or low-back problem.

Using a treadmill. Using a treadmill is a lower-body impact-loading exercise that is excellent for most people. Running on a treadmill has a higher impact than walking on one, but has possibly a little less than outdoor running. Use a treadmill for running, especially in poor weather, just as you would incorporate regular running into your program. Avoid a treadmill if you have poor balance or if you have foot, ankle, knee, or hip problems.

Using an EFX elliptical trainer. This machine provides a unique combination of motions. It feels a bit like running, but with less impact. By adjusting resistance and incline, you can change which muscles are targeted. Muscles trained include the buttock region, hip flexors and extensors, quadriceps, and hamstrings. It is excellent for general conditioning and for hiking, climbing, snowshoeing, or cross-country skiing. Potential problems include the possible strain of hip muscles, due in part to a wide foot position, and an aggravation of back or knee problems.

Using a treadwall. This machine is actually a vertical treadmill/climbing wall with hand- and footholds attached. The rate of climb and the angle of the wall are adjustable to make it harder or easier. Climbing is intended to be predominantly a leg exercise. Instead of pulling up with your arms, push your weight up with your legs. As the wall angle becomes more of an overhang, you use your arms more in the workout. There is some technique required to use this machine well (see Figure 9). Possible injuries include finger and forearm strains, and tendonitis in the upper body.

Using a stationary cycle. Several types of stationary bicycles are available in gyms. Muscles trained include hip flexors, quadriceps, and, with proper mechanics, hamstrings and gluteals. Upright bikes mimic the traditional cycle with a small saddle. Recumbent bikes offer a slightly reclined body position on a chairlike seat with back support. Adjust the seat position so that your knee is flexed about 15–30 degrees at the end of your pedaling stroke. Stationary cycling offers several advantages, including reduced joint compression of your hips, lower impact, and a minimal need to balance your body on the cycle. Cycling can also be used when one ankle, knee, or hip is recovering from an injury. Stretch your hips and legs thoroughly after a bike session. Potential problems on a bicycle are aggravation of low-back pain and occasionally of kneecap or iliotibial band disorders. Bicycles can also be used to stimulate kneecap cartilage when healing from a knee injury or chronic knee problem.

FIGURE 9

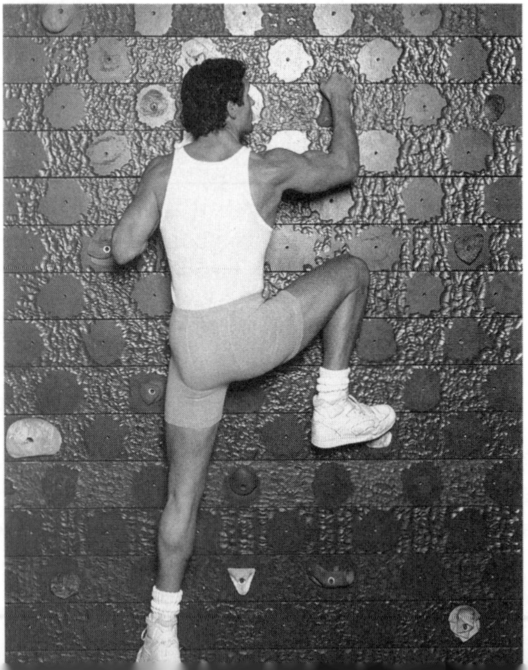

Taking a spinning class. Spinning classes are classes that use upright stationary cycles at high intensity. They often incorporate interval training and they are excellent cardiovascular workouts. They are a good way to burn calories for stress and weight management. Avoid spinning classes if you experience pain while riding a bicycle or if you have active knee or cardiac problems.

Using a rowing machine. Rowing is an excellent total-body motion involving your legs, shoulders, arms, and back. Range of motion in your ankle, knee, hip, and back is challenged in this activity. Begin with a controlled range of motion and see how your body responds. On an indoor ergometer, use a lower flywheel resistance. The stroke power is in the pull. Keep your strokes per minute in the mid-20s. Use the return movement as a time to recover for your next pull. Good back positioning is important on this machine. The excessive use of low-back muscles may cause low-back pain or aggravate existing problems. Kneecap problems can also be aggravated.

Doing aerobics classes. Aerobics classes are excellent training tools for both your lower and upper body. It is best to talk with an instructor to find out the duration of the target heart rate period and whether there are sprinting intervals, upper-body exercise, or moves that might compromise an area of your body that you are concerned about. Many aerobics classes are more like calisthenics or dancing, depending on the instructor, and should be classified as either high- or low-impact. They can be used as part of a cross-training program for most activities done in a standing position. Aerobics may cause a shoulder, back, or knee problem to flare up.

Doing step aerobics. This class format uses a step at the height of your choice. It develops coordination and balance. Much of the effort comes from calf muscles, quadriceps, and hip muscles. It is good indoor training for hiking, climbing, mountaineering, snowshoeing, and so on. This format is considered moderate- to high-impact. Possible problems include kneecap problems, low-back pain, and ankle sprains from stepping on or off the bench improperly.

Doing Tae Bo aerobics. Tae Bo aerobics involves many different arm and leg motions, including kicking and punching. It is excellent for general conditioning as well as for hiking, climbing, running, skiing, or snowshoeing. Tae Bo can aggravate knee, hip, back, or shoulder problems.

Doing aerobics with weights. These classes typically use handheld weights and can help build tone while giving you a cardiovascular workout. Make sure that the nonstop aerobic portion of the class is at least 30 minutes long or that you can maintain a heart rate in your training zone. Avoid such classes if you have an active shoulder problem.

Walking. Walking is the most natural movement pattern for the human body. Walking at a brisk pace is often enough to achieve and maintain a good functional level of aerobic fitness for people over the age of 55–60 and to reduce body fat. For fit individuals, walking on level ground is not usually intense enough to achieve a training effect. Walk with a good heel strike and roll through your foot, keeping your hips level. Walk on alternate days until you can walk continuously for 30–50 minutes at a good pace. To increase intensity, walk uphill. Don't use hand or ankle weights, as this throws off your gait and balance. Walking downhill may cause a knee problem to flare up.

In-line skating. This aerobic activity requires a moderate level of balance and coordination to be done safely. It helps develop your thigh, hip, and buttock regions. You can get an excellent aerobic workout with a variety of outdoor scenery. It is good for general aerobic conditioning as well as for cross-country skiing. Wear protective gear, and if you are a beginner, avoid hills and uneven surfaces. The risk of falling is very high and is most likely to occur when you are trying to stop, going downhill, or on uneven terrain.

Circuit Training. This mode employs stations of weight-lifting and aerobic equipment for approximately 30 minutes of exercise time to achieve both aerobic and strength training fitness. Although circuit training can improve aerobic fitness, it seems to bring about less improvement compared to other more standard aerobic options. Ideas for outdoor circuits are described in chapter 8.

The Impact of Aerobic Options

The impact of an exercise is measured by the amount of force that is transferred to your joints, bones, ligaments, tendons, nerves, discs, and other important body structures. This is important, because low- to moderate-impact exercise has been shown to be a significant factor in slowing the loss of bone density in women at risk for osteoporosis. It is also important because overuse injuries, including stress fractures, can be related to excessive accumulated impact in which your bone or other structure is not able to rebuild, repair, or remodel in a positive way.

Impact from aerobic exercise is usually thought of in terms of its effect on your feet, knees, hips, and low back, but the repetitive motion of aerobics can also lead to injuries of your upper back, neck, shoulder, and arms, especially from activities such as crew or ergometer rowing. If you are starting to feel pain from your back down, minimize the impact by decreasing the duration, frequency, or intensity of the activity. You might be able to minimize the impact of an activity by varying how you do it, such as by avoiding downhill running or by slowing down the pace of downhill hiking. If this is not effective, go to a lesser-impact activity; consult a physician if the pain persists or if you are having difficulty walking.

Higher-impact options:

- Running or jogging, especially with intervals of sprinting or downhill running
- Stair climbing or stair running
- Step, tae Bo, or high-impact aerobic dance classes
- Basketball, volleyball, or soccer
- Racquet sports, including squash, racquetball, handball, and tennis
- Hiking, backpacking, and glacier mountaineering (especially with a heavier pack and going downhill)
- Downhill skiing, especially over moguls, and snowboarding

Moderate-impact options:

- Skating and in-line skating
- Cross-country and telemark skiing, and ski machines
- Walking outside and on treadmills
- Stair-climbing machines

Lower-impact aerobics classes

- Circuit training
- EFX elliptical trainer

Minimal-impact options:

- Cycling
- Kayaking and canoeing
- Rowing machines and rowing (but these activities can lead to a higher impact on your upper back and shoulder regions)
- Swimming
- Water aerobics classes

Establishing Aerobic Goals

Match yourself up with one of the following goals. After each goal comes the action that will initiate your aerobic conditioning program.

1. **Goal:** Achieve some increase in stamina and some health benefits (I am presently not exercising or am rarely exercising).
   Action: Start any form of aerobic exercise at a mild exertion, and gradually work up to the minimum aerobic program described earlier in this chapter, if you are medically cleared.
2. **Goal:** Increase your likelihood of achieving the basic minimal health benefits.
   Action: Do the minimum aerobic program.
3. **Goal:** Achieve the full benefit of coronary artery risk reduction.
   Action: Gradually build up your program until you are burning 2,500–3,500 calories a week by doing longer and more frequent aerobic sessions, and/or add one longer-duration, lower-intensity (LILD) session per week.
4. **Goal:** Lose weight.
   Action: Work out at intensities of 55–70% max HR for 45–50 minutes per session, for 5–6 sessions per week. Start at 15 minutes per session and add 1 minute per session until you are up to 45 minutes. Do short exercise sessions, such as walking for 10–15 minutes, whenever you have a break. Choose types of exercise that are pain-free and allow at least two variations in order to avoid overuse injuries. Stationary cycles, EFX elliptical trainers, walking, and water aerobics are good choices for most people.
5. **Goal:** Increase your stamina for endurance activities that last longer than 1 hour.
   Action: Start incorporating 1 longer day of continuous aerobic activity at or slightly higher than the intensity level required for your desired activity. For example, training for backpacking, hiking, scrambling, or mountaineering would involve longer workouts of 50–65% max HR for up to 1 hour of an exercise activity. This would lead into hikes of increasing length and elevation as the season begins, increasing distance by 10–15% per week.
6. **Goal:** Achieve goal 5, but also be able to

do brief spurts of high-intensity activity such as a very difficult trail section or snowfield, or a kayak sprint in high waves.
Action: Do the actions for goal 5, but add intervals to your training that simulate the intensity and difficulty of your desired short bursts. Add a pack if it will be a pack-carrying activity (see Interval Training earlier in this chapter).

7. **Goal:** Train for moderate-intensity distance races.
   Action: Increase the intensity of some of your aerobic workouts to an intensity that is similar to the intended races, and gradually increase the distance/duration of your training on 1 day a week. Consider adding interval training to your workouts to increase power and speed.
8. **Goal:** Maintain your aerobic fitness with decreased boredom.
   Action: Vary your activities and cross train, or work out with other people.

Evaluating Your Aerobic Fitness During Your Conditioning Period

There are many methods for evaluating the progress of the aerobic component of your conditioning program. Keep a record of your resting heart rate; as you improve, it should decrease gradually down to a certain level (usually between 45 and 60 beats per minute). Have a standard self-test aerobic activity that is relatively consistent in aerobic demands, one for in the city and one for out of the city. Do each periodically to see how you feel on a rating of perceived exertion (RPE) scale. In-city activities could be a 3- to 5-mile walk or run, a 15-mile bike ride, or a particular aerobics class or stair-climber routine. Outside-the-city activities could be a particular hike, ski, or kayak trip. If the standard self-test activity is getting easier and you can do it more quickly, then you are making progress. You can expect the gains to be gradual at first and related to your consistency, specificity, volume, and variety of training.

Setting Up an Aerobic Conditioning Program Based on an Activity Goal

In order to effectively design an activity goal–oriented aerobic part of your conditioning program, do the tasks listed below:

Identify your activity goals.

Assess your target activity in regard to the aerobic continuous and interval requirements.

Evaluate your current fitness level, especially in regard to your ability to comfortably meet the aerobic duration and intensity requirements of your planned activity.

Determine the time you have for conditioning both in the city and for a longer outdoor aerobic day.

Divide your training into periods for building an aerobic and strength training base and for developing higher-intensity aerobic fitness according to the demands of your activity. (See Periodizing Your Conditioning Program in chapter 7 for more information on training periods.)

Monitor and write out your training plan week by week by using the Aerobic Conditioning Calendar (Figure 10) or the Aerobic Conditioning Log (Figure 11). You can make blank copies of the forms to record what and how you are doing over time.

The basic Aerobic Conditioning Calendar is a good place to start. Record your daily aerobic activity, the time spent doing it, and your heart rate. If you skip a day, make a note describing why you did not exercise.

The more detailed Aerobic Conditioning Log is especially useful as you progress and if you choose to periodize your training (see chapter 7). Record your activities, expected duration, and intensity as rate of perceived exertion (RPE) or percentage of maximum heart rate (% max HR). If you are planning intervals, record the duration, intensity, number, and rest-period duration. It is important to record details, such as the intensity of your aerobic exercise, as either the % max HR or as a particular training zone (1–5). The following abbreviations make it easy to record using the log: aerobic regular sessions (AR); lower-intensity, longer-duration (LILD); intervals (I).

Evaluate your progress based on how you are feeling in your mind and body at the end of each aerobic session, at the end of each week, and especially at the end of each training period.

Make adjustments to your plan as appropriate.

Consult a health or fitness professional for any special problems or health concerns.

To meet your goals, you can do a very basic program that combines gradually building your aerobic and strength base with increasing LILD activity. You can add interval training for improved performance and ability to do spurts of high-intensity activity, if your goal demands it or for improved aerobic fitness. You can also plan a program around a heart-zone periodization approach (see chapter 7).

FIGURE 10. AEROBIC CONDITIONING CALENDAR

Name: ______________________________

Date: ______________________________

I want to (check each desired benefit):

- ☐ Reduce my risk for fatal heart attacks by as much as half
- ☐ Reduce my risk of strokes by as much as 40%
- ☐ Improve my cholesterol
- ☐ Improve strength
- ☐ Decrease my blood pressure
- ☐ Reduce my risk for injuries
- ☐ Decrease my risk of colon cancer
- ☐ Build muscle
- ☐ Improve my immune system
- ☐ Improve my bone density
- ☐ Unload daily stress
- ☐ Slow down my aging process
- ☐ Improve my sleep
- ☐ Improve my performance in a sport
- ☐ Improve my mood
- ☐ Improve my tone and look better
- ☐ Improve my endurance
- ☐ Lose weight

My maximum heart rate is: 220 – age = ______.

My heart-rate training zone is a pulse rate per minute of ______–______.

The suggested length of an aerobic session in my heart-rate training zone is ____________________.

The suggested **frequency** of my aerobic sessions is ______________________________.

My **exercise options** are ______________________________.

On the calendar, record your daily aerobic activity, time spent doing it, and your heart rate. If you skip a day, note why.

SUN	MON	TUES	WED	THUR	FRI	SAT

FIGURE 11. AEROBIC CONDITIONING LOG

Name:________________ **Periodization phase:**________________ **(Week:____)**

Long-term goal: Maximum Heart Rate 90% 80% 70% 60% 50%

Short-term goals: Beats/Min Beats/Min

1) 2) 3)

	SUN	MON	TUES	WED	THUR	FRI	SAT
WEEK 1 ACTIVITY							
Time/Distance							
Exercise Activity							
Intervals							
Heart Rate							
Comments							
WEEK 2 ACTIVITY							
Time/Distance							
Exercise Activity							
Intervals							
Heart Rate							
Comments							
WEEK 3 ACTIVITY							
Time/Distance							
Exercise Activity							
Intervals							
Heart Rate							
Comments							
WEEK 4 ACTIVITY							
Time/Distance							
Exercise Activity							
Intervals							
Heart Rate							
Comments							

chapter 4 WARM-UP AND STRETCHING

By Maria Zanoni, P.T., and David Musnick, M.D.

THIS CHAPTER WILL HELP YOU:

- Understand the principles of warming up.
- Learn how to safely stretch and maintain flexibility.
- Learn how to do active as well as passive stretches.
- Develop a warm-up and stretching program.

Stretching, although commonly regarded as a warm-up, does not in itself increase muscle temperature or enhance coordination. Stretching is important, but stretching alone is not an adequate warm-up. This chapter introduces the components of a more dynamic warm-up, as well as techniques to improve and maintain your flexibility.

THE WARM-UP

Increasing muscle temperature can improve flexibility as well as muscle contractile force and speed of movement. Warm-ups also stimulate balance pathways. You can warm up in several ways, but most warm-ups should include an aerobic activity (using large muscle groups: legs, arms, or both) done at low intensity for 5–10 minutes.

After the brief aerobic session you can add functional or conventional strength-training exercises at low resistance and high repetitions, or you can combine the above and add some agility or balance drills to prepare yourself for an activity.

It is best to do a warm-up that matches the demands of your activity. Think about the movement patterns and joint ranges of motion required in your shoulders, hips, and knees, and use some active stretches as well as functional exercises (see chapter 5) in your warm-up.

An activity that requires more strength, balance, and coordination requires a longer warm-up period. For example, a hike starting off on level ground without any immediate river crossings or boulder fields would require only a gradual increase in hiking speed as a warm-up. A hike or mountaineering day on scree, snow, or boulder fields with high requirements for shoulder-leg integration, balance, and full joint range of motion would benefit from some active stretches and agility drills.

The Aerobic Warm-Up

The aerobic warm-up is a good beginning for any activity. It is adequate for health-club workouts as well as for most hiking, bicycling, running, cross-country skiing, and water sports. Exercise aerobically 5–10 minutes at a low intensity (50–65% max HR). Start slowly, and gradually increase your intensity. You can do this with any aerobic activity, but it is best to use an activity that uses the same muscles as your workout. When preparing for an outdoor workout, your warm-up could be a brisk walk, jog, or cycle.

Your aerobic warm-up could also be the same as the activity you will be doing, but at a lower intensity level. An easy kayak before engaging rough water, gently jogging before running, or hiking at an easy to moderate pace before hiking quickly or steeply are all good aerobic warm-ups.

> **PRACTICAL POINT**
>
> You can make a warm-up walk more effective by doing it at a quick pace and with variations in arm motions. Your fast walk could include exaggerated arm swings, forward and rotational punches, rowing motions, or virtually any functional arm motion.

The Weight-Lifting Warm-Up

You can do an aerobic warm-up to prepare for weight lifting. A rowing machine or an arm/leg cycle are ideal because they use the arms and legs. In addition, you could also do a few lower-weight, high-repetition sets of some of your intended strength training exercises. Try to do a few that use larger muscle groups and go through a full range of motion. Consider a few functional shoulder-hip-leg combination exercises (see Exercises 20–22).

The Functional Exercise Warm-Up

In a functional exercise warm-up, pick a number of functional exercises (3–5) that best simulate the motion patterns and balance demands of the activity you are preparing for. You can choose these exercises from chapter 5, Functional Core and Strength Training, or use the dynamic warm-up suggestions in the outdoor activity chapters in Part III. It makes sense to precede a functional exercise warm-up with a 5-minute aerobic period. You can keep the warm-up aerobic by doing the functional exercises quickly in 30- to 45-second sets, but without any added resistance except your body weight. Such a warm-up more adequately prepares your muscles and joints in different planes of motion.

The Agility and Balance Warm-Up

If your activity requires balance challenges and quick responses to changes in terrain, it can help to do balance or agility drills as part of your warm-up. Such activities include skiing (all types), snowboarding, climbing (including scrambling and mountaineering), and whitewater kayaking. Start with a 5- to 10-minute aerobic activity, then add a few balance and agility drills. For standing balance, do Exercises 59 and 60. For an agility component, do Exercises 59–61 and/or follow the agility circuit guidelines in chapter 8 or chapter 20. You can make a simple agility drill by walking quickly or jogging for 1–3 minutes while making quick changes in direction.

The Outdoor Activity Warm-Up

It is a good idea to do a warm-up before you begin your outdoor activity. If that activity requires strength, balance, and agility, it is good to integrate these components after a brief aerobic period. The outdoor activity chapters in Part III have specific warm-up programs for the different activities covered. The dynamic warm-up discussed below is a good generic warm-up for many activities.

Dynamic Warm-Up Drills

Dynamic warm-up drills work on coordination and can be done prior to sports or outdoor activities. You can do these after a brief aerobic period or as part of your aerobic warm-up. Each one can be done for 30–90 seconds. They can be linked together or done individually.

Carioca: Run sideways to your right, with your left foot crossing in front of your right foot on the first step, and behind your right foot on the next step. Reverse direction, moving to the left, with your right foot crossing first in front of and then behind your left foot.

Crazy Legs: Run forward along an imaginary line, with your left foot crossing to the right side of the line, and then your right foot crossing to the left side of the line.

Shuffle Run: Stand with the front of your

shoes about 6–8 inches apart. Using quick motions, take a 2- to 3-foot step forward with your right foot, making initial contact with your heel. Then bring the toes of your left foot forward to meet the heel of your right foot, making sure not to make heel contact with your left foot. Repeat this movement pattern quickly for 3–5 strides, then change your forward leg.

Horse Gallop Side Shuffle: Stand sideways to your direction of travel, with your feet shoulder-width apart and knees slightly bent. When moving to your right, push off your left leg and land on the ball of your right foot. Quickly bring your left foot next to your right foot, lightly tapping your feet together so that it sounds like a horse galloping. Move sideways rapidly for several strides, and then switch direction.

Dynamic Warm-Up

For a generic dynamic warm-up, start with brisk walking for 2 minutes, then either continue walking for 5 more minutes, or jog. This leads into a walking lunge exercise with alternate shoulder/arm raises, such as Exercise 30. Next do the warm-up drills above (Carioca, Crazy Legs, Shuffle Run, and Horse Gallop Side Shuffle). Finish up with Exercises 1, 3, 7, 8, 9, 13, and 19. A dynamic warm-up should generally last 5–15 minutes. Try experimenting with dynamic warm-up routines to see which works the best for you.

STRETCHING AND FLEXIBILITY

Flexibility is related to the range of motion in a joint or a series of joints, as well as the length of muscle and tendons. It is related to age, gender, activity level, and genetic factors. Stretching can improve flexibility. If your joints are very tight, stretching alone may not be adequate; you may need manual treatment to improve flexibility. The degree of flexibility in your body can almost always be improved by stretching.

The primary goal of stretching is to lengthen muscles and tendons. Contractile tissue is more elastic; therefore, muscles and tendons respond better to stretching than do ligaments and joint capsules. Even so, stretching does increase the elasticity of both the contractile and noncontractile tissues. A tight and stiff joint capsule may also be loosened through stretching.

The most effective stretching techniques involve postures that stabilize one end of the muscle in order to stretch the other end. Stretching can be done at any time, but in order to improve flexibility it is best done when your body is well warmed up. When stretching a cold muscle, use caution because it is much easier to injure a cold muscle. Stretching is often done too quickly and/or with poor positioning. This will not improve flexibility.

If your goal is to increase flexibility, for indoor workouts do the majority of your stretching after an aerobic exercise period. For outdoor activities, a few stretches at the end of your warm-up are advised. It is important to note that a stretching program needs to be accompanied by a balanced strengthening program for the best flexibility.

For definition of anatomy terms related to stretching, see Basic Anatomy in chapter 9.

Flexibility Improves Performance

Limited flexibility has been shown to decrease the efficiency of an activity; that is, the body must expend more energy to complete a task. Increased flexibility can improve performance. For example, full hip flexibility along with adequate strength allows a climber to make moves that require full rotation of the hip, and the mountaineer to take long, high steps.

Correcting Muscle Imbalances

Occasionally, stretching will not improve flexibility or alignment in a particular muscle or body region because there is too much imbalance of muscle strength. For example, stretching your pectorals (pecs) may not be enough to decrease your chances of injury. If your back muscles are significantly weaker than your chest muscles, you can stretch all day long, but the stronger muscles will take over. In this example, it is more important to strengthen the weaker muscle group (in this case, your back) than only to stretch your tight pecs.

Tight Muscles Can Alter Joint Position

Muscles have an optimum length that allows for optimum strength and function. It has been shown that muscle strength and function change with a change in length. Muscles that are excessively shortened or excessively lengthened may change joint position and predispose you to injury. A common example of this is the weight trainer who likes to train the large muscles of his chest and deltoids more than his back. His pecs become shortened and his shoulder bone (humerus) actually begins migrating forward in the shoulder joint. This is a very common muscle imbalance and a real culprit in shoulder injuries. The shoulder joint does not function normally when the humerus is too far forward.

Another example of altered joint position actually involves more than one joint. Tight hamstrings that attach to your pelvis pull your pelvis down and can change the position of your back. Your back is then in a more flexed position and loses its optimal alignment. This can increase forces to your low back and raise the chances of injury.

Common Tight Muscles

There are common patterns of tight muscles and weak muscles in the human body. This is due to the way our body is designed. Muscles prone to tightness are usually those that span more than one joint.

Tight pectorals are usually the result of poor sitting posture and the tendency to overtrain the pecs as compared to the upper back. The hamstrings (back of the thigh), iliotibial band (side of the thigh), quadriceps (front of the thigh), and hip flexors (front of the hip) are all large muscle groups that are commonly tight. General inactivity can lead to muscle tightness, but so can a lot of training with heavy weights. This shortens muscles and decreases flexibility.

The calf and Achilles tendon are also commonly tight, especially if you are involved in running or jumping sports. These activities demand power from the calf muscle group, and increased use of this muscle group creates an environment in which the muscles tend to stay shortened. People with high arches in their feet also tend to have tight heel cords. Stretching can maximize the length of the muscle, but stretching cannot change a skeletal alignment condition.

Reasons for Tight Muscles

Chronic bad posture. Probably the most common reason for tight muscles is poor posture. For example, sitting for extended periods of time with a slumped, forward head posture and a forward shoulder posture leads to tight pectoral muscles. Furthermore, sitting for extended hours can lead to shortened hip flexors, as well as shortened hamstrings.

Spine problems. Back and neck problems can lead to tight muscles due to an area of irritation in the spinal joints or nerve roots. Muscles related to these joints can stay tight for a prolonged period of time. An example is persistently tight hamstrings; frequently, there is an associated low-back problem.

Joint injury. In the event of an injury, a muscle reflexively tightens around the injury to guard the joint from further injury. A common example is a low-back strain. In an injury of the disc or ligaments, the low-back muscles tighten to protect the area.

Joint dysfunction with hypomobility. A muscle might be tight if a joint cannot move through a full range of motion for a prolonged period of time. The muscle attached to the joint may then shorten. Two examples are when the latissimus tightens after a prolonged frozen shoulder (adhesive capsulitis) and when the iliopsoas tendon and muscles tighten in the setting of hip arthritis, resulting in decreased ability to extend the hip.

Joint dysfunction with hypermobility. If the ligaments in a joint are significantly lengthened and the joint is loose, surrounding muscles can get tight or go into spasm. This is because the muscles may have to work excessively to stabilize the joint. When this is occurring there can be areas of tenderness or tender points in a muscle. There can also be trigger points that are sensitive fibrous areas in the muscle. The best way to deal with this is to train the muscles to stabilize the joint, with help from a trainer or physical therapist. If this is not effective and the joint is deemed to be loose, then seek medical advice regarding methods of treatment, including ligament injections.

Imbalances in training. Imbalances in strength training can lead to muscle tightness in some regions. An example is a very tight, strong chest area with a weaker upper-back area. In this case, the commonly tight area is reinforced by overtraining the pecs and neglecting to strengthen the back. Another example is overtraining the quadriceps in relation to the hamstrings with resultant quad tightness and greater likelihood of hamstring injury.

Methods of Stretching

There are many ways to promote flexibility, including passive and active stretching as well as hands-on techniques by health professionals to loosen muscles and joints. Methods used by professionals, such as massage therapy and joint mobilization/manipulation techniques, are most appropriate for chronically tight muscles and joints. Of the several methods of stretching, this chapter focuses on passive and active stretching.

Passive Stretching

Passive stretching is the common technique in which your body is positioned appropriately to increase the distance between the origin (beginning) of a muscle and its insertion (end), and the position is held for a specific amount of time (usually 15–20 seconds). The stretch can be repeated 2–3 times. It is usually safe if proper positioning is used.

Some muscles cover one joint, like the soleus (deeper calf area), while other muscles cover two joints, like the gastroc (surface of the calf). The one-joint mover lends itself to a more simplified stretch. If you are stretching two-joint muscles, you must consider the position of both joints in order to maintain an optimum stretch.

The key to passive stretching is to be certain that you feel a slight pull in the muscle group. For example, if during a hamstring stretch you feel the pull in your back instead of your hamstrings, you should reposition yourself.

Use your breath to maximize your stretch in the following manner: When in the stretch position, take a deep breath in, relax, then slowly breathe out and slightly increase your stretch.

Active Stretching

Active stretches work more on dynamic flexibility, which refers to the muscle and joint tissue forces that resist motion throughout the range. The benefit of an active stretch is that it teaches the body to lengthen muscles and improve joint motion. Actively working on range of motion may be helpful in improving your performance.

One type of active stretch, the paired muscle active stretch, takes a body region through a full range of motion with a muscle contraction while stabilizing surrounding joints. This type of stretch takes advantage of muscle agonist/antagonist relationships to get a relaxation and stretch of one muscle during contraction of another muscle. An example is the active hamstring stretch done by straightening your knee while sitting. This type of stretch can be held briefly at the end of the contraction and then repeated 5–10 times.

Another type of active stretch (or active flexibility exercise) uses more than one muscle in a body region to bring joints through a full range of motion and muscles into more-lengthened positions. This type of stretch is usually repeated numerous times and may be finished with a hold of position. An example of this is the hip swing in which you stand on one leg and swing your knee in full circles.

Try a few active stretches to get used to them, and then use them with your passive stretches, depending on your activity goals. Note that many of the functional strength exercises in chapter 5 take your joints into a wide range of motion and may have active stretching benefits as well.

Stretching Precautions

Protecting Your Low Back

This chapter's exercise descriptions use the term *neutral spine* (see chapters 14 and 25). In the low back, the neutral spine position is a slight arch. The degree of the arch is unique to each individual. In a neutral spine, the low back is not too extended (arched) or too flexed (slouched). A wall mirror can be very useful in helping you become aware of the position of your spine during stretching.

In general it is good to position your low back in a neutral posture during your stretching session, unless of course the stretch requires a different position. You should monitor your back and be aware if you have any back pain or thigh, leg, or foot tingling or burning during a stretch. If you do, stop the stretch immediately. Also, if you hear a pop or feel a clunk during a stretch you should modify or stop the stretch.

If you have a low-back problem with your discs or with your facet or sacroiliac joints, use caution while stretching. Stretching your hips or hamstrings with too much spine flexion can put your discs under excessive stress. Also be careful during any stretch done in a sitting position with spine side bending. Your low back's facet joints can be injured during excessive side bending, extension, or rotation. Stretching exercises with side bending include the sitting adductor stretch (Exercise 8), the iliotibial band stretch (Exercise 5), as well as any hamstring stretch done in a sitting position with spine side bending.

If you have a sacroiliac problem and are under the care of a physical therapist or a physician you will need to consult your health-care provider to learn how to protect your sacroiliac joint during stretching. Certain stretches can easily irritate this joint, such as those with any prolonged asymmetrical stress in which the pelvis rotates on the sacrum or a muscle pulls on the sacrum. Be careful or consider avoiding piriformis (buttock), hip flexor, adductor, and iliotibial band stretches.

Stretching While Injuries Are Healing

It is possible to overstretch, particularly if you have an injury. One of the most common mistakes is stretching too hard too soon. Wait several days before stretching an injury, because you don't want to tear the healing tissue. An injured muscle or tendon needs to be stretched very gently and definitely not pushed into pain. Any stretching program after a muscle-strain injury should usually be accompanied by low-resistance, high-repetition (20–30 reps per set) range-of-motion exercises for the first few weeks to help heal the injured muscle. This type of exercise involves contracting muscles and moving joints through a range of motion that is pain-free.

WARM-UP AND STRETCHING EXERCISES

This section includes certain active stretches and some of the most popular passive stretches, because they are often done improperly. When stretches are described for one side of the body, remember to switch and repeat on the opposite side. Most passive stretches can be held for 20–30 seconds and repeated 2–3 times per stretching period, 2–3 times per week. Active stretches can be repeated 5–10 times.

LOWER-BODY STRETCHES

1 HAMSTRING STRETCH

Equipment: 12- to 18-inch-tall stool or chair.

Purpose: Stretch the large muscle group located on the back of your thigh. Tight hamstrings can contribute to back dysfunction because of the hamstring insertion on the pelvis.

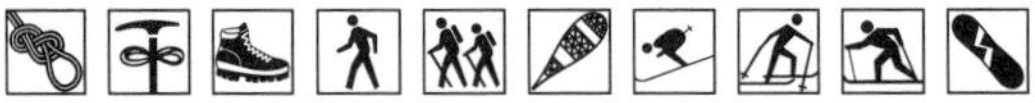

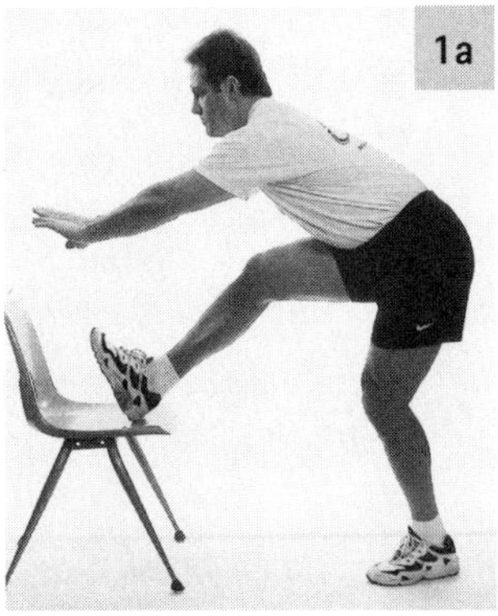

1a

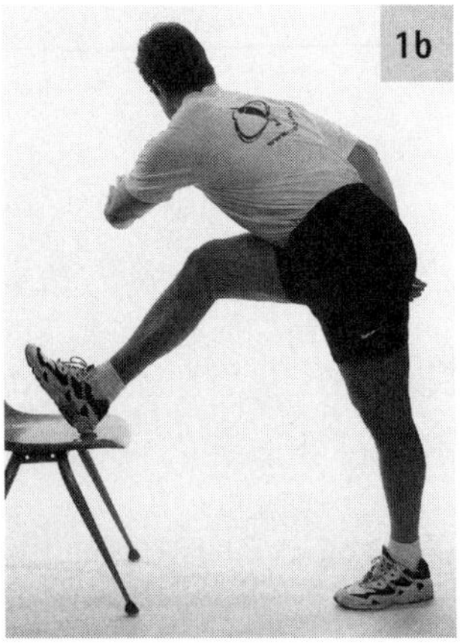

1b

Technique: While standing, position your heel on a stool or chair, with your toes pointing toward the ceiling, and bend forward at your hips (not your waist) with your arms extended straight in front of you, until you feel the stretch in the back of your knee and thigh. Keep your back neutral or slightly extended. Look straight ahead as you bend from the hips, not from the back. Think of yourself as projecting your chest forward. Try a stretch with your elevated knee slightly bent (1a) and one with it completely straight. To increase and improve the stretch, try modifying your foot or hip and leg position. For example, flex your elevated foot to move your toes toward your face. Or rotate your elevated leg and hip inward so your foot points inward, and hold that position, then rotate it outward and hold. You can also rotate your mid back and point to the left and then the right with one or both arms (1b). Do 2–3 reps.

Variation: 1.1. Sit on the floor with your right leg extended straight out in front of you, with your toes pointing up toward the ceiling. Bend your left leg and place the sole of your left foot against the inside of your right thigh. Keep your back in a neutral position. Flex at your hips, bringing your chest toward your right knee. If you can, grab the outside of your right foot with your left hand to include the left latissimus and upper back in this stretch.

Precautions: These exercises are usually done with excessive spine flexion; remember to maintain a neutral low-back position throughout the stretch.

2 SITTING AND SUPINE ACTIVE HAMSTRING STRETCH

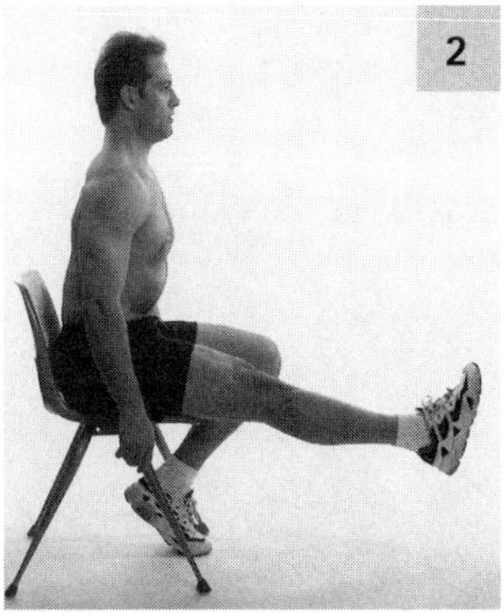

2

Equipment: Chair or other surface above ground level.
Purpose: Actively stretch the hamstring. Use this stretch if you have tight hamstring and back problems.

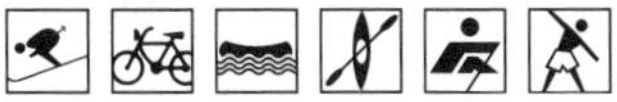

Technique: Sit on a surface that is high enough that your feet don't touch the ground when you have your low back slightly to fully arched. Slowly straighten one leg while keeping your low back in the arch position. The endpoint of this stretch is when you feel it in the back of your thigh. Hold the stretch for 5 seconds. Do 6–10 reps.
Variation: 2.1. A similar stretch can be done lying on your back. Hold the back of one thigh just behind your knee and slowly straighten your knee until you feel the stretch in your hamstrings.

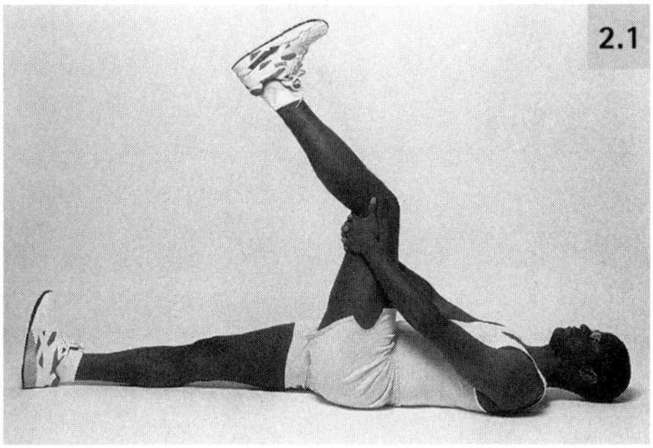

2.1

Precautions: This active stretch is often done too quickly, so that people don't realize that their spine is moving into a rounded position. This exercise demands awareness of spine position, so do it slowly. Be sure your knee does not rotate in or out while doing this stretch.

3 QUADRICEPS STRETCH

Equipment: None.
Purpose: Stretch the large muscle group in the front of your thigh. Lack of flexibility may contribute to knee pain as well as back problems.

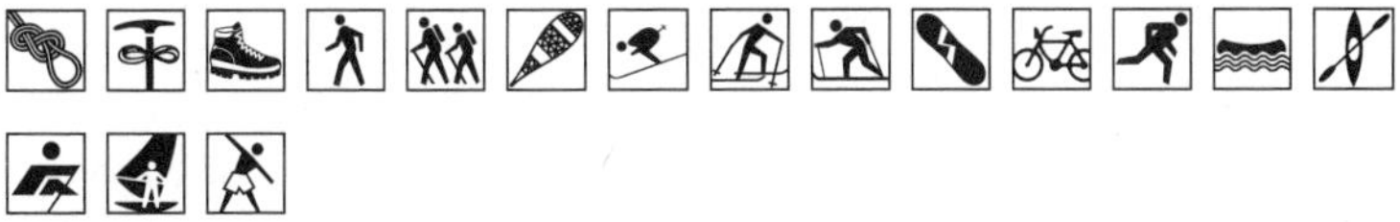

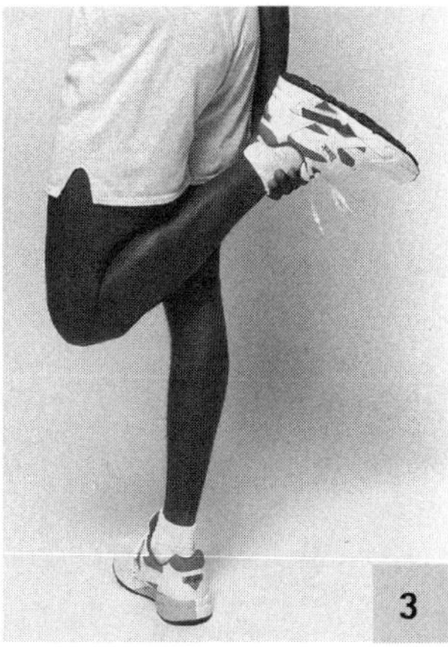

3

Technique: This is a two-joint muscle, so it requires attentiveness to both joints. The quadriceps both extend (straighten) the knee as well as flex (bend) the hip. The hip must be in extension, that is, slightly behind you, while the knee is bent. All the while, keep a neutral spine position. Stand on one leg with your knee slightly bent, and raise the heel of your other leg toward your back. Using your same-side hand as your raised leg, grab your ankle or something attached to your ankle, such as your pant leg or a towel, and pull it toward the

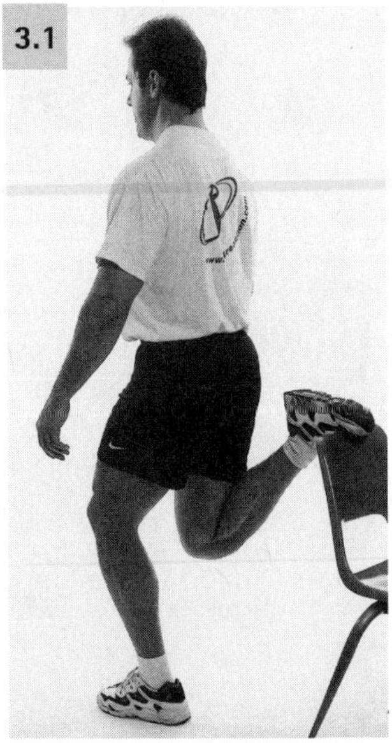
3.1

same-side buttock until you feel a stretch on the front of your thigh. The stretch will be better if you bring your pelvis in a posterior direction (flex your low back). Do 2–3 reps. Also try using the opposite hand to bring your heel toward the opposite buttock (photo 3). This stretch also stretches your hip flexors.

Variation: 3.1. To stretch your quad and hip flexors at the same time, stand about $2\frac{1}{2}$–3 feet in front of a chair, high bench, or other surface that is at the same height or up to $1\frac{1}{2}$ feet higher than the height of your knee. Place the top of one foot on the surface and have your other foot far forward enough of the chair so that when you bend your forward knee, you can feel a stretch in the front of both your thigh and your hip. Make sure your back is in a slightly flexed position.

Tips and Precautions: Optimal range of motion is heel to buttock without compensating by hyperextending your back, bending your hip, or allowing your knee to go out to the side. Make sure you don't hyperextend your low back (don't arch your back). Your knee should not migrate out to the side; keep it close to your other knee.

4 ACTIVE QUADRICEPS STRETCH

Equipment: None.

Purpose: Stretch your quadriceps if you have difficulty with balance or have problems extending your hips.

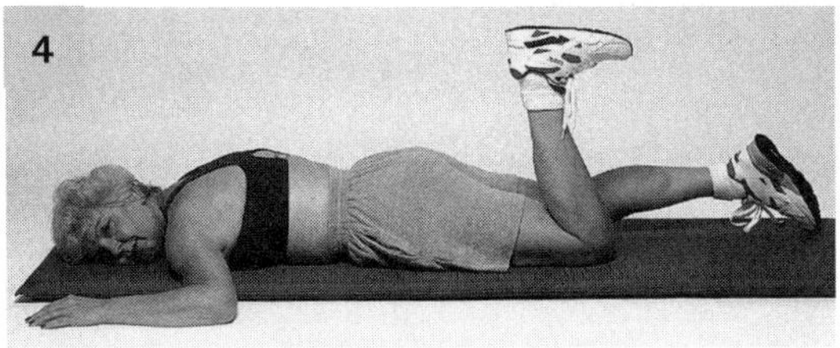
4

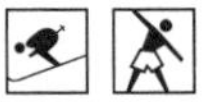

Technique: Lie on your stomach. Tighten your abdominal muscles so your pelvis won't move during this exercise. Bend one knee and move your heel toward your buttock, but don't let your spine arch. Do 6–10 reps.

5 ILIOTIBIAL BAND (ITB) STRETCH

Equipment: Wall, tree, boulder, or other vertical support.

Purpose: Stretch the muscle and fascia tissue on the side of your hip and thigh.

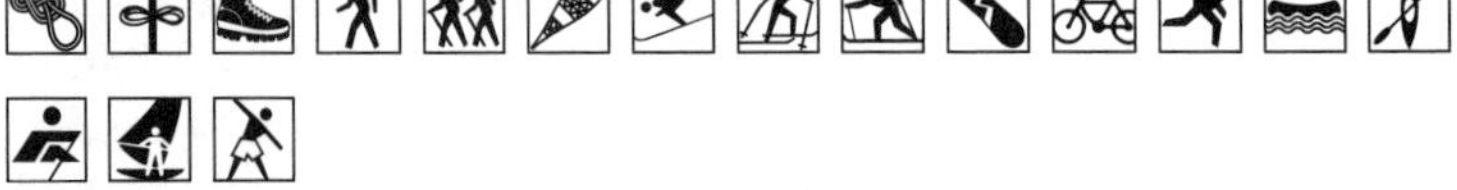

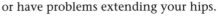

Technique: Stand with your left side facing a wall, tree, or boulder, and touch it with your left hand. Have your left knee in front of you and slightly bent. Position your right leg behind your left leg and closer to the surface you are touching. The outside edge of

your right foot should be touching the ground, bearing most of your body weight. Side-bend your spine to the left while you move your right hip slightly to the right. The right side of your body should be in a C-shaped curve. Do 2–3 reps.
Variations: 5.1. You can also do this with your right hand extended over your head, elbow bent, and pointing to the wall. **5.2.** Stand with your right side facing a wall or vertical surface, and balance on your right leg with your knee slightly bent. Place the toes of your left foot behind your right heel, and your right hand above your head on the vertical surface for balance. Move your right hip toward the wall until you feel a stretch along your right hip and lateral thigh. For additional stretch, move farther away from the wall and reach your hand farther above your head.

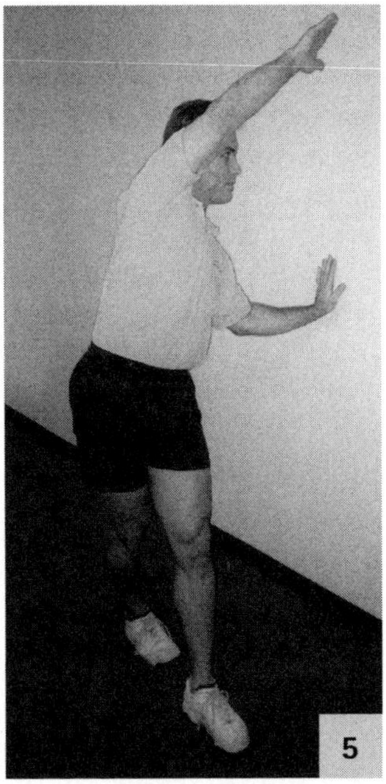
5

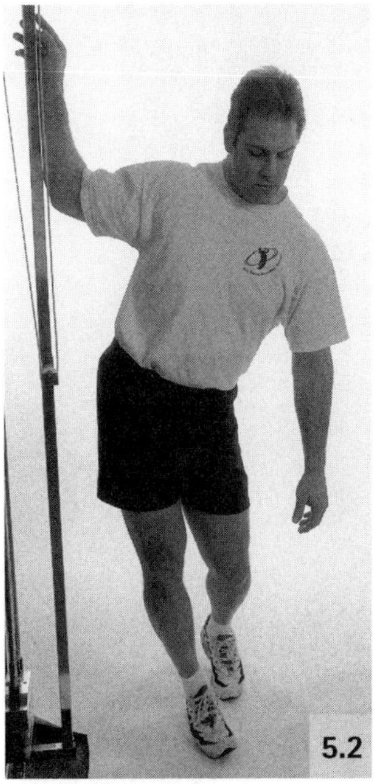
5.2

6 HIP FLEXOR STRETCH

Equipment: Chair or bench.
Purpose: Stretch the muscles that bring your knee toward your chest. These are tight in almost everyone, because most people spend a significant amount of time sitting. These muscles extend from the low back to the front of the hip.

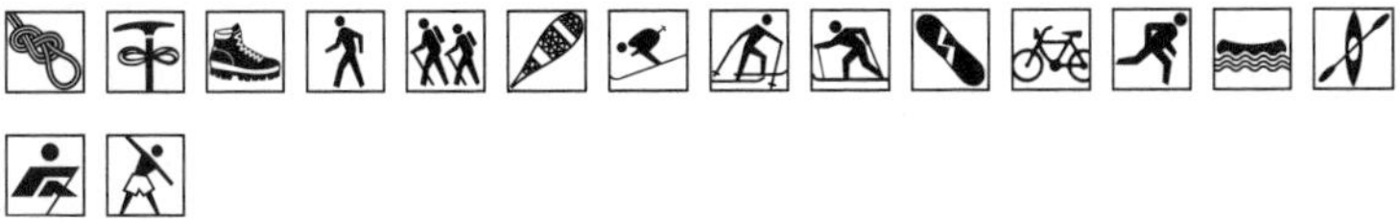

Technique: Kneel on the floor on one knee, with your other foot in front of you. Your hip on your kneeling side should be slightly extended, with that knee in back of your buttock. Hold onto a chair or bench while you shift weight onto your forward leg, allowing that forward knee to bend more. This will move your kneeling-side hip into a more extended position. Do 2–3 reps.
Precautions: Be careful that in the process your back is not hyperextended (don't arch your back). Also be careful that you achieve a neutral spine position, or the stretch will not be very effective.

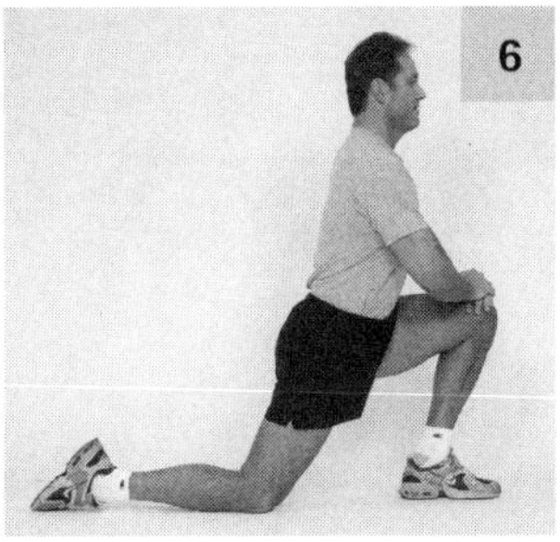
6

EXERCISE 7 8 9 10

7 ACTIVE HIP STRETCH

Equipment: Vertical surface.

Purpose: Actively stretch your hip joint capsule and surrounding musculature.

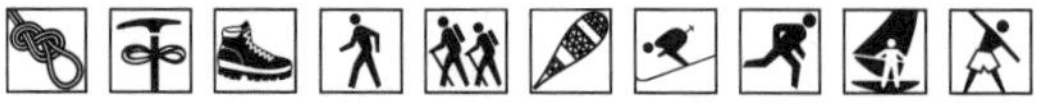

Technique: Stand on your left leg and bend it slightly; with your right hand, touch a vertical support surface. Move your right knee into a flexed position (bend it 90 degrees) and bring it toward your abdomen. Imagine you have a pen on the front of your right knee and move it around clockwise to draw the largest circle that you are comfortably able to. Your right knee should rotate outward (with your right foot pointing inward) when it is on the outer half of the circle (7a), and rotate inward (with your right foot pointing outward) when it is on the inner half of the circle (7b). Tighten your abdominal muscles to stabilize your back. Do 5–10 circles and then switch to the other leg. You can also move your knee counterclockwise.

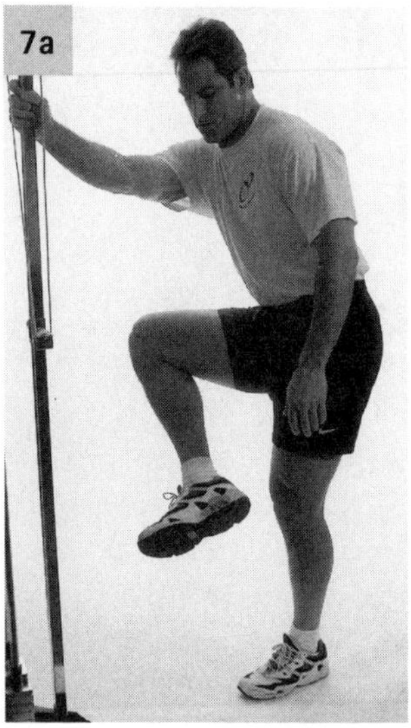
7a

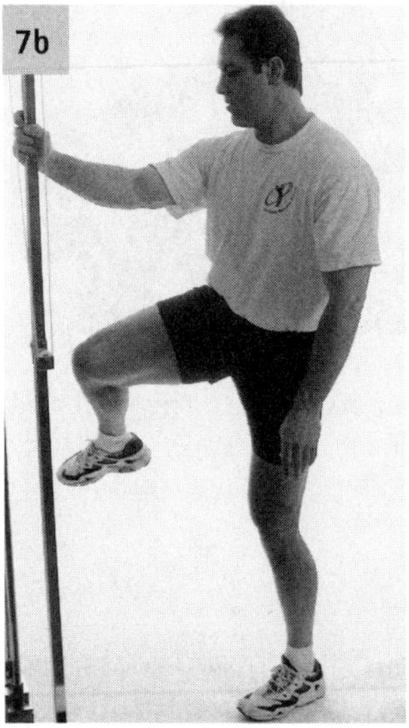
7b

Precautions: People often allow for too much movement in the leg on which they are standing. Keep that leg stable so most of the motion goes into the leg that is raised.

8 ADDUCTOR STRETCH

Equipment: None.

Purpose: Stretch the muscles of your inner thigh.

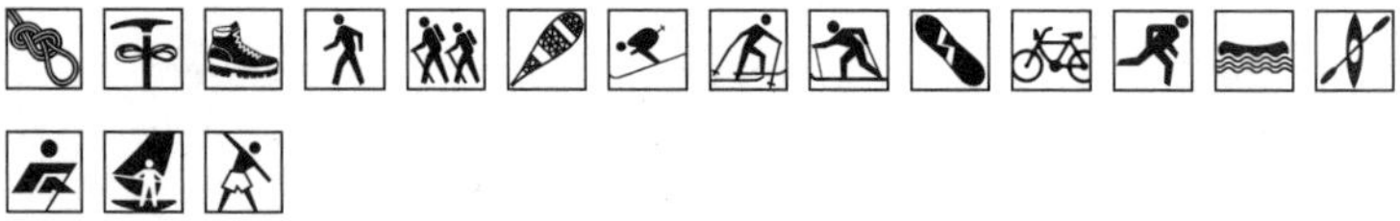

Technique: Sit on the floor with your legs spread apart and knees slightly bent. Lean forward at the waist, keeping your back straight, until you feel a pull in your inner thigh.

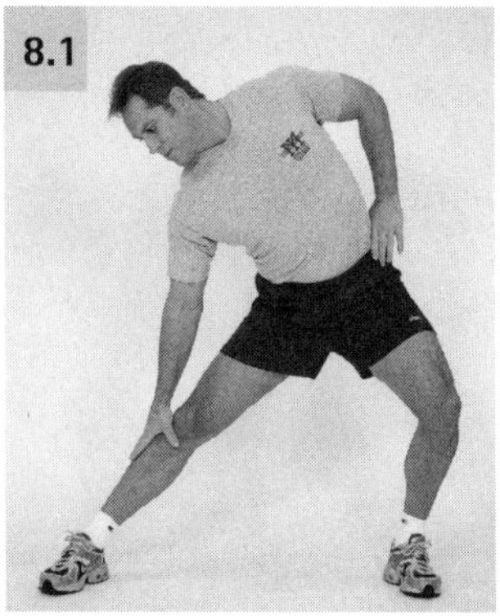
8.1

Variation: 8.1. Stand with your feet spaced very widely apart. Bend your left knee and side-bend your back to the right while you slide your right hand down the outside of your right leg. Bend your left

knee and move your pelvis to the left to feel a stretch on the inner side of the right groin. Extend your left arm over your head toward the right to get a stretch in your left side at the same time.
Precaution: Don't round your back when you do this exercise while sitting.

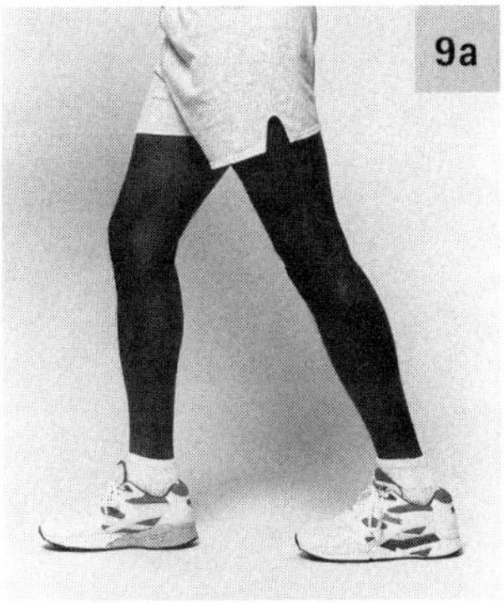

9a

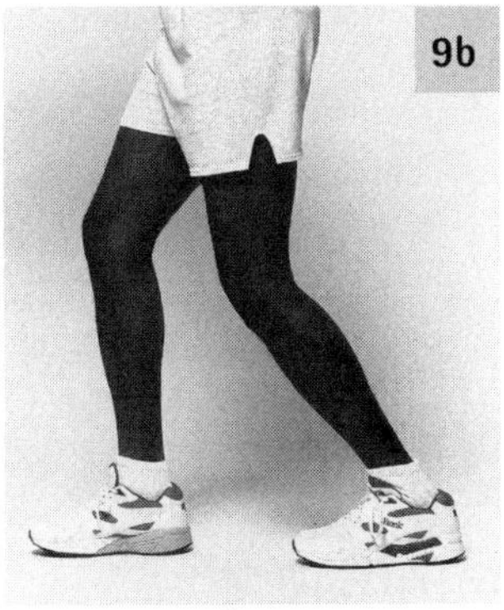

9b

9 HEEL CORD (ACHILLES) STRETCH

Equipment: Vertical surface.
Purpose: Stretch your heel cords and calf muscles.

Technique: Stand in front of a vertical surface such as a wall, tree, or side of a car; position your feet shoulder-width apart and touch the surface to stabilize yourself. Then place one foot $1/2$–$1\,1/2$ feet behind the heel of your front foot. Slightly bend your front knee while keeping your back knee straight. Transfer weight to your forward knee until you feel a stretch in the back of your leg (9a). Hold this for 20 seconds, then bend your back knee slightly and repeat the weight transfer (9b).
Tips and Precautions: This stretch is even more effective if you put your weight onto the outside of your foot. Be sure your toes are pointed straight ahead or even a little bit inward. The tendency is to allow the foot to turn outward, and this is not an effective stretch. Furthermore, try to maintain an arch in your foot. Make sure you bend at the ankle and keep your heel on the floor.

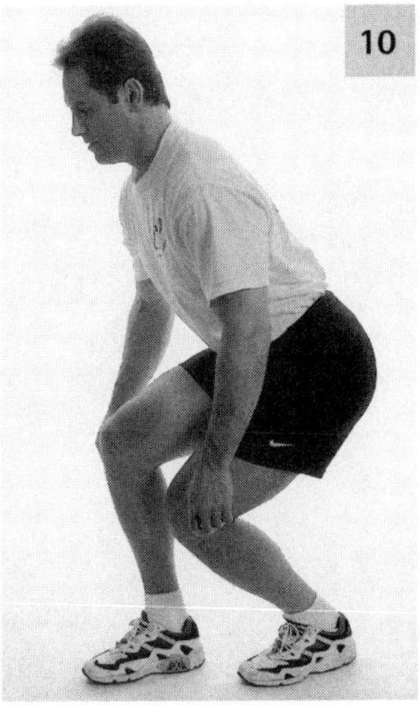

10

10 ACTIVE SQUAT STRETCH TO THE HEEL CORD

Equipment: Pole or door handle.
Purpose: Stretch your heel cord and ankle joint into the functional squat position. The ankle joint's normal range of motion includes performing a full squat with your heels on the ground. Most people lose this range of motion and don't realize it.

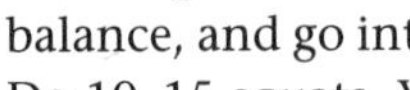

Technique: Hold onto something like a pole or a door handle for balance, and go into a squat while keeping your heels on the ground. Do 10–15 squats. You also can do this stretch without holding onto anything, with your feet parallel or with one foot in front of the other.
Precaution: To avoid jamming your ankles, do not do this too quickly.

UPPER-BODY STRETCHES

11 CHEST STRETCH

Equipment: Doorframe or pole.
Purpose: Stretch your pectoralis and anterior shoulder.

Technique: Stand in a doorway or by a pole. Extend your right arm straight out to your right side at 45 degrees above horizontal, and grasp the doorframe or pole. Rotate your body to the left to feel the stretch in your chest. Do 2–3 reps.
Precaution: Don't do this stretch if you have pain down your arm.

12 RHOMBOID AND POSTERIOR SHOULDER STRETCH

Equipment: Doorframe.
Purpose: Stretch the muscles between and on the back surface of the shoulder blades.

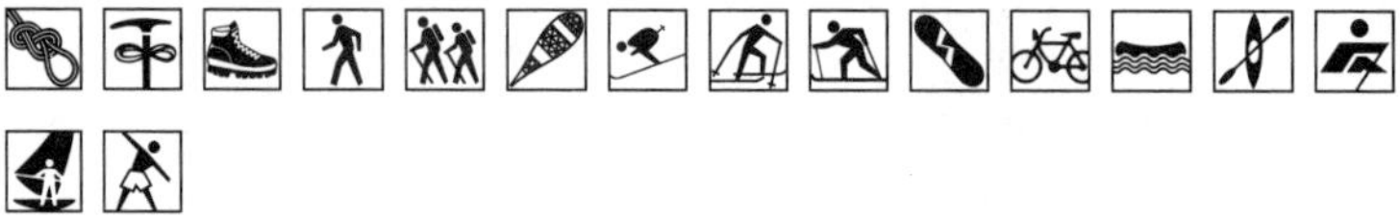

Technique: Stand in a doorway with your toes at the front of the doorframe. Grasp the left outside edge of the doorframe. Rotate your torso to the right until you feel a stretch on your right shoulder blade. Hold for 20 seconds and reverse sides. Do 2–3 reps.

13 ACTIVE SHOULDER STRETCH

Equipment: None.
Purpose: Actively stretch the shoulder capsule and surrounding musculature. This is a good stretch for climbers, skiers, and boaters.

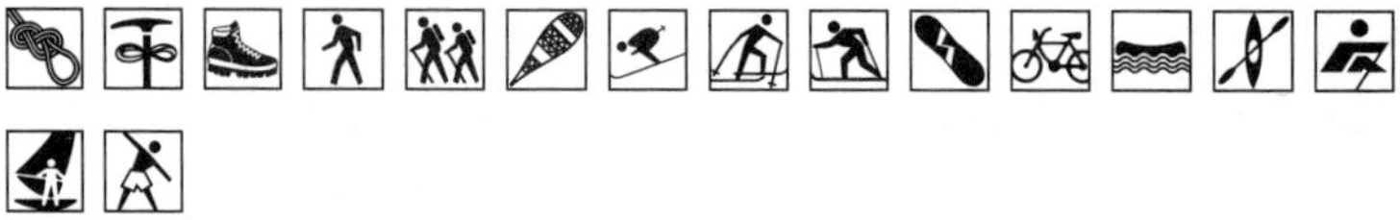

Technique: Standing with your feet shoulder-width apart, bend your right elbow to 90 degrees and point in front of you. Initially, have your elbow touching the side of your rib cage. This is the starting position. Move your arm and shoulder in a clockwise circle. You can do this for 4–6 circles on one side, gradually moving into larger circles, before you switch to the other side. After you complete this motion,

move your right hand (with a straight elbow and your palm facing toward the midline of your body) in a clockwise forward arc motion, until you are pointing toward the ceiling or sky. Then move your arm in a reverse arc so that your fingers point behind you. Do 6–10 reps.
Precautions: Don't do this exercise if you have tendonitis of your biceps or rotator cuff, or if it is painful in your shoulder, neck, or arm.

14 ROTATOR CUFF AND SHOULDER CAPSULE ACTIVE STRETCH

Equipment: 1- to 2-pound weight or can of food, rolled towel, pillow.
Purpose: Stretch the rotator cuff muscles and ligaments that surround your shoulder joint. A tight rotator cuff can lead to shoulder joint problems. This is an important stretch if you can't achieve full shoulder motion.

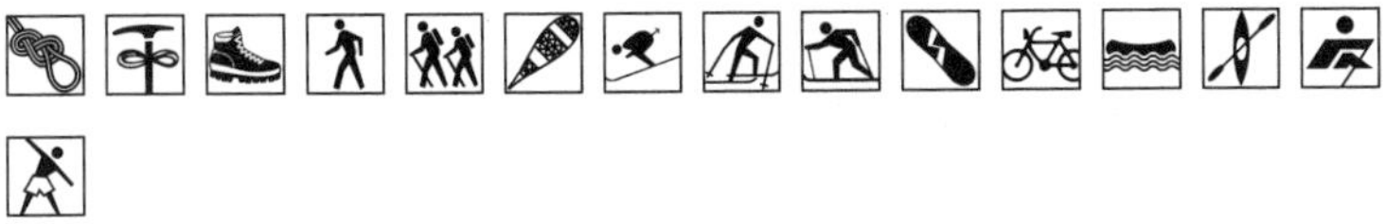

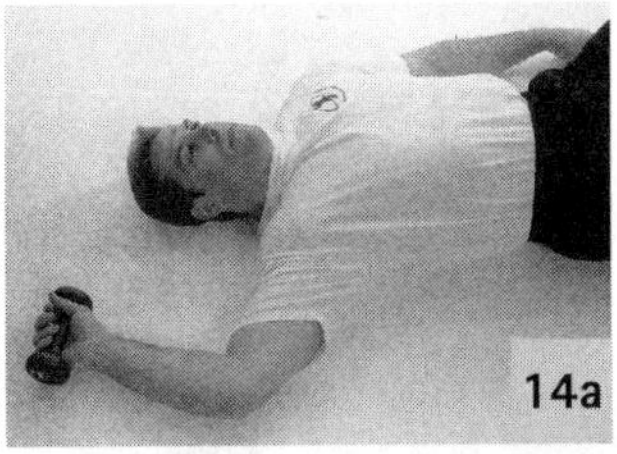

14a

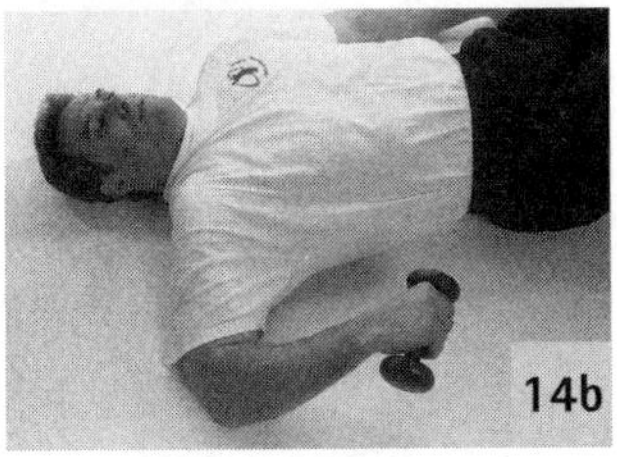

14b

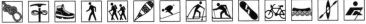

Technique: Lie on your back. Support your shoulder with a small towel roll under your shoulder blade. You also may need a towel or a pillow to support your hand if it will not lie flat on the ground. Use a can of food or a weight for slight resistance; the weight should not be too heavy. Place your right arm extended out to your side at shoulder level and elbow bent to 90 degrees, so that your hand faces the ceiling. Allow your shoulder to rotate externally so that your forearm points straight up parallel to your head (like a holdup position in an old western movie) (14a). Hold this position for 30–45 seconds. Keeping your elbow on the floor, raise your forearm by rotating at your shoulder, moving your hand toward your feet until it is a few inches off the floor near your waist. Your goal is a 20-degree angle measured from your hand to the floor (14b). If you feel the front of your shoulder moving forward, you have gone too far. Hold it for about 30–45 seconds. Next, straighten your elbow and raise your arm to 90 degrees so that your fingers are pointing toward the ceiling. Bring your straight arm back toward the floor until you feel a stretch in your shoulder and latissimus. Your shoulder is loose enough if the back of your hand touches the ground. Do 2–4 reps.
Variation: 14.1. Stand with your feet shoulder-width apart. Hold a towel with your right hand and place it over your shoulder, above waist height. Put your left hand behind your back, above waist height, and grab the towel; gradually pull up with your right hand. Hold when you feel a stretch. Repeat this stretch on the other side.
Precautions: In the floor version, don't allow your arm to migrate toward your body. Don't let your shoulder lift off the ground.

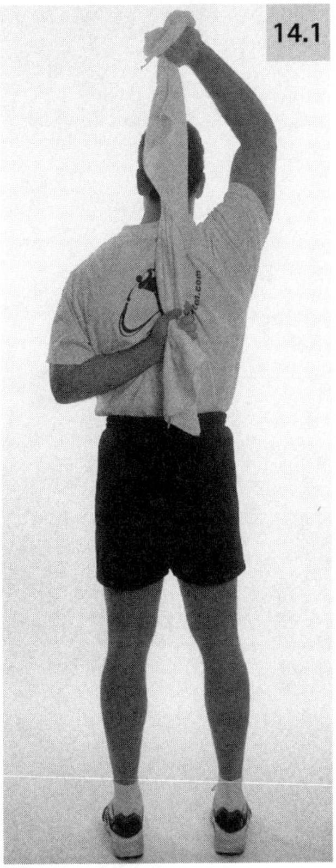

14.1

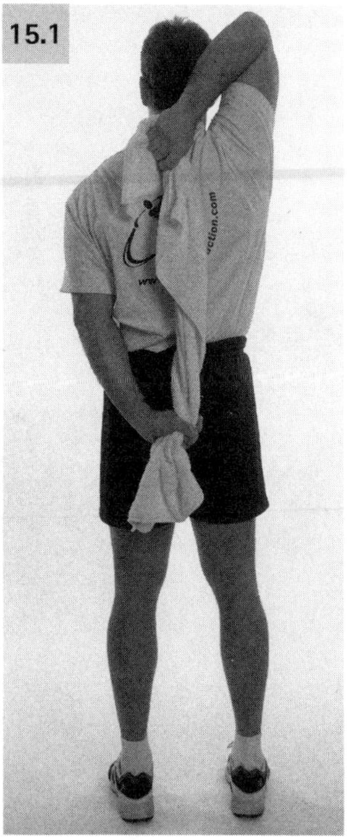

15.1

15 TRICEPS STRETCH

Equipment: Towel.
Purpose: Stretch the back of your arm.

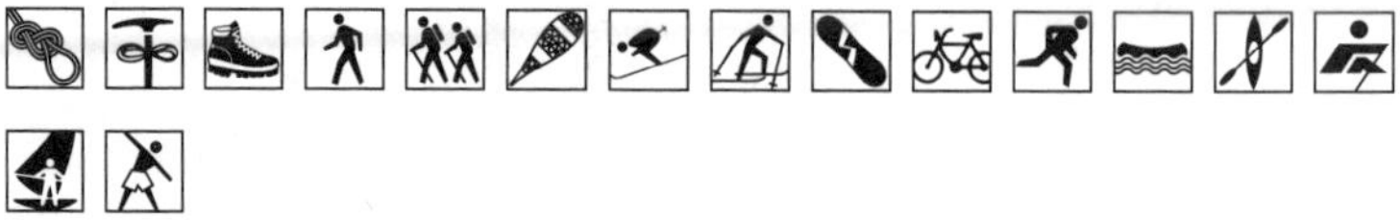

Technique: Standing with your feet shoulder-width apart, lift your right arm over your head; bend your elbow so that your right hand is behind your neck. Hold your right elbow with your left hand and pull gently toward the back of your neck. You can also stretch your torso at the same time by side-bending your torso to the left. Do 2–3 reps.
Variation: 15.1. Set up as for the stretch described in Exercise 14.1, but pull down on the towel with your left arm.
Precaution: Don't let your right arm migrate out to the side.

16 FOREARM STRETCH

Equipment: None.
Purpose: Stretch the muscles of your forearm; this is particularly useful for those who do racquet sports, climbing, or kayaking.

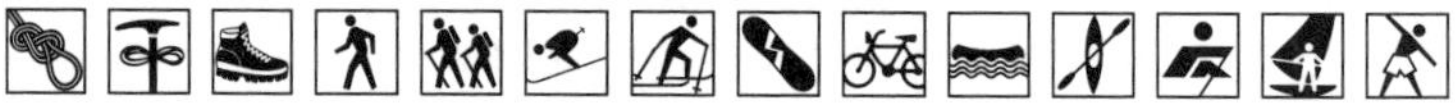

Technique: Extend your right arm straight out in front of you, with your arm, wrist, and fingers parallel to the floor. Now move your wrist and fingers toward the floor. Rotate your hand so your fingers point out away from the right side of your body, and hold it. You can increase the stretch by grasping your left hand with your right hand and gently pulling on your hand (photo 16). Then point the fingers of your right hand down and gently pull them back toward the middle of your body with your left hand. Do 2–3 reps.
Variation: 16.1. You can also stretch your forearm flexors by holding your arm straight out in front of you, parallel to the floor, with your elbow extended (straight). Bend your fingers back toward your body so that they are directed toward the ceiling.
Precaution: Don't bend your elbow.

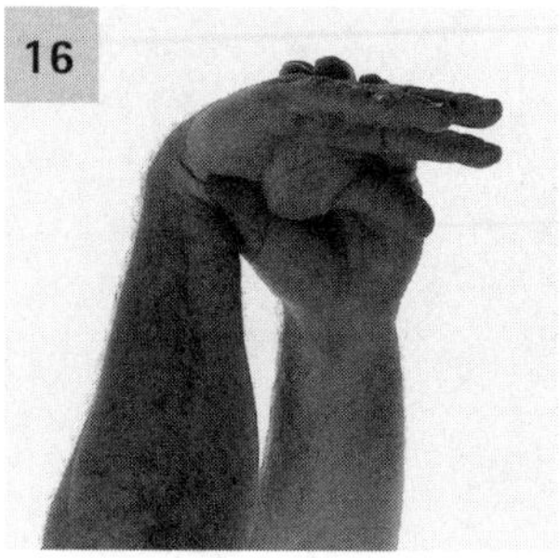

16

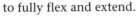

SPINE STRETCHES

17 CAT/CAMEL STRETCH

Equipment: None.
Purpose: Maintain and improve the flexibility of your back and neck to fully flex and extend.

Technique: Start on your hands and knees on the ground, with your hips and knees bent at about 90 degrees. Initiate an extending arch in your low back by moving your pelvis forward and bringing your belly button slightly closer to the ground in an arched-back position. Gradually extend up your spine until your neck is extended and you are looking straight ahead (17a). Hold this position for a few seconds. Next, initiate a flexing action in your low back by moving your pelvis back and raising your belly button up toward the ceiling. Gradually move the flexing all the way up your spine to create a humped back and until you are looking downward (17b). Hold this position for a few seconds. Repeat this sequence 5 times.

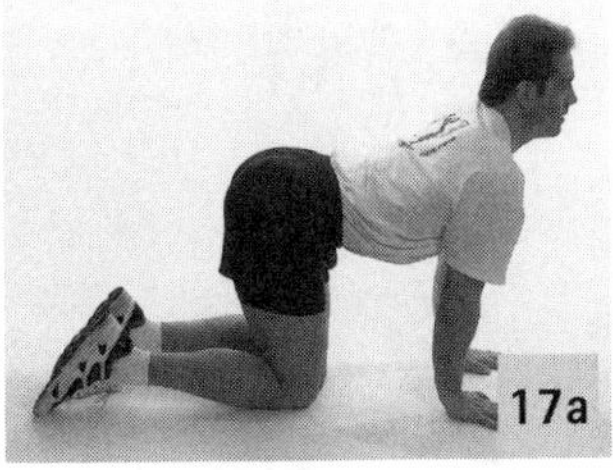
17a

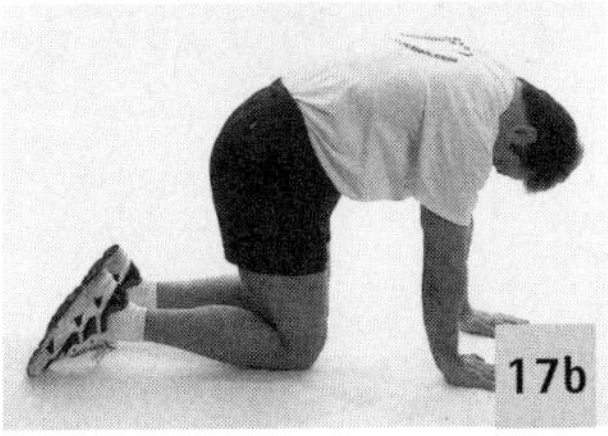
17b

18 PELVIC CIRCLES

Equipment: None.
Purpose: Prepare the mid and low back for rotational motions.

Technique: Stand with your hands on your hips and your knees slightly bent (or sit on a chair). Move your pelvis from side to side, then tip it forward (back arching) and back (back flexing).Then combine these movements to move your pelvis and hips in a smooth, circular motion (to the left, then forward, then to the right, then back). This will require you to shift your center of gravity while your pelvis circles underneath your unmoving upper body. Perform this motion for 4–6 revolutions to the left and then to the right.
Precaution: Be cautious if you have a lower-back problem.

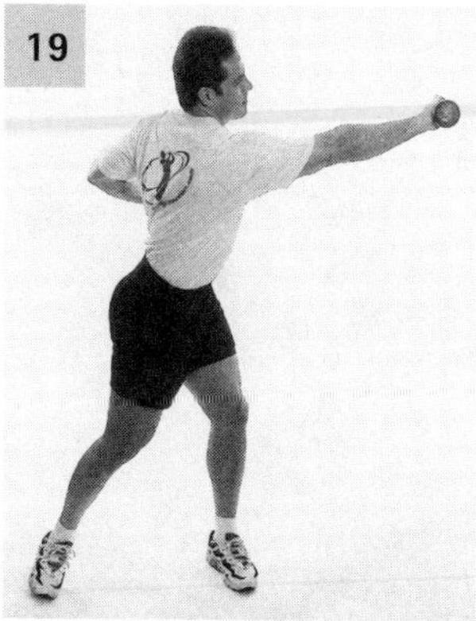

19 ACTIVE SPINE ROTATIONS

Equipment: None.
Purpose: Maintain the rotation in your spine.

Technique: Start with your knees slightly bent in a mini squat position, with your feet spaced wider than shoulder-width apart, and with your right elbow in a flexed position and your right arm drawn back so your hand is close to your shoulder. Initiate a punch across your body with your right shoulder and arm extending to the 10:00 position, and at the same time push off with your right buttock and foot, thus extending your right hip, straightening your right knee, and weight-shifting to the left foot. Pivot on the ball of the right foot and end on the toes of your right foot with your heel up at the end of the punch. Then repeat the punch with the left hand, punching in the opposite direction to the 2:00 position. One rep is a punch to the right and a punch to the left. Perform 2–3 sets of 15–30 reps.
Variations: **19.1.** Position your feet so that one foot is a running-stride length in front of the other, with both heels on the ground and your knees slightly bent. Punch in a forward direction, 12 times with each arm, then add rotational punches as described above but keep the same stance position. After 12 rotational punches, switch your forward leg with the backward leg and repeat. **19.2.** Try the exercise while sitting. This will take your knees and hips out of the motion and focus the rotational demands on your spine. **19.3.** Try this exercise with small free weights starting at 3 pounds. This will improve your neck and shoulder strength.
Tips and Precautions: In the standard version, punches can be performed in any direction, and either high or low, but are usually performed at shoulder height. You can punch as far as your spine can rotate after you have done it well to the 10:00 and 2:00 range. This exercise should initially be done in a slow and controlled manner so as to not injure your spine or shoulders. Increase the speed gradually and be cautious if you have a shoulder or back problem.

chapter 5 FUNCTIONAL CORE AND STRENGTH TRAINING

By Mark Pierce, A.T.C., David Musnick, M.D., and Michael Hansen, P.T.

THIS CHAPTER WILL HELP YOU:

- Understand the benefits of strength training.
- Understand the various strength training methods and equipment options.
- Understand the difference between traditional and functional strength training.
- Identify and learn how to use the various types of equipment used in resistance exercise.
- Learn specific functional strength exercises.

The basic strength training concepts in this chapter will help you choose and evaluate which strength training options are most appropriate for your goals. Strength training can be used for:

- Bone density maintenance and improvement.
- Enhancing metabolism and hormone function.
- Preserving and increasing lean body mass.
- Preserving and improving muscular function with aging.
- Weight management.
- Injury prevention.
- Muscle hypertrophy.
- Toning and shaping.
- Core strengthening.
- Sport and activity-specific training.

In this chapter, we discuss conventional and functional strength training. Conventional strength training usually focuses on isolated muscular development. It is best used for toning, shaping, and hypertrophy. Functional exercises use your muscles and body regions in patterns that are closest to how your body functions in real life, and can improve your strength, coordination, speed, power, and balance significantly. Functional training is an important component of any activity-specific and injury-prevention program. In order to design or modify your strength training program it is helpful to understand some basic concepts.

The term *strength* implies the maximum tension or force generated by a muscle or muscle group at a specified velocity.

The term *one repetition maximum* (1 RM) is often used to define the ability of a muscle to produce a single repetition (rep) of a movement with maximal resistance. In strength training and outdoor activities, we are usually using a percentage of 1 RM.

Strength training can be defined as any form of active exercise in which a muscular contraction is resisted by an outside force. Outside forces include gravity, free weights, balls, pulleys, resistance tubing, and exercise machines. Such machines have made exercise easier, but their carryover to sport-specific function is sometimes questionable, and they should not be the sole basis of a strength training program.

Strength endurance refers to the time limit of a muscle's ability to perform a strength exercise repeatedly. Exercise programs designed to increase muscular endurance emphasize doing sets with higher reps (15–35) and thus lower amounts of resistance.

Power refers to the product of force exerted

and the velocity (speed) of the exercise, and thus the rate of performing the work of the exercise. When exercising, the force is a given resistance, that of a weight or the weight of your body against gravity. Your power can increase in one of two ways. (1) You can increase the number of reps in a given time. (2) You can do the same number of reps in a shorter time. This is important for a number of reasons. We usually are instructed that it is important to lift heavier loads with fewer repetitions. In fact, we function in most of our activities with lower loads and higher reps (for example, the kayaker's stroke). In certain outdoor situations, you may need to perform a movement with high resistance at quick speeds (a quick high step on snow or rock, a jump off a boulder or across a river, a quick climbing move, or a kayak roll). To be prepared for these challenges, you should train at both ends of the power spectrum.

If your activity requires brief periods of moving your body rapidly, incorporate some higher-speed training into your routine.

BENEFITS OF STRENGTH TRAINING

The benefits of strength training are numerous. Resistive exercise creates adaptive changes in the muscle as it is progressively overloaded. These changes include hypertrophy (increase in size) of muscle fibers, as well as an increase in the recruitment of muscle fibers, creating an improvement in muscle tone. Bone, ligament, and tendon density also improve, helping to stabilize your joints. As the strength of muscle continues to increase, the cardiovascular response to the muscle also improves, which results in an increase in muscular endurance and power. Strength training improves your physical capacity to do your activities with less fatigue and less risk of injury. It can improve your physical appearance in regard to your level of muscle tone and aid in shaping your body. In addition, strength training can improve your mental outlook and sense of physical well-being.

Strength training can also enhance your body composition and metabolism by increasing the ratio of muscle mass to fat. It can also stimulate growth hormone release, which is helpful in maintaining muscle. Both of these benefits make strength training a necessary part of any antiaging program (one of the most significant signs of aging is sarcopenia, which is a loss of muscle mass). For a discussion of achieving specific benefits through strength training, including stimulating hormone and metabolic responses, see Strength Training Goals and Prescriptions toward the end of this chapter.

DETERMINANTS OF STRENGTH

People of all ages can increase their muscle size and strength as a result of progressive strength training. Strength gains decline 7% per decade after age 30. Studies show that we lose a half pound of muscle every year of life after age 25 unless we perform regular exercise. The rate at which skeletal muscle can adapt to vigorous exercise is reduced as we age, but adaptations still take place and improvements in performance can occur.

A person's strength is related to many factors, including gender, distribution of muscle fiber type, muscle and bone anatomy, genetics, body frame, nutrition, hormone levels, injuries, and training.

The *length tension* relationship of the muscle is another important factor in determining strength. When a muscle is at its resting length, a maximal number of sites are available for muscle fiber contraction. However, when the muscle is shorter (contracted) or longer (stretched) than its resting length, there are fewer available sites. Thus, the muscle can generate the most force around its resting length in a midrange position and less force when it is in a stretched or shortened state. Training programs should include both exercise of a muscle at midrange for maximal force generation and through all ranges for functional full-range strength and balance.

Neural control (nerve control) of the muscles also affects strength by influencing the maximal force of a muscle. It is directly related to coordination of the simultaneous use of different muscles and recruitment of fibers within a muscle. Neural control is a function of how many and how fast muscle fibers are involved in a contraction. It is also a function of the time elapsed between a stimulus and the beginning of the muscular reaction to it. An increase in muscle size takes 6–8 weeks to occur, yet people improve strength performance in 2–3 weeks of training. Much of the improvement in strength evidenced in the first few weeks of resistance training is attributable to neural firing adaptations.

MUSCLE FIBER TYPES

Our musculoskeletal systems possess two different types of muscle. This was discovered in 1873 by a scientist named Ranvier, who reported differences in muscle color within and among species. His initial observation was the coloring of the two muscle types, red and white. The explanation for the color differences is pretty simple and has a basis in physiology.

The darker-colored muscle type is red or *slow-twitch* muscle. The lighter-colored muscle type is white or *fast-twitch* muscle. They are differently colored because the slow-twitch muscle fibers have more mitochondria (full of red-pigmented cytochrome complexes) and more myoglobin packed within the muscle cells. This gives them a darker, reddish color. Some of our muscles, like the soleus in the lower leg, are almost all slow-twitch fibers. Others, such as those controlling eye movements, are made up of only fast-twitch fibers. Function dictates form for our specialized skeletal muscles (muscles that attach to the skeleton).

The majority of our muscles contain a mixture of both slow and fast fiber types. On average, we have about 50% slow and 50% fast fibers in most locomotory muscles, with substantial intraindividual (muscle-to-muscle) variations. It is these variations that make sports and outdoor activity performance training interesting.

The exact composition of each muscle is genetically determined, so if you want to win an Olympic medal in the 100-meter dash, you had better be born with about 80% fast-twitch fibers, and the opposite if you have aspirations of winning a marathon. The fast-twitch fibers benefit the sprinter because they reach peak tension much faster than their slow-twitch counterparts. Gram for gram, the two types are not different in the amount of force they produce, only the rate of force production. So, having a lot of fast-twitch fibers only makes a difference when the time available for force production is very limited (milliseconds), like the brief time the foot is in contact with the ground during a sprint or a long jump. It makes no difference to the power lifter.

For the pure endurance athlete, slow-twitch fibers are needed. These fibers trade lightning speed for fatigue resistance. Plenty of mitochondria and more capillaries surrounding each fiber make them more adept at using oxygen to generate ATP without substantial lactate accumulation. This aids in exercise that requires repeated muscle fiber contractions, as in a 2,000-meter rowing race, a long hike, or in a 10K run or marathon.

Skeletal muscles respond to chronic overload (training) by trying to minimize the cellular disturbance caused by the training. With intense endurance training, fast-fiber muscles can develop more mitochondria and surrounding capillaries. So can the slow fibers. Therefore, training improves your existing fiber distribution's ability to cope with the exercise stress you create. Even among a group of elite endurance athletes, fiber type alone is a poor predictor of performance. This is especially true in the intermediate duration events. There are many other factors that go into determining success. In fact, evidence suggests that a mixed fiber composition is ideal for success in an event like the mile run or for good performances across a range of strength and endurance events.

You cannot change the percentage of fast- and slow-twitch fibers you were born with. If you have more fast-twitch fibers it may be easier for you to increase the speed of your exercises and to make progress in doing plyometric exercises (discussed under Strength Training Methods below). You can somewhat compensate for a low percentage of fast-twitch fibers by training with speed and plyometrics, especially if you are involved in an activity in which fast-twitch fibers would help (such as mountain biking, mountain and rock climbing, high-level alpine skiing and snowboarding, and white-water kayaking).

TONIC AND PHASIC MUSCLES

Tonic muscles have a certain amount of tone at all times. They are the muscles responsible for maintaining joint integrity and for keeping our bodies upright and erect. They include the deep flexors of the neck, the abdominal obliques, the transverse abdominous, the multifidi in the back, the middle and lower trapezius, and to a slightly lesser extent, the serratus anterior and posterior fibers of the gluteus medius in the buttocks. Lesser-known tonic muscles live close to the spine and stabilize minute changes in joint motions. Put simply, these are the muscles that stabilize the spine and provide strength to control your center or core.

Phasic muscles work primarily to move our arms, legs, and torso. In other words, when you are performing an activity such as lifting a weight, paddling, or climbing a mountain, the phasic muscles kick in to move the trunk or limb.

Unfortunately, what often happens is that through poor posture or excessive performance of a movement (as in a particular sport or exercise program that does not address core stability), we exercise the phasic muscles until they start to dominate and act like tonic muscles. A common example is the erector spinae muscles of the low-back region. As long as the phasic muscles are doing their job, everything should be OK, right? For a while, sometimes it is. However, as the phasic muscles get stronger and stronger, the tonic muscles get weaker and weaker. The spine becomes unprotected, unstable, and vulnerable to injury. Ensuring an overall efficiency in the operation of our bodies is why learning and exercising proper balance and maintaining strong core musculature will benefit anyone—from athletes who need to react to stimuli from all directions with speed and agility, to people doing garden-variety tasks such as walking to the mailbox.

Good tone in postural muscles is necessary for spinal stability. Our modern sedentary lifestyle uses postural muscles more than the phasic, "use-on-demand" muscles. If we have poor tone in postural muscles, muscle imbalances occur. There are a number of problems that lead to imbalance between phasic and tonic muscles. These include (1) poor posture and ergonomics during sitting, standing, and recumbent positions (see discussions in chapters 14 and 27); (2) inadequate understanding and practice of how to engage postural muscles of the core in all of the above positions (see chapter 14); and (3) lax ligaments and hypermobile (loose) joints from either poor posture, injuries, or one's genetic tissue makeup (see chapter 9).

Emotional stress, sedentary lifestyle (deconditioning), and improper exercise training also play their part in eroding the health of our musculature and in creating prolonged muscle imbalance, such as tight tonic muscles and weak phasic muscles, which leads to dysfunction and pain.

MUSCLE ACTIONS

Strength training puts the types of muscles and muscle fibers to work by engaging several different kinds of muscle action.

Isotonic muscle action is that which is carried out against a constant load and variable speed as the muscle contracts. Most exercise machines involve isotonic muscle action.

An *isometric* muscle action is a static muscle contraction in which there is no change in the length of the muscle fiber. Functionally, it is a stabilizing contraction. This type of contraction occurs if you hold a position without allowing any motion, as when you hold one position in a dip, squat, or a pull-up. Such training is useful if you are involved in an activity that requires you to maintain a position for prolonged periods.

In a *concentric* muscle action, the muscle shortens and joint motion occurs; for example, flexing your elbow while holding a 10-pound weight (an exercise called a curl) causes the biceps to shorten and brings your hand closer to your shoulder.

Eccentric muscle action occurs when the muscle lengthens while developing tension, because the contractile force is less than the resistive force (e.g., in the second half of the curl exercise, lowering the weight from a position close to your shoulder to a straight elbow position). In the biceps curl, the eccentric action of the biceps muscle prevents you from dropping the weight. Eccentric muscle action decelerates joint motion and is a very important function of muscles.

Many of your lower-extremity muscles (buttocks to feet) function eccentrically to control your legs from collapsing forward or inward. Your quadriceps have to work eccentrically to prevent your knees from flexing and are subject to greater loads when you are going downhill. Many acute or gradual overuse injuries are due to inadequate eccentric strength. You can emphasize training eccentrically by having the eccentric part of the exercise take twice as long as the concentric. Eccentric muscle action in the lower extremities can be enhanced by performing exercises in standing positions that simulate the eccentric demands of standing activities. Such exercises can be made more challenging by performing them on one foot, by orienting the movement in various directions, or by adding weights.

Econcentric muscle action combines both concentric (at one joint) and eccentric (at the other joint) contraction in a muscle that spans more than one joint. Examples of this include (1) a biceps curl performed while your shoulder moves into extension (backward movement of the elbow); and (2) when walking, prior to your heel rising, your calf muscle acts to both slow down the progression of forward ankle motion while assisting your upper leg muscles in extension (straightening) of your knee. Jumping exercises like those discussed under Plyometric Training below and in chapter 11 will work your muscles in this fashion.

STRENGTH TRAINING METHODS

There are many strength training methods that involve the various muscle actions. In fact, one classification of strength training is by the type of muscle action, being either isotonic (moving) or isometric (not moving). Other methods include circuits and plyometrics.

Isotonic Training

As described above, isotonic resistance exercises are carried out against a constant load and variable speed as the muscle contracts. Isotonic training includes free weights, pulleys, and most exercise machines.

Isometric Training

Because isometric exercise involves static muscle contraction, it is most important for people participating in rock climbing, mountaineering, skiing and wind surfing or any other activity that requires the ability to maintain static positions. Strength gains are specific for the joint angle held, but may have benefits within a range of approximately plus or minus 20 degrees. The exercise should be done in a few different joint positions as close as possible to the positions that you will be using in your activity. See Exercise 57 in chapter 6 for an example of an isometric exercise.

Isometric training is particularly applicable to climbers, and the climbing athlete should incorporate some such exercises into his or her routine. Maintaining a climbing hold on rock or ice could be trained by an isometric hold on a climbing wall, boulder, or fingerboard, or by a pull-up. You could start off with holds of 6 seconds and repeat each minute for 5–10 reps. You could increase the hold times of some of the reps to simulate the expected hold times in your climbs. See chapter 18 for climbing-specific isometric exercises.

Circuit Weight Training

Circuit weight training includes weight stations mixed with aerobic stations. The workout emphasizes muscle endurance. If the circuit consists solely of machines it may aid in weight loss and in building a base of tone. If you are just starting to work out you might make some moderate initial strength gains in a circuit training format. For people with a base of strength conditioning, circuit training is not efficient for making significant strength gains. The aerobic part of circuit training might be helpful if you are just beginning to do aerobic workouts and if you need a significant structure for your workout. The aerobic workout is only effective if you are able to elevate your heart rate consistently and stay in a heart-rate training zone.

Plyometric Training

Plyometric exercises are a type of strength training that incorporates rapid muscle contraction and often explosive movements as in jumps and hops. Such exercises are usually done with the legs but can be done with the arms, as in a plyo push-up (see chapter 8, Exercise 77). Plyometrics can be done singly or in combination, and can be done on different sloped surfaces indoors or outdoors. Plyometric exercises are used in addition to a training program and never before establishing and continuing a solid base of strength training for at least 6 weeks. Its advantages are (1) preparation for activity-related demands for jumping, hopping, and speed; and (2) improved reaction times to unpredictable surfaces.

Plyometrics can be helpful for mountain biking, alpine skiing, snowboarding, mountain and rock climbing, whitewater kayaking, windsurfing, or any sport that requires jumping. Plyometrics are also beneficial for activities such as basketball, football, soccer, track and field, tennis, volleyball, and any other sports that require explosive motions. Climbers can do modifications of plyometrics on climbing walls by doing quick motions with legs and arms to reach for a particularly difficult hold. Plyometric exercises in this book include:

Upper body: chapter 8, Exercise 77.

Lower body: chapter 8, Exercises 70 and 71; chapter 11, Exercises 100 and 101; chapter 20, Exercises 159 and 161–167; and chapter 22, Exercises 176–178.

Plyometric equipment. You can purchase or make plyometric equipment. Most of the equipment available simulates jumping or hopping over various barriers. Plyo Boxes are available in sizes from 6 to 36 inches. You can jump on and off these at various angles. If you are planning your own training, use a 12-inch box to start with and then use higher boxes depending on your size, abilities, and the demands of your sport. If you are working with clients, have a number of Plyo Boxes that are 6, 12, and 18 inches. Banana Steps can be set up for progressive jumping and are available in 6- and 12-inch sizes. Side-jump boxes are available for the advanced skier or

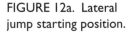

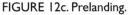

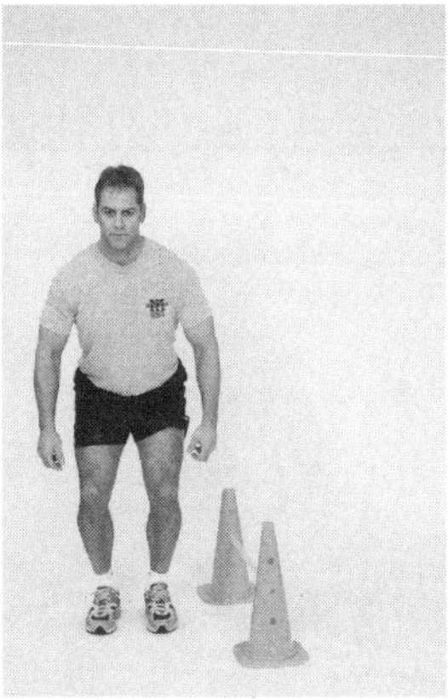
FIGURE 12a. Lateral jump starting position.

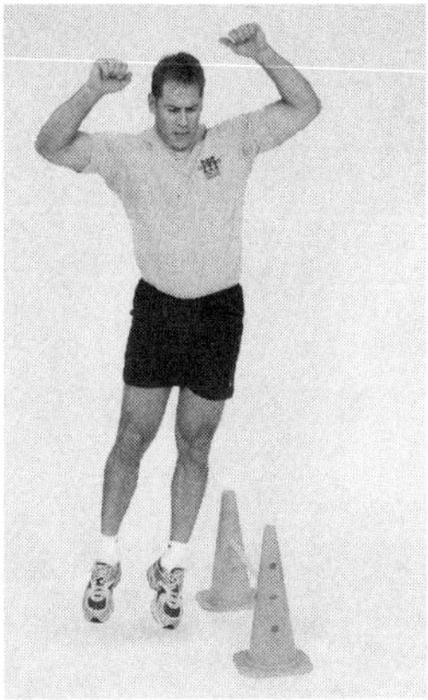
FIGURE 12b. Take-off.

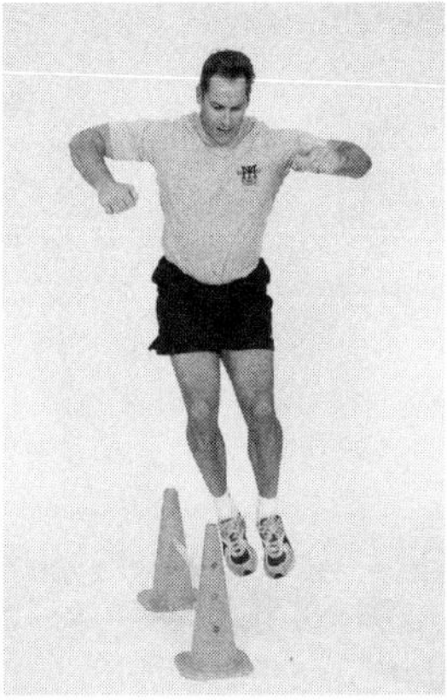
FIGURE 12c. Prelanding.

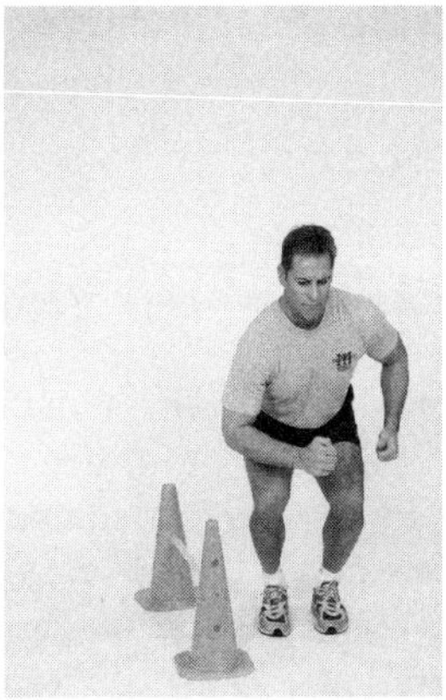
FIGURE 12d. Landing.

snowboarder. Hurdle poles and cones are available for jumping training. They are perhaps the lightest, most economical equipment and are quite adjustable. Gorilla agility hurdles are also very portable and inexpensive and are useful for forward or side jumps and hops.

Refer to the websites in Selected References for online pictures and descriptions of plyometric equipment. A side-jump exercise with cones is shown in Figures 12a–d.

Plyometric precautions. There is an increased risk of injury with plyometric exercises, so be careful and consider doing a supervised session. Don't engage in plyometric training if you have any active or chronic painful conditions in your feet, ankles, knees, hips, low back, neck, or shoulders. If you have lax ligaments and loose joints in your ankles it is important to wear stable athletic footwear. You might even consider wearing an ankle brace or taping your ankle prior to your workout. Please see chapter 11 for further plyometric jumping techniques and precautions.

WEIGHT, RESISTANCE, AND GOOD FORM

The amount of resistance that you use when strength training is related to a number of factors, including your goals, your injury status, how long you have been strength training, and the number of reps in your sets. Use as much weight (resistance) as is comfortable to complete a set pain-free and with good form. The last 1–2 reps in a set should fatigue your muscles so that the reps are difficult but are still done in good form. This means having good posture, safe spine positioning with your core engaged, and good movement patterns.

Good form is a key to injury prevention. You are using too much resistance if (1) you are fatiguing before the last 2 reps in a set; (2) your movement patterns are poorly coordinated or done with poor balance; or (3) you have pain in the muscles while you are exercising or in other muscles or joints in your body.

There are different reasons and methods to increase the resistance used in an exercise. You would increase the resistance in a particular set when you are no longer fatigued in the last 1–2 reps in a set. You would usually increase the resistance if you are doing lower-rep sets to build hypertrophy or to work on power and strength. In general, it is safe to increase the resistance used in a set by 5–10% of what you are currently lifting. If you are doing consistent strength training, you can go to lower-rep sets and make

FIGURE 13. 1RM CONTINUUM

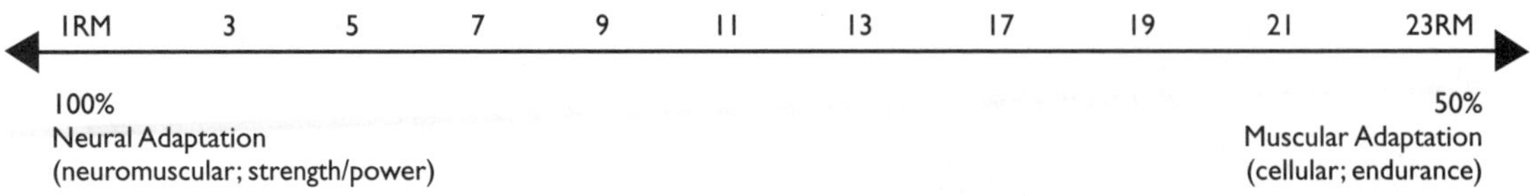

higher-percentage increases in the resistance. If you have just injured a region, it is important to decrease the resistance for 4–6 weeks while your tissues are repairing. During that time you can consider doing higher-rep sets with lower resistance to improve circulation in the injured muscle and then gradually building back to the preinjury resistance.

Neuromuscular adaptations are very specific to the intensity of your exercise. Intensity can be described in terms of a repetition maximum (RM). The maximum that a person can perform once in a resistance exercise is called 1 RM. The maximum weight that you can correctly lift 5 consecutive times during a particular exercise, without significant rest, would be 5 RM. Lifting at 1 RM is not recommended because it increases your risk of injury, especially if you don't have appropriate training and spotting.

The relationship between reps and the 1 RM is known as the 1 RM continuum (Figure 13). Higher-resistance, lower-rep exercises elicit neural adaptations (fiber recruitment). Neural adaptation is when all the motor nerve units needed to meet the intensity of a task fire in response to that task. Basically, our physiology works in the conservation mode all the time. It will only use energy as it is needed. If a task or exercise immediately requires many muscle fibers for a 1 RM effort, then your neuromuscular system will respond and recruit as many fibers as are available to perform the task. Strength and power are developed by training the musculoskeletal system to adapt neurologically. This is done by performing repetitions in the 1–3 RM range.

PRACTICAL POINT

Train with higher weight and lower repetitions for greater gains in maximal strength. For greater gains in strength endurance, train with lower resistance and higher repetitions. See Figure 14.

On the other hand, lower-resistance and higher-rep exercises (14–17 RM) emphasize muscular adaptations. Muscular adaptation occurs on the cellular level when muscles are stressed. If muscles or groups of muscles are stressed submaximally—for example, doing a set of squats with a weight that produces fatigue in 9 reps—then our muscular physiology adapts in a number of ways. More capillaries are formed to supply needed oxygen, the cellular mechanisms that produce energy required for muscle contraction are heightened, and the muscle cell itself hypertrophies and grows in size. Lower resistance and higher repetitions (14–17 RM) elicit an endurance response from muscles, creating the cellular mechanisms needed to produce prolonged levels of muscle contraction, such as that required in cycling, rowing, or running.

REPETITIONS AND SETS

A repetition is the number of times you repeat an exercise in a set before a rest period or before you exercise different muscles. The number of reps in your sets should be based on your exercise goals. When you are working with machines or free weights in conventional exercises, consider beginning with 15 reps in a set for the first 2–3 weeks to avoid injuries, develop muscle capillary networks, and to put your muscles and joints through a full range of motion.

FIGURE 14. TRAINING EFFECTS OF REPS AND RESISTANCE

Reps in Set	Training Effect	Useful For
3–5	Maximum power and strength	Rock climbers, competitive lifters
6–8	Strength with hypertrophy	Skiers, snowboarders, high-level athletes
9–12	Hypertrophy (best range)	Body building, toning, shaping
14–17	Strength endurance	Endurance athletes
20–30	Endurance with improved circulation	Injury healing, range of motion exercises

Note: *The average person may incorporate sets of different numbers of reps to accomplish a number of goals for the exercise session.*

For maximum benefit, you should feel fatigue during the last 1–2 reps of a set. When you have been strength training consistently 2–3 times per week (working all body regions), consider adding 1–2 sets of 8–12 reps, which will emphasize strength more than endurance. Gradually build up the resistance used with this number of reps. After 3–4 weeks you can add lower-rep sets (4–6) to build maximum strength and promote hypertrophy. As you progress through your training program, consider incorporating sets of different lengths to achieve a diversity of training effects: 1–2 sets of 15 reps, 1–2 sets of 8–12 reps, and 1 set of 4–6 reps.

For functional exercises that work on strength, balance, and coordination (see the exercises at the end of this chapter), start with 8–12 reps and do them slowly enough to establish your movement pattern. Remember that functional exercises can be more difficult and you may need to use less resistance as compared to a traditional exercise. For instance, you will likely to be able to use more weight in a simple biceps curl (chapter 15, Exercise 125) than when you do a biceps curl with a lunge (Exercise 28 in this chapter). As you feel stronger and more able to do a particular functional exercise, you might consider doing a set on a timed interval such as within 30–60 seconds. Don't increase speed unless you can maintain good form with your core engaged. If you do a set in a timed interval and are able to increase the speed of each rep, benefits include improved balance, reaction time, and coordination (for a further discussion of speed see Overloading and Strength Training Options below).

Specific Sets and Reps

Improve your physique, increase muscle size, and build some strength at the same time: 2–3 sets of 9–12 reps, and 1–2 sets of 6–8 reps per set with higher resistance.

For women, improve basic toning, shaping, and strength without building too much muscle mass: 2 sets of 14–17 reps and 2 sets of 9–12 reps.

For endurance athletes: 2 sets of 9–12 reps, then continue with at least 2 sets of 15 reps. You could consider a third set of 9–12 reps and a fourth set of 6–8 reps.

For strength/endurance athletes, such as downhill skiers, mountain bikers, rock and mountain climbers, and windsurfers: 3 sets of 14–17 reps, 2 sets of 9–12 reps, and 1 set of 6–8 reps.

For seniors (over 60), slow age-related muscle loss and build some strength: 2 sets of 15 reps and 1 set of 10 reps.

Augment growth hormone release to slow age-related muscle loss and decrease sagging and wrinkling: 3–5 sets of 10 reps working large muscle groups, including your thighs, buttocks, upper back, and chest. This could include doing squats, lunges, lat pulls, and bench presses.

PRACTICAL POINT

Rest at least 1 minute between each set and before doing a different exercise that targets the same muscle in a similar fashion. This will allow your muscle to regain the energy it needs for further contraction. Instead of doing nothing for 1 minute, you can do strength training in a circuit, moving to an exercise that uses different muscles.

If you are doing machine exercises or isolated muscle free-weight exercises, you can pair your exercises so you are exercising one muscle group, then its opposite (e.g., biceps then triceps, quads then hamstrings, chest then back). You may then find it unnecessary to take 1-minute breaks between sets. You can also alternate between an upper-extremity and then a lower-extremity exercise. Rest a full minute between each functional exercise that pairs exercises of the hips and legs with the shoulder.

OVERLOADING AND STRENGTH TRAINING OPTIONS

Overload, simply stated, means applying stress to a muscle or group of muscles. If you overload a muscle in the way you want it to perform, the muscle will adapt and remodel in that fashion. As adaptation occurs, increased loading and modification of your training regime needs to occur. There are numerous methods of overloading muscle, each with its own advantages and disadvantages. A number of these have been listed with various goals in mind (see Specific Sets and Reps above). Other methods of overloading muscle include:

Light weight to heavier weight, same number of reps: If you are doing 3 sets of 12, in the first set you would use about 75% of your known or predicted max, in the second set 85%, and in the third set 100%. Perform all three sets for 12 reps.

Light weight to heavy weight, lower reps: With this overload method, you progressively increase the load with fewer reps for each successive set. For example, if you can bench press 100 pounds 10 times, follow that with 8 reps of 120 pounds for the second set, and finish with 6 reps of 140 pounds for the third set. This method is used frequently for achieving increased strength, power, and mass, and could be used if you have already established your strength foundation or after 4–6 weeks of consistent base training.

Increased speed or rate of movement: This overload method is useful if you're trying to perform motions at faster speeds, such as fast paddling in whitewater kayaking, crew rowing, any racing activity, or climbing. After you have established a good strength workout with at least 4 weeks of 2 sets at 15 reps, you can try increasing the speed of your exercise. You may have to do this with the same resistance or slightly less resistance if using weights or machines. Safety during this type of overload method must be observed. With increased speed during any resistance movement comes increased risk of injury. Always maintain control of the resistance and increase the speed only in the concentric phase of the motion. This is the phase of motion you use to move the resistance against gravity. This method also increases coordination, especially with functional exercises, after you can perform the motion patterns well. There is some physiological carryover from one training speed to another, so it is beneficial to cross train at multiple speeds.

PRACTICAL POINT

In general, rest approximately 48 hours between training sessions of a specific muscle area or region to allow the muscles to adapt and heal from the overload.

STRENGTH TRAINING GUIDELINES

Warm-Up

Always warm up your muscles and joints with 5–10 minutes of aerobic exercise. Preferable methods are biking (especially bikes with moving handlebars), cross-country skiing, skipping rope, or rowing, because they use your arms and legs. Walking, running, or stair climbing are also acceptable for a warm-up.

Frequency

During the initial stages of your exercise progression, exercise each body region 2–3 times per week. The intensity of each workout and your current level of fitness will determine the amount of time needed for proper recovery. Allow at least 48 hours between strength training sessions that target particular body regions. Performing resistance exercise of a particular body region without adequate time for recovery can lead to injuries and excessive soreness.

Range of Motion

Use as full a range of motion of the joint as possible to allow the muscle to strengthen at different lengths. Try to control the speed at the end ranges of a joint (especially the shoulder and knee) to avoid jamming it at its end range. Stay in a pain-free range of motion. This may mean limiting your range of movement if you have an injury. For example, if you are exercising with rotator cuff tendonitis, you may want to decrease the range of motion of a lat pull to decrease the repetitive work that is above 90 degrees of shoulder abduction (see Function and Anatomy in chapter 15). If you have a back problem, you may want to decrease certain ranges that will move your pelvis forward or backwards, for example in exercises that involve significant hip and spine flexing such as Exercise 31. If you have active tendonitis in your knee or kneecap pain, you may want to decrease the flexing of your knee during a deep squat.

Work Larger Muscles First

In designing your strength training program, try to work large muscle groups first. Your larger muscles are your thighs (quads and hamstrings), your gluteals, your latissimus, and your chest. Your smaller muscles are your biceps, triceps, rotator cuff, calves, and so on. If you fatigue your small muscles early in your workout, they will not be efficient at assisting with movements using larger muscle groups.

> PRACTICAL POINT
>
> Don't hold your breath while lifting weights. Exhale upon the greatest exertion. For example, when performing a bench press, exhale as you push the weight upward and inhale as you lower it to your body.

Engaging and Exercising Your Core (Torso)

There has been a great deal of press concerning the concept of the *core* (see chapter 14 for a full discussion of the anatomy and function of your core muscles). It is important to understand and engage your core during your exercises so that you can protect your low back during strength training. Such attention is also important during your outdoor and sports activities.

Engaging your core translates into activating the following muscles: multifidus (low-back extensors), transverse abdominus (part of your deeper abdominals), and the muscles of your pelvic floor. This can be done while you are in any posture, including lying down, sitting, and standing. You can think about this type of exercise as part of good posture, back alignment, and movement patterns to protect your body during exercise.

In this book we use the term *expanded core* to describe the core muscles along with other muscles important for protecting your low and mid back. These include your core muscles, described above, abdominals (all of them), buttocks, hamstrings, spine erector group, and your latissimus.

For spine protection, it is important to do exercises to keep your expanded core functional.

The muscles of the expanded core are decelerators, initiators of movement, and stabilizers. A strong set of expanded core muscles can support strengthening of your extremities. Expanded core exercises include Exercise 72 (abdominals); Exercises 23, 31, 35, 70, and 110 (buttocks); and Exercises 60, 73, 107, 108, 119, and 120 (low back, upper back, and latissimus). Save specific abdominal exercises for last because you will need your abdominal strength to stabilize your body during all other activities. In addition, there are other types of workouts that can exercise your core, including Pilates mat workouts.

Practice Safe Spine Postures and Movements

In general, try to lift with your buttocks and your legs as opposed to your back. Assume neutral spine positions (see chapters 14 and 27) when using seated equipment or in standing exercises, unless otherwise indicated. Avoid excessive spine flexion and extension. When you move into spine extension and flexion, be careful and make sure to engage your core.

You can think of your body as having a number of places to move or hinge. You can flex at your hips rather than in your low back. If you flex in your low back, especially while lifting weights or equipment, you are putting your low-back discs and your sacroiliac joint at risk of injury. Flexing and rotating your low back at the same time as you lift can be even more dangerous to your low back.

In general it is important to keep your back in a neutral position during most of the exercises in this book. Some of the exercises will ask you to flex at your hips. This is in general much safer than flexing or bending in your low back. You can initially try flexing at your hips while you are in a chair. Put your low back in a neutral position as in Exercise 180, Sitting Arcing Exercise. Keep the neutral spine position while flexing or hinging at your hips, trying to bring your chest closer to your knees. This will give you the feeling of hinging at your hips rather than your low back. You can try this in a standing position as well (Exercise 110, Waiter's Bow).

Try to always maintain a neutral spine position whenever you are attempting to lift, move, or carry objects. If you consistently do this throughout your daily activities and exercise routines, you will decrease your risk of injury to your low back.

Avoid Maximum Lifts

A maximum lift is usually defined as 1 RM, or what you can do only once. We recommend against ever doing this unless you are a competitive lifter or you have been training consistently for 1–2 years and have a good spotter and no present back or other active injuries. Even doing a set of 2–3 reps to failure (until you can't do any more) can be risky. With a new exercise or when you have taken a break from your regular strength training program, initially use a weight or resistance lower than you think you can do. This will help you avoid injury. Be especially careful with new shoulder exercises when you are raising your arm to the front or side, as the rotator cuff muscles are prone to straining with heavier weights.

Muscle Symmetry

Workouts should be designed to maintain muscle symmetry. This can be thought of as exercising muscles that do opposing actions in a body region, that stabilize a region, or that are prone to weakness.

Opposing muscles include quads/hamstrings; abdominal muscles and hip flexors/gluteus maximus and spine extensors; pectorals/rhomboids and trapezius; biceps/triceps; wrist and finger flexors/wrist and finger extensors. Think of giving attention to muscles on the front and back of your body. To provide stability, exercise muscles that stabilize a region along with the muscles that move it.

PRACTICAL POINT

It is important to maintain the strength of all of your major muscles. You may want to place more emphasis on some for strengthening and others for stretching. To maintain muscle balance, it is important to maintain flexibility of overused muscles and to maintain strength and endurance of underused muscles. Focus some of your strengthening on muscles commonly prone to weakness, and make sure you include stretches for muscles commonly prone to tightness (e.g., Achilles, quads, iliotibial band, psoas, upper trapezius, levator scapulae).

In the majority of people, certain muscles are prone to weakness and are a good focus for strength training. These include hamstrings, gluteus maximus and medius, abdominal obliques, spine extensors and rotators, middle and lower trapezius, rotator cuff of the shoulder, and wrist and finger extensors.

Repetitive activity can promote imbalances in muscle strength and length/tightness and lead to musculoskeletal injuries and pain.

Plateaus and Varying Your Routine

You may have plateaued in your strength training when you experience any of the following: (1) You feel bored with your workout and you start not wanting to go to the gym. (2) You are not gaining strength and are not able to progress to higher-weight, lower-rep sets. (3) You are getting injured with your strength program.

Reaching a plateau can happen for a number of reasons, and varying your routine in the following ways can help avoid this problem: (1) Vary how you exercise a muscle or a group of muscles. (2) Vary the speed of the exercise. (3) Vary the number of reps per set. (4) Vary the sequencing of your sets. (5) Vary the order of your exercises. (6) Vary who you work out with. (7) Vary where you work out. (8) Vary the time of day that you work out (you may find that you have the greatest energy and strength at a certain time of day; this is the best time for strength training and for increasing resistance and the intensity of your workouts).

Muscle Inhibition and Recruitment Problems

There may be intermittent changes in the strength of one or more muscles secondary to problems with recruitment of muscle fibers. This can be due to many different reasons. Postural alignment during an exercise may cause a particular muscle group to increase or decrease in strength; if lower-trapezius strength is less than upper-trapezius strength, abnormal scapular rhythm can result; or a low-back disc might inhibit normal recruitment of the hamstring. You may also notice changes in your strength during activities and during strength training workouts. Please see chapter 9 for a detailed look at these issues.

Muscle Soreness

You may experience delayed-onset muscle soreness the day following a strength training workout. This is a normal, slight amount of pain in the muscles you were exercising, especially if you increased the resistance. It is helpful to do some low-impact aerobic exercise with the same aching muscles to decrease the muscle pain and improve the elimination of muscle metabolism products.

Periodizing Your Program to Meet Activity Goals

Periodization in strength training is the planning of time periods of strength training options in regard to resistance, reps, and speed to meet certain activity goals. Periodized use of functional exercises, plyometrics, and sport-specific skill training will prepare you for activities or race goals.

We know that muscle adapts to stresses it is exposed to and strength gains will reach a plateau unless the stress is continually increased. With periodization, you change the training schedule so that when your goal activity begins, you will be maximally prepared. Periodization in strength training can include many plans, depending on your goals. For example:

The first stage might be a preparation stage in which you exercise with low resistance and higher reps (15–20) for 2–4 weeks while you are getting used to the equipment, movement patterns, and proper postures.

In the second phase, you become more specific with your exercises, increasing resistance and adding higher-resistance, lower-rep sets. Add functional exercises during this stage. This phase could be 3–4 weeks. Start your activity-specific skill and balance work by the end of this phase.

In the third phase, add more speed and power to your program. Consider doing certain exercises in 1–2 sets with higher resistance at 4–6 reps if you have significant strength and power goals. Consider adding speed to some of the exercises, especially the functional exercises. Add plyometrics at this stage if appropriate.

The final stage is your goal activity or competition, in which you are trying to maintain your strength while primarily performing your activity. Decrease the total volume of strength training and decrease frequency to 2 days a week. Also include a core of functional or free-weight exercises with 2 sets of 8–12 reps, and avoid strengthening sessions 1 day prior to goal activity sessions.

STRENGTH TRAINING EQUIPMENT

Selection of strengthening equipment can be confusing because of the diversity and variety of equipment available. Your choice should be made based on individual needs, but the best choice—based on function, economics, and space—is still free weights. In addition to the equipment listed below, assorted training aids such as slide boards and push-up handles can also be used for strength training (see chapter 6 for a description of these).

Dynamic Variable-Resistance Equipment (Machines)

Machines such as the Cybex, Hammer, Nautilus, and Technogym are designed to provide variable resistance to load the muscle throughout range of motion. Their advantages include safety, isolated guided movements, and quick and incremental adjustment of loads. They also help build muscle tone and general muscle strength. Disadvantages include limited training movements and no balance or combination of body motions involved.

Machines that allow independent, multi-planar arm motion are more challenging and are best used along with free weights once you have built up a base of strength.

Dynamic Constant-Resistance Equipment (Free Weights)

Dynamic constant resistance refers to fixed loads and variable speeds. Examples are free weights, weighted balls, or anything you can lift, such as a rock or log. Advantages include low cost of equipment, similarity to most functional work and exercise, and unlimited variety of training movements. Constant resistance is easily quantifiable, more functional, and is often closed-chain for the lower extremity (see Closed-chain vs. open-chain below). Disadvantages include inconsistent matching of resistive forces with muscle forces throughout the exercise, so your whole muscle does not get exercised with the same intensity. The weakest part of your muscle gets the greatest workout.

Ankle weights can help simulate the hip work needed in going uphill, in snow travel, or when wearing heavy footwear.

Pulleys

Pulleys are excellent for shoulder, back, rotator cuff, and sitting or standing abdominal exercises. Many functional exercises can be done with pulleys in a gym or with tubing at home or outdoors. The best pulleys are adjustable so they can be pulled at different heights, depending on your activity. Most pulleys can only be pulled from the ground or from overhead, but some are fully adjustable on a vertical axis. The fully adjustable pulleys are best to use for rotator cuff and other shoulder and upper-back exercises.

Versatile pulley machines are available in some gyms and physical therapy clinics. The FreeMotion machines by Hydra Fitness and Cybex are examples of pulleys that can be put in many different angles to allow use of one or both arms or legs in many different standing, sitting, or recumbent exercises. These machines allow you to change the resistance in smaller increments. You can also position these pulley systems at different angles for people of different heights and for people experiencing injuries or with particular exercise needs. With this equipment, you can incorporate balance and core work with your shoulder/arm or lower-body exercises. See Exercise 21 in this chapter as well as exercises in chapters 10, 14, and 15.

Elastic Resistance Equipment

Tubing comes in variable widths and resistance. Advantages are low cost, portability, and simulation of pulley motions. They are reasonable tools for the climbing, skiing, or paddling athlete. Disadvantages include a resistance increase as the tubing is stretched. This can lead to excessive force on some muscles at the end of the joint range and when the muscle is usually the weakest. **Note:** Attach elastic tubing to closed doors by tying a large knot in the tubing and closing the door, or by tying it to a doorknob or other attachment. Outside, tie tubing to trees, bleachers, poles, and so on. Be careful to anchor the tubing securely. You can buy tubing in different widths at most physical therapy clinics.

Medicine or Weight Balls

Weighted balls of various sizes are excellent for the balance reach exercises shown at the end of this chapter. They are also helpful for standing functional abdominal exercises. **Precautions:** Be careful with them if you have an active problem in your shoulder, neck, or low back.

Large Inflatable Balls

Physioballs or stability balls come in various sizes and can be used for strengthening your abdominal muscles and for sitting balance training. They are available through most physical therapy clinics.

Choose a size that allows you to sit with your knees and hips at 90 degrees and your feet flat on the floor for seated exercises. For nonseated stability ball exercises, choose a size that allows you to perform your exercise in control with minimal motion of the ball. If you are doing an exercise while lying on your abdomen, make sure the ball is sized so that you can touch the floor with your fingers and toes.

You can use your stability ball in many different positions. Sitting, standing, lying on your back with your ankles on the top of the ball, or lying on top of the ball are examples. The larger the ball, the easier it is to stabilize against it. The smaller the ball, the more difficult it is to maintain control.

Precautions: Lying on your back or prone (on your abdomen) on a stability ball puts you at risk for falling off the ball or for straining a muscle.

Steps

Steps are used to simulate a stepping motion and can be real steps, wooden boxes, or step platforms used in aerobics classes. Try to avoid such things as telephone books, as these are unsteady surfaces. Outdoors you can use steps, bleachers, rocks, and logs.

FUNCTIONAL VS. NONFUNCTIONAL EXERCISE

Muscles do three basic things:

1. They decelerate or slow down the body (and its joints) against the pull of gravity.
2. They stabilize the body.
3. They accelerate the body (and its joints) against gravity.

The body has three basic planes of motion: the *sagittal plane* (forward-backward movements), *frontal plane* (sideways movements), and *transverse plane* (rotation movements). All joints and muscles have some component of movement in all three planes. Some joints and muscles are dominant in one plane versus another, but they all move three-dimensionally. This is called *triplanar motion*.

Function is a combination of motions in one or more joints at the same time. Performing an exercise within three planes of motion can make it more functional and true to real life.

From the Weight Room to the World: What Muscles Really Do

The functional demands of your outdoor activity relate to the following factors:

- Movement patterns and the planes of motion of your trunk, arms, and legs
- Postures you must maintain
- Loads you are carrying
- Balance and coordination requirements
- Endurance requirements of muscles used
- Combination of movements of your body regions
- Speed and power of the motion
- Closed-chain vs. open-chain requirements of muscles and joints

Closed-chain vs. open-chain. It is important to view the body as an interlocking chain, each link dependent upon the others. *Closed-chain* activity is when the end segment (e.g., foot or hand) of the chain is fixed to a relatively stable surface (e.g., the ground or a wall). *Open-chain* movement is when the end segment is not fixed to a stable surface. Lower-body muscles usually function with the foot fixed to the ground, a closed-chain movement, while the upper-extremity muscles function primarily with the arm and hand free off the ground or other surfaces, an open-chain movement. The upper extremity is used in closed-chain movements during certain outdoor activities, such as climbing.

If you need to use a muscle group in a closed-chain function during your activity, it is important for some of your strength training exercises to use that muscle in a closed-chain way. For example, a sitting leg extension is not adequate to strengthen your quad region because it is an open-chain exercise. Closed-chain exercises for the quad region include squats, lunges, step-ups, step-downs, jumps, hops, and so on. In preparation for climbing, scrambling, cycling, windsurfing, skiing, and snowshoeing, it is appropriate to do closed-chain upper extremity exercises. These would include dips, pull-ups, push-ups, using Ab Rollers, and so on.

Interrelationships of body regions. A weakness in a link may affect the rest of the chain. Muscle performance in your upper extremity and trunk may depend on the muscle function of your lower extremity, and therefore the two are interrelated. For example, a traditional exercise to strengthen your shoulders might be a barbell overhead press in a sitting or standing position, or sitting in a machine with a controlled fixed load. Traditionally, we are taught to stabilize the trunk of the body and press the load straight overhead using only arms and shoulders. In real life, if you were loading a bicycle onto the top of the car, you would use your whole body, including your ankles, knees, hips, back, and shoulders, to push the load overhead. In function, the shoulder is usually dependent on the opposite leg and hip. If you don't train your hip extensors (gluteals) with overhead shoulder presses, and direct these presses in different planes, you are failing to train a very important part of your body for this functional movement. Some of your exercises should therefore work combinations of body regions.

When looking at an outdoor activity, it is helpful to decide what is the most challenging or difficult movement you will have to do. An exercise can then be done or designed around that challenge.

Functional Self-Tests

You can test yourself on functional strength and balance with some very simple tests. Try balance self-test (BST) Exercises 44, 46, and 48 in chapter 6. How far did you reach with your left foot as compared to your right foot? Was there any pain? Are there directions of motion with your leg or arm reach that feel unstable or less symmetrical? Do you feel wobbly or unsure? How strong do your abdominal muscles feel in their ability to control motion? How strong does your thigh and hip region feel in controlling motion after a set of 12?

Try BST Exercises 54–56. Can you do multiple lunges, flexed enough to simulate your activity needs, with good spine position and without knee wobbling or pain?

Try Exercise 35 without the overhead press (also see Exercise 98). How far can you confidently step up and down without knee pain or wobbling? How well can you control the motion, especially toward the end of the set?

These are good exercises for self-testing, but any of the functional exercises can be used. Most people find that they cannot initially transfer their strength on machines to functional exercises and that they are sore in their buttocks and thighs for the first week after beginning a functional exercise program. Don't get discouraged by your initial performance on these self-tests. You will definitely improve quickly if you practice these exercises.

Functional Exercise Guidelines

- Always begin workouts with a proper aerobic warm-up to increase the core muscle temperature.
- Engage your core to stabilize your low back.
- Do functional exercises before your individual machine exercises.
- Practice each exercise slowly, to get the movement pattern and balance down, before increasing speed.
- Exercise in sets of 4–6 repetitions initially, to get the form and movement pattern, then gradually increase to 12–15 reps in a set.
- Do exercises without resistance or with low resistance (weights, pulleys, or tubing) before you increase resistance.
- Do any standing exercises successfully with two feet on the ground and equal weight distribution before doing them with only one foot on the ground or toe touching.
- In some exercises, challenge your balance by placing more weight on one leg than the other, progressing to a toe touch and then only one foot on the ground. You may have to decrease the resistance you are using when doing an exercise on one leg. You will likely be able to do fewer reps if you are doing an exercise on one leg only.
- Try variations on an exercise, such as those listed in this book's exercise descriptions, to see which exercise challenges you the most and works best for you.
- For some exercises, you can vary the environment to prevent boredom or increase the challenge. After you have done them indoors and have the movements down, try them outdoors on hills. This is especially important within 2–4 weeks of your activity.
- Breathe properly.
- Exercise in strong, pain-free directions before exercising in weak planes.
- Don't do a particular exercise if you feel pain or significant weakness.
- Modify the exercises related to any injuries

you have or based on your knowledge of the body region or your functional needs. You may initially want to try an exercise with much less range of motion to feel comfortable with it.

- Use good footwear with orthotic supports, if necessary.
- Train with a partner to improve the challenge and increase your motivation.
- Consider increasing an exercise's speed to see how many reps you can do within a 30- to 60-second period, especially if speed is important in your activity.

Workout Frequency and Integration of Functional Exercises

How often you train depends on the workout you choose and your goals. You can accomplish most functional strength goals with 2–3 periods of training per week of each muscle group. Two training sessions per muscle group per week are enough to maintain a level of strength, while 3–5 are needed to boost performance. You could decide to do all of your strength exercises on one day or split them up by body regions (lower extremity one day and upper extremity another day). You can do your functional exercises on the same day as you do other exercises, such as machine exercises. You should do them before your machine exercises because most functional exercises use larger muscles and may incorporate challenges to balance. You don't want to be too fatigued before doing them, so you can maintain your form and avoid injury.

Whichever you choose, rest a minimum of 48 hours and not more than 96 hours between workouts of the same muscle groups.

STRENGTH TRAINING GOALS AND PRESCRIPTIONS

Bone Density Maintenance and Improvement

This goal is especially important for peri- and postmenopausal women. It is also important if you are a man over age 60, as men can have bone-density issues as they age. If this is your goal, try loading your arm and leg bones as described in chapter 28. The program described there should be adequate, but you can add to it by using an assisted dip (Exercise 127) and other upper-body exercises that work the biceps and upper back (e.g., rows). Use any of the exercises in this chapter that load your arms and legs (see especially Exercise 28). Use squats and lunges to load your legs, as well as an aerobic activity that loads your legs (e.g., walking, hiking, or using stair climbers, treadmills, EFX machines, etc.)

Managing Aging, Preserving/Increasing Lean Body Mass, and Improving Hormone Function

One of the most significant things that goes on in the human body as we age is a loss of lean body (muscle) mass, a process called *sarcopenia*. If you don't strength train, enough muscle can be lost to contribute to the following problems: (1) A higher risk of injuries. (2) Less ability and lower performance in sports and outdoor activities. (3) Declines in balance and agility. (4) A higher risk of falling and fracturing your hip, arm, or spine. (5) Changes to metabolism as fat increases and muscle decreases. (6) Decrease in your resting metabolic rate, making it easier to gain fat weight and more difficult to lose it.

FIGURE 15. AGE-RELATED CHANGES AND EFFECTS OF STRENGTH TRAINING

	Aging	Strength Training
Body Fat	Increases	Decreases
Bone Density	Decreases	Increases
Muscle Endurance	Decreases	Increases
Muscle Fiber Size	Decreases	Increases
Muscle Mass	Decreases	Increases
Muscle Strength	Decreases	Increases
Resting Metabolic Rate	Decreases	Increases
Growth Hormone	Decreases	Increases
Testosterone	Decreases	Increases

Growth Hormone

Growth hormone is necessary for growing to a normal height during the first 16–19 years of life, after which it is important in the maintenance of muscle mass. It can be measured by a blood test. Among the physiological effects of growth hormone are that it: (1) Increases protein synthesis in muscles. (2) Increases utilization of fatty acids and promotes fat breakdown (important in keeping body fat down). (3) Increases collagen synthesis and stimulates cartilage growth and repair. (4) Enhances immune cell function.

Growth hormone decreases with age, but there is some evidence that resistance training might increase growth hormone release. This appears to be more true in men than in women. Do exercises with large muscle groups in sets of 10 (3 sets minimum), with short rest intervals between sets (30–60 seconds).

Testosterone

Testosterone is usually 10 times higher in men than women, but it is an important hormone for both sexes and it serves as a marker for anabolic status. Testosterone has a number of functions, including: (1) Increasing muscle tissue synthesis. (2) Possibly promoting growth hormone release. (3) Increasing the size of the neuromuscular junction and possibly improving the force production capabilities of a muscle.

If blood levels of free and total testosterone are low, a person (especially a man) may have difficulty making significant strength and hypertrophy gains. If it is significantly low, it can be replaced with gels, injections, and so on.

If your testosterone is in a reasonable range, we don't recommend augmenting it with anabolic steroids. These supplemental hormones can lead to an increased risk of heart attacks, strokes, and liver cancer. Strength training, however, may be able to increase testosterone levels. Methods include: (1) Strength training with large muscle groups (e.g., squats, dead lifts, power cleans). (2) Heavy resistance exercise for large muscle groups with low-rep (3–5) sets. (3) Moderate- to high-volume exercise (6–10 sets) with multiple sets and exercises of the same large muscle groups (e.g., thighs, chest, and upper back). (4) Short rest intervals between sets. Testosterone will also increase with prolonged training (i.e., greater than 2 years of consistent resistance training).

Enhancing Metabolic Function

Obesity, diabetes, and the metabolic syndrome are all health problems associated with how you metabolize insulin (i.e., insulin resistance). The metabolic syndrome actually describes several health problems acting together in varying combinations; these can include hypertension, hyperlipidemia (high total and LDL cholesterol), and glucose intolerance or diabetes. Even if you are not diabetic, insulin resistance is a concern because it puts you at risk for heart and blood-vessel diseases.

To reduce your risk of such conditions or to improve your health if you do suffer symptoms, aerobic exercise is very important because it improves the sensitivity of insulin, thereby decreasing insulin resistance. Strength training is also important in improving insulin sensitivity; exercise sessions 2–3 times per week using large muscles are recommended.

Weight Management

If you increase your body's muscle mass and decrease the fat mass (especially if you have been overweight with adipose tissue), several improvements can result: You can improve your body's metabolism. Your insulin sensitivity can improve. Your resting metabolic rate can increase if there are significant increases in your muscle mass. Note that muscle does weigh more than fat so that if you are losing fat and gaining muscle you cannot measure your progress simply by your weight. You may wish to measure progress with more-specific metabolic measurements, including changes in your body mass index (BMI), your percentage of body fat, and in your resting metabolic rate. (See chapter 29 for more information on BMI.)

Injury Prevention

Strength training can decrease your risk of strains, sprains, and joint injury. It can do this by changing your threshold of tissue failure in regard to particular stresses that you may encounter in your activities. If you find that you are getting injured in the same muscle or body region, it is important to tune up your strength training. It is also important to consider any of the factors discussed in chapter 9 related to injuries and to seek professional advice.

Muscle Hypertrophy

If your goal is to increase the size of various muscles, you will need to do a base of strength training for at least 4–6 weeks with higher-rep sets. You can then incorporate at least 2–3 lower-rep sets of 9–12 reps, making sure you are working to fatigue. Use a spotter to help you lift to fatigue. Vary the exercises you use to strength-train a particular muscle or region. Use shorter rest intervals. Consider having a snack with protein within an hour of your strength training workout. It is important to get adequate sleep (at least 8 hours), because sleep is essential for tissue repair and growth hormone release.

Toning and Shaping

For toning and shaping, both aerobic exercise and strength training are essential to promote fat burning and fat loss. (See chapters 3 and 29 for details on fat loss and aerobic exercise). You cannot dictate where you will lose fat by which muscles you strength-train, but you can help to shape and tone those "problem" areas. Try starting your workouts with 1 higher-rep set of 15 and then do 2 sets of lower reps (9–12). Do a balanced program of biceps (Exercise 125), triceps (Exercises 126, 127), upper back (Exercises 118, 120), chest (Exercise 114), abdominals (Exercises 79 or 92, and 80, 83), buttocks (Exercises 97, 98), and thighs (Exercise 102).

Sport and Activity-Specific Training

For strength training for outdoor activities, refer to Part III. For strength training for sports that are not listed in this book, you can create a dynamic and specific program using the exercises in chapters 5, 8, 10, 11, 14, and 15 that can improve your performance and decrease your risk of injury.

USING A STRENGTH TRAINING LOG

Make a master copy of the chart below (Figure 16), and use it to record your short- and long-term goals and to track your progress toward your activity goals. In the spaces provided in the right column, list your exercises and record the date, reps, sets, and resistance for each workout during the week. Try rearranging your workout every 3–4 weeks for best results. You can do this by changing the order of the exercises within each body region or by changing the order of body regions every workout session.

FIGURE 16. STRENGTH TRAINING LOG

Name: ______________________ **Periodization Phase:** ______________ **Week:** ________

Long-term goal: ____

Short-term goals: 1) ____

2) ____

3) ____

		exercise dates __/__/__	__/__/__	__/__/__	__/__/__	__/__/__	__/__/__
Body Part or Exercise Type	**Sets/Reps**	**Day 1**	**Day 2**	**Day 3**	**Day 4**	**Day 5**	**Day 6**
Warm-Up/Stretch							
1. ________	___/___	____	____	____	____	____	____
2. ________	___/___	____	____	____	____	____	____
3. ________	___/___	____	____	____	____	____	____
Upper Body							
1. ________	___/___	____	____	____	____	____	____
2. ________	___/___	____	____	____	____	____	____
3. ________	___/___	____	____	____	____	____	____
4. ________	___/___	____	____	____	____	____	____
5. ________	___/___	____	____	____	____	____	____
Lower Body							
1. ________	___/___	____	____	____	____	____	____
2. ________	___/___	____	____	____	____	____	____
3. ________	___/___	____	____	____	____	____	____
4. ________	___/___	____	____	____	____	____	____
5. ________	___/___	____	____	____	____	____	____
Abdominals							
1. ________	___/___	____	____	____	____	____	____
2. ________	___/___	____	____	____	____	____	____
3. ________	___/___	____	____	____	____	____	____
4. ________	___/___	____	____	____	____	____	____
Functional Strengthening							
1. ________	___/___	____	____	____	____	____	____
2. ________	___/___	____	____	____	____	____	____
3. ________	___/___	____	____	____	____	____	____
4. ________	___/___	____	____	____	____	____	____
5. ________	___/___	____	____	____	____	____	____
Balance/Agility							
1. ________	___/___	____	____	____	____	____	____
2. ________	___/___	____	____	____	____	____	____
3. ________	___/___	____	____	____	____	____	____
Plyometrics							
1. ________	___/___	____	____	____	____	____	____
2. ________	___/___	____	____	____	____	____	____
3. ________	___/___	____	____	____	____	____	____

Record your reps per set, resistance, and/or rest period in the day column for each exercise.

STRENGTH TRAINING AND FUNCTIONAL EXERCISES

In addition to the functional exercises in this chapter, you'll find body region–specific function exercises in Part II. In this chapter we have included those exercises that are more functional and that integrate body regions. If you are just beginning strength training it is best to do exercises from the body-region chapters for at least a month before trying these exercises. Remember to read chapter 14 and to practice Exercise 108 to activate your core muscles while doing functional exercises. If you are a physical therapist or an athletic or fitness trainer, this chapter's functional exercises can be integrated into a performance or rehab program.

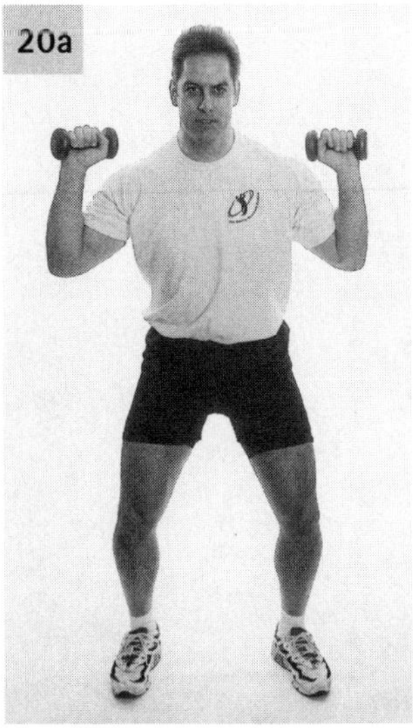

20a

FUNCTIONAL CORE EXERCISES

These are exercises that will improve core strength and stability while strengthening your arms and legs.

20 X-COMBO

Equipment: 2- to 5-pound free weights.

Purpose: Strengthen your leg, trunk, shoulder, and arm muscles in the same fashion you use them in activities that involve reaching overhead.

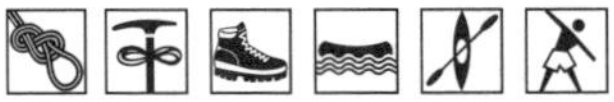

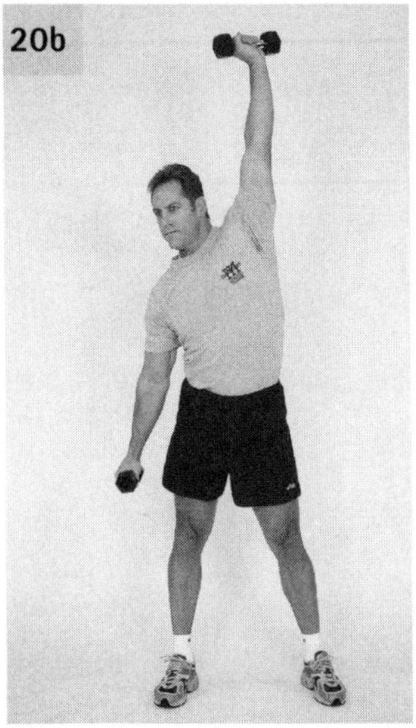

20b

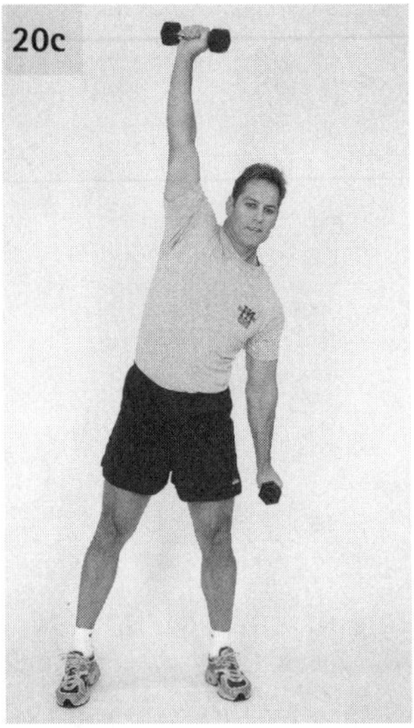

20c

Technique: Start in a standing position with your knees bent slightly and your feet shoulder-width apart, with your elbows flexed to about 90 degrees and your hands at about the height of your ears or top of your shoulders (20a). Start with a light free weight in each hand, and reach for the ceiling with your left hand while pushing off from your left leg and left buttock (20b). Elevate your left shoulder, extend your left elbow, and shift your weight over your right leg. With your right arm and hand, reach for the floor and side-bend your trunk to the right. Repeat this movement on the opposite side, bending your knees in transition

(20c). Do one set of 12–15 repetitions and progress to 2–3 sets.
Variation: 20.1. Balance on one leg with your knee slightly bent. Reach one arm toward the ceiling and the opposite arm toward the floor (20.1a) and alternate (20.1b). You can do this with unequal weights to challenge your balance. After 30 seconds, switch legs and repeat for 30 seconds. This works your hips and challenges your balance.
Precautions: Inappropriate weight of free weights causes abnormal compensation patterns in the spine and shoulders. Start light and determine what your muscle endurance is for this movement.

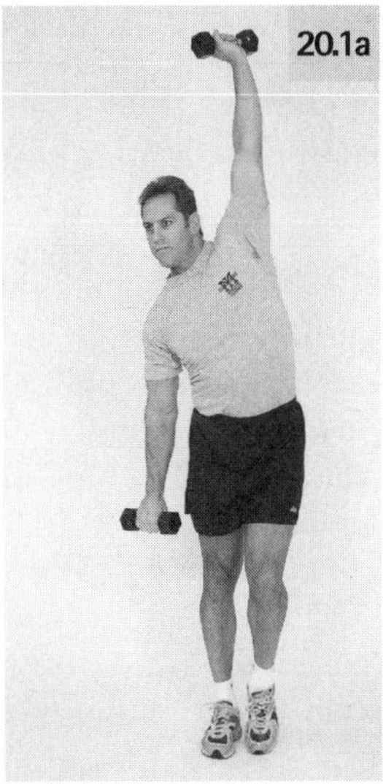

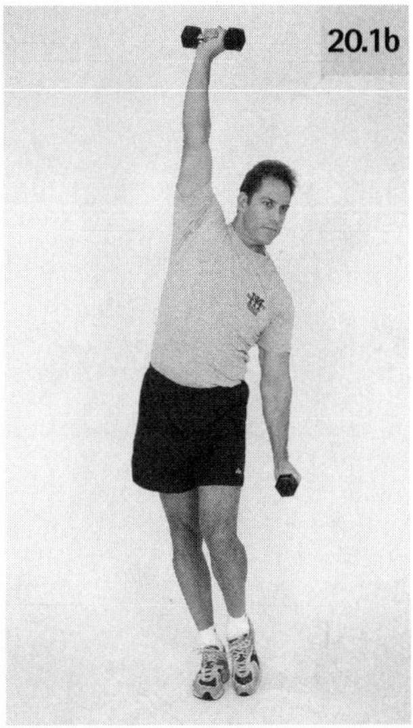

21 CORE CABLE FLYS

Equipment: FreeMotion, Cable Cross, or other similar pulley system.
Purpose: Strengthen your chest, shoulders, and abdominals and improve your balance.

Technique: Adjust the arms of the pulleys at shoulder height. If you can adjust the range setting, bring it out one setting. Face away from the body of the machine and grasp a handle with each hand. Get into a straddle position with your right foot forward, knee slightly bent, and your left foot simply toe-touching to help maintain balance. Activate your core. Keeping your elbows slightly bent and below shoulder level, bring the handles together in front of your body. You can think of the ending position like hugging a big barrel. Return to the starting position slowly and in control, not allowing your hands to pass behind your shoulders. Alternate your sets with your other leg forward. Note that you will have to use your abdominals to prevent your body from moving off balance in a posterior direction. In other words, you will have to use your abs to control against quick extension motions of your back. Do 2–3 sets of 12–15 reps. (See Exercise 25 for another variation.)
Variation: 21.1. Seated Physioball cable flys: Chose a Physioball that will allow you to sit with your hips at 90 degrees with your feet flat on the floor. Position the pulleys so that they are at shoulder height when you are seated. Hinge at your hips in flexion and assume a slight forward lean position to help you maintain your balance. This

exercise will work sitting balance and core stability while sitting. This will challenge your abdominals even more than the basic exercise.
Precaution: Don't perform this exercise if you have an active problem in your low back, knee, or shoulder.

22 DYNAMIC CORE: CHEST-ABDOMINAL EXERCISE

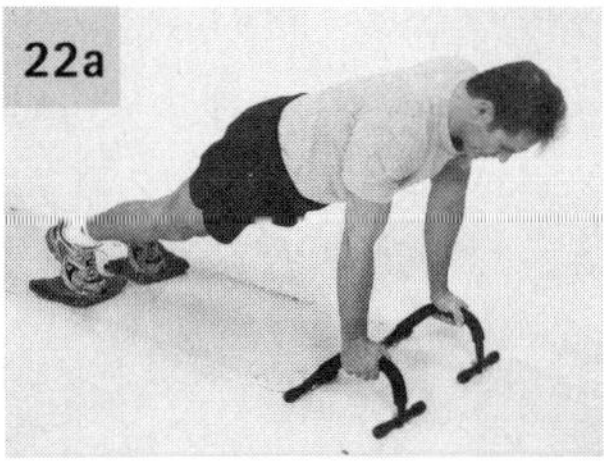
22a

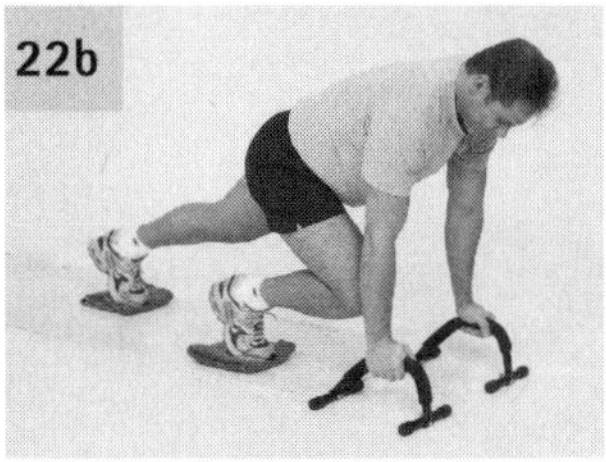
22b

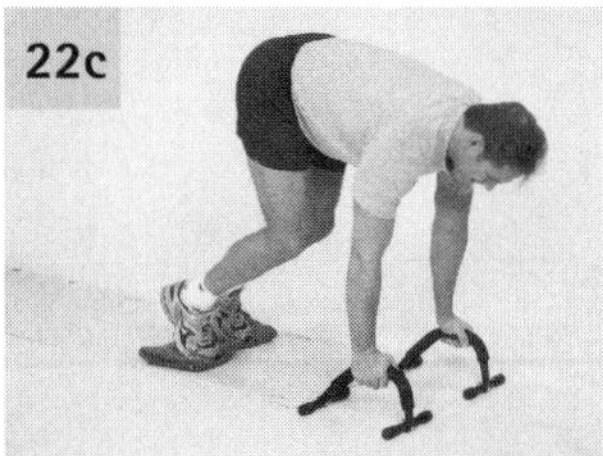
22c

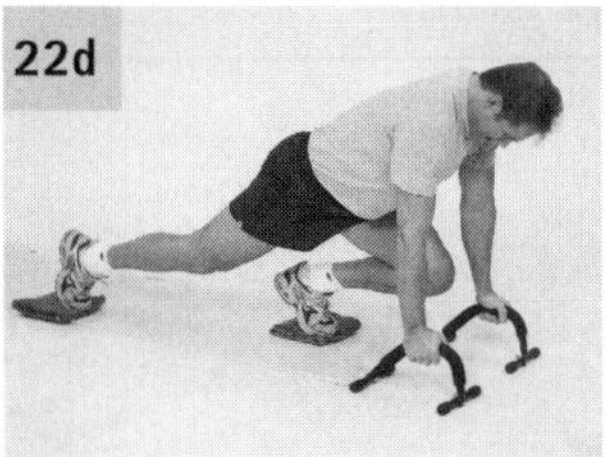
22d

Equipment: A slide board or a slick floor, booties or socks, 2 hand towels and push-up handles.
Purpose: Strengthen and condition your chest, shoulders, arms, abdominals, and hip flexors for core strength, stability, and improved flexibility.

Technique: Place your push-up handles at the end of the slide board or anywhere on an open slick floor. Put your booties or socks on your bare feet or over your shoes, and place your feet on top of the hand towels. Assume a push-up position, grasping the handles in a straight body position. You should be supporting yourself on the balls of your feet with your arms fully extended and grasping the handles (22a). Slide your foot along the floor or slide board to bring one knee close to your chest with the other leg fully extended (22b). Keeping your arms straight, switch leg positions by raising your hips high toward the ceiling (22c), bringing your feet parallel, and sliding your other leg behind you while bending the front knee (22d). Repeat this in a controlled, quick fashion, raising and lowering your hips every time you change your foot position. Perform 3–4 sets of 15–20 reps for each leg.
Precautions: Keep your low back and neck in a neutral position at all times during this exercise. Don't do this exercise if you have an active problem in your shoulder or low back (especially your sacroiliac joint).

FREEMOTION INTEGRATED CORE STABILITY PROGRAM

FreeMotion cable machines feature two independent arms that move 180 degrees vertically (rotation angle). Some of the FreeMotion machines can also move 45 degrees horizontally (reach angle). These weight machines challenge and strengthen muscles in real-life patterns with unlimited variations. Each single cable can travel more than 12 feet, which is applicable for sport-specific movements such as lunging, stepping, and swinging. Standing and seated exercises allow for increased awareness of your core in relation to your legs, arms, feet, hands, and head.

23 STANDING AND SEATED TORSO ROTATIONS

Equipment: FreeMotion machine or a pulley system that is vertically adjustable.
Purpose: Functionally strengthen your core, integrating your arms and legs for improved performance during sports and recreational activities. This exercise will also aid in increasing thoracic spine rotation.

Technique: Adjust the rotation settings of the movable arms so the pulley is at chest height and adjust the reach settings to about 45 degrees away from the body of the machine. Grasp a handle with both hands, keep your elbows close to your sides (bent at 90 degrees), and center your hands in the midline of your body. Center yourself between both pulleys so that you are facing away from the body of the machine. Stand with your knees slightly bent and your feet shoulder-width apart (23a). Keeping your hips and head still, rotate inward (toward the pulley arm not in use) as far as possible without allowing your head or hips to move (23b), then rotate outward (toward the pulley arm you are using), controlling the resistance through a full range of motion (23c). Perform 2–3 sets of 12–15 reps on both sides.
Variations: 23.1. Seated torso rotation: This same exercise can be done while seated on a Physioball. Choose a ball size that allows your hips and knees to be at about 90 degrees with your feet flat on the floor. Adjust the pulleys to the height of your chest in the seated position. Place the stability ball in the center of the two pulleys. Grasp the handle with both hands (in the above-mentioned arm position), sit on the ball facing away from the body of the machine, and place both feet flat on the floor (23.1a). Do this seated variation in the same manner as the standing, keeping your elbows by your sides and rotating your torso and shoulders inward (23.1b). Perform 2–3 sets of 12–15 reps on both sides. **23.2.** Seated diagonal pattern rotation: Sit on the stability ball with your hips and knees at

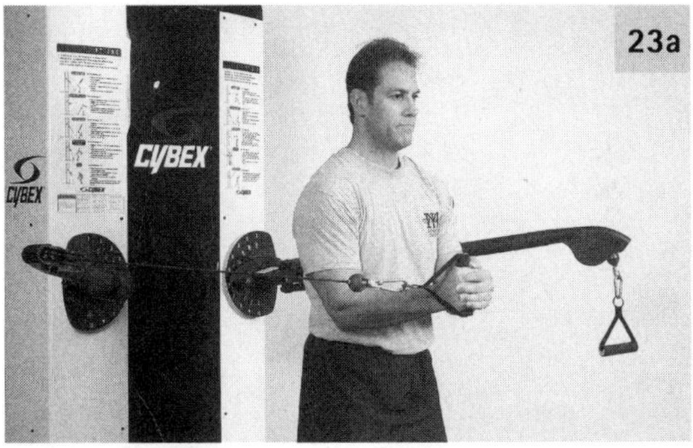

23a

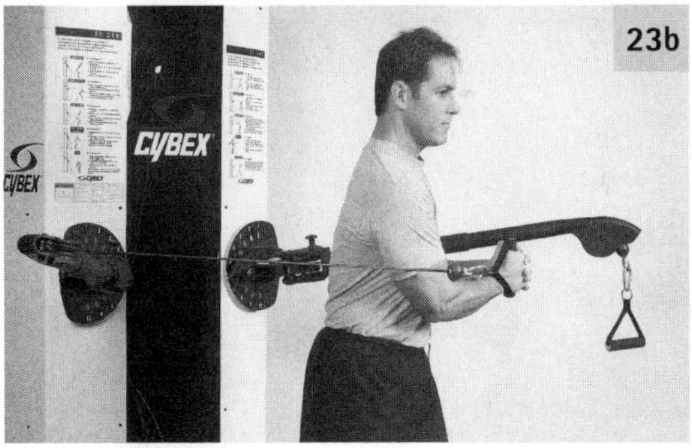

23b

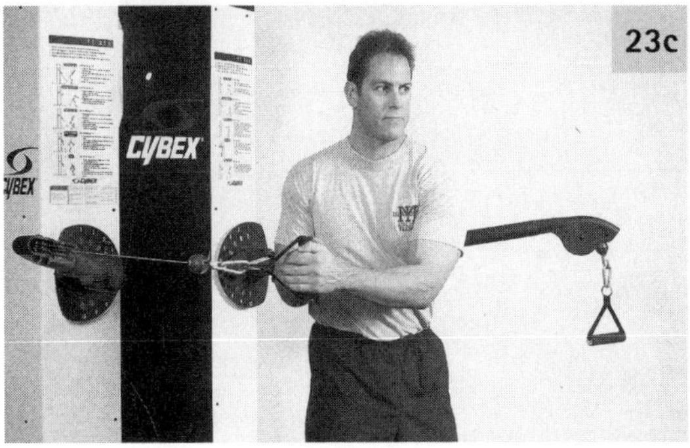

23c

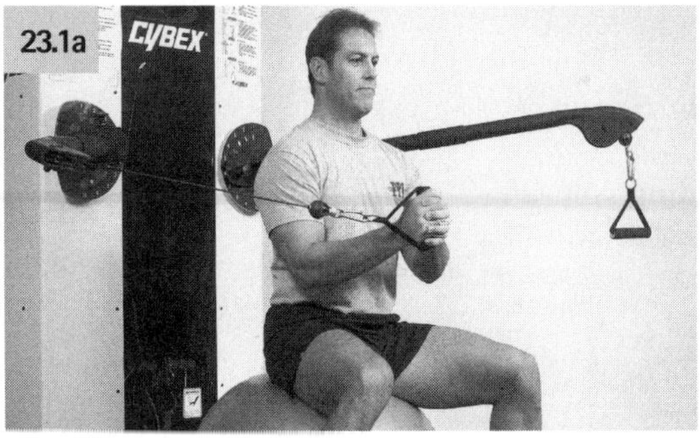

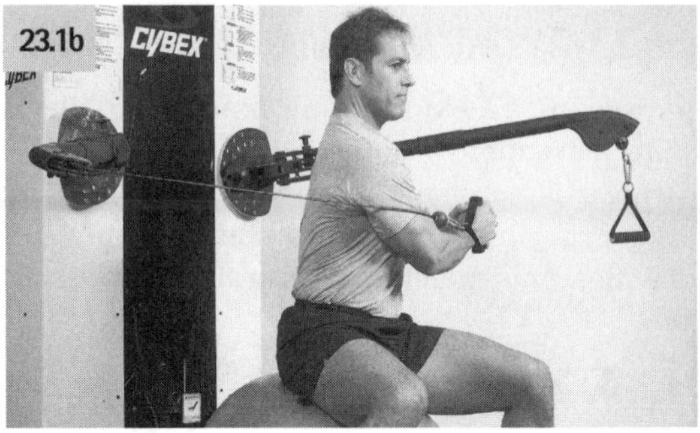

about 90 degrees with your feet flat on the floor. Starting on your right side, position the FreeMotion arm or a vertical pulley so that the pulley is behind you, overhead and to the right side. Pull the handle to your right shoulder with both hands. Then, move the handle toward your opposite hip while moving your spine into rotation and flexion toward that opposite hip (a diagonal pattern) at the same time. Use your spine and abdominal muscles to slowly return your trunk to an upright position and the pulley to your right shoulder. Perform 2–3 sets of 12–15 reps on both sides.

Tip: Maintain a neutral low-back position and a wide foot stance.

24 STANDING PUSH-PULL CORE ROTATIONS

Equipment: FreeMotion machine or a pulley system that is vertically adjustable.

Purpose: Challenge your standing and seated balance while strengthening your core, shoulders, and arms for pushing and pulling activities. This is similar to Exercise 39 but is easier to set up and offers constant resistance rather than the variable resistance of a sport cord.

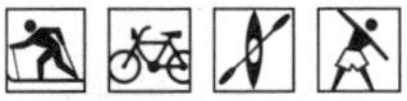

Technique: Position the rotational setting of the arms so the pulley arms are at chest height with the reach position at about 45 degrees.

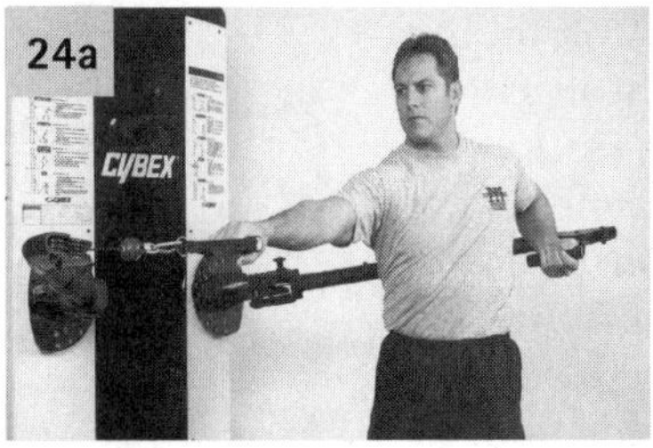

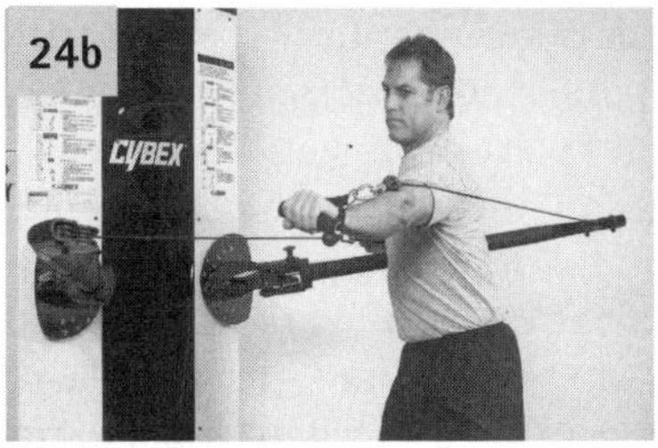

Stand in the center of the machine (at a 90-degree angle to it), holding one of the handles with one elbow bent at 90 degrees and the other handle with your opposite arm straight and extended in front of you (24a). Engage your core muscles and initiate the exercise with a row motion, pulling the extended arm to your rib cage and pressing forward with your other arm (24b). Repeat this on the opposite side and perform 2–3 sets of 12–15 reps per side.

Variation: 24.1. Seated push-pull core rotations: Center the stability ball in front of the machine, grasp the handles as described above, and position yourself at a 90-degree angle to the machine (24.1a). Move your arms against the resistance in the same manner described in the standing version (24.1b). Perform 2–3 sets of 12–15 reps on each side.

Tip: Keep your feet on the floor and maintain stability of your core while pushing and pulling against the resistance.

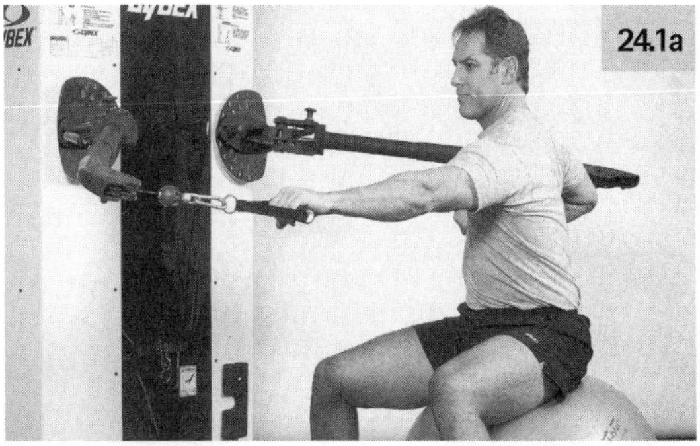

24.1a

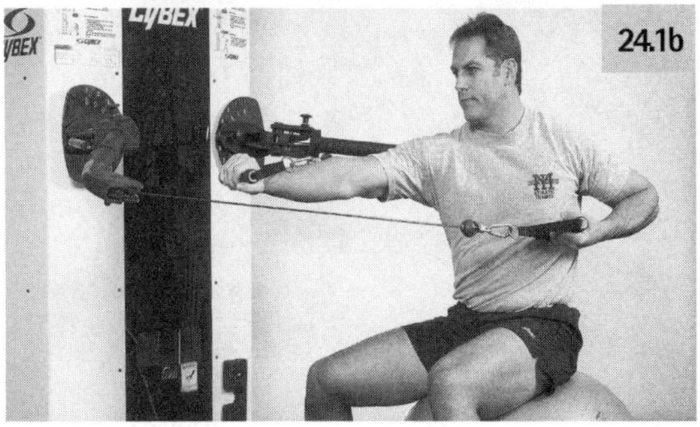

24.1b

25 STAGGERED STANCE OVERHEAD DIAGONAL ARM CROSSES

Equipment: FreeMotion machine or a pulley system that is vertically adjustable.

Purpose: General core stabilization with chest and shoulder strengthening. Strengthens your core against arm motion and loads, common to climbing athletes. Also good for upper-back strengthening and upper thoracic mobility.

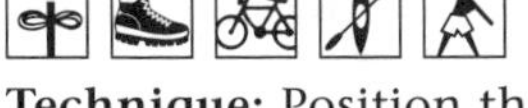

Technique: Position the rotational setting of the arms to an angle just outside vertical (the arms should form a sharp V). Set the reach position at its highest point (this should be the first reach setting). Face away from the machine, reach overhead, and grasp the handles. Step slightly forward until you feel resistance with your arms diagonally overhead. Position yourself in a staggered stance with most of your weight on your forward foot (25a). Maintaining a slightly bent elbow, bring your hands to the opposite hips, crossing the cables in front of you (25b). Return to the start position in a controlled, smooth manner, being careful not to reach back too far. Try to prevent your arms from going behind your ears. Perform 2–3

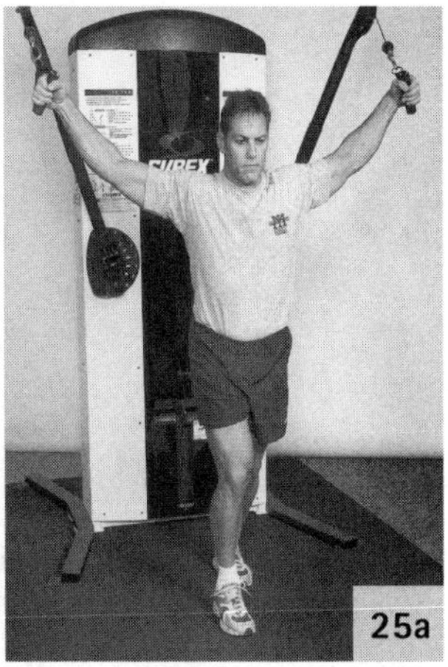

25a

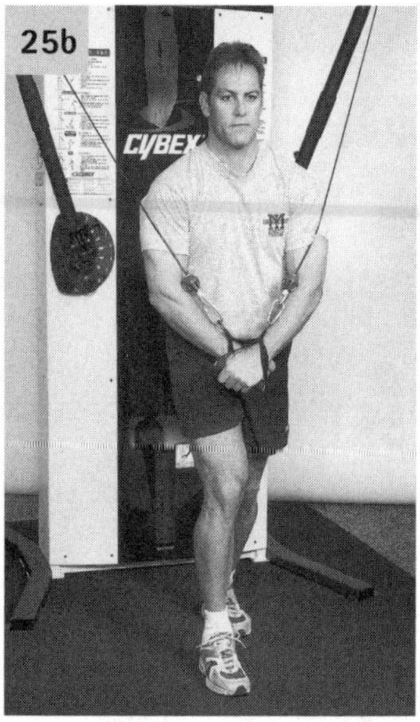

25b

sets of 12–15 reps. (See Exercise 21 for another variation.)

Precautions: Avoid this exercise if you have an active problem in your neck or shoulder, including rotator cuff problems.

26 SQUAT WITH ALTERNATE FORWARD-OVERHEAD PRESSES

Equipment: FreeMotion machine or a pulley system that is vertically adjustable.

Purpose: Strengthen your core, arms, and legs for climbing, lifting, reaching, and carrying activities.

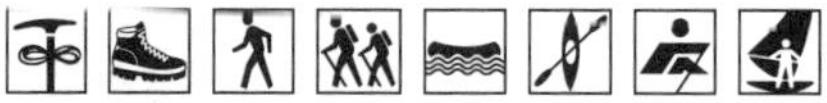

Technique: Position the rotational setting of the arms so that the pulleys are down by the floor, with the arms not quite vertical. Face away from the body of the machine, in the center. Reach down and grasp the handles, with your feet about shoulder-width apart. Stand up and bring the handles to shoulder height (26a). Squat to a level that you can control (26b) and stand back up, reaching one handle to a slightly forward and overhead position with your arm fully extended (26c). Squat again while bringing the overhead handle back down to your shoulder, then stand back up reaching the other handle to the slightly forward and overhead position with your arm fully extended. Repeat this squat-to-reach combination, alternately

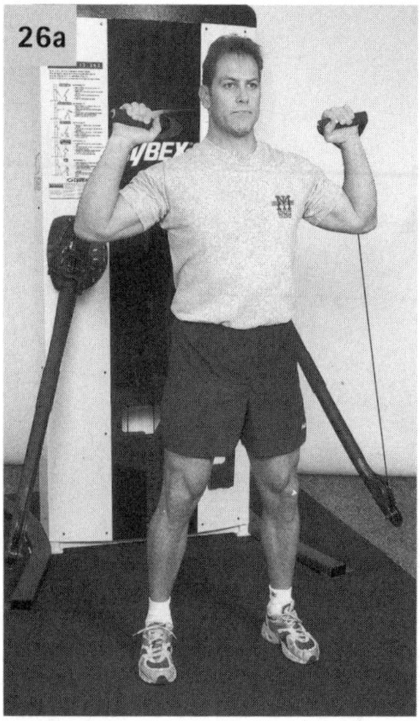
26a

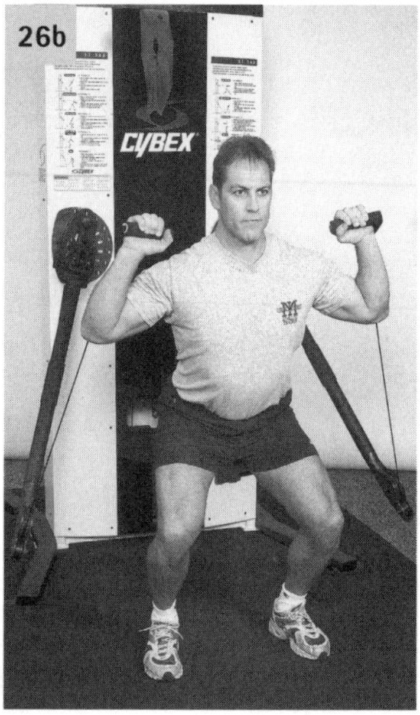

26b

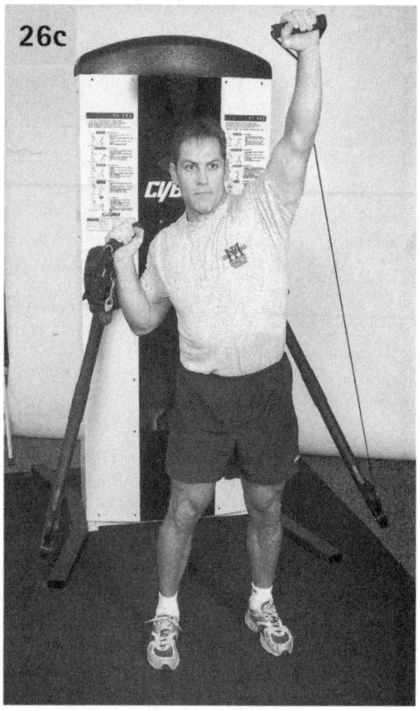
26c

from side to side, for 2–3 sets of 10–12 reps on each side.
Precaution: Don't do this exercise if you have an active problem in your shoulder or cervical spine.

27 SINGLE-LEG BALANCE ALTERNATE BICEPS CURL

Equipment: FreeMotion machine or a pulley system that is vertically adjustable.
Purpose: Strengthen your biceps while challenging your core and balance.

Technique: Position the rotational settings of the pulley arms as in Exercise 26. Reach down and grasp the handles with your feet about shoulder-width apart and return to the standing position with your arms extended, palms facing to the rear, and balance on one foot. Alternately, curl one handle toward your chin while maintaining balance on one foot (27a). Keep the curling motion continuous. As you raise one handle toward your chin, lower the other down to your side and face your down hand toward the rear (27b). Perform 2–3 sets of 15 reps on each leg.
Tips and Precautions: To challenge your balance further, speed up the alternate curl motion for a time interval of 30 seconds on each leg. If your goals are to develop bicep and core strength, add resistance and move at a slower tempo. Don't do this exercise if you have an active shoulder problem.

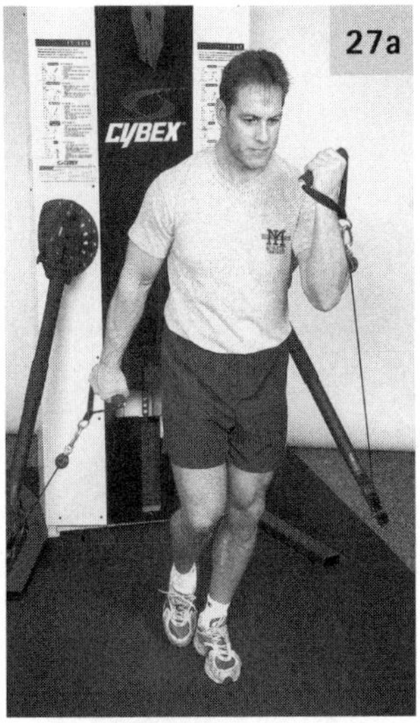

27a

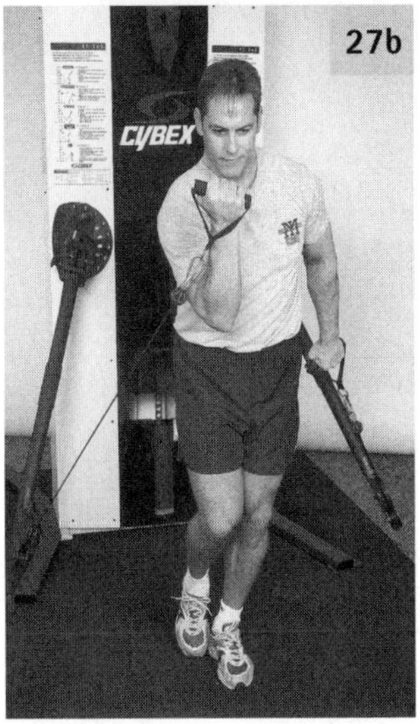

27b

LUNGES WITH ARM AND SHOULDER CHALLENGES

These lunges combine arm and shoulder motions. They exercise the thighs, buttocks, arms, shoulders, and core. You can do any lunge in place or move around on a surface in a walking lunge. You can also do lunges on hills to increase the challenge. See Exercise 97 in chapter 11 for the basic lunge technique with several other variations.

28 FORWARD LUNGE WITH A BICEPS CURL

Equipment: Free weights.

Purpose: Strengthen leg, trunk, and arm muscles that are involved in controlling lunging movements in the forward direction. Add challenges to your balance and strengthen your spine. Save time by combining biceps curls with lunges.

Technique: Grasp a pair of hand weights and position them at your sides (photo 28). Lunge in a forward direction with one leg, while flexing the opposite elbow and curling the weight to the shoulder. Return to standing. Repeat the movement with the opposite leg and arm. Perform 2–3 sets of 12–15 reps.

Variations: 28.1. Curl the elbow on the same side as the lunging leg. **28.2.** Vary the amount of flexing of the lunge knee. **28.3.** Start with both elbows flexed (28.3a) and lower them simultaneously as you lunge on one leg (28.3b), especially if you want to save time or to strengthen your back. Your forearm and hand position can vary at the bottom of the lunge. Initially try lunging with your fist and palms facing forward. Progress to ending with your palms facing inward (toward the midline of your body) and, eventually, ending with your palms facing to the rear. Changing the position and direction of your hands during the lunge will incorporate an important function of the biceps (supination). **28.4.** Starting with both hands at your sides, do a simultaneous curl with both hands while you lunge (28.4), for less stress on your back as well as to save time.

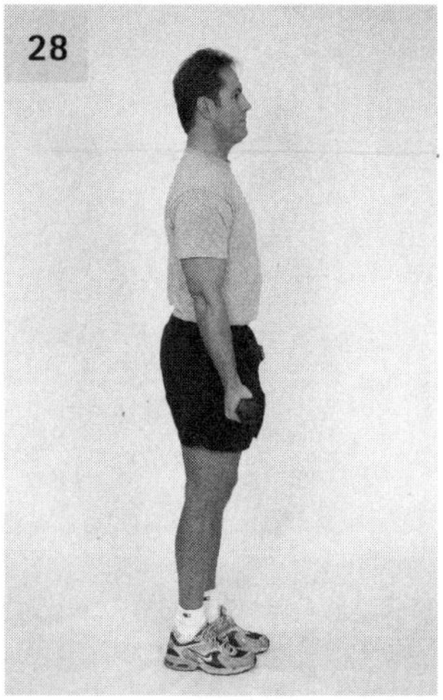

28

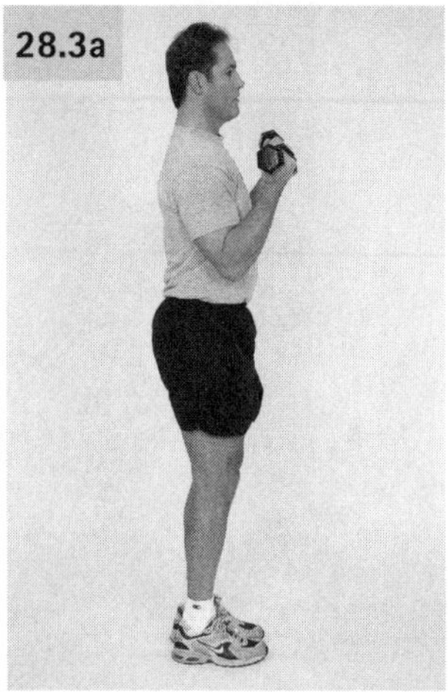

28.3a

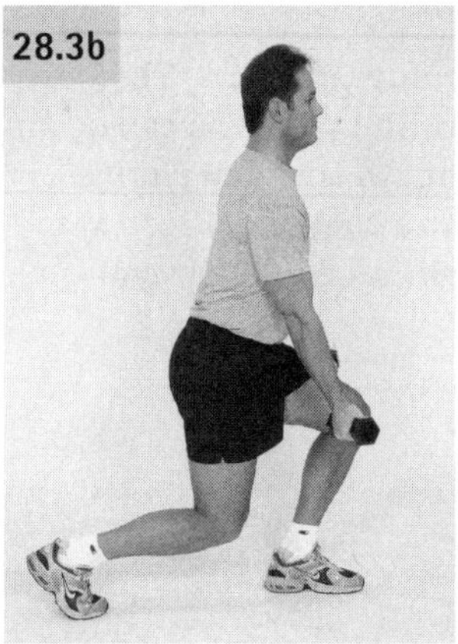

28.3b

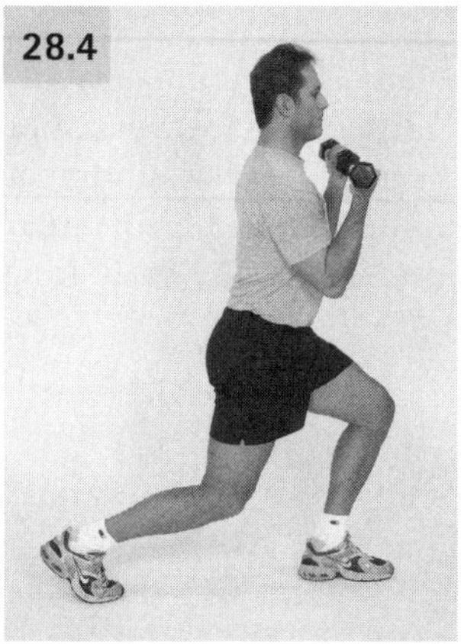

28.4

29 ANTERIOR LUNGE WITH OPPOSITE KNEE REACH

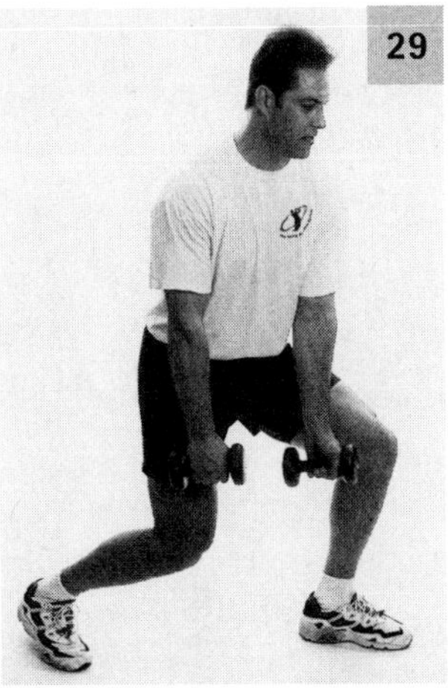

Equipment: Free weights.
Purpose: Strengthen leg, trunk, shoulder, and arm muscles involved with lunging leg movements, with a weight/gravity challenge toward the midline of the body. This is good for skiers, especially telemark and cross-country.

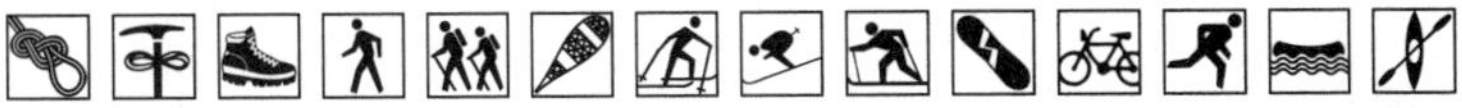

Technique: Stand with weights in each hand and your hands at waist height, with the weights pointing up in the air. Your knees should be just slightly bent and within 2–4 inches of each other. Lunge forward with the left leg while bringing the weights above your right knee. Your spine will rotate to the right slightly. Try to keep your left knee pointing forward, and use the muscles of your leg and hip to keep it from rotating inward. Go back to the starting position and repeat the lunge with the same knee, or do the lunge with the opposite knee. Increase the weight of the hand weights to increase the challenge of the exercise. Perform 2–3 sets of 12–15 reps.
Variation: 29.1. If you are a telemark skier, try holding the position long enough to simulate a turn.
Precaution: Do this slowly at first to develop control and decrease the stress on your knees.

30 LUNGE MATRIX/COMBOS

Equipment: 3- to 15-pound free weights.
Purpose: Increase your entire body's strength, coordination, and endurance in multiple directions. Integrate every body region by incorporating lunging, reaching, bending, twisting, and lifting overhead in combination.

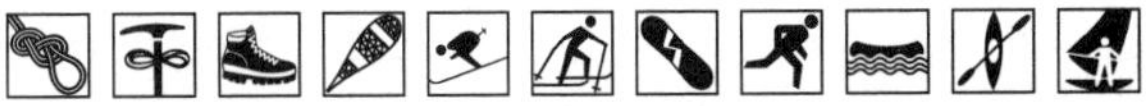

Technique: Stand inside a giant imaginary clock, with 12:00 located directly in front of you, 6:00 directly behind you, and 3:00 and 9:00 to your right and left, respectively. These are the directions for each sequence of the lunge matrix. After each lunge, return to the start position with your feet close together, standing in the center of the imaginary clock and facing the 12:00 position. Each time you perform a lunge, reach the hand weights toward the lunge foot. This will require you to bend your hips, knees, and mid back as you reach for the lunge foot.

Start the **first sequence** with your hand weights at hip height (30a). Lunge with your left foot toward 12:00 while reaching the

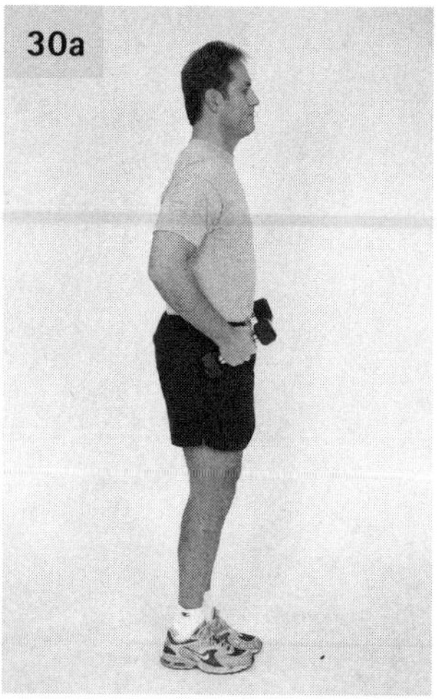

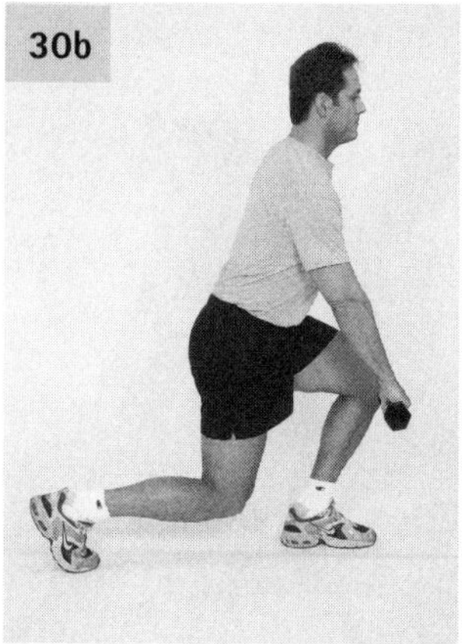

hand weights toward your left foot (30b). If this is too difficult, reach the weights to knee height. Once you have lunged and reached to a safe level, return to the start position (the center of the giant clock), with your hand weights returned to hip height. Repeat this lunge maneuver in the same direction with your right leg, again reaching your hand weights toward your right foot or knee, and returning to the start position in the center of the clock. Once you have completed 3 lunges and reaches, alternately on each leg, you are ready to change directions.

The **second sequence** is performed with a side-to-side motion. Stand in the center of the clock with your hand weights at hip height, and lunge toward 9:00 with your left leg while reaching the hand weights toward your left foot (30c). Once you have lunged and reached to a safe level, return to the start position in the center of the clock. Repeat the same lunge maneuver with your right leg lunging toward 3:00 while reaching your hand weights toward your right foot. Perform 3 lunges to each direction, alternately. With each lunge, return to the upright position in the center of the clock.

For the **third sequence,** position yourself in the center of the giant clock and locate 5:00 (to your right and slightly behind you) and 7:00 (to your left and slightly behind you). Start by lunging toward 7:00 with your left foot while pointing the toes of your left foot at the 7:00 position (30d). Remember to pivot on your right foot so that you don't hurt your knee. Again, during your lunge, reach your hand weights toward your left foot, bending your knees, hips, and back. Once you have lunged and reached to a safe range, return to the start position in the center of the clock and face the 12:00 position. Repeat this lunge-and-reach maneuver toward 5:00 with your right foot while pointing your right toes toward the 5:00 position. Perform 3 alternate lunges and reaches in each direction.

One set consists of performing all three sequences (with 3 lunges and reaches for each leg in each direction). Start with 1 set and work up to 2–3 sets over 2–3 weeks.

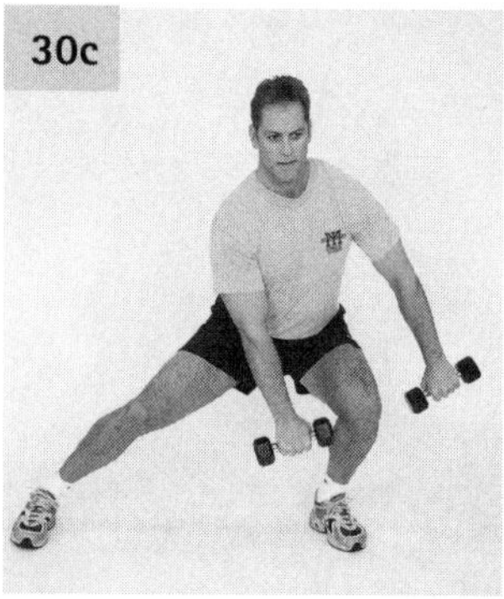

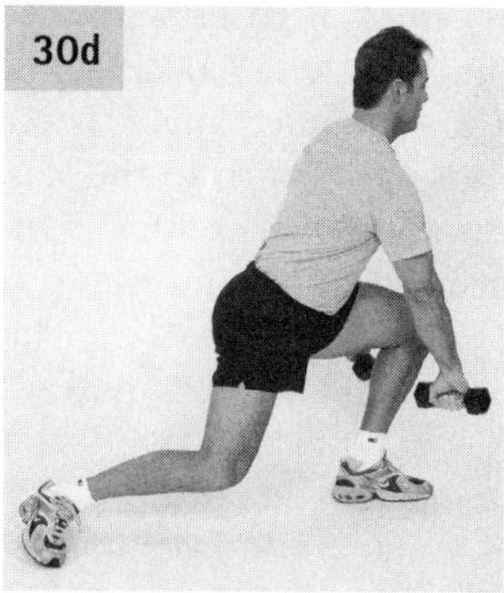

Variations: Progress to each variation in the order given here. Each variation is more difficult than the previous one. **30.1.** Start with your hand weights at ear height (30.1). Lunge and reach as described above. Make sure that when you return to the start position in the center of the clock the hand weights return to shoulder height. This variation incorporates your arm and shoulder flexors and adds additional loads to your legs and back. **30.2.** Start as before, facing the 12:00 position. Extend your arms and hold the hand weights overhead (30.2). Perform the same sequence of lunge and reach. When reaching toward the lunge foot, allow the hand weights to pass close to your chest on the way toward the floor and upon your return to the start position. **30.3.** Try an assortment of arm movements during your lunge and reach. For instance, when reaching toward the lunge foot with your hand weights, turn the hand weights so that your knuckles are facing each other at the bottom of the lunge. Then return to the start position, turning the hand weights so that your palms are facing each other. During the second-sequence side-to-side lunge and reach, raise the hand weights out to your sides so that they are at shoulder height when you are in the center of the clock, then reach the hand weights toward the lunge foot as usual.

Tips and Precautions: The start position for this exercise is always in the center of the clock, facing the 12:00 position. Make sure to use your knees during the lunge. Don't overtax your back by bending too far at your waist. If you have a history of low-back, knee, or shoulder problems, move in a pain-free range of motion in the direction you are lunging and reaching. Stick with the main exercise rather than the variations if you have any unresolved injuries. Don't lunge to low positions if your kneecap area is hurting. Use lighter weights, especially when first trying this and for variations 30.1 and 30.2.

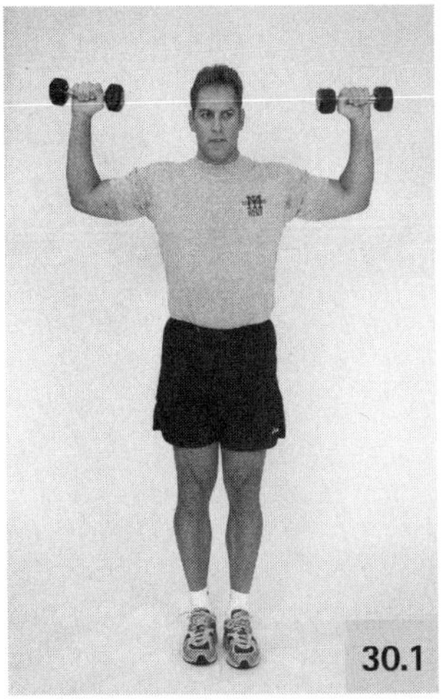
30.1

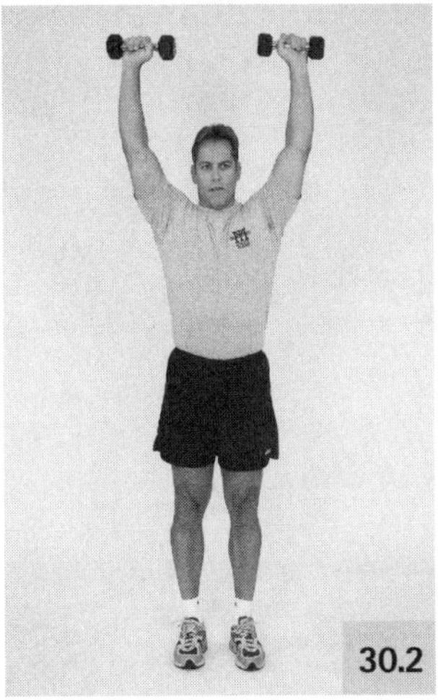
30.2

ROW/LATISSIMUS EXERCISES

These exercises strengthen the shoulder region in pulling, rowing, and rotational patterns. When doing these with tubing, make sure the tubing is securely attached. Start with lower resistance when using pulleys or smaller-diameter tubing.

31 LAWNMOWER PULLS TO A ROW OR AN EXTERNAL ROTATION

Equipment: Free weights or vertically adjustable pulley.

Purpose: The free-weight variations improve dynamic buttock strength and coordination of combined shoulder and hip movements, exercising all the muscles of the legs, trunk, upper extremity, and neck that help you pull or lift an object off the ground. The adjustable pulley variation strengthens and challenges your balance on one leg and improves your buttock, hamstring, and low-back strength while improving your upper back strength in a diagonal pattern.

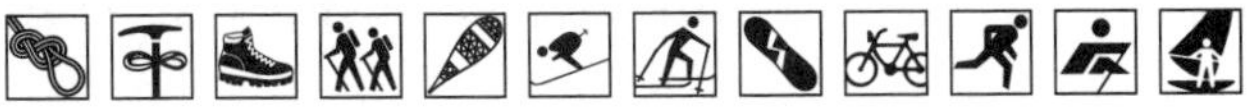

EXERCISE 31

31a

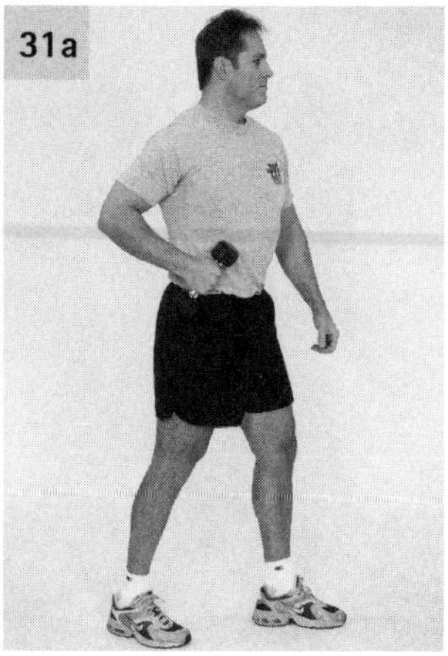

31b

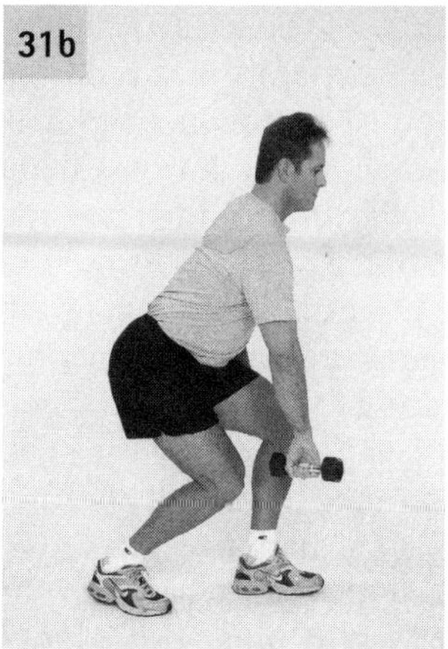

Basic Technique: Stand upright in a forward stride position with your left foot forward and body weight equally distributed over both feet. Hold a free weight in your right hand at about hip height with your elbow bent (31a). Activate your core and abdominal muscles to stabilize and protect your back. Keeping your upper body fairly erect and bending at both your knees, hips, and ankles, lower the weight toward your left heel to about knee height while turning your right palm outward so that your thumb faces to the rear at the bottom of the motion (31b). Return to the starting position by standing up and returning the hand weight to your hip with your palm facing inward. Perform 2–3 sets of 12–15 reps on each side.

Intermediate Variation: 31.1. Assisted single-leg stance lawnmower row: Stand in a forward stride position with your left knee forward and slightly bent and your right knee back and almost extended (31.1a). Most of your body weight should be on the forward leg, with your toes of the back foot providing assistance in balancing. Start with a slight forward lean to your torso (flexing at your hips). Hold a free weight in your right hand at about waist height. Lower the weight toward the left foot, to about midway between your left foot and left knee, while flexing your left knee, hips, and back slightly (31.1b). Pull the weight back to your waist while extending your front knee and return to the starting position. Your trunk rotates slightly as you pinch the shoulder blade of your pulling arm back and extend your shoulder. The movement resembles that of someone starting a lawnmower. Perform 2–3 sets of 12–15 reps on each side.

31.1a

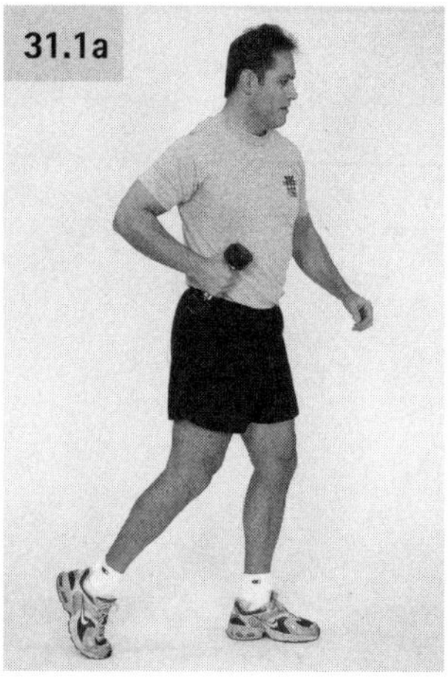

31.1b

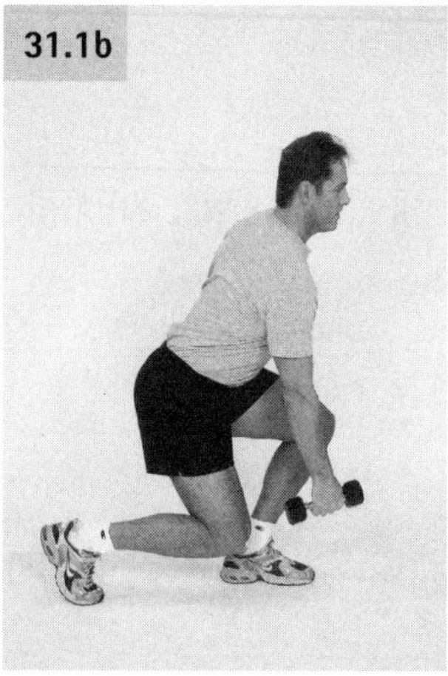

Advanced Variation: 31.2. Single-leg balance lawnmower rows: This most difficult variation increases buttock and hamstring strength while working your balance. Start by picking up a dumbbell off the rack with your right hand. Balance on your left foot. Position the weight so that your arm is horizontal to the ground, your elbow flexed to 90 degrees, and your hand gripping the weight, pointing straight up in the air (31.2a). If your shoulder will not easily move into a position with the weight pointing directly vertical, rotate it only as far as it will comfortably go. Bring your right elbow toward your right hip and then reach the weight toward the inside of your left foot (31.2b). Do this carefully, while hinging in your hip and flexing in your back. Then bring the weight in a controlled manner to the starting position using your thigh and buttock muscles rather than your back muscles. Perform 2–3 sets of 12–15 reps on each side.

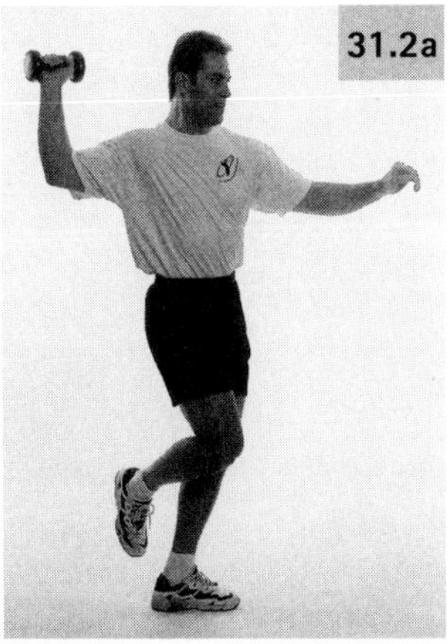
31.2a

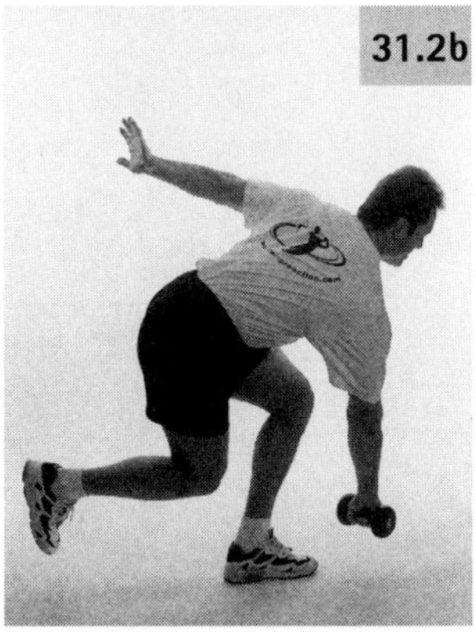
31.2b

Adjustable Pulley Variation: 31.3. This variation is slightly different from the single-leg balance lawnmower row. Instead of using a hand weight for resistance, use a low pulley, such as a vertically adjustable pulley machine or a FreeMotion machine. To start, set the pulley to the height of your knees and select a weight that you can confidently lift with one arm. Get into position by assuming a staggered stance with your left foot forward, facing the pulley. Hinging at your ankles, knee, and hips, grasp the pulley handle with your right hand and stand up with the pulley handle, bringing it to your right hip. Start the exercise by placing most of your body weight and balance on your forward left leg and the pulley handle at your right hip. Keeping your weight primarily on your left leg, reach the pulley handle toward the pulley, hinging at your ankles, knees, and hips. Then return to the start position with your body weight primarily over your left leg and the pulley handle at your right hip. Perform 2–3 sets of 10–12 reps. Each set, change your forward leg position.

Tips and Precautions: Don't do the free-weight variations if you cannot balance easily for 10 seconds on one leg. First, make sure that you can pass the peripheral balance and reach sagittal plane test (BST Exercise 44 in chapter 6); it is also helpful if you can do a deep lunge (BST Exercise 54). Avoid the free-weight variations if you have any active low back or sacroiliac problems, especially if you have loose ligaments. For the pulley variation (31.3), start slowly with 3–5 reps and get a feel for the movement pattern. Try to maintain most of your body weight over your forward leg. As your balance and strength improve, try variation 31.3 solely on one leg. Make sure to bend or hinge at your ankles, knees, and hips, not your low back; a good tip for this is to look forward while doing this variation and not at the floor or your feet.

32 DOUBLE-ARM COMBINATION ROW SQUAT

Equipment: Resistance tubing, cord, or pulley.
Purpose: Strengthen muscles associated with pulling/rowing movements in your legs, trunk, shoulders, arms, and neck. This can be helpful for paddlers as a substitute for dynamic bent-over rowing machines if a gym is unavailable.

Technique: Tie a large knot in the center of resistance tubing or cord and attach it on top of a closed door. You can also use a high pulley. Stand with your feet at slightly more than shoulder-width apart. Grab each end of the tubing or cord (or pulley handles) and move into a squat position so that your elbows are relatively straight (extended) and are at eye level at the start. Pull the tubing (or pulleys) to your chest with both hands simultaneously as you straighten both knees. Your hands should start in a palm-down position when your elbows are extended and finish in a thumb-up position as your elbows flex, thus bringing your hands to your chest. Perform 2–3 sets of 12–15 reps.
Variation: 32.1. Eye level combo row squat: Grasp the tubing so that your arms are straight and your elbows are at eye level. Back away from the door until you feel tension in the resistance tubing or cord. Balance on your left leg (32.1a); you can assist your balance by toe-touching your right foot to the ground. Simultaneously pull the tubing toward your chest and perform a single-leg squat (32.1b). Return to the single-leg balanced position while straightening your arms.
Tips: The pulley or tubing can be attached in a low, middle, or high position. Securing the tubing or pulley at waist height is better for the crew athlete. Securing the tubing or pulley in an overhead position is better for the climbing athlete. Both positions are beneficial for the windsurfer.

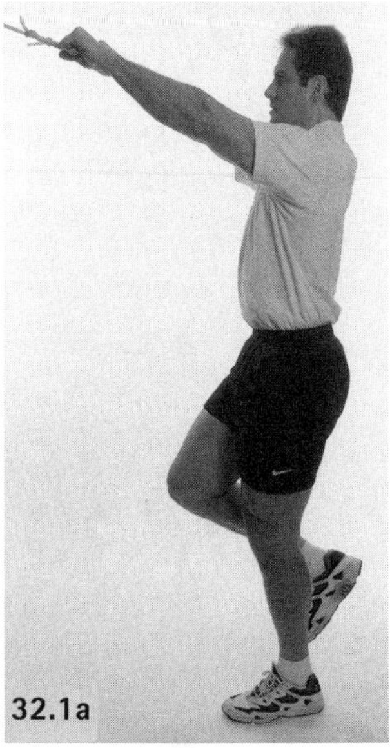

32.1a

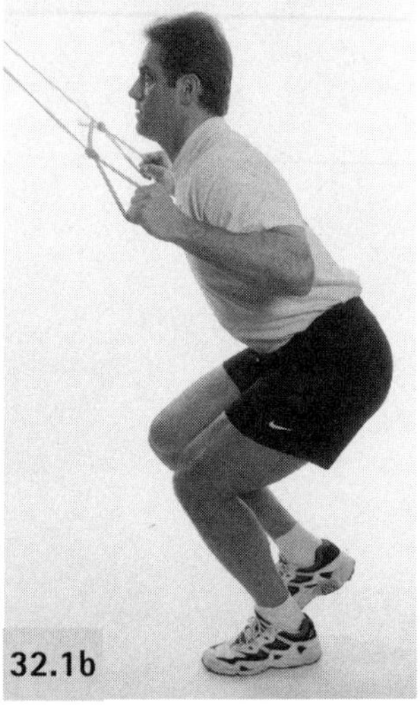

32.1b

33 SINGLE-ARM PULLEY ROWS

Equipment: Resistance tubing, cord, or pulley.
Purpose: Improve flexibility of and strengthen muscles associated with rotational pulling movements in your legs, trunk, shoulders, arms, and neck, especially if you don't have access to a gym or have back problems.

Technique: Start as in Exercise 32 but with only one hand on the tubing. Pull the tubing or pulley handle to your chest with one hand. Your hand should start in a palm-down position, with your elbow extended, and finish in a thumb-up position with your elbow flexed, thus bringing your hand to your chest. You can do this with very little or a lot of spine rotation. For water sports (especially kayaking, sweep rowing, and canoeing), do it with a moderate amount of spine rotation. Perform 2–3 sets of 12–15 reps.
Variations: **33.1.** Single-leg opposite arm pulley row: Start by standing on your left leg with your knee slightly bent. Pull down with your right arm as you extend your left knee. Do this 10–12 times, then switch your standing leg. **33.2.** Single-leg same-side arm pulley row: Pull down with the arm on the same side as the extending knee. **33.3.** Single-arm variable angle pulley row: Change the angle of the tubing or pulley to simulate different angles of climbing holds. **33.4.** Single-arm rotational pulley rows: Face 90 degrees away from the original starting position, holding the tubing so it crosses your chest when performing the row motion.
Tips: The pulley can be attached in a low, middle, or high position. The pulling motion can be performed with or without a squatting motion of the legs.

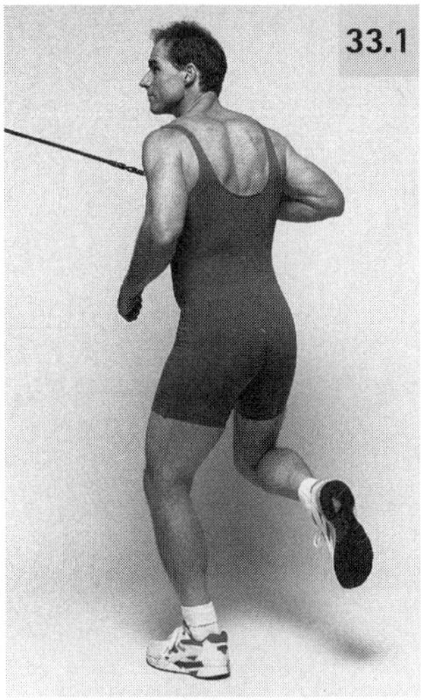
33.1

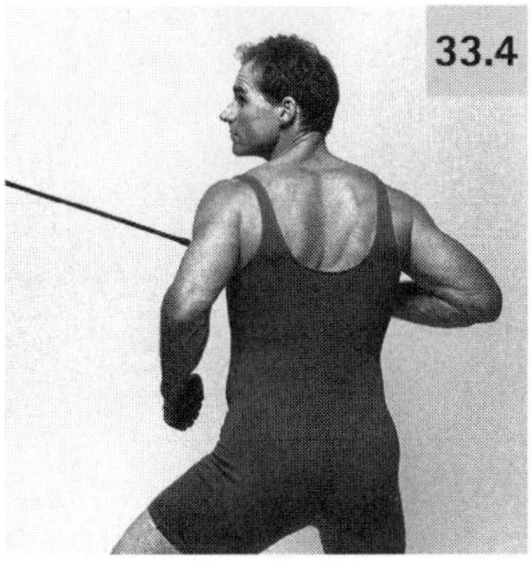
33.4

34 STANDING LATISSIMUS (LAT) PULL-DOWN

Equipment: Lat bar and lat machine.
Purpose: Train your lats, buttocks, abdominals, and legs together. An excellent challenge for your standing balance.

Technique: Stand in a squat position with your feet shoulder-width apart, in front of a lat pull-down machine. Hold the ends of the lat bar and pull the bar to your chest at the same time that you are straightening your knees and pushing off with your buttocks. Use a light amount of weight, definitely less than you would use in a sitting lat pull-down. Do 1–2 sets of 8–12 reps.

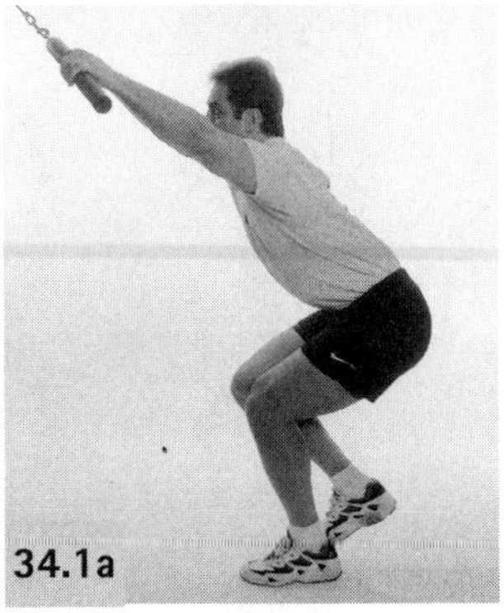

34.1a

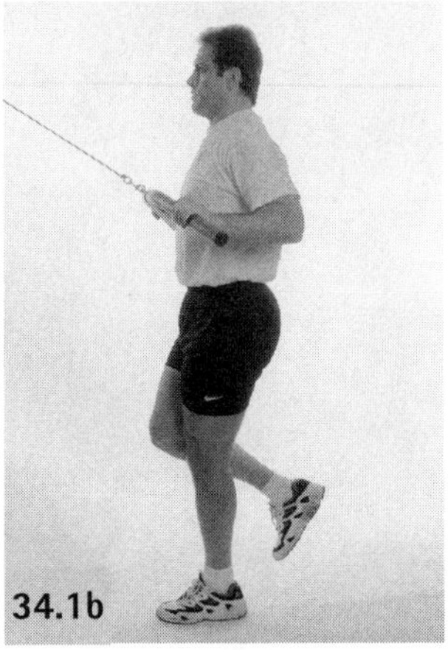

34.1b

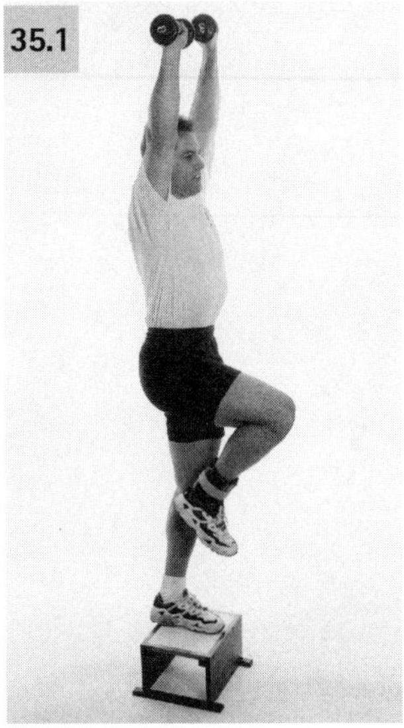

35.1

Variation: 34.1. Single leg lat pull-down: When you can do this easily with both legs on the ground, do it with only one leg on the ground, for a balance challenge. (For starting position, see 34.1a; for ending position, see 34.1b.) Do a set of 10–12 reps on one leg, then alternate to the other leg.
Precaution: This advanced exercise should be avoided by anyone with neck, low back, or shoulder problems.

STEP-UP ARM/LEG COMBINATION EXERCISES

These exercises strengthen and coordinate the step-up motion with arm/shoulder motions (including pushing and pulling). These are especially good for climbing, backcountry skiing, and snowshoeing.

35 ANTERIOR STEP-UP WITH OVERHEAD SHOULDER PRESS

Equipment: 6- to 12-inch step, free weights.
Purpose: Improve the strength of knee and hip muscles used to climb hills and rocks, and increase the strength of trunk, shoulder, and arm muscles used for pushing loads overhead. This exercise will increase balance and coordination for hiking.

Technique: Standing 6 inches from a 6-inch-high step, with free weights held at your side, step forward up onto the step with one leg and straighten your knee while pressing the weights overhead, and then bring your opposite foot up. Then step down with the same leg that initiated the step up, lower the weights, and return the opposite leg to the initial starting position. Repeat the same sequence of steps so that the same leg always leads stepping up and down. Perform 2–3 sets of 12–15 reps, then switch to the opposite leg.
Variations: 35.1. Step-up with overhead press and hip flexion: Do this exercise with the nonstepping hip and knee rising in a flexing fashion in the air in front of you, with or without an ankle weight (35.1). The ankle weight is helpful to simulate the weight of backcountry skies, snowshoes, or heavy boots. **35.2.** Step-up with straight-arm raise: Do Exercise 35 with an arm elevation (raising a straight arm in front of your body to an overhead position), which is better for telemark skiers, instead of a press up. **35.3.** Side step with overhead press: Do Exercise 35 to either side as a side step instead of a forward step. This is good for cross-country skiers or climbers.
Tips: Step height can be varied depending on your strength and needs to do higher stepping in your activity. Climbers, scramblers,

and glacier mountaineers should work with progressively increasing step heights. Start with a 6-inch step and work your way up to 12–14 inches (or higher).

36 ANTERIOR STEP-UP WITH RESISTED SHOULDER EXTENSION

Equipment: 6-inch step, resistance tubing, or pulley.
Purpose: Improve the strength of knee and hip muscles used to climb hills and rocks, and increase the strength of trunk, shoulder, and arm muscles used for pulling down as in climbing. Also increase balance and coordination for hiking and climbing.

Technique: Standing 6 inches from a 6-inch-high step, and holding two ends of resistance tubing (or a pulley) in each hand overhead or at shoulder height, step forward up onto the step with one leg (36a) while pulling the resistance tubing backward behind your waist. Then step up with your opposite leg (36b). Then step down with the same leg that initiated the step up. Allow your arms to return to the original position, with hands over your shoulders, and return the opposite leg to the initial starting position. Repeat the same sequence of steps so that the same leg always leads stepping up and down. After a set, switch the leading leg. Perform 2–3 sets of 12–15 reps.

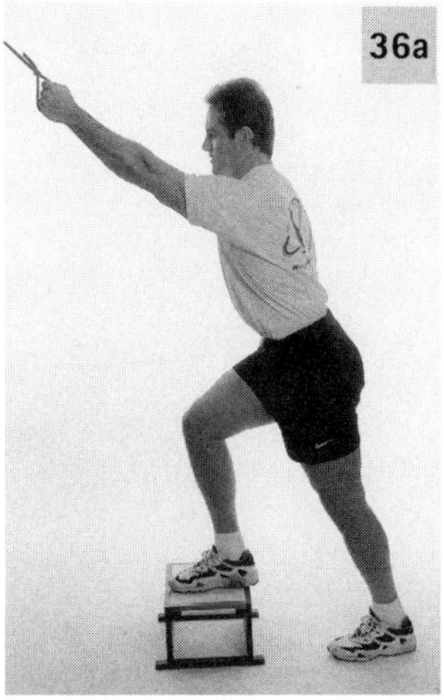

36a

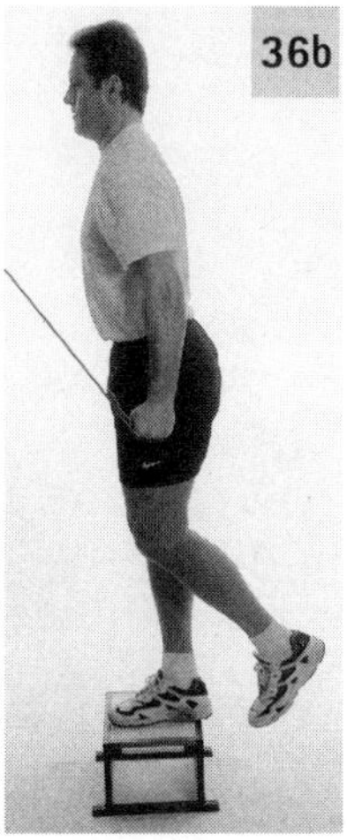

36b

Variations: 36.1. Single-arm resisted shoulder extension step-up: Try Exercise 36 with one leg and one arm, especially if you are a climber. Start by holding the tubing with your right shoulder and arm in an elevated or close to overhead position, to simulate a reach for a climbing hold. Step up on your left leg and straighten your left knee at the same time as you pull down with your right arm. Do this 12 times, then switch legs and arms. You can also do the same-side leg and arm. **36.2.** Cyclists' resisted shoulder extension step-up: For cyclists, have your handholds in cycling positions and the direction of the tubing at waist height.
Tips and Precautions: The basic technique is a good simulation for scrambling and climbing. Vary the step height depending on your strength and activity demands. The angle of the tubing or pulley can be varied to better simulate your activity. If you increase the step height or the resistance of the tubing, slow down the exercise and decrease the number of reps.

SITTING BALANCE PULLING AND PUSHING EXERCISES

These exercises enhance sitting balance and strengthen muscles used in pulling and pushing for water sports. When preparing for canoeing, sit with your feet slightly ahead of your knees. When preparing for kayaking, sit with your knees slightly bent as if in a kayak. When preparing for crew, sit on the floor with your knees bent and, if possible, sit on a plastic bag or something that will allow you to slide as you extend your knees when you pull back.

37 MAKE YOUR OWN ROWING ERG

Equipment: Resistance tubing, cord, or pulleys, and/or 4-foot wooden dowel or kayak paddle; Physioball or chair.
Purpose: Strengthen muscles associated with pulling movements in your trunk, shoulders, arms, and neck. Do this for aerobic training if you are unable to get out on the water.

Technique: Attach the center of resistance tubing or cord to a door, or use a pulley. Grab each end of the tubing (or pulley handles), or attach the ends to a paddle or a dowel. While sitting on a Physioball, on a chair, or on the ground, pull the tubing to your chest in a rowing type of motion with both hands (for crew), or simulate a kayak or canoe stroke. Try doing it at first with both feet firmly on the ground, then try it with only your toes touching the ground. Do this with lower-resistance tubing for 20–30 minutes.
Tips and Precautions: The tubing or pulley should be attached below waist height, where you would expect the water level to be. Be careful to balance and keep your feet on the ground.

38

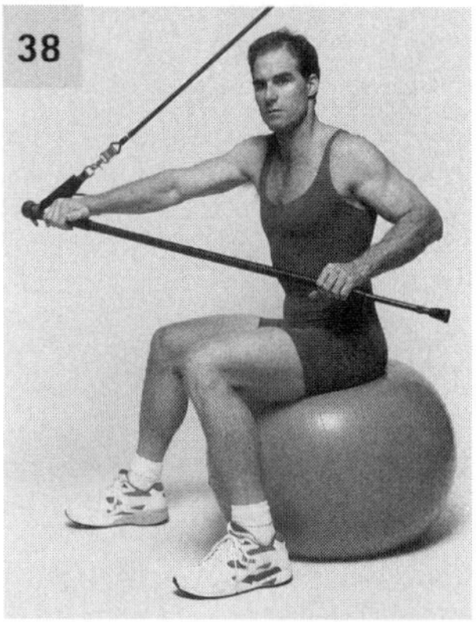

38 SEATED SINGLE-ARM PULLEY PUSHES

Equipment: Resistance tubing, cord, or pulley, and/or 4-foot wooden dowel or kayak paddle; Physioball or chair.
Purpose: Improve the strength of muscles associated with rotational pushing movements in the legs, trunk, shoulders, arms, and neck.

Technique: Attach the end of resistance tubing or cord to a door and the other end of the cord to a paddle. Sitting on a ball or chair facing away from the attachment of the resistive tubing, reproduce the same pushing motion you use in kayaking or canoeing. Perform 2 sets of 20–30 reps. Switch hand positions after each set.

39 SEATED PUSH-PULL DOUBLE-ARM PULLEY ROWS

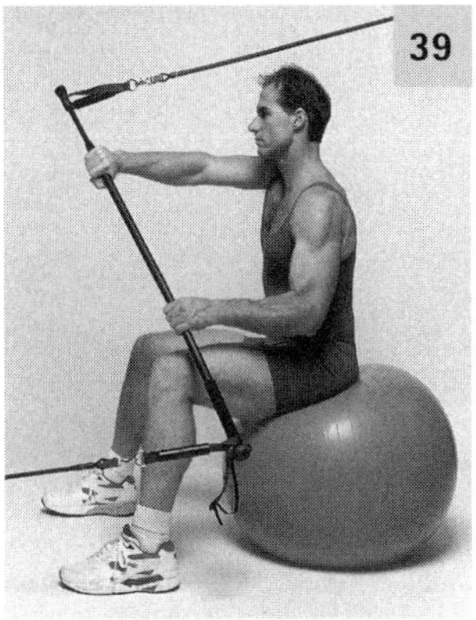

Equipment: Resistance tubing, cord, or pulleys, and/or 4-foot wooden dowel or kayak paddle; ball or chair.
Purpose: Strengthen muscles associated with rotational pushing and pulling movements in your legs, trunk, shoulders, arms, and neck associated with kayaking or canoeing.

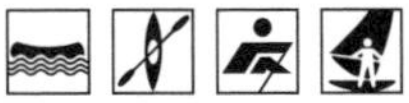

Technique: For canoeing training, attach one larger-gauge piece of resistance tubing or cord to a door in front of you and fix the other end to the neck of a paddle or dowel. Attach a smaller-gauge piece of resistance tubing or cord to a door or solid object behind you and fix the other end to the paddle grip. For kayaking training, use two pieces of equal-gauge cord and attach the free ends to the opposite ends of the paddle shaft or a dowel. Sit on a Physioball or chair with your knees only slightly bent. Emphasize the push-pull motion of kayaking on the tubing (photo 39 shows the midrange position). Switch the resistance cord to the other ends of the paddle after you fatigue, and exercise the opposite side. Allow your torso to rotate during this exercise. Perform 2 sets of 20–30 reps in 30–60 seconds.

DESIGNING YOUR OWN FUNCTIONAL EXERCISES

Believe it or not, all of the exercises that you could be doing have not already been designed or written about. Exercises can be individually designed for you, or for groups of people who do your activity, based on the demands of your activity. The number of exercise variations are endless if you follow a few basic rules:

- Analyze your most difficult activity movement challenges.
- Try a functional movement that simulates a part or all of the movement.
- Combine body regions that you will use together in your activity (think in terms of what your shoulders/hands and thighs/legs will be doing).
- Perform the motion slowly to learn the movement pattern before increasing the speed.
- Engage your core and maintain safe spine technique.
- Add resistance with weights and tubing or pulleys after you have done the exercise without resistance for a number of sets.

Functional exercises are practical, creative, and fun. The key is to look at the type of functional activity you are trying to train for and the type of movements required to accomplish this task. Then you can break the task down into components of movement and test yourself to determine the thresholds of how far and well you can move in these components of movement, and then expand these thresholds with training. Many exercises are provided here in this chapter, and they indicate which activities they are good for. The body region chapters in Part II have many functional as well as conventional exercises. In addition, the activity chapters in Part III combine functional exercises with conventional exercises in strength programs.

chapter 6 BALANCE AND AGILITY TRAINING

By Mark Pierce, A.T.C., and David Musnick, M.D.

THIS CHAPTER WILL HELP YOU:

- Understand the definitions of balance, agility, and coordination.
- Understand the planes of motion of balance present in everyday life and high-level activity.
- Design a balance and agility enhancement program that meets you at your current level of proficiency and prepares you for your specific activity goal.
- Design a balance program that will decrease your risk of falling and help prevent injuries.
- Understand how improving balance, agility, and coordination will contribute to the success of your activity.
- Self-test your present balance thresholds and abilities.

There are inherent physical challenges in any type of activity. The ability to negotiate slope, speed, and surface change is the functional defining rod of our success during outdoor and athletic activities. These challenges are mediated by a set of skill-related components of fitness called *balance, coordination,* and *agility*. Balance, coordination, and agility go hand in hand to create a synergy of critical musculoskeletal responses, which enable us to become proficient and to enjoy our activities with decreased risk of injury.

In athletic pursuits, if your balance is not sufficient, you are more likely to sustain injury because you are less able to use your core and your arms and legs to react quickly to changes in your environment. This could result in an ankle or back sprain during a hike or walk or an easily avoidable fall while skiing. If your sitting balance is not adequate, you are more likely to roll your kayak or canoe or fall off your mountain bike on a challenging trail.

Balance training is also important in everyday life, especially for the older adult. As we age, we lose lean body (muscle) mass, and as we lose muscle we become more susceptible to falling and becoming injured. You can slow the rate of muscle loss by doing strength training. If you are over the age of 60, you should emphasize balance training along with strength training because you are at higher risk for falling and breaking a wrist or a hip during walking or outdoor activities.

In order to improve your balance, you must improve not only the strength of your muscles, but your ability to use the strength and responsiveness of your muscles in response to specific balance challenges. Incorporating exercises into your program that challenge your balance, agility, and coordination will decrease your likelihood of injuries, increase the rate of your strength gains, and make you more successful at your chosen activities.

BALANCE

Balance is the ability to maintain equilibrium while in a stationary position or in motion, or in other words, it is your ability to react quickly to gravity or environmental challenges. Balance is important in standing as well as sitting positions. Sitting balance is especially important in boating and mountain biking activities.

Balance is the first and most fundamental component of human biomechanical function, and there are different aspects of balance. The most rudimentary is *static balance*, or the ability to maintain equilibrium while balancing on one foot. This is sometimes referred to as "central balance." The second aspect is called *peripheral balance*, or the ability to balance and reach away from your center of gravity with either your arm(s), leg(s), or your torso. This can be thought of as your "balance bubble," or how far you can reach with an arm or leg on one or two feet while maintaining control of your balance. The third component is *dynamic balance*, which is the ability to maintain equilibrium while moving. All three aspects of balance apply in all planes of motion common to your activity.

Balance can be trained during an exercise in a number of ways:

- Moving your arms or legs away from your torso (for example, Exercises 58 and 59 at the end of this chapter)
- Moving your torso away from your center of gravity or your base of support (for example, Exercise 31 in chapter 5)
- Standing, walking, or sitting on an uneven or unstable surface such as logs, rocks, foam rolls, large Physioballs, or specialized balance equipment

Climbing, windsurfing, skiing, snowboarding, snowshoeing, and mountaineering athletes can benefit the most from standing balance exercises. Walking on rocks or logs in parks or other outdoor environments will help train balance. Agility drills such as those described below can also be helpful. Exercises 20.1, 23, 28, 29, 31.2, 33.1, 34.1, and 57 are excellent balance exercises. Other standing balance exercises are those in chapter 8 and 80.1, 81, 82.1, 84, 84.1, 85, and 86. Besides the exercises and balance tests mentioned in this chapter, Exercises 37–39 and 62 are good for sitting balance if done on a large ball with less weight on your feet. Other sitting balance exercises are Exercise 94 and the balance and agility drills in chapter 21. Depending on your goals, your exercise program can be designed to work on muscle strength, endurance, power, balance, agility, or all of these.

It is important to identify where your current balance threshold is before starting an activity-specific exercise program. You can do this by performing the balance self-tests (BSTs) in the exercise section of this chapter.

COORDINATION AND NEUROLOGICAL CONTROL

Coordination can be defined as the ability to use multiple regions of your muscles and joints simultaneously, with skill in performing motor tasks smoothly and accurately.

When we first engage in an unfamiliar activity, our neuromuscular and musculoskeletal awkwardness limits our abilities to be efficient in that specific activity. Our reactions and movement patterns are sometimes clumsy and fatiguing, until we perform the activity numerous times. After a while, we become more familiar with the task or activity and develop very efficient and economical movement patterns to facilitate our objectives.

It takes numerous repetitions for a given task to become "second nature." Coordination is the result of many such activity-specific repetitions and complements other sports-related skills such as speed, agility, reaction time, and balance. Training any one of these skills independently or in combination will enhance your coordination. Usually, through trial and error and keen awareness, we develop proficient biomechanical strategies toward excellence that allow us to spend the least amount of energy while enjoying our activities to the fullest.

AGILITY

Agility is the ability to rapidly change position of the entire body in space with speed and accuracy. It can be thought of as maintaining balance and good body positioning while responding quickly to changes in your environment while you are moving. Climbing, windsurfing, skiing, snowboarding, snowshoeing, and mountaineering athletes all require a fair amount of agility to react to unstable surfaces or to bound, leap, and react to a jump or potential fall. Cyclists and mountain bikers, in particular, require agility in and out of the seat to respond to various road and trail conditions. Being agile allows you to move quickly, change direction, cut, jump, hurdle, glide, and slide rapidly.

Training your agility can range from doing controlled footwork drills around obstacles and over differing terrain to performing plyometrics exercises over boxes. An adequate base of fitness and conditioning is required before starting to train your agility. This type of training can be very intense and places large loads on your joints, connective tissues, and tendons. If you are beginning an exercise program or have not exercised regularly for more than a month, be sure to condition aerobically and engage in a balance and strengthening program for 3–4 weeks before starting any agility drills. Then start easy with drills you can safely perform. Try doing the Shuffle Run or Carioca (dynamic warm-up drills in chapter 4). The drills you eventually choose should reflect identifiable, sport-specific movements. This will enable you to easily relate the training to the sport.

Agility circuits are an ideal way to add variation to your exercise program. They are designed to improve your reaction times, coordination, and balance. When designing an agility circuit or program you must take into consideration the planes of motion (discussed below) and intensity demands of your activity. Move slowly at first and develop your coordination for each movement, then speed it up. Develop a competent base before adding more intense or complex challenges.

The following exercises and circuits can be used in conjunction with your daily exercise program or independently during the week as a substitution to a workout.

Skiers, snowboarders, and snow-sport athletes: Do Exercises 153–157 in chapter 20.

Boating athletes: Do chapter 21's on-the-water exercises and, in this chapter, BST Exercise 43 and the seated variations for BST Exercises 45 and 51.

Road cyclists: Do Exercises 171–173 in chapter 22.

Mountain bikers: Try Exercises 174–178 in chapter 22.

Runners: Do BST Exercises 49, 51, and 53 in sequence, and then BST Exercises 54–56, all in this chapter.

PLANES OF MOTION

There are three cardinal planes of motion with numerous vectors within each plane. At any time during your activity or daily life you are moving in these three planes simultaneously. In many activities there are times in which you will be emphasizing one plane more than another and thus might want to do exercises and train in that dominant plane. Balance and functional exercises can be biased toward one, two, or all three planes of motion. If you understand planes of motion in general and those specific to your activity, then you can train accordingly.

It is also important, when doing your balance self-tests in this chapter, to determine if you have balance deficits in any particular plane. You can then decide to do balance exercises that emphasize this plane along with balance exercises that target the planes specific to your activity.

Sagittal Plane

The *sagittal plane* is motion forward, backward, up, and down. This is the dominant plane of motion during most activities. Examples of dominant sagittal plane activities include cross-country skiing, running, snowshoeing, and walking. Include both functional strength and balance exercises that emphasize the sagittal plane in your exercise program.

Strength training exercises in other chapters that emphasize this plane (listed from easiest to more difficult) are squats, lunges (forward and walking), step-ups, step-downs, jumps, and hops.

Sagittal plane balance exercises are in this chapter and other chapters. The following programs will help in sagittal plane training.

Beginning sagittal plane exercises: This program is good for anyone that would like good balance. It is appropriate for all athletes as well as seniors. It is good for backpackers, hikers, snowshoers, and walkers.

Start with a leg balance like BST Exercise 43 or 44. Then add the balance and arm reach in Exercise 58 (avoiding all variations except 58.3a) and the leg reach in Exercise 59. When these become easy, progress to the basic forward lunge, Exercise 97.

Intermediate sagittal plane exercises: This program is good for cyclists, cross-country and skate skiers, and runners.

You can progress your basic lunge to Exercise 97.6, which adds a biceps curl, and Exercise 97.9, which adds walking. You can also do exercises with a rocker board (see Balance Equipment Exercises later in this chapter).

Advanced sagittal plane exercises: This program is good for mountain and rock climbers, skiers, snowboarders, and competitive runners.

Start with a walking lunge with weights, Exercise 97.6. Then, add Exercise 99, step-downs, if you have the equipment. Progress to a basic jump, Exercise 100, then to a hop, Exercise 101.

Sitting sagittal plane exercises: These exercises will be helpful for boaters and mountain bikers.

Start with the Exercise 62, a sitting ball toss. You can substitute Exercise 93 if you don't have Physioballs. You can then add Exercises 88, 92, and 94. See chapters 21 and 22 for specific balance and agility suggestions for boaters and cyclists, respectively.

Frontal Plane

The *frontal plane* is considered side-to-side motion. This plane of motion dominates sports such as canoeing, cycling, kayaking, mountain biking, mountaineering, rock climbing, skate skiing, and snowboarding.

Beginning frontal plane exercises: Start with the leg balance in BST Exercise 44. Add a side bend with weight by doing Exercise 84. Progress to a side lunge in Exercise 97.3.

Intermediate frontal plane exercises: Start with lateral step-ups in Exercise 98.3 and progress to the sidestep walking lunge in Exercise 97.11.

Advanced frontal plane exercises: Start with lateral jumps, Exercise 100.5, and then progress to lateral hops, Exercise 101.2.

Sitting frontal plane exercises: Start by sitting on a Physioball as described in BST Exercise 43. Progress to Exercise 62, the sitting ball toss, and then to Exercise 94, which is especially geared for boaters and cyclists.

Transverse Plane

The *transverse plane* is considered rotational motion. This plane is used during our everyday lives and many activities and yet appears to be the most neglected plane of motion during most exercise programs. Transverse plane motion allows us to accelerate and decelerate while running or walking. This plane of motion dominates throwing and swinging activities such as golf, softball, racket sports, soccer, and volleyball. It is also very important in kayaking, skiing, and snowboarding.

Beginning transverse plane exercises: Start with the leg balance in BST Exercise 48 and the leg reach in Exercise 59.

Intermediate transverse plane exercises: Start with the balance with chopping motions in Exercise 60. Then add lawnmower pulls in Exercise 31. Progress to the abdominals with rotation, Exercise 83 (do this exercise with your back foot toe-touching for assistance).

Advanced transverse plane exercises: Start with the lawnmower pull that has external rotation, Exercise 31.1. Then add the transverse plane jump in Exercise 100.3 and progress to transverse plane hops in Exercise 101.5.

Sitting transverse plane exercises: Start by sitting on a Physioball, doing the pulley pushes in Exercise 38. Then progress to the push-pull pulley rows in Exercise 39. For cyclists, perform these two exercises with toe-touch balance on both feet. For boating athletes, do them with your heels touching the floor.

Tri-Planar Function

Tri-planar function describes how our muscles and joints perform during everyday life. Every muscle and joint in our body contracts or moves in all three planes simultaneously. Even when we walk down the street or up a mountain trail, in the sagittal plane, our musculoskeletal system is moving and responding to stresses in the other two planes of motion. This physiological adaptation is the product of being bipedal and dealing with gravity, ground reaction forces, and momentum.

Our musculoskeletal system reacts in three different ways. For example, let's take a look at our musculoskeletal strategy as we lift an object off the floor. First, our muscular system slows us down through eccentric contraction while we control our collapsing joints against gravity and ground reaction. This action occurs as we lower ourselves to the object resting on the floor. This controlled collapse is called *pronation*. Our joints during pronation are flexing, rotating, and side bending, basically moving in three different planes all at once, with the sagittal plane being dominant. This collapse happens via numerous muscular contractions, which control the descent in all three planes. Second, the muscles around the moving parts of our body isometrically contract to momentarily stop and stabilize each moving joint while we grasp the object and ready our return to the standing position. This is called *stabilization* or *transformation*. Third, our muscles concentrically contract to move our body and limbs with the object in our hands against the force of gravity back to an upright position. This is called *supination*. This concert of muscular contractions and limb movements occurs simultaneously in all three planes of motion, requiring balance and control at every joint and muscle involved with the task or activity.

It is therefore helpful for anyone to do balance exercises in all three planes of motion. Certain activities would especially benefit from balance and functional exercises to train all three planes. These include backpacking, cross-country (especially backcountry) skiing, hiking, scrambling, snowboarding, and windsurfing. Participants in most school, professional, and team sports would similarly benefit.

BALANCE EQUIPMENT

You can use balance equipment for a number of reasons: (1) To improve your reactions on a less stable surface (especially helpful for skiers and snowboarders, mountain and rock climbers, windsurfers, and boaters). (2) To improve the dynamic functional use of your core muscles.

Balance equipment creates balance challenges in multiple planes of motion. It is good to start with one that moves forward and back or side to side before you try the multidirectional equipment. You can do exercises on this equipment by simply trying to maintain your balance or by moving on a piece of equipment with or without hand weights. Use poles for additional support when you are starting to use this equipment. To determine your comfort level and ability, you might slowly and carefully try various exercises on balance equipment. Successful completion of the balance self-test exercises (Exercises 40–56) might also indicate that such equipment is right for you. Use special caution with this equipment if you have a current injury (especially of your foot, ankle, or low back) or if you tend to have loose ligaments (see chapter 9).

If you belong to a health club, it is a good idea to ask a trainer to help you. You can also order this equipment from any of the websites listed in the references for this chapter.

Sagittal/Frontal Plane Equipment

Foam Rolls and Half Rolls

Foam cylinders can be used cut in half lengthwise or as cylinders. The balance challenge increases as you go from standing on the curved surface of a half roll to standing on the flat side of a half roll. Make sure the foam is firm. It is good to use 1- to 2-foot rolls. You can use these rolls to do Exercise 58 or to simulate log crossings or walking on rocks. You can stand on the curved or the flat side of a half roll to challenge your balance with any functional exercise done while standing on one or both feet (see Figure 17).

Balance Beams

These beams are usually made out of wood, foam, or polyvinyl and they vary in size. They are designed to improve your self-confidence, balance, and spatial awareness. You can walk on them or balance on one or two feet, and they can improve your dynamic balance.

Rocker Boards

These devices are 15- to 20-inch rectangular or square platforms with a wooden or plastic fulcrum that attaches to the bottom (Figure 18). Rocker boards can be used for either sagittal or frontal plane balance work depending on which way you stand on them.

The Fitter

The Fitter is a frontal plane, dynamic piece of equipment that rocks side to side to simulate a skiing motion. It has resistance cords that change the resistance of the moving platform. You can use this with or without ski poles. To use it you would assume a skiing position and transfer your weight from one side to the other. This equipment is appropriate for snowboarders, skiers, and high-level rock climbers. (The Fitter is pictured in Exercise 68.)

Slide Board

A slide board is available at most health facilities or fitness stores. It emphasizes the frontal plane. It is approximately 8 feet long and made of plastic. You will need shoe covers or very thick socks to slide back and forth in a motion similar to skating. It helps challenge balance while you are decelerating and accelerating your body. It also improves hip, quad, buttock, and groin strength. Initially stand on one end of the slide board with your foot against the edge. Get in a position so that your knees and hips are flexed. Push off the edge and slide across to the other side's edge. You can initially try this for 45–60 seconds per set, doing 4–5 sets. This is especially helpful for cyclists, mountain and rock climbers, skiers, snowboarders, and windsurfers.

Body Blade

The Body Blade is a piece of graphite metal shaped like a bow, with small weights at each end. It can be held with one or two hands and oscillated while balancing on one or both legs. You can use it while standing on the floor or on other balance equipment. It is expensive and is more commonly found in physical therapy clinics than in gyms (Figure 19).

Multiplanar Balance Equipment

Wobble Boards

These are circular platforms with a hemisphere base that creates multidirectional instabilities to challenge your balance. You can stand, sit, or kneel on these wood boards. The base tilts and rocks to challenge your balance and proprioception. Increase the difficulty of wobble boards by using a smaller board with a larger hemisphere. Wobble boards usually come with three height adjustments.

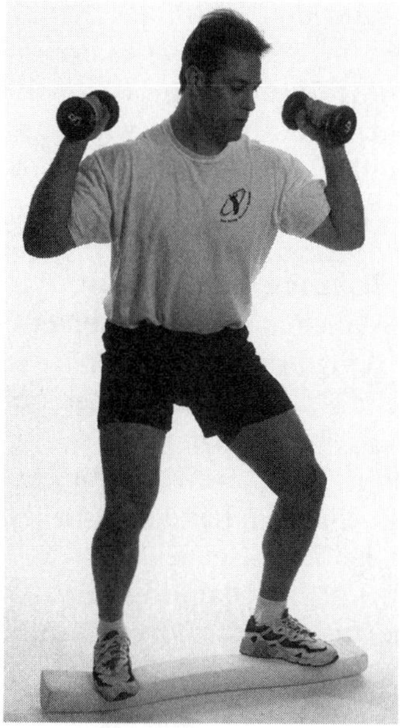

FIGURE 17. Foam roll.

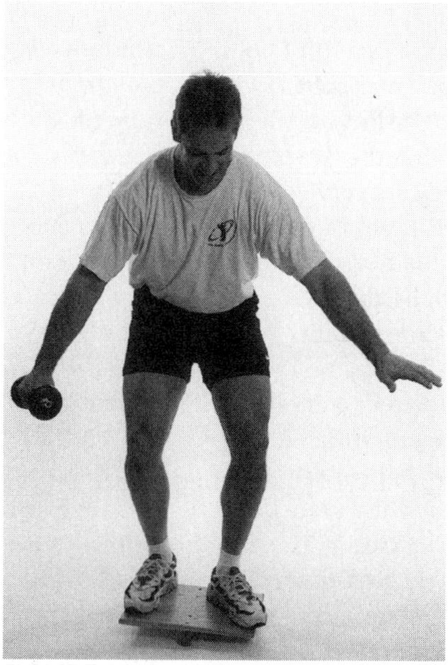

FIGURE 18. Rocker board.

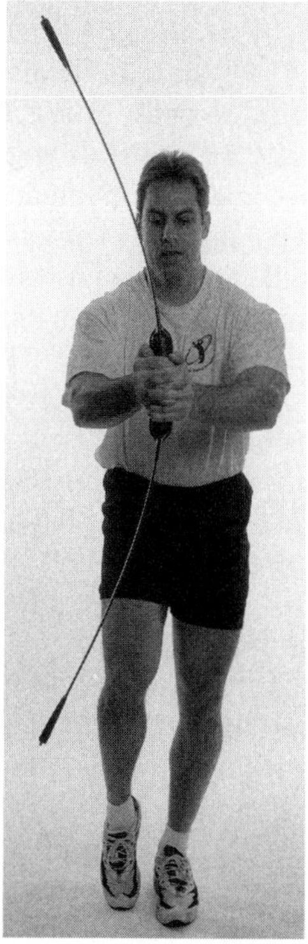

FIGURE 19. Body Blade.

Disc Pillow

These are air-filled plastic discs that come in various sizes that allow you to challenge your standing balance. They are inexpensive and easy to transport. You can get these in pairs—one for each foot to stand on—or you can use a larger size that will accommodate both feet. (See Exercise 66.1 for a picture of a disc pillow.)

Bosu Balance Trainer

This device looks like a stability ball (Physioball) with a flat bottom. It is moderately expensive and is often found in gyms and physical therapy clinics. It is a very versatile training device for balance, core stability, and proprioception training. With the "bubble" side up, you can sit, stand, lie, or kneel on it. With the platform side up, this training aide can be used for push-ups or you can stand on it for an advanced balance workout. More air makes the Bosu more stable.

Balance Pads

These devices are mildly firm foam pads that can be used in a similar fashion to discs. Your body weight causes you to sink into the soft mat, creating instability. These help retrain your lower-extremity function. You can stack two pads or use a pad on top of a larger mat for greater instability.

Balance Steps

These are relatively inexpensive, small, air-filled domes. They are excellent all-around tools for improving agility and balance. They are especially good for hikers and backpackers who want to improve their ability to cross rivers; try setting the steps up at varying distances to simulate rocks in a river.

Physioball

Physioballs are also known as stability balls, exercise balls, fitness balls, balance balls, Swiss balls, gym balls, or yoga balls. The Physioball has become a very popular tool within the fitness and rehabilitation community. They are very versatile and can be used for numerous types of exercises in standing, seated, or prone positions Like most balance equipment, Physioballs create an unstable surface that challenges core stability while using your arms and/or legs. They come in various sizes and are usually color-coded based on their circumference when properly inflated.

Selecting a ball is simple. A properly sized ball will allow you to sit on it with your knees and hip at 90 degrees. However, using different-size balls will allow you more flexibility and variation in your exercises. Try not to use any type of support or anchors for supporting limbs when training with a Physioball. The whole idea is to train in an unstable environment. When using hand weights, use lighter loads. While spotters are recommended when using external resistance equipment, if you are using appropriate loads and form, minimal supervision is needed. Body alignment of the spine when using a Physioball should be kept in a neutral position with your core engaged.

Homemade Balance Equipment

You can make balance challenge equipment at home and shake it vigorously in multiple directions while standing on one or both feet, on a foam roll, on a rock, or on a log.

- Partially fill two canning jars with beans or rice, and hold one in each hand and shake them while balancing on one leg.
- Fill a beach ball with 16–64 ounces of water and shake it vigorously side to side and front to back.
- Half fill a 2-liter plastic bottle with water and shake it.
- Balance or walk on a 2×4 or 4×6 for a static or dynamic challenge.

SELF-TESTING YOUR FUNCTIONAL BALANCE

Balance testing is the functional testing of your successful thresholds in all appropriate planes of motion and positions relative to your particular sport (seated or standing). Each balance self-test below is designed to identify your balance strengths and weaknesses relative to your particular activity. Determining your balance thresholds in each particular plane of motion and position will give you a starting point to begin your balance program.

The function of balance is measured in three ways: static, peripheral, and dynamic. As discussed earlier in this chapter, static balance is the ability to maintain your standing or seated equilibrium on one leg without motion; peripheral balance is the ability to balance and reach away from your center of gravity with either your arm(s), leg(s), or your torso; and dynamic balance is the ability to maintain equilibrium while moving.

Static balance is important for activities such as skiing or rock climbing that require prolonged periods of static positioning. Peripheral balance is important for any activity that requires your arms or legs to move away from your core. Dynamic balance aids in any activity that requires your body to be in motion.

The goal of these self-tests is to measure your abilities with static, peripheral, and dynamic balance relative to each plane of motion (sagittal, frontal, and transverse). In addition to doing these self-tests to assess balance, you can use any self-test as an exercise to strengthen an area of deficit. You can also do other functional exercises that target a particular plane of motion in order to improve your planar abilities.

As with any type of physical test or challenge, a few rules will help you to safely make progress in your balance efficiency.

Rule 1: Be safe and pain-free. Make your static position or movement patterns safe and pain-free, aiming for a maximum time of 30 seconds for all static tests. Your balance foot must maintain its position on the floor without your heel rising.

Rule 2: Stay in control. Be centered and coordinated with your movements. Evidence that you have reached your threshold of balance includes:

- Wobbling of your legs.
- Quick uncontrolled movements of your pelvis, hips, back, arms, or your non-weight-bearing leg.
- Pain in your muscles and joints.

Reaching your threshold indicates that you may need more work on that plane of balance, especially if you can surpass that threshold on the other side (i.e., when working your right as opposed to your left leg). If you find yourself wobbling or about to lose your balance, make your movements smaller or slow down. If you are unsteady balancing on one foot, use your opposite foot to assist by toe-touching it next to your balancing foot during any single-leg balance challenge.

Rule 3: Challenge yourself but be smart about it. Be as aggressive as you can without breaking rules 1 and 2. Initially, start with the easiest balance challenge and become successful at it before moving on to more difficult or aggressive balance challenges. Start with slower motions before moving faster and with shorter ranges of motions before moving to longer ones.

Rule 4: Record your results to determine if you have deficits in the sagittal, frontal, or transverse planes when comparing your right and left sides. Record your results in regard to how many seconds and at what level you are able to do the test.

Rule 5: Work to correct imbalances. If you cannot do 30 seconds of a self-test at any particular level, consider doing the self-test as an exercise until you are successful at it for 30 seconds before moving to the next level. Also consider doing other exercises that incorporate that plane of balance.

Further guidelines are the following:

Footwear: Do these tests while wearing an athletic or walking shoe. If you have orthotics, use them during these tests.

For cycling and boating athletes: Perform the balance self-tests in standing and sitting positions. When performing the self-tests while seated, use a Physioball or some other unstable surface to simulate the balance challenges of your sport or activity (see Balance Equipment in this chapter for a description of Physioballs). You can start your seated versions of the self-tests with both feet firmly on the floor. Then, to increase the challenge, try placing both feet with just your toes touching for cyclists and just your heels touching for boaters.

Precautions: If you are at a high risk for falling, perform these tests carefully, with at least one foot bearing weight and your other foot bearing partial weight. If you have a shoulder problem, be careful with arm swings. If you have a low-back problem, be careful with leg swings and start a test at a low level to avoid abrupt movements of your back and pelvis.

STATIC BALANCE SELF-TESTS

Equipment: A clock with a second hand or a stopwatch and a hard level surface to stand on. A homemade test vector (Figure 20). On the surface that you will be conducting your self-test, make a test vector using tape to mark a big + sign. Make each line of the + about

8 feet long. Use the center of this + as the starting reference point for each of these tests. The perpendicular lines represent the sagittal plane (forward and backward) and frontal plane (side to side) vectors. The forward spaces between the lines represent the anterior frontal and transverse planes, and spaces to your rear represent the posterior frontal and transverse planes. From the center of the +, if you look and rotate your body, without moving your feet, 90 degrees to your left or 90 degrees to your right down the frontal plane vectors, you will have moved your back and neck into the transverse plane. Correspondingly, if you are standing in the center of the + facing relatively forward (anterior sagittal plane) and rotate to reach or point your foot and lunge down the frontal plane vectors, you will be moving into the transverse plane proper. Figures 20 and 21 help illustrate this and show examples of planar stepping motions.

Purpose: To test your ability to balance on one foot compared to the opposite side with challenges in three planes of motion. Seated tests challenge core stability in the plane tested. Good for all activities and for general conditioning.

FIGURE 20. HOMEMADE TEST VECTOR

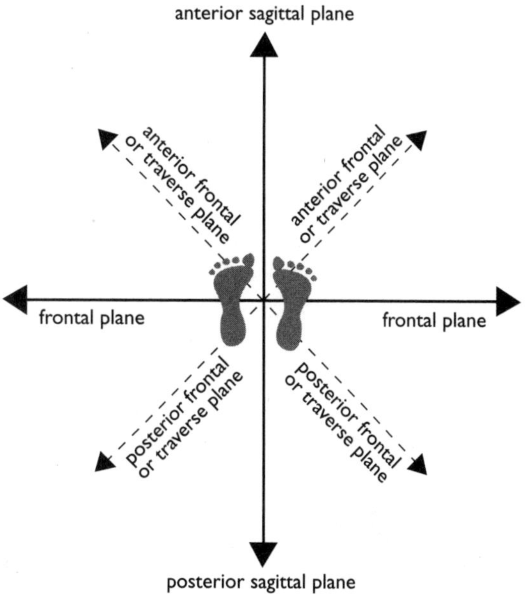

FIGURE 21. PLANAR STEPPING MOTIONS. Examples of movement into planes of motion referencing and testing the left leg. The left leg/foot is stationary, while the right leg/foot moves along the test vector. Comparisons are made of the weight-bearing lower extremity/leg using the non-weight-bearing leg/foot to impose the challenge.

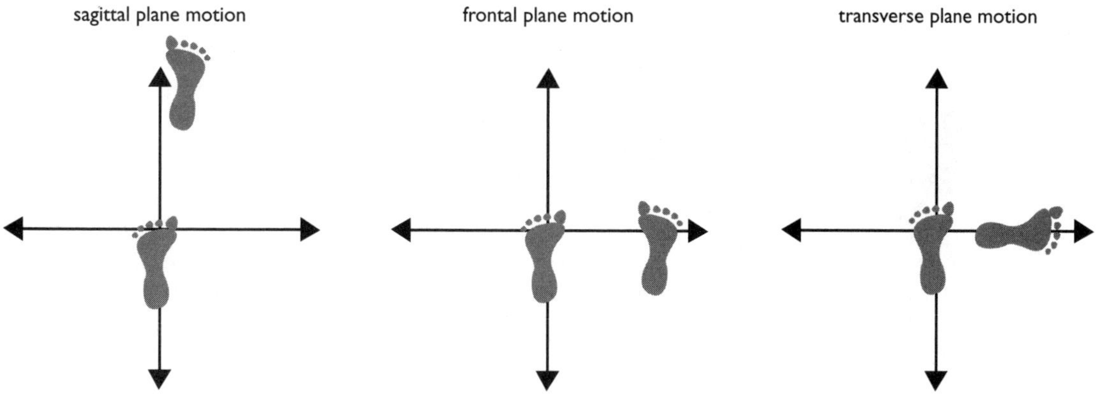

Measurement: The time you are able to balance on one foot compared to the other for a maximum of 30 seconds on each side. If you have a comparative deficit of 10 seconds on one side, use the test as an exercise to equalize your balance capacities in the plane tested.

General Technique: If you find that you cannot do a balance test with only one foot bearing weight, then start with your toes just touching beside your balance foot. One of your goals is to eventually do the balance self-test with only one foot bearing weight. When you record your results, note if you did the test on one foot or if you used your other foot to assist.

BASIC STATIC BALANCE SELF-TESTS

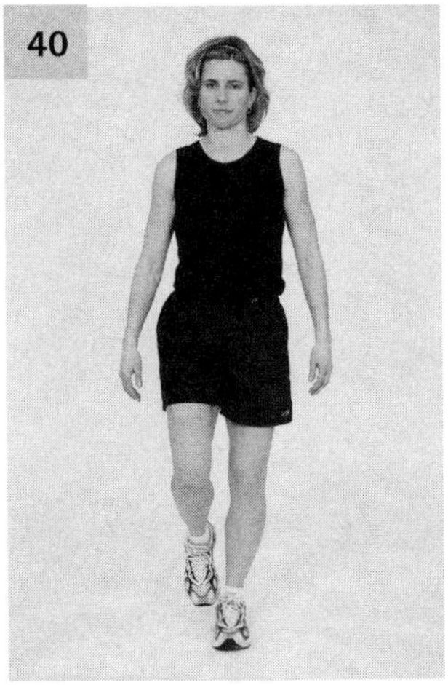
40

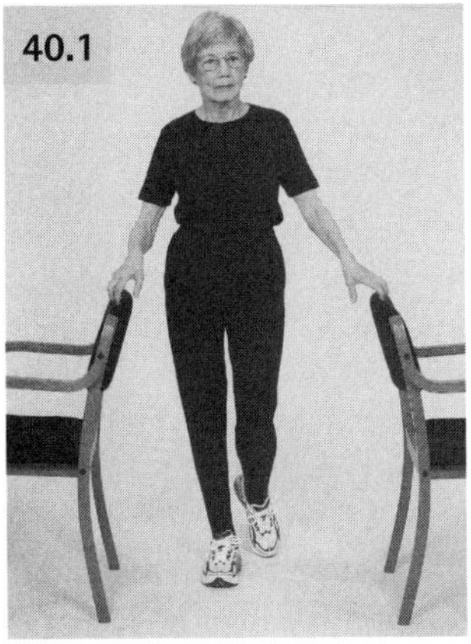
40.1

40 (BST) BASIC SELF-TEST

Technique: Stand on a firm, predictable surface with your arms by your sides. Bend both knees slightly to engage your quadriceps and raise one foot off the floor. Measure the time you can maintain balance on one foot without touching the floor with the raised foot and compare that to the opposite side.

Variation: 40.1. Assisted basic self-test: If you have recently sprained your ankle or are a senior with leg weakness, you may want to do this self-test by holding onto a chair or ski poles with one or both hands. You can increase the challenge by gradually gripping the top of the chair with less force until your balance improves. At that time you can progress to not holding on.

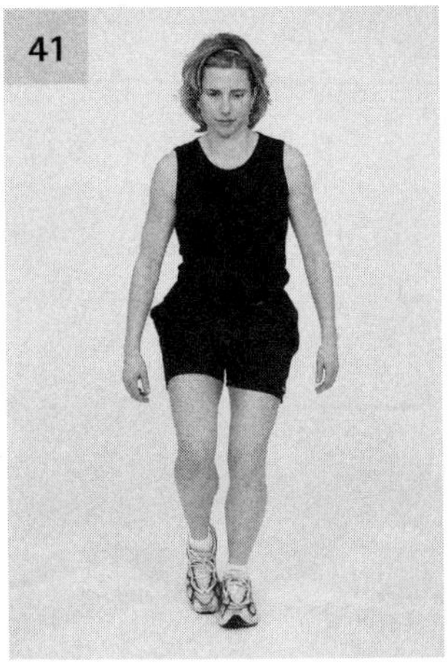
41

41 (BST) BENT-KNEE BASIC SELF-TEST

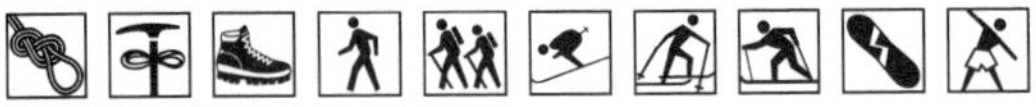

Technique: Assume the same position as BST Exercise 40, but bend your support knee or flex it to 60 degrees and maintain that position. This is a great way to test and exercise your static balance for skiing and other activities that require adequate prolonged positioning.

STATIC BALANCE: SAGITTAL PLANE

42 (BST) SAGITTAL PLANE BALANCE WITH ARM SWING

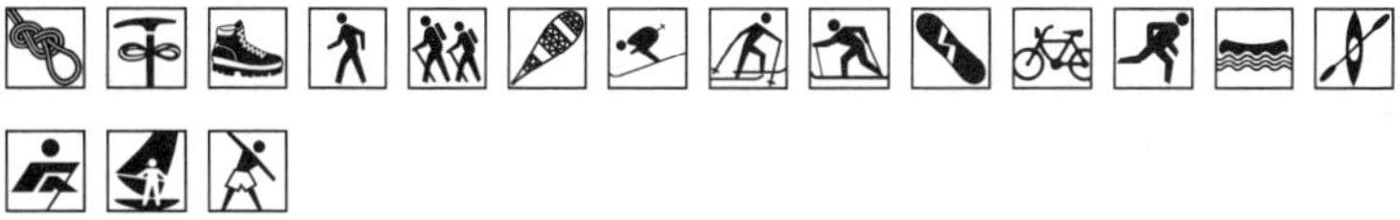

Technique: Start by balancing on one foot with your knee slightly bent and your opposite foot raised or toe-touching the floor beside your balance foot. **Level 1.** Swing your arms together, forward and backward in short ranges of motions, initially up to 45 degrees in front of you (42a and 42b). **Level 2.** Swing your arms in front of you so that your arms reach an angle of 90 degrees to the floor. **Level 3.** Do level 2 and swing your arms faster to increase your momentum and challenge in the sagittal plane.

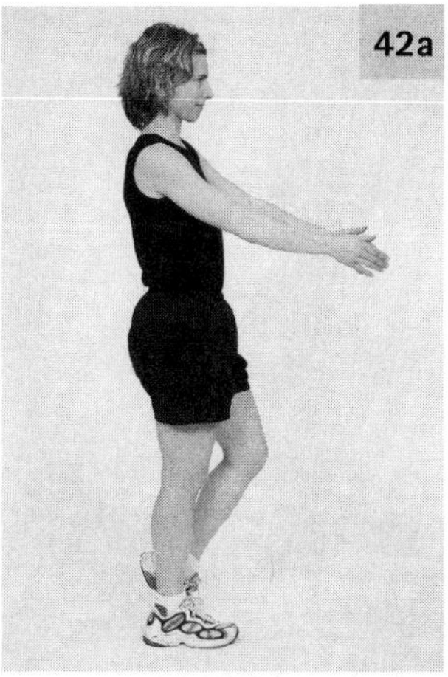
42a

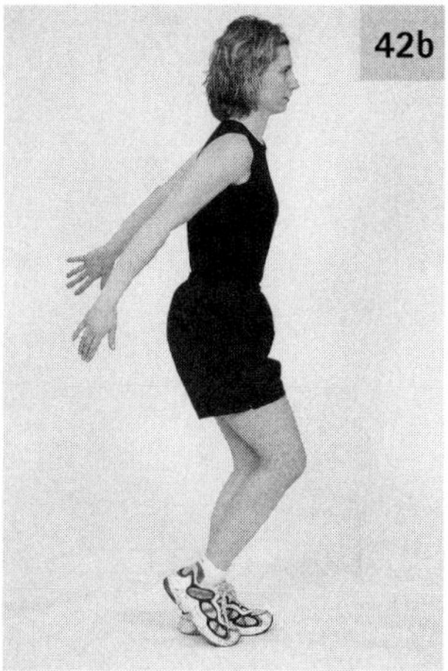
42b

43 (BST) SEATED SAGITTAL PLANE BALANCE WITH ARM SWING

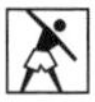

Technique: For boating and cycling athletes, perform the forward and backward arm-swing tests described in BST Exercise 42 while seated on a Physioball. **Level 1.** Place both feet firmly on the floor. **Level 2.** Place both feet on the floor with only your heels touching the ground (43a and 43b). **Level 3.** Place one foot firmly on the floor and lift the other foot off the floor (43c and 43d).

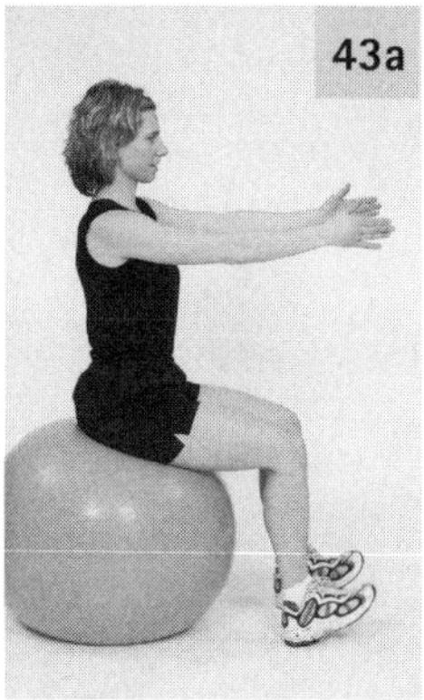
43a

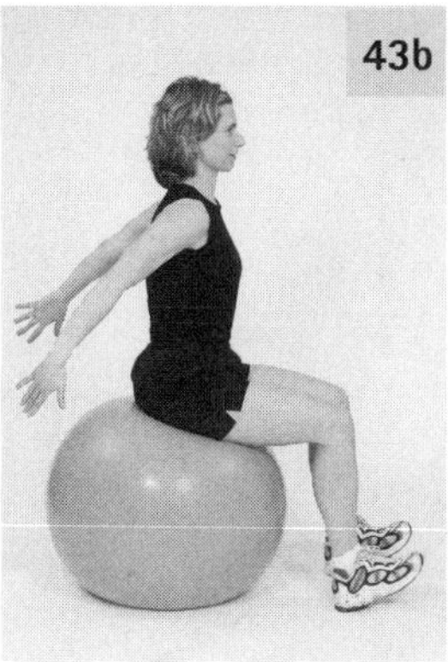
43b

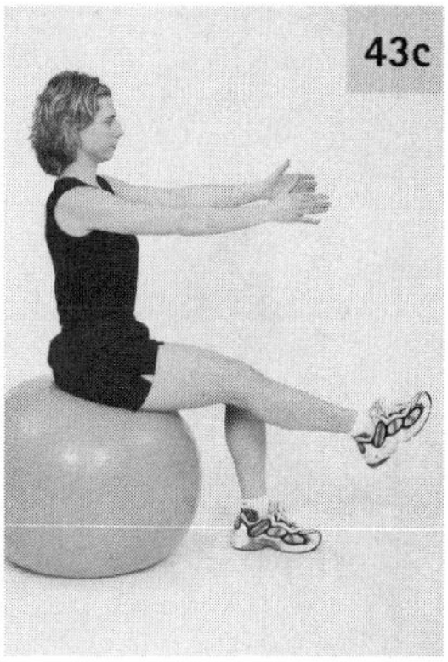
43c

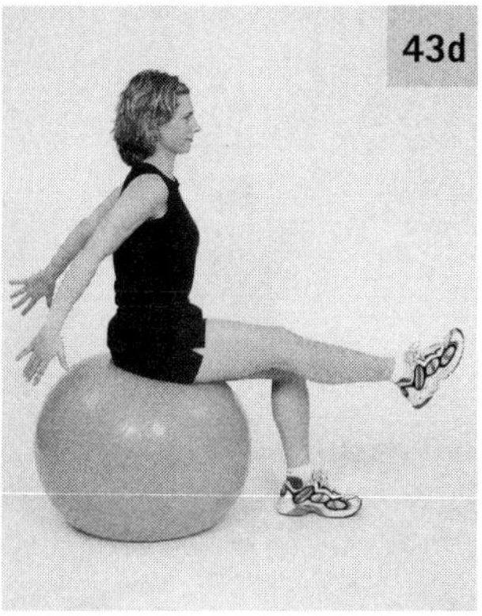
43d

EXERCISE 44 45 46 47

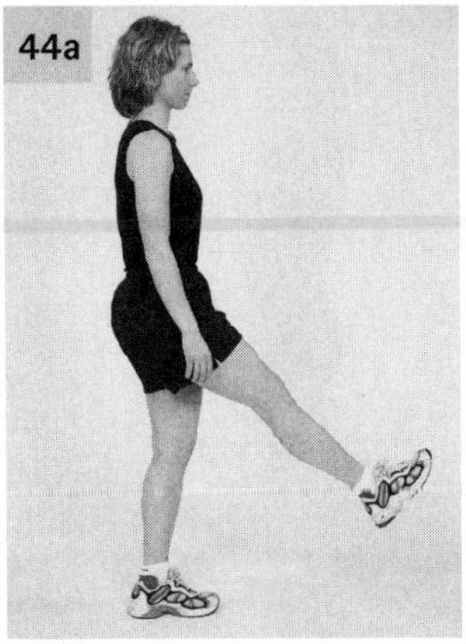

44a

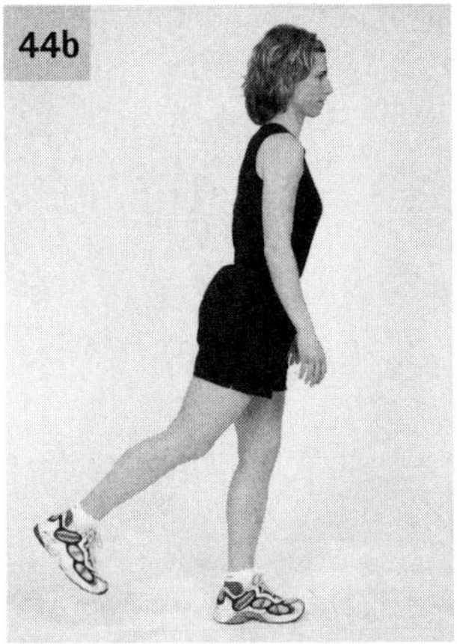

44b

44 (BST) SAGITTAL PLANE BALANCE WITH OPPOSITE-LEG SWING

Technique: Balance on one foot with your standing-leg knee slightly bent and your opposite foot raised. **Level 1.** Bring your non-weight-bearing leg out in front of you (with a straight knee), to an angle of about 20 degrees (your heel should be about 4 inches above the ground). Try to balance for at least 2–3 seconds. **Level 2.** Next, move your leg to about 30 degrees (with your heel about 10 inches off the ground; 44a). When you are doing the test with a leg swing this will be the forward ending position. **Level 3.** Now take your leg and bring it behind you to a comfortable position, with your knee either straight or just slightly bent (44b). This will be your ending position. **Level 4.** When you have mastered these positions, swing your leg forward and backward in short ranges at first, then in longer ranges as you become more successful. This will test your ability to balance against a forward and backward challenge.

STATIC BALANCE: FRONTAL PLANE

45 (BST) FRONTAL PLANE BALANCE WITH ARM SWING

Technique: Start by balancing on one foot with your knee slightly bent and your opposite foot raised or toe-touching the floor beside your balance foot. **Level 1.** Swing your arms together, side to side, in short ranges of motions initially up to 45 degrees across your body (45a and 45b). **Level 2.** Do level 1 and swing your arms faster to increase your momentum and challenge in the frontal plane.

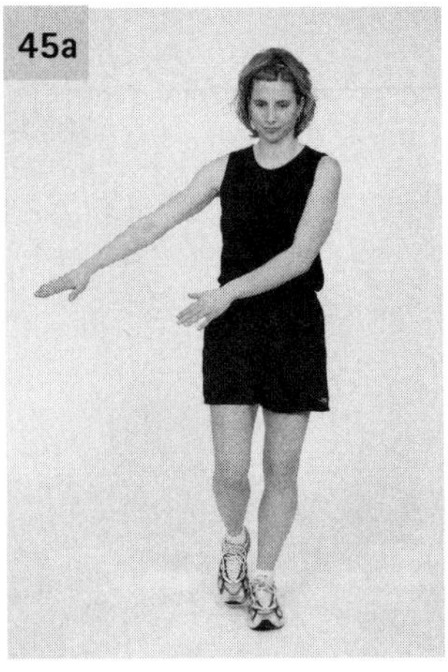

45a

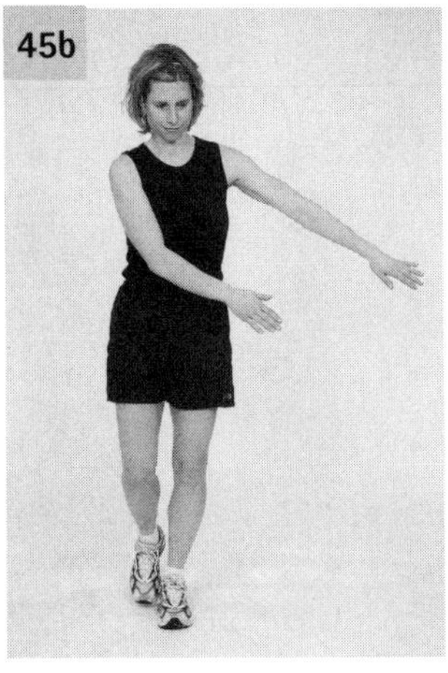

45b

46 (BST) FRONTAL PLANE BALANCE WITH OPPOSITE-LEG SWING

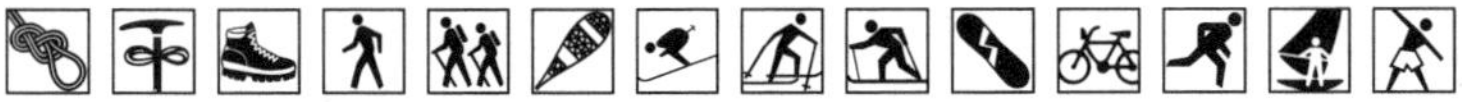

Technique: Balance on one foot with your opposite foot raised. Swing your non-weight-bearing leg side to side, crossing it in front of your balance leg (46a and 46b).

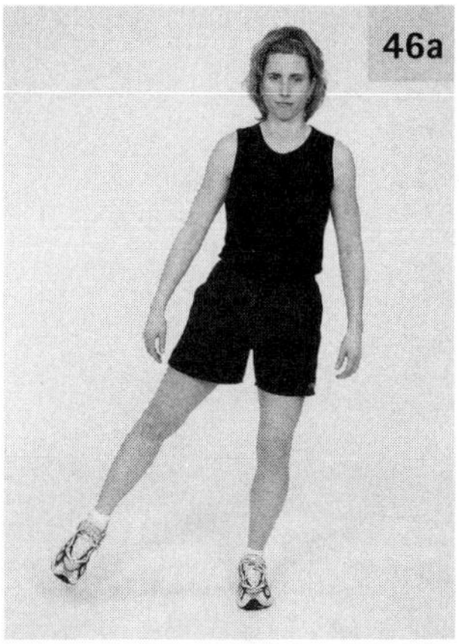

46a

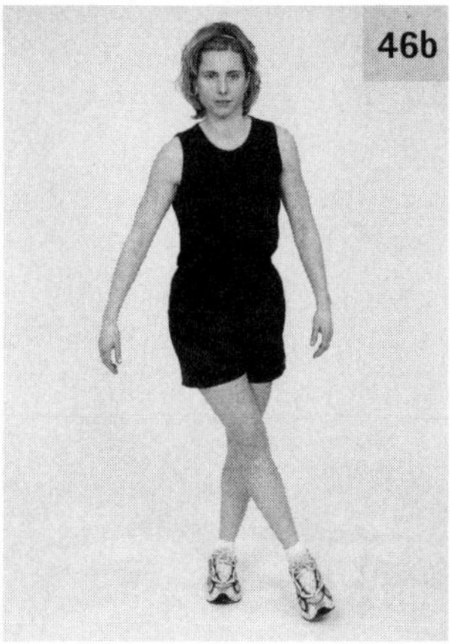

46b

STATIC BALANCE: TRANSVERSE PLANE

47 (BST) TRANSVERSE PLANE BALANCE WITH ARM SWING

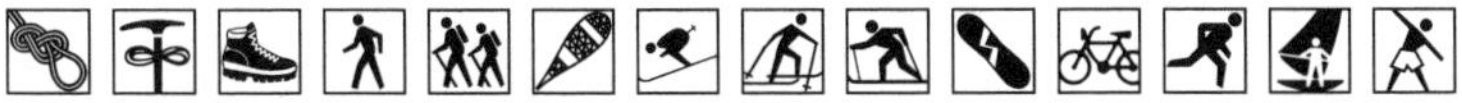

Technique: Balance on one foot with your opposite foot raised or with your opposite toe touching the floor beside your balance foot. Bend your elbows to a 90-degree position and swing them together to the left, then the right, in front of your body (47a and 47b). This will test your ability to balance against a basic rotational challenge.

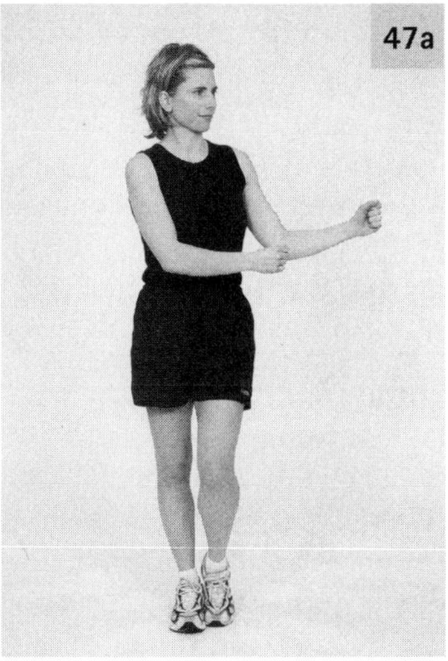

47a

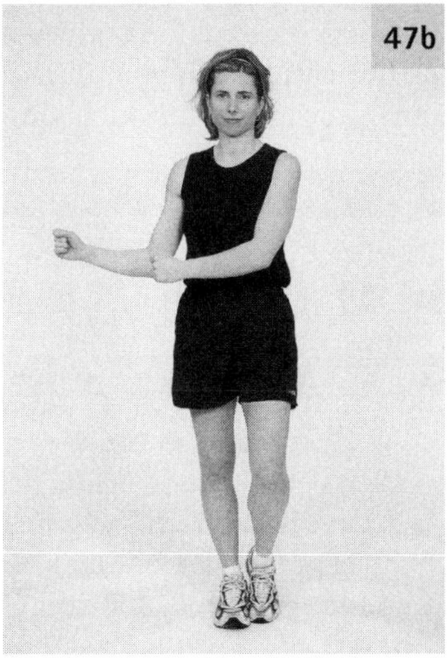

47b

48a

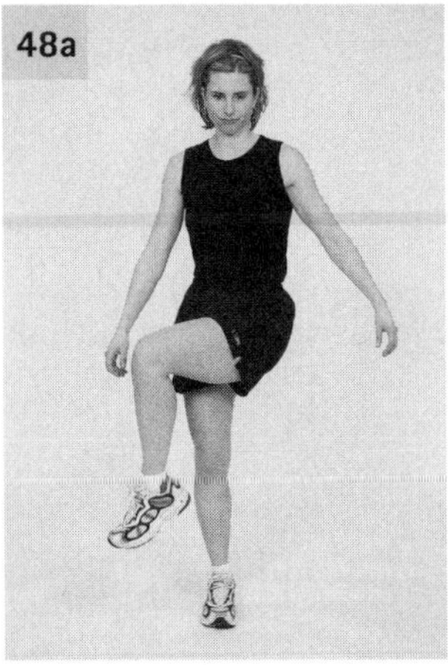

48b

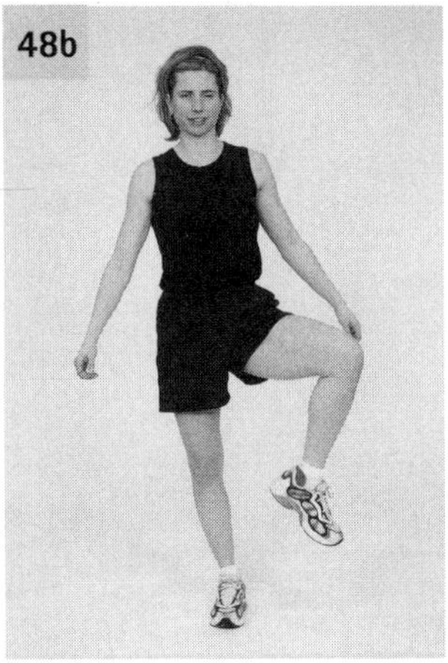

48 (BST) TRANSVERSE PLANE BALANCE WITH OPPOSITE-LEG/ KNEE SWING

Technique: Balance on one foot with your opposite knee raised to hip height. Swing your raised knee to the right, then the left, in controlled smooth motions (48a and 48b). This will test your abilities to balance against a basic transverse plane challenge.

PERIPHERAL BALANCE SELF-TESTS

Equipment: The homemade test vector; measuring tape; and for the arm-reach tests, a pole or a broomstick. A partner is helpful for marking the distances you reach on the test vector and for using the measuring tape for side-to-side comparisons.

Purpose: To test your ability to balance, and balance and reach on one foot compared to the opposite side with challenges in three planes of motion.

Measurement: For leg-reach tests, the distance from the toe of your balance foot to the toe of your reach foot. For arm-reach tests, the distance from the toe of your balance foot to where your fingertips reach along the plane tested. If you have a comparative deficit of 6 inches between sides, use the self-test as an exercise to equalize your balance and reach capacities.

General Technique: Stand in the center of the test vector facing what would be the 12:00 position on the test vector. Keep your balance foot flat on the floor, maintaining its position during all peripheral tests, and don't raise your heel. Reach as far as you can down the test vector with your non-weight-bearing foot and return to the starting position without losing balance.

PERIPHERAL BALANCE: SAGITTAL PLANE

49 (BST) SINGLE-LEG BALANCE AND REACH WITH OPPOSITE FOOT

Technique: Stand in the center of the test vector, facing the 12:00 position with the toes of your balance foot behind the horizontal line. Place your non-weight-bearing reach foot next to, but not touching, your balance foot or leg (49a). Keeping your back straight and bending at your ankle, knee, and hips, reach your non-weight-bearing foot down the sagittal plane vector as far as you can while maintaining control and balance, and without raising your balance foot heel. Touch the tape with your reach toe and maintain that position for 1 full second (49b), then return to the start position in a balanced and controlled fashion. Note your full reach position and mark it on the tape (or have a partner mark it). Do this reach 3 consecutive and successful times and record the farthest successful distance. Perform the test the same way on the opposite foot and compare the results.

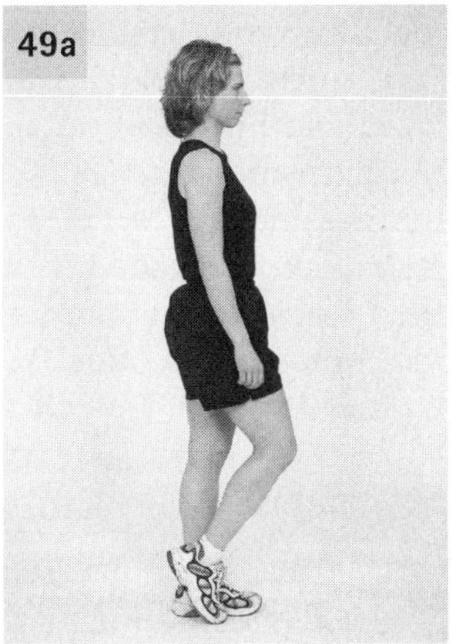
49a

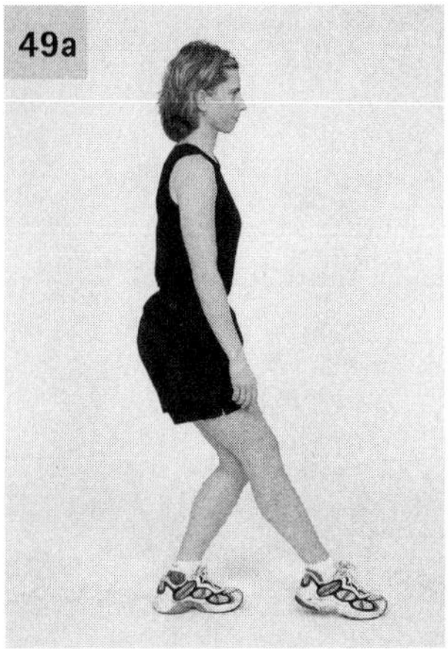
49a

50 (BST) SINGLE-LEG BALANCE AND REACH WITH BOTH ARMS

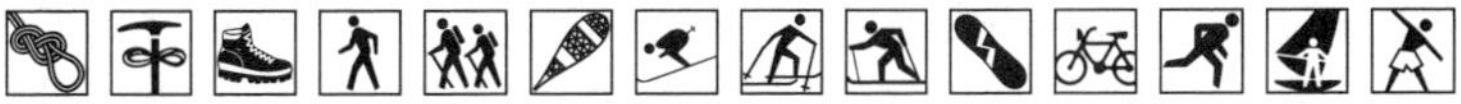

Technique: Stand in the center of the test vector, facing the 12:00 position with the toes of your balance foot behind the horizontal line. Position your non-weight-bearing reach foot next to, but not touching, your balance foot or leg. Keeping your back straight and maintaining slightly bent ankle, knee, and hips, reach both arms down the sagittal plane vector as far as you can at hip height while maintaining control and balance and without raising your balance foot heel. Maintain that position for 1 full second, then return to the start position in a balanced and controlled fashion. Have your partner mark your distance reached with a pole or broomstick. Do this reach 3 consecutive and successful times, and record the farthest successful distance. Perform the test the same way on the opposite foot and compare the results.

PERIPHERAL BALANCE: FRONTAL PLANE

51 (BST) FRONTAL PLANE BALANCE AND REACH WITH OPPOSITE FOOT

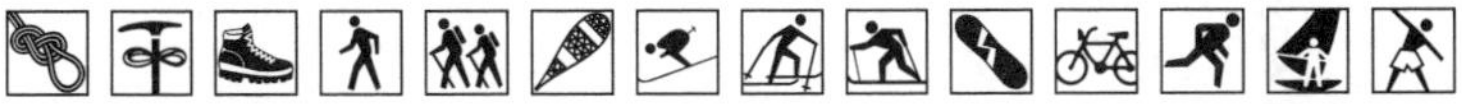

Technique: Stand in the center of the test vector, facing the 12:00 position with the toes of your balance foot behind the horizontal line. Position your non-weight-bearing reach foot next to, but not

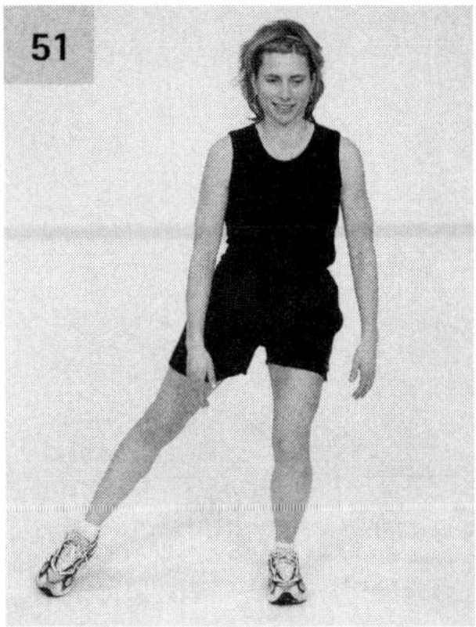
51

touching, your balance foot or leg. Keeping your back straight and your reach foot parallel to your balance foot, bend at your ankle, knee, and hips, and reach your non-weight-bearing foot down the frontal plane vector as far you can while maintaining control and balance and without raising your balance foot heel. Touch the tape with your reach toe and maintain that position for 1 full second, then return to the start position in a balanced and controlled fashion. Note your full reach position and mark it on the tape (or have a partner mark it). Do this reach 3 consecutive and successful times and record the farthest successful distance. Perform the test the same way on the opposite foot and compare the results.

52 (BST) FRONTAL PLANE BALANCE AND REACH WITH BOTH ARMS

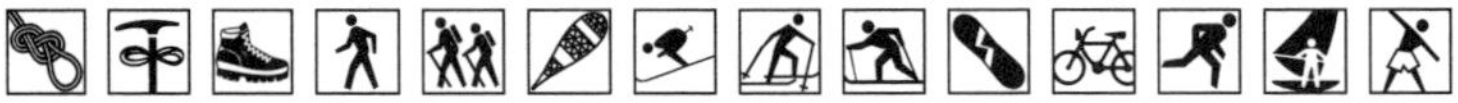

Technique: In this exercise, you measure your ability to balance on each foot while reaching both directions on the frontal plane (90 degrees to your left and 90 degrees to your right). Stand in the center of the test vector, facing the 12:00 position with the toes of your balance foot on the intersection of the horizontal and vertical lines. Position your non-weight-bearing reach foot next to, but not touching, your balance foot or leg. Keeping your back straight and with slightly bent ankle, knee, and hips, reach both arms down the frontal plane vector 90 degrees to your left as far as you can while maintaining control and balance and without raising your balance foot heel. Maintain that position for 1 full second, then return to the start position in a balanced and controlled fashion. Have your partner mark your farthest distance reached with a pole or broomstick. Do this 3 consecutive and successful times and record the farthest successful distance. Perform the test the same way on the same foot, reaching to the right. Then switch balance feet and perform 3 reaches to the left and 3 reaches to the right. Compare the reach distances achieved on one balance foot versus the other.

PERIPHERAL BALANCE: TRANSVERSE PLANE

53 (BST) TRANSVERSE PLANE BALANCE AND REACH WITH OPPOSITE FOOT

Technique: Stand in the center of the test vector, facing the 12:00 position with the toes of your balance foot on the intersection of the horizontal and vertical lines. Position your non-weight-bearing reach foot next to, but not touching, your balance foot or leg. Keeping your back straight and bending at your ankle, knee, and hips, turn your body and your reach foot 90 degrees, and reach down the transverse plane vector as far as you can while maintaining control and balance and without raising your balance foot heel. Touch the tape with your reach toe and maintain that position for 1 full second, then return to the start position in a balanced and controlled fashion. Note your full reach position and mark it on the tape (or have a partner mark it). Do this reach 3 consecutive and successful times and record the farthest successful distance. Perform the test the same way on the opposite foot and compare the results.

DYNAMIC BALANCE SELF-TESTS

Equipment: The homemade test vector, a measuring tape, and a partner to mark and record the measurements.

Purpose: Test and challenge your lunge balance in the three planes of motion.

Measurement: The distance measured from the toe of the fixed foot to the heel of the lunge foot. If you have a comparative deficit of 6 inches between sides, use the self-test as an exercise to equalize your lunge balance capacities in the plane tested.

General Technique: Stand in the center of the test vector with your feet close together but not touching and your toes behind the horizontal line. Let your arms hang normally at your sides and lunge down the test vector with one foot, bending your ankles, knees, and hips, keeping your back upright. The heel of nonlunge (fixed) foot may rise during these tests, but must return to the flat, forward-facing start position upon return from the lunge.

DYNAMIC BALANCE: SAGITTAL PLANE

54 (BST) SAGITTAL PLANE LUNGE

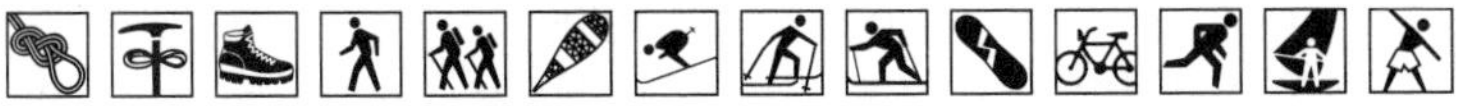

Technique: Stand in the center of the test vector with your feet parallel, your toes behind the horizontal line, and with your arms hanging normally at your sides. Lunge forward down the sagittal plane vector with one foot, bending your ankles, knees, and hips, keeping your back upright. In a safe and controlled fashion, push off your lunge foot and return to the start position behind the line. Perform 3 consecutive lunges on one side safely and in good control, and

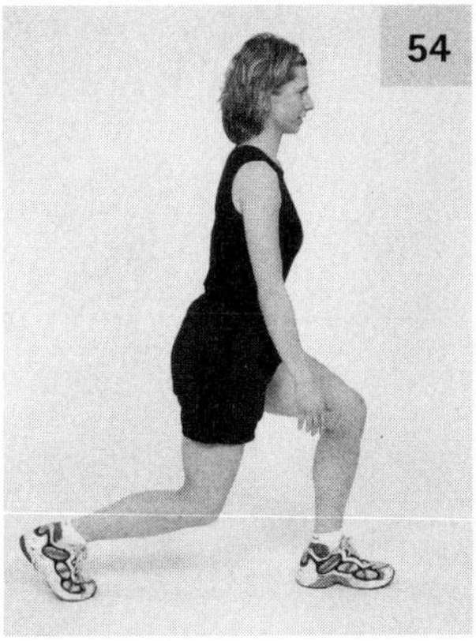

have your partner measure the best distance. Perform this test on the opposite leg in the same fashion and compare the findings.

DYNAMIC BALANCE: FRONTAL PLANE

55 (BST) FRONTAL PLANE LUNGE

Technique: Stand in the center of the test vector with your feet parallel, your toes behind the horizontal line, and with your arms hanging normally at your sides. Lunge down the frontal plane vector 90 degrees to your right with your right foot, keeping the lunge foot parallel to the nonlunge (fixed) foot while bending your ankles, knees, and hips, and keeping your back upright. In a safe and controlled fashion, push off your lunge foot and return to the start position behind the line. Perform 3 consecutive lunges on this side safely and in good control, and have your partner measure the best distance. Perform this test on the opposite leg in the same fashion and compare the findings.

DYNAMIC BALANCE: TRANSVERSE PLANE

56 (BST) TRANSVERSE PLANE LUNGE

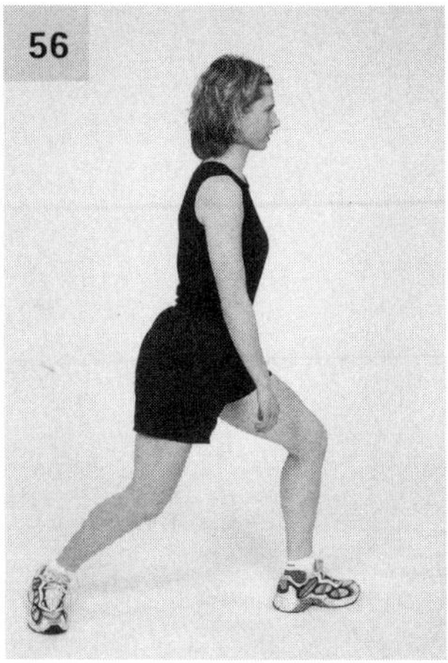
56

Technique: Stand in the center of the test vector with your feet parallel, your toes behind the horizontal line, and with your arms hanging normally at your sides. Rotate your torso 90 degrees to the left, keeping your fixed foot pointing forward, and lunge down the horizontal line with your left foot, turning your lunge foot so that its toes are pointing down the line. In a safe and controlled fashion, push off your lunge foot and return to the start position, with your feet parallel and facing forward. Perform 3 consecutive lunges on this side safely and in good control, and have your partner measure the best distance. Perform this test on the opposite leg in the same fashion and compare the findings.

BALANCE EXERCISES

These exercises are designed to challenge your standing balance and to increase the strength of your trunk, buttocks, and legs. In addition, try outdoor balance exercises in chapter 8, and abdominal Exercises 84 and 85 in chapter 10, which also train balance.

57 SKIER/CLIMBER/CYCLIST/WINDSURFER POSITION HOLDS

Equipment: None.
Purpose: Strengthen your quads, hamstrings, and gluteal muscles in skiing, climbing, and windsurfing positions. Consider doing these within 1 month of starting your activity.

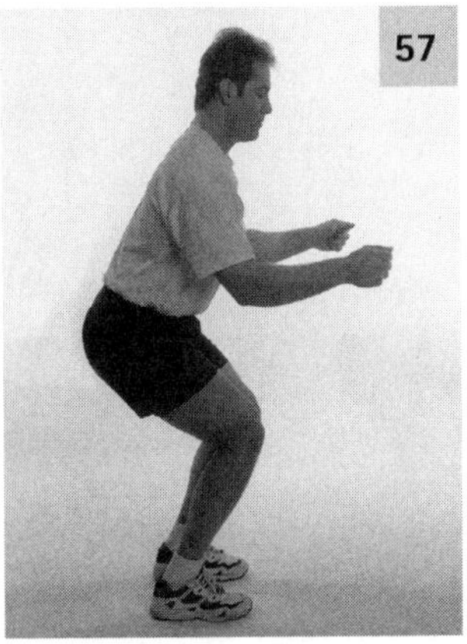

57

Technique: Ski position: Stand in a squat position and position your arms and hands as if you were holding poles. Keep your back from flexing excessively. Hold this position for 30 seconds at first and try to gradually work your way up to 2–3 minutes. If you can only hold it for 30 seconds before fatiguing, then try to return to this position 5 or more times for 30 seconds.
Variations: 57.1. Downhill knee oscillations: When you get into the skiing position, try slightly dropping down into your knees (flexing), then slightly extending them in a rhythmical pattern (bouncing) as if skiing. Also try weight-shifting from your left to your right leg rhythmically. Try this on a foam half roll (flat side up) to challenge your balance. **57.2.** Cross-country position holds and weight shifts: For cross-country skiing, try getting into a turning position and try weight-shifting from your right to your left leg. **57.3.** Telemark lunge position holds: For telemark skiing, try all of the above in a telemark position (a lunge). When in the telemark position with your right foot in front, move your hands and rotate your trunk toward your left knee for 10 seconds, then go back to the starting position. After 60 seconds, reverse your leg position. **57.4.** Climber position holds: For climbing, assume a position on a climbing wall or against a regular wall with legs farther than

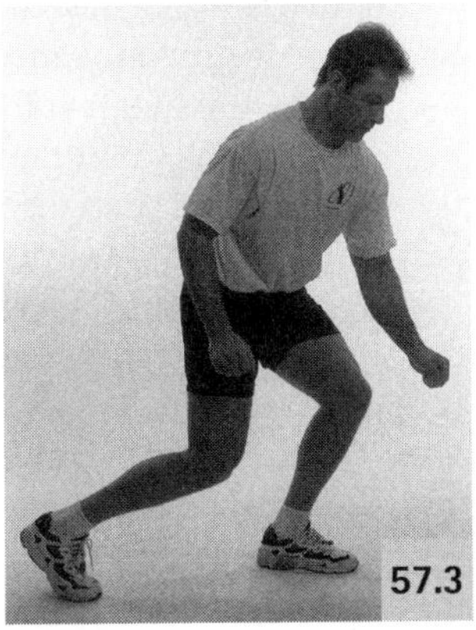

57.3

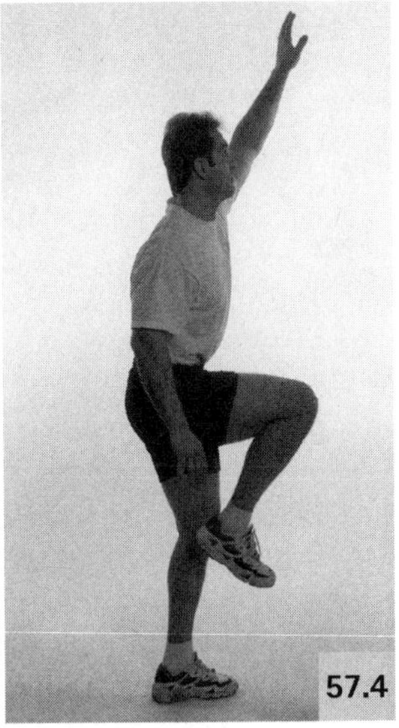

57.4

shoulder-width apart. Try your feet in various positions, including parallel or perpendicular to the wall. Put your hands at varying heights. From this position, try weight-shifting from foot to foot or slight bobbing motions in your knees. This could also be done in a gym while holding two overhead pulleys at different heights above your head and with different weight resistance. You can also do the climber's variation while standing on a foam roll. **57.5.** Cycling position holds: For cycling, get into a lunge position as if you are on a bike going down a hill. Bounce slightly in this position for about 30–45 seconds. **57.6.** Windsurfer position holds: For windsurfing, get into your board position. From there try weight-shifting from your left to right foot with a rhythmical side-to-side squat.
Precaution: This exercise can aggravate kneecap pain problems.

58 ARM AND LEG BALANCE AND REACH

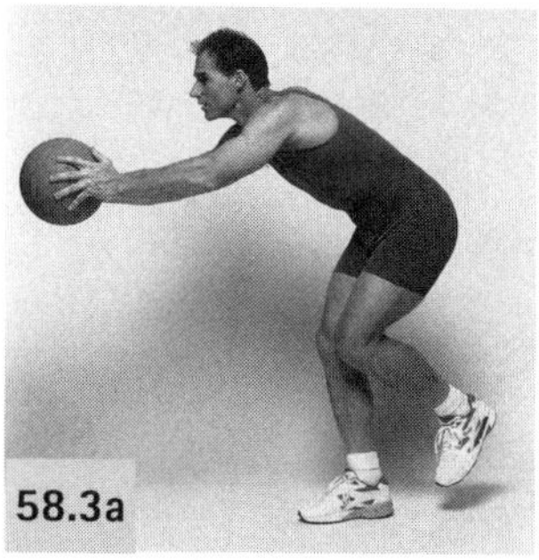
58.3a

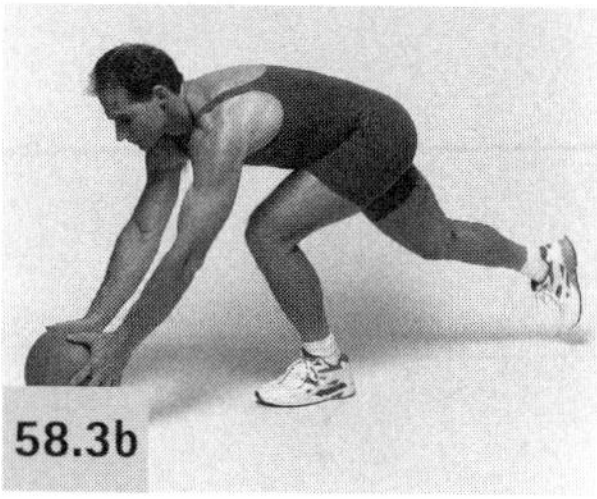
58.3b

Equipment: None.
Purpose: Emphasize balance and strengthening of your gluteal and hamstring muscles, posterior trunk, abdominals, shoulders, arms, and neck.

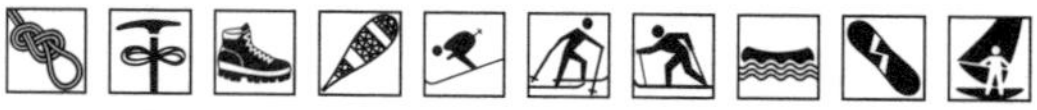

Technique: Start with your feet shoulder-width apart and your knees slightly bent. Position your hands in front of your body and at waist height with your elbows straight. Start your forward reach by bending at your hips, keeping your back slightly arched. Reach forward approximately 6 inches, then return to your start position. Keep your reaches pain-free and move with good control. To monitor your progress, assume your starting position, with your fingertips touching a wall. While maintaining this position, back up 6 inches from the wall without changing your posture. Reach and touch your fingertips to the wall. As you become more successful at this distance, increase the speed of your reach before increasing the distance. You can also hold a ball while performing this exercise. Try 5–10 reps initially, then progress to 1–2 sets of 12–15 reps.
Variations: 58.1. 45-degree angle reach: Reach not only forward but also at 45 degrees to the right and then to the left. **58.2.** Frontal plane wall reach: Stand on one leg with your knee slightly bent, approximately 1–$1\frac{1}{2}$ feet from a wall; reach overhead and touch the wall at imaginary 12:00, 10:00, and 2:00 positions. Do 12–15 touches and then switch the standing leg. **58.3.** Bent knee reach: Try the main version of Exercise 58 while balancing on one leg with your knee slightly bent (58.3a). Counterbalance reach: You can start with your other leg behind you for counterbalance, but then progress to plac-

ing your raised foot next to your standing foot. Try reaching down toward the floor with a ball or weight (58.3b). Opposite leg counter-balance reach: Switch to your other foot after 30–60 seconds. If you have had knee problems, do this with a bent knee. **58.4.** Bilateral balance with foam roll: Try doing the main version of Exercise 58 while standing with both feet on a foam half roll or with one foot on the roll.

Tips and Precautions: Start with no resistance and control your body weight first. Avoid this exercise if you have a back problem, unless you are supervised by a physical therapist or a physician.

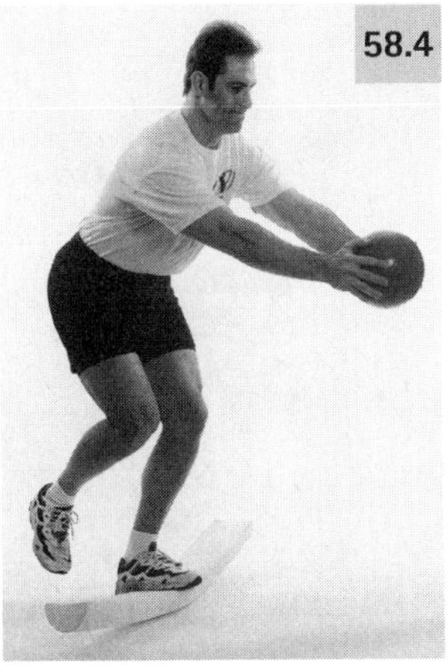
58.4

59 CLOCK LEG REACH

Equipment: None.

Purpose: Emphasize balance and strengthen your gluteal, hamstring, and trunk muscles. This is a good, basic balance drill.

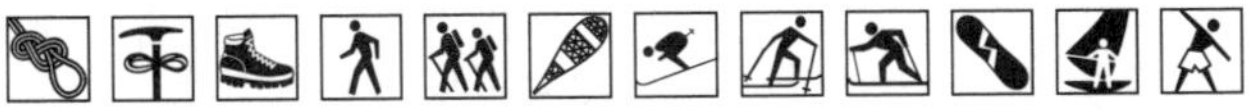

Technique: Make believe you are in the center of a large clock. Balance on your left leg and bend your knee slightly. Initiate a single-leg squat with your standing leg, squatting enough to touch the toes of your other foot to the ground in the 10:00 position; do 2 mini squats and toe touches. Then do the same at the 11:00 position, and then touch around the clock until your right foot gets to the 7:00 position. After you have mastered the basic exercise, try placing your toe touch randomly to do quick directional changes. For example, try this sequence: 12:00, 4:00, 11:00, 5:00, 1:00, 7:00. For an extra challenge, have a partner call positions out randomly. Switch to standing on your right leg and repeat the sequence in the opposite direction. Each time around the clock on a leg is 1 set. Perform 2–3 sets on each leg.

Variations: 59.1. Leg and arms reach: To make this more challenging, add a reaching motion with both of your arms in the same direction as the motion of your toe-touching foot. **59.2.** Weighted reach: Reach with a free weight or medicine ball to increase the challenge. **59.3.** Foam roll reach: Do this exercise while standing on a foam half roll.

Tips: Progress this exercise initially by increasing the speed and randomness of your toe touch before increasing the distance. Add the arm reach when you feel comfortable with the random toe touching.

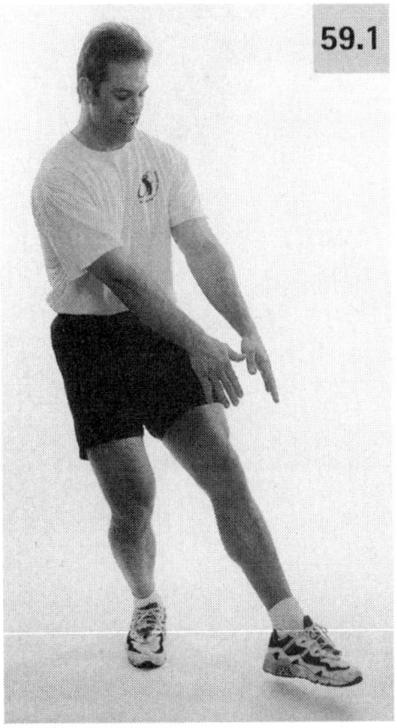
59.1

60 SINGLE-LEG STANCE UPPER-EXTREMITY CHOPPING PATTERN

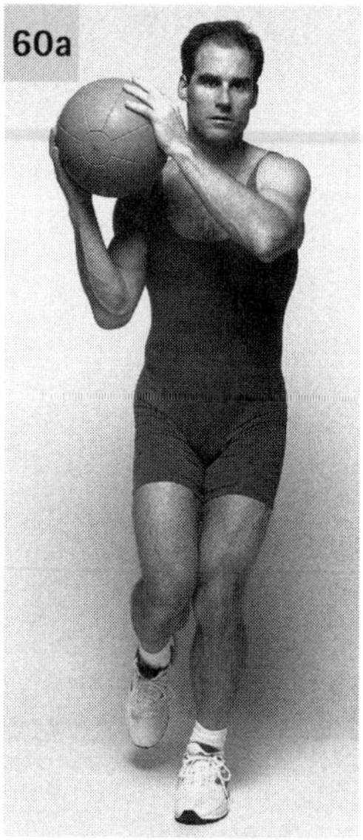

60a

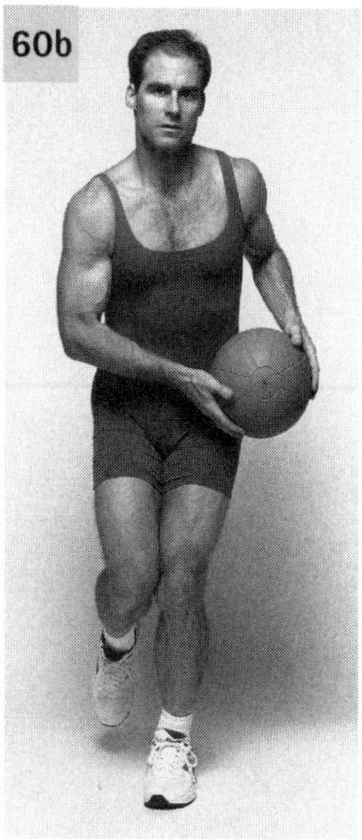

60b

Equipment: Medicine ball or free weight.
Purpose: Emphasize balance and strengthening of your leg, trunk, shoulders, and neck.

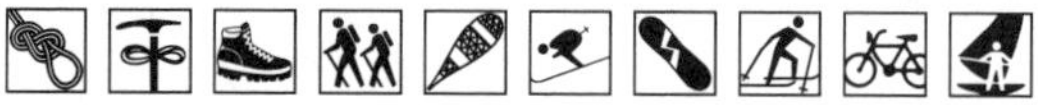

Technique: Balance on your left leg with your knee slightly bent. Hold a medicine ball or a free weight above your right shoulder (60a), and move it toward your left hip (60b) and then back to an overhead position. Stabilize your spine with the movement by tightening your abdominals and minimizing the amount of spinal movement. As you become familiar with this exercise, you can incorporate more spine and hip motion. After doing a set of 12–15 reps, repeat the sequence but start with the weight over your left shoulder while standing on your right leg and bring it to your right hip.
Variation: 60.1. Chopping pattern with hip flexion: Try bringing your right hip and knee toward your hands. Do this with an ankle weight to increase your hip flexion work, for climbing, telemark skiing, and snowshoeing. For water sports, do this sitting in an appropriate position without moving your hips.
Tip: This exercise is designed to improve your balance, so try to avoid contacting the ground with the lifted, nonbalance foot.

61 SINGLE-LEG BALL TOSS

Equipment: Small to medium-size lightweight ball.
Purpose: Challenge your balance quickly and in multiple directions.

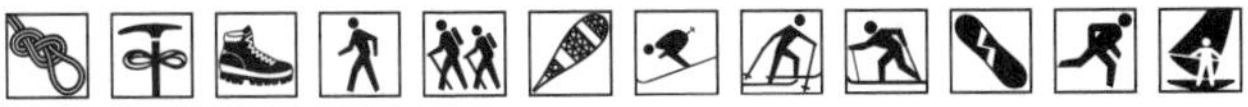

Technique: Stand on one foot with your knee slightly bent. Sagittal plane ball toss: If you have a partner, ask him or her to throw you the ball, initially directly to you at your chest level (61a). Transverse plane ball toss: Catch the ball with both hands (61b). When this is easy and you are not too wobbly, ask your partner to throw the ball to you anywhere in a half circle from the 9:00 to 3:00 positions (61c). You can do this exercise by yourself by throwing the ball against a wall.
Variation: 61.1. Unstable surface ball toss: For an increased challenge, stand on a half foam roll or ankle balance equipment as found in health clubs.
Precautions: Be careful with this exercise if you have had a knee injury. Don't rotate excessively on a fixed foot to catch the ball. Always feel free to put your other foot down if the ball is thrown poorly.

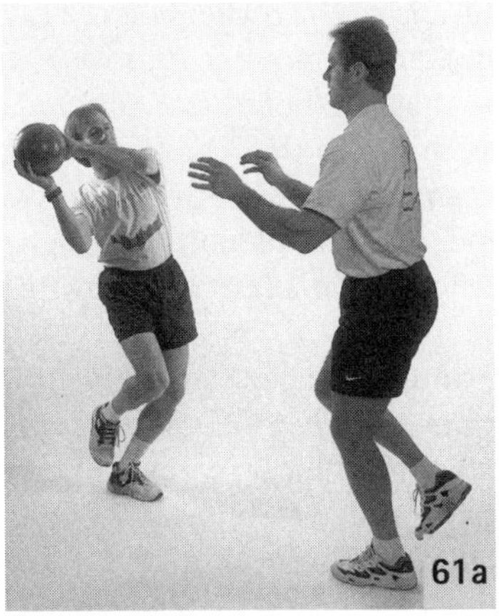
61a

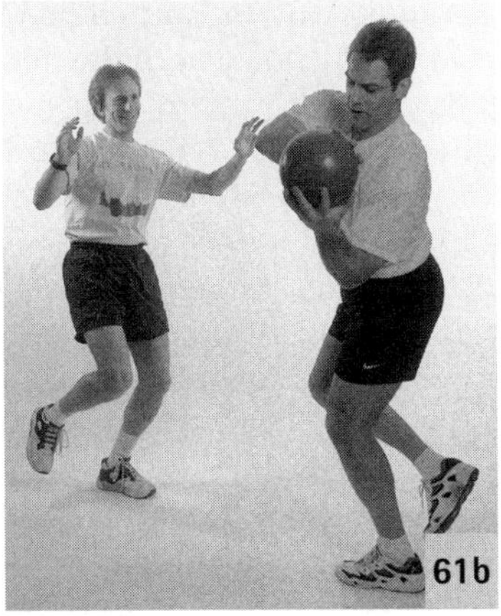
61b

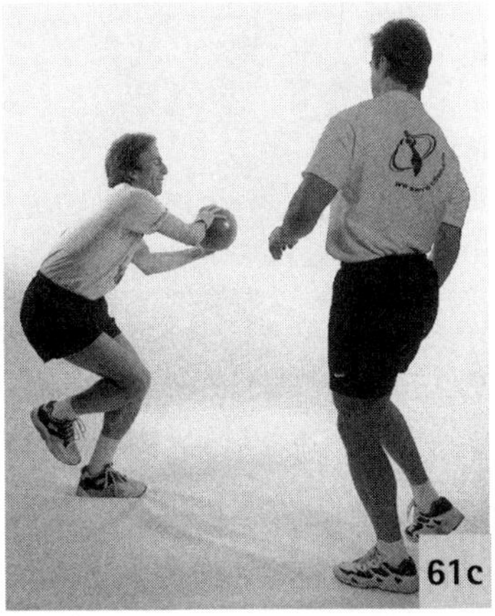
61c

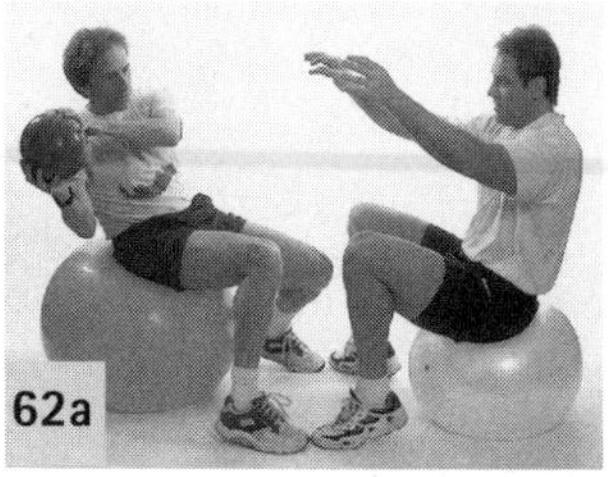
62a

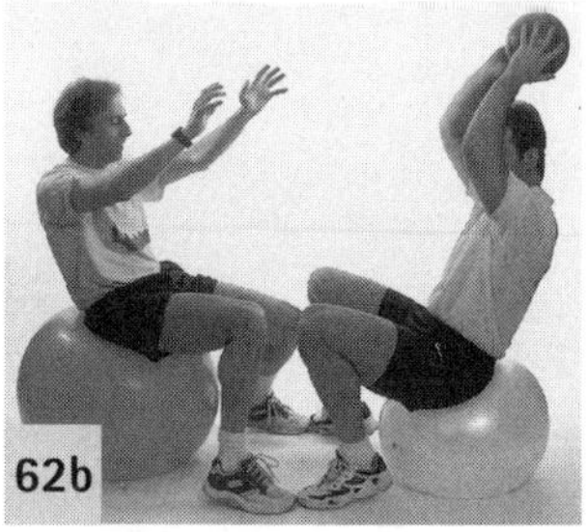
62b

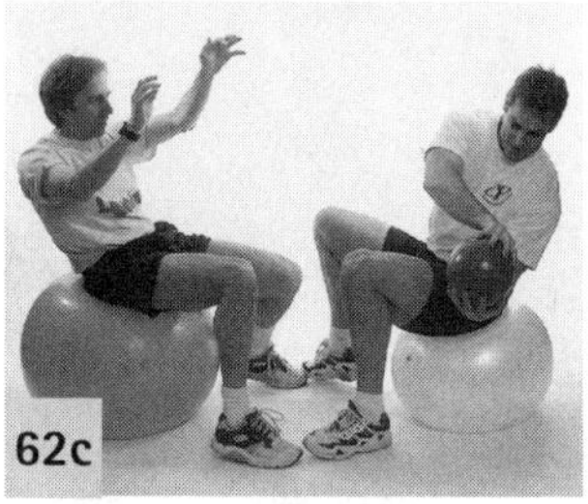
62c

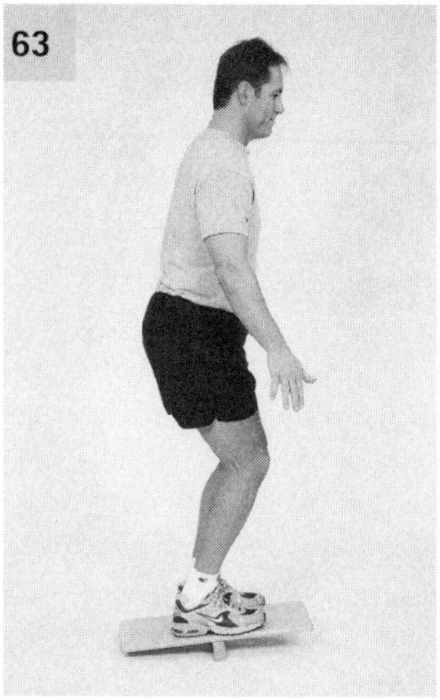
63

62 SITTING BALL TOSS

Equipment: Physioball to sit on, small ball or medicine ball to throw.
Purpose: Improve sitting balance and strengthen your abdominals for boat and cycling activities.

Technique: Sit on a Physioball with your toes just touching the ground. Face a partner or the wall (62a). Throw the ball in multiple directions to your partner so that he or she has to move forward, to the side, or overhead to catch it (62b and 62c). Try to keep a minimum amount of weight on your toes. To increase the challenge, catch the ball with both hands.

BALANCE EQUIPMENT EXERCISES

63 ROCKER BOARD SAGITTAL PLANE STATIC BALANCE

Equipment: Rocker board.
Purpose: Improve your ability to balance in a sagittal plane.

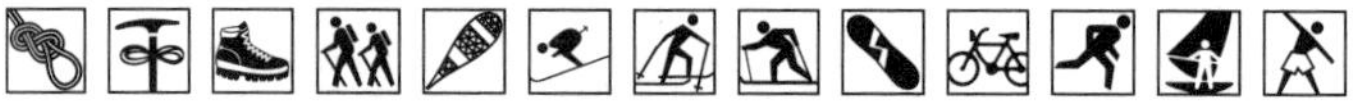

Technique: Position yourself on the middle of the rocker board with your feet perpendicular to the fulcrum. Start by moving your weight slightly forward, toward your toes, so that the board tips forward. Then transfer your weight toward your heels so that the board tips backward (photo 63). Now try to maintain the board perfectly in the middle, controlling the motion with your abdominal, buttock, thigh, and leg muscles. Now try to include a slow, then a faster, arm swing forward and backward.
Variation: 63.1. Sagittal plane balance and reach: Now try doing BST Exercise 50 on the rocker board, balancing on one foot and reaching down the sagittal plane (forward) with the other. Be careful to engage your core and to move in a slow, controlled fashion.
Precaution: The balance and reach variation should not be done if you have an active back problem.

64 ROCKER BOARD FRONTAL PLANE STATIC BALANCE

Equipment: Rocker board.
Purpose: Improve your frontal plane balance abilities.

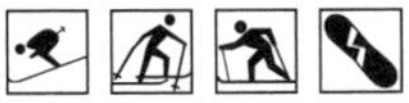

Technique: Position yourself sideways, with your feet on the end of the rocker board so that your feet are facing in the same direction as the fulcrum. Slightly flex your knees and ankles (see photo 64). Do a weight transfer so that the board moves first to the left and then to the right, and then try to maintain your balance in the middle for about 10 seconds. Now try to include a side-to-side arm swing or hold a weight in one hand.
Variation: 64.1. Frontal plane balance and reach: Try BST Exercise 51 while standing on the rocker board, balancing on one foot and reaching down the frontal plane (to one side) with the other. This is an excellent exercise for snowboarders and skiers.
Precaution: Avoid the balance and reach variation if you have an active back problem.

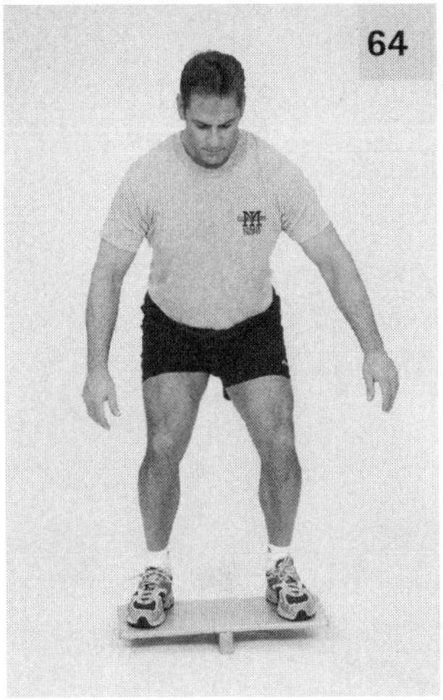

64

65 WOBBLE BOARD STATIC MULTIPLANAR CHALLENGE

Equipment: Wobble board.
Purpose: Challenge and improve balance in all planes.

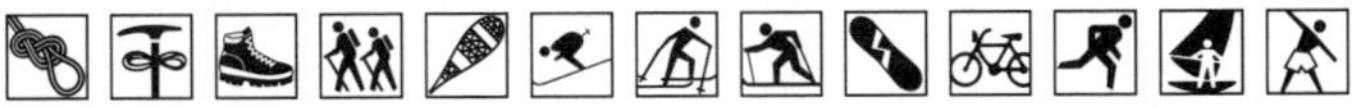

Technique: Stand on the wobble board, placing your feet on the outside borders with your knees and hips flexed slightly. Weight-shift onto your right foot slightly, then your left foot, then toward your toes, and then toward your heels. Then roll on the wobble board, shifting your weight to create a circular motion.
Variation: 65.1. Wobble board squat: Try a basic squat while you maintain your balance so that you don't allow the side of the board to touch the floor. Do this slowly at first and then speed it up.
Precaution: If you have an acute ankle, knee, or hip injury, avoid this exercise for 3–4 weeks.

EXERCISE 66 67 68 69

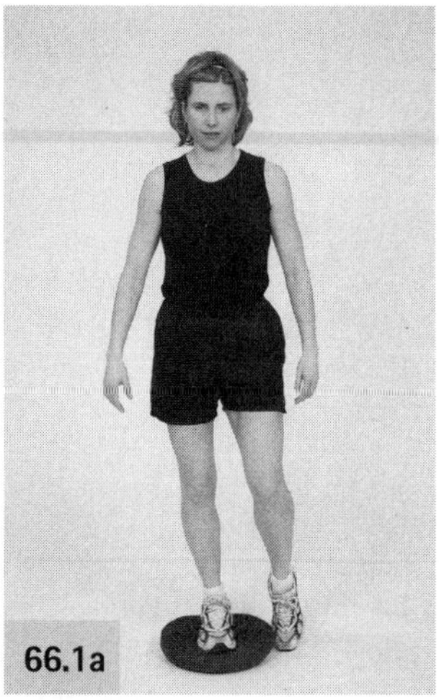

66.1a

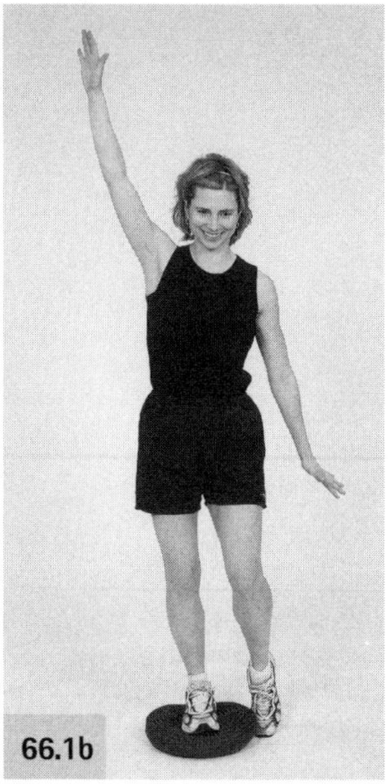

66.1b

66 DISC PILLOW STATIC BALANCE

Equipment: Disc pillow.
Purpose: Challenge and improve your balance in all three planes on a low-cost, unstable device.

Technique: Stand on a disc pillow with both feet. Once you feel relatively stable, try doing a forward and backward arm swing as in BST Exercise 42. You can then try a side-to-side arm swing (BST Exercise 45) or a rotary arm swing (BST Exercise 47).
Variation: 66.1. Disc pillow ceiling-floor reach: Start by standing on the disc pillow with only your right foot. Have your left foot touching the floor with your toes only (66.1a). Once you have your balance, try simultaneously reaching for the ceiling with your right hand and the floor with your left hand (66.1b). Continue this exercise by alternating your ceiling-to-floor reach directions.

67 BOSU BALL SQUAT

Equipment: Bosu ball.
Purpose: Challenge your balance in all three planes of motion while performing static or dynamic exercise variations.

Technique: Stand on the Bosu ball with your feet slightly off-center and your knees slightly bent. Engage your core, flex at your hips slightly, and lower yourself in a pain-free and controlled motion into a squat. You can use your hands to balance by stretching them out in front of you. A weighted ball adds to the challenge. Return to the starting position maintaining good balance and control throughout the squat. Try 5–10 of these.

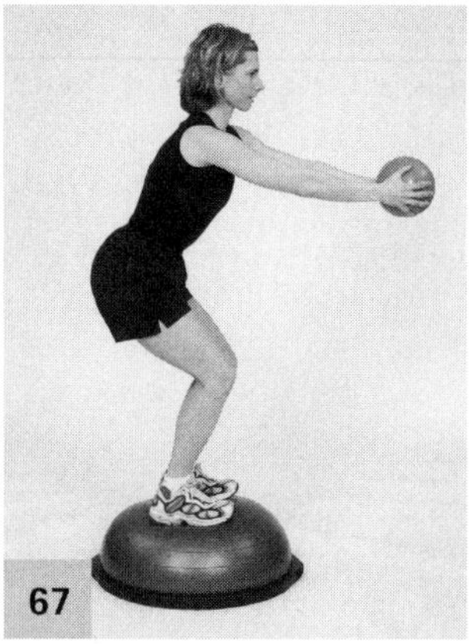

67

68 THE FITTER SKIING AND FRONTAL PLANE DYNAMIC BALANCE

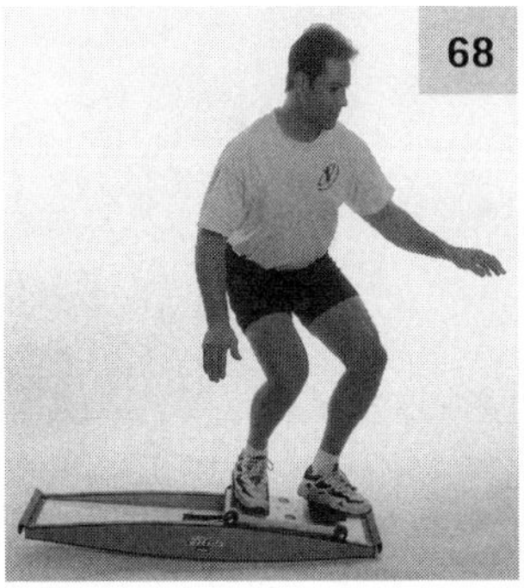

Equipment: The Fitter and ski poles.
Purpose: Simulate skiing and snowboarding motions to improve your dynamic frontal plane strength and balance.

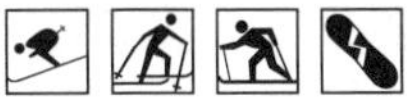

Technique: Carefully stand on the Fitter's platform with both feet. Get into a ski-ready position, with hips and knees flexed and your buttocks counterbalancing you. Go from a flexed-knee position and quickly rise up and shift your weight to the right side of the Fitter, ending in a ski-ready position. Then quickly push off and move to the left side of the Fitter, and end in a ski-ready position. Continue this until you feel some leg fatigue.

69 BODY BLADE SINGLE-LEG MULTIPLANAR CHALLENGE

Equipment: Body Blade.
Purpose: Improve your balance in all planes of motion by externally challenging your core to react quickly to rapidly changing arm motions.

Technique: Grasp the Body Blade handle by lacing your fingers together with the thin edge of the blade facing you. Stand on your left foot and toe-touch the ground with your right foot. Activate your core muscles. Move the blade about $1\frac{1}{2}$ feet away from you with your elbows bent about 45 degrees. Oscillate the Body Blade side to side while maintaining your balance. Once you can do this with your toe touching, lift your left foot off the floor completely. Perform this same exercise on the other foot.

chapter 7 TRAINING CONCEPTS, CONDITIONING GOALS, AND PROGRAM PLANNING

By Carl Petersen, P.T., and Darcy Norman, P.T., A.T.C., C.S.C.S.

THIS CHAPTER WILL HELP YOU:

- Set goals and evaluate your progress.
- Become familiar with smart training principles.
- Understand how to plan the progression of your conditioning program based on your time and scheduling (periodization of training).
- Understand principles of energy sequencing training.
- Learn principles and sequencing of strength training.
- Learn recovery techniques to facilitate training.
- Use a daily log and monthly calendar to plan and evaluate your progress.

If you have a particular physical or activity goal, designing a training program can aid you in achieving it. Physical training is very specific, producing physiological adaptations in the musculoskeletal and cardiorespiratory systems that progress if you are giving your body the proper gradual training stimulus. You will benefit the most from this chapter if you have read chapters 3 and 5. If you have any musculoskeletal or medical conditions that may limit your exercise, consult a physician before embarking on a training program.

GOALS

Goals for conditioning should be realistic and reasonable in light of the time you have available, your body frame, your age, and any medical conditions you have. Conditioning goals should also be a good fit with the goals you have for the other parts of your life. Try to set specific goals for your aerobic and strength training, as well as for flexibility, agility, balance, and skill development. Goals for conditioning may not be achieved for many reasons. The following are some tips to help you achieve your fitness goals:

- Give yourself adequate time to prepare for your activity.
- Assess equipment you have available before planning.
- Make a program based on equipment that is easily accessible.
- Be thorough in your planning.
- Keep track of evaluation numbers and objective numbers that will show you progress.
- Focus on good technique while exercising.
- Take any necessary precautions or time to take care of any injury or conditions that may hinder your training activity.
- Plan out all your sets and reps so you know what you are doing before you do it.
- Be as specific as possible; it will make your program that much easier to follow.
- Give yourself adequate time to recover from exercise sessions.

When assessing your goals, make sure to have long- and short-term goals for every aspect of your training program. First, start with your activity goals. Identify the most difficult parts of your activity and when you would like to achieve them. Then, plan to develop your flexibility, balance, agility, strength, and aerobic goals to meet the overall activity demands. Next, modify your program to meet the most difficult demands during a particular part of the season. If there is a particular challenge associated with the activity, use an exercise (or design your own) to prepare to meet that challenge using the periodization technique described later in this chapter.

This chapter and the activity chapters in Part III should give you a base of information to help you along the way. You need to set realistic objectives, allow enough time, and evaluate your progress.

Are Your Objectives Reasonable?

Your objectives are the action elements that help you achieve your goal. They need to be well defined. For aerobic training, you should know what, how much, at what intensity, and for how long you will be training. For strength training, you should know what number of sets, reps, and amount of resistance to use. Write them down ahead of time and be as specific as possible so that on the day of your activity, you don't have to do any significant planning or decision making. Of course, you can modify things depending on how you feel when you are working out.

How Much Time Will It Take?

The amount of time it takes to achieve your goals depends on your present level of fitness and skill, as well as your build, present health, age, equipment available, and quality of your program planning. If you already have a base of aerobic and strength fitness, you may be able to move into the second stage of a program quickly. If not, you will likely have to spend a minimum of 4–6 weeks building that base.

Most activities that have a long race or a high-endurance component, such as a marathon or a 2-day mountaineering climb, can require 3 or more months of preparation. In order to finish a race, you have to be quite close to doing the race distance in your workouts a few weeks prior to the race. Many activities take a minimum of 2 months of preparation, such as a difficult run or telemark skiing, downhill skiing, rock climbing, or glacial mountaineering.

Shorter-duration goals can take less time. The average person could be ready within a month for a full day of hiking. Evaluate your progress before undertaking difficult activities. If you try an activity before you are ready, you will be more susceptible to injury or to not completing the activity. As a rough estimate, figure that you will increase aerobic distances by 10–15% per week and will need to achieve at least half to three-fourths of the distance of your goal. You should be able to simulate most of the moves requiring strength and balance numerous times and under various conditions.

Evaluating Your Progress

Evaluating your progress means many things. Are you doing what you had planned? Is it enough or too much? Modify your plans depending on your outcomes. How will you measure your progress? You can use measuring devices such as simply doing what you set out to do, or you can quantify the ease and time it takes you to accomplish an aerobic activity.

For your aerobic component, have a sport-specific activity that you do intermittently to judge your effort, time, and how you feel in general. This could be a 30-mile bike ride with hills, a 4- to 6-mile run, a 6- to 8-mile moderately steep hike, and so on. This activity should be the same or directly related to your goal activity. If it is getting easier or it takes you less time to do it, you are making progress. You could also use an indoor aerobic activity to see if you can accomplish the same intensity and duration of activity with less effort.

In evaluating your strength, use your progress in increasing the weight or resistance on particular exercises. For functional exercises, see how many reps you can do in 45 seconds. You can also use a functional measurement; for example, how much effort it takes to lift something such as a full pack, your ease of performing a climbing move, or the effort required to maneuver your boat in rough conditions.

Overtraining

Being smart about your training means recognizing nonadaptive responses to training such as prolonged fatigue, poor endurance, elevated resting heart rate, sleep disturbances, frequent infections, and pain.

Occasionally exercise and outdoor or other sporting activities can be done to such an extent that your body cannot adapt well. In the early stages of excessive training, you might have some mild fatigue and decreased stamina or performance. You may initially have more overuse injuries involving the musculoskeletal system, such as tendonitis or stress fractures. If excessive training continues, you might develop all of the symptoms and signs of overtraining syndrome, including increased muscle soreness, greater susceptibility to minor illnesses, decreased appetite, decreased motivation, poor performance, fatigue, and possibly a fast resting heart rate.

Establish a baseline for your resting heart rate by checking your pulse when you first wake up. Keep a chart to make sure your resting heart rate is not elevating more than 7–10 beats per minute above your baseline during your training. If you have an elevated resting heart rate or have a persistence of any of the above symptoms, you may be overtraining.

Short-duration fatigue is common and can be associated with long exercise days, temporary illness, high altitude, and so on. Prolonged fatigue, especially with the other symptoms, is something to be concerned about. If these symptoms occur, cut back on your training schedule by decreasing the duration and intensity of your exercise. Take a number of rest days. Try to decrease your regular aerobic session to 40 minutes or less. Eliminate interval training for at least a few weeks. As you get back to your regular exercise, try to schedule no-exercise or light-exercise days after heavy days such as interval training, long-day activities, or 3 consecutive aerobic days. Avoid exercising 7 days a week. Try to get adequate rest and adequate nutrition. Try to decrease stress in the rest of your life.

COMPONENTS OF A CONDITIONING PROGRAM

Proper Warm-Up

A 5- to 10-minute warm-up should precede your workout. See chapter 4 and the activity chapters in Part III for more details.

Flexibility Goals

Maintaining flexibility is an important goal, especially as we get older. Hips, knees, and ankles are key areas. Static and active stretching can be done with every workout, even if only briefly. If you have had an injury or an arthritic condition, you may decide to devote more time to your flexibility program. Stretching is best done after a warm-up or at the end of your workout.

Strength Training Goals

Strength training is now recommended for every individual as a part of a minimum conditioning program. In addition to a basic strength program, you can design exercises to build specific strength for your activities to allow you to do them with less effort and less likelihood of injuries.

Agility and Balance

Establish agility and balance goals, especially if you are kayaking, boulder hopping, skiing, snowboarding, windsurfing, climbing, or over 60 and wish to prevent injuries. For this you can do short periods of balance and agility activities 2–3 times a week and gradually increase the challenges. (See chapters 6 and 8, as well as the activity chapters in Part III, for more details on exercises.)

Aerobic Stamina Goals

Aerobic endurance should be developed before anaerobic high-intensity interval endurance. A solid base of aerobic endurance facilitates recovery and allows training at higher intensity levels. A solid aerobic base will help improve anaerobic and strength training because it promotes faster recovery.

If you do aerobic stamina training more than 4 days a week, alternate hard and easy days. This is necessary because hard days deplete muscle glycogen, which takes 48 hours to replenish. Hard days are those of interval training, races, or longer-duration aerobic activity.

The minimum aerobic program in chapter 3 will help you achieve basic health benefits. You may increase your aerobic endurance by training at lower intensities for longer duration (LILD), for example at 50–65% max HR, to be able to do longer-duration activities (see chapter 3).

Gradually increasing your duration by 10–20% per week can get you to the endurance you will need. Add brief intervals of high-intensity training to improve your ability to do short bursts of difficult, high-intensity activity if you have first built your aerobic base with 4–6 weeks of basic low- to moderate-intensity training. See chapter 3 for interval training details.

Proper Cooldown

Cool down at the end of your aerobic workout by gradually decreasing your level of intensity for 2–5 minutes. See chapter 3 for details.

PERIODIZING YOUR CONDITIONING PROGRAM

Periodization is the process of structuring and planning training programs around blocks of time to provide optimum performance at a required time. This is done by dividing up the time available for training into smaller, more manageable periods of training with specific objectives in each segment. Periodization is appropriate if you are conditioning to prepare for a season of moderate- to high-level activity or a particular event such as a race or a climb. You can also use these concepts to guide you in progressing your fitness program.

One-month blocks of time work well when setting up the periodization plan, as this allows a gradual increase in training volume over the first 3 weeks of the cycle, followed by 1 week with decreased volume. The 3-week buildup positively stresses your body and the 1 week of decreased volume allows for recovery and adaptation to the imposed physiological demands. This improves overall conditioning.

Ideally, your training plan should be divided into phases or periods. The length of each phase depends on the amount of time you can devote to training. The periods are:

Phase A: General preparation or aerobic base building

Phase B: Intensity building

Phase C: Sport- or activity-specific fitness

Phase D: Maintenance, competition, or time of maximum activity participation

Phase E: Recovery and active rest period

If you have a certain amount of time in which to reach your activity goal, then divide your time between the first three periods (phases A–C) in preparation for your activity. Periodization allows you to move from general activities to more sport-specific conditioning one phase at a time. Using this system optimizes your physical skills, leading to faster adaptations, improved performance, and decreased injury potential.

Phase A: General Preparation Period (Aerobic Base Building)

Phase A is approximately the first one-third of a training program. It can last 4–12 weeks, depending on how many training activity goals you have. Generally, this period lasts 6–8 weeks. The objectives of this phase are to improve flexibility, stamina (general aerobic endurance conditioning), general strength endurance, and coordination.

In this phase, most of your aerobic training is of low to moderate intensity, and you don't do any interval training until possibly the end of this period. Build up your aerobic sessions to a duration of 30–50 minutes at 60–75% max HR for 4–6 sessions a week. During this phase, 60–70% of your time is devoted to aerobic endurance training.

Perform your strength training with higher reps (15) and lower weight (resistance). You can build up the resistance gradually at about 5–10% per week, or as your strength improvements allow. During this phase, plan on strength training each body region approximately 3 times per week. A general whole-body strength workout is recommended, and it does not have to be very sport-specific. You could do a short period of balance exercises toward the end of this period if you do an activity requiring a moderate amount of balance.

Phase B: Intensity Period (Increasing Exercise Volume)

This period lasts from 4–12 weeks, with an average of 4–6 weeks for most of the activities described in this book. The general objectives of this phase include improving specific stamina and increasing maximum strength. This stage involves a greater volume (number of hours and caloric output) of exercise and more aerobic, moderate- to high-intensity work.

To maintain your aerobic base, devote about 50–60% of your time to low- to moderate-intensity aerobic endurance activities, including LILD activities. Gradually increase your 1-day-a-week LILD workout. Do 5 other aerobic sessions per week. These should be sport-specific activities with 2 sessions lasting 40–50 minutes. You may wish to include a cross training session 1 time each week. Two of your aerobic sessions could incorporate interval training if your activity requires brief high-intensity periods—such as for climbing, mountaineering, scrambling, snowshoeing, cross-country or telemark skiing, paddle sports, cycling, running, or windsurfing.

Initially start with 30- to 120-second intervals of 2–5 repetitions at moderate intensity. Gradually increase the number (progressing to 8 intervals), duration (some intervals to 3–4 minutes), and resistance (grade of hill, rough water, etc.) of your intervals. Remember to avoid excessive-speed workouts to avoid overtraining or injuries early in the season. You may try some short races if your activity goal involves racing.

Focus more on strengthening exercises pertinent and functional to your activity; do some sets with 12–15 reps and some with decreased reps (4–8) and increased weight to improve maximum strength. Add appropriate functional strength training to the rest of your strength workout during this period.

Phase C: Sport-Specific Fitness Period

Phase C is approximately the final third of the training program and is 4–8 weeks long. The general objectives of this phase are to build stamina and strength particular to your activity and to improve skill and coordination.

About 40–50% of the training time should be in aerobic, LILD workouts if you will be doing an activity requiring long-duration aerobic stamina. Consider some cross training to avoid boredom and overuse. Decrease total training volume during this phase. You can continue the interval training, but add higher-intensity and shorter intervals and some with more resistance (hills), if applicable.

Your strength training should include some functional exercises and focus on the body regions you will be using the most. Increase the speed of your functional exercises (see chapters

5, 8, 10, 11, and 15) prior to adding more resistance. An example would be to perform as many repetitions as possible safely in a 45-second period. For your regular resistance exercises, perform some sets of 4–6 reps for maximum strength along with sets of 12–15 reps for strength and endurance. You might add some plyometrics (such as jumping) and power work if your activity requires it (downhill or telemark skiing, snowboarding, windsurfing, rigorous climbing, and mountaineering). Add balance training early in this phase for water, climbing, and snow-based activities.

Phase D: Maintenance, Competition, or Maximum Activity Participation Period

The maintenance phase is the time during your competition or maximum activity period. The general objectives of this phase are to maintain all the component aerobic and strength gains while allowing optimal performance and activity enjoyment.

During this time, there is less total volume of exercise. Continue your basic aerobic endurance, and use cross training intermittently. Decrease or eliminate interval training. Maintain strength training, but with little attempt to increase strength. Eliminate your low-rep (4–6 reps) sets. Include ample time for rest in this phase, especially after a race or a multiday activity.

Phase E: Recovery and Active Rest Period

The transition phase is the off time between the end of your activity season and the start of the next training cycle. The general objectives of this phase are recovery from the previous activity season, including injury rehabilitation, rest, and maintenance of general strength and endurance.

Recovery means giving your body the rest it needs to adapt to the stresses you have put it through during an intense training season. Note: This can also be a brief period lasting a few days to a couple of weeks to recover from overuse injuries or overtraining during a training period.

Use active rest activities to recover from high-intensity or long-duration activities or races. Recovery periods are days of lighter or no exercise. After big events, give yourself a few days of rest or minimal activity, then begin a period of 2–4 weeks of low- to moderate-intensity aerobic and strength workouts to maintain what you have gained. Try some cross training or other sports to prevent burnout and to use your muscles differently.

THE PERIODIZATION PLAN

Always start a training program with a clear idea of what it is you hope to accomplish. The periodization plan gives direction to training and must be continually revised to ensure optimum benefits. Consider reviewing your plan each month throughout your training schedule.

To devise your plan, list your goals (as indicated earlier in this chapter) and the amount of time you have. Determine as well as you can what the demands of your activity are in the categories of aerobic (lower-intensity, longer-duration —LILD—and higher-intensity intervals), strength, flexibility, balance, and skill. Is it an activity such as hiking that requires stamina for long periods of time, or is it helicopter skiing, which requires anaerobic power and strength with long breaks in between? Write down in clear terms what you would like to be able to do in these categories. Remember, the plan you make is tailored to your needs based on your present fitness level, age, build, and the demands of your activity. The amount of time you spend doing low-intensity, long-duration interval training and strength, speed, and power work can vary considerably depending on your needs and comfort level. Certainly, if you are conditioning for general hiking or backpacking, you don't have to do much except for regular aerobic and LILD sessions.

Break the time you have into the five phases of periodization and into monthlong blocks. Use a special training log or a regular calendar with enough room to fill in your training schedule and your remarks on your progress and how you feel. Plan out the first 3–4 weeks of a period and give yourself at least 1 rest day and 1 lighter day per week (after a long or intense workout). Evaluate your progress every 2 weeks and modify your program as needed. Approximately 1 month before your activity season or event, plan a test activity of shorter duration than your expected activity. This should give you feedback as to whether you have any major deficits in your fitness so you can modify your program in the remaining month.

Recording Your Daily Program on a Calendar or Daily Log

Using calendars and daily logs is an excellent way to monitor your aerobic conditioning and strength training progress. Chapter 3 contains an Aerobic Conditioning Calendar (Figure 10, p. 62) and an Aerobic Conditioning Log (Figure 11, p. 64). Chapter 5 contains a Strength Training Log (Figure 16, p. 103). Use them as thoroughly as you want. They can be used by themselves but are better used as a monthly calendar. Use them in a basic way and record the amount of time you spend in each activity. Or use them as a more detailed planning tool and plan out your predicted time in each activity from your monthly and yearlong periodization plans. It is important to record details in the boxes.

Each log covers 4 weeks. Your phase can consist of 1 week or all 4. If it is 6 weeks, just fill in another sheet for the remaining 2 weeks and leave the last 2 weeks blank. Recording your morning heart rate is one method to monitor for overtraining. Recording your resting heart rate at another time of day can assess your cardiovascular training response in regard to pumping efficiency. The more-accurate records you keep, the easier it will be to stick to your program. If your program at any particular time does not include agility training, just cross out that portion. Evaluate your progress every 2 weeks, then modify and plan your schedule for the following 2 weeks.

Planning Your Own Program

Programs can be planned from the top down or from the bottom up. The top-down planning process can seem complex and difficult and is most useful for competitive athletes. Top-down planning involves looking at a whole year, or parts of a year, and planning phases and varying volumes of different types of activities. Use guidelines based on sample templates from this book and other sources to choose the number of sessions and the amount of time per week or month that you devote to a type of conditioning activity. Top-down planning is possible for anyone to do if they have particular goals and don't mind the time involved. For further information on developing a periodization plan or a yearly plan, or to see more templates, see the activity chapters in Part III and Selected References (especially Sleamaker) at the back of this book.

The planning process can be modified for outdoor athletes into the bottom-up version. Simply assess your present level of fitness in regard to your expected activity demands or conditioning goals, and start planning for actions to meet them. You can go at a gradual pace as you improve your aerobic and strength base. After you have improved your base level fitness for 4–6 weeks, you can add aerobic interval training and speed and plyometric training if you have a need for bursts of higher intensity. Add balance, agility, and activity-specific functional exercises within 6 weeks of the desired activity.

chapter 8 CREATIVE USE OF THE OUTDOORS IN TRAINING

By Peter Shmock, C.S.C.S.

THIS CHAPTER WILL HELP YOU:

- Understand the benefits of training in an outdoor setting.
- Become familiar with the most important outdoor training exercises, such as hill running, jumping, and agility drills.
- Develop balance skills using logs, rocks, and hills.
- Design training programs with simple equipment outdoors.
- Choose outdoor conditioning exercises for your upper body, lower body, and torso.

Outdoor environments offer unique advantages to help you train for balance, agility, and power, especially when utilizing hills, logs, and so on. Training outdoors can also add variety to your workout and decrease boredom. Training under the open sky has additional benefits. In skiing, climbing, mountain biking, and any other outdoor sport, it is essential to be able to respond quickly to the unexpected that can be encountered outdoors.

When training outdoors there is a lot of room for creativity. It is best to scout around for locations that provide many different options, such as schools, parks, or a diverse area of land. Here are some things to look for:

- Stadium steps, bleachers, stairs, park benches, and tables for step-up exercises
- Trees on which to anchor tubing
- Hills with varying degrees of incline to practice lunges, jumps, interval training, and agility drills for skiers, climbers, and mountain bikers
- Snowfields for simulation of balance challenges
- Sand (a beach or a long-jump sand pit) to practice jumps
- Playgrounds with objects to balance on
- Logs, low fences, and rocks for balance drills
- Boulders for variable-level push-ups or dips with one or two hands while standing and for climbing practice

In addition, the following simple, transportable, and affordable training tools are easy to take outdoors.

- Weight balls for throwing; large Physioballs (approximately 3 feet in diameter, available from physical therapy departments) for sit-ups
- Free weights for resistance exercises
- Traffic cones, ski poles, garden poles, and other markers for agility drills
- Rope placed on the ground or from tree to tree to step over and under
- Tubing or webbing for resistance in row and balance exercises
- Ankle weights to use in step-ups or hill lunges to simulate the weight of snowshoes or telemark skis and boots

CONDITIONING IN OUTDOOR SETTINGS

Strength

Strength can be increased in outdoor environments by adding weight or gravity as resistance. For example, you can improve strength in your lower body by doing gradually progressive step-ups on bleacher steps, park benches, logs, rocks, and boulders. You can improve your jumping and hopping ability by using hills and sand pits.

Balance

Standing balance, the ability to maintain your body core and extremities in a safe and well-functioning position despite challenges from the environment, is most important for climbers, backpackers, snowshoers, snowboarders, and skiers. Exercises to improve it are best done in outdoor areas with slopes and surfaces that challenge you in ways similar to your activity. Identify equipment that could be challenging to balance on—a fallen log, rocks, a low log fence, tires in a playground, a snowfield, and so on. Plot out a course of walking on these surfaces. Try it initially without a backpack and then with a backpack.

When doing any balance exercise, make sure your center of gravity is slightly forward so you are not leaning backward. When walking on logs, your steps should be a normal stride length, but you can increase your stride to challenge your balance more. When walking from rock to rock, land with a forward momentum on the largest surface of the rock. If there are a lot of rocks in an area, try varying which rocks you walk over, to change your direction and stride length. Try these balance challenges:

- Walk a narrow log.
- Walk from rock to rock as if you were crossing a river.
- Walk from post to post or tire to tire in a playground.
- Place a 25- to 75-foot string on the ground and anchor it so it will not move much when you walk on it. Walk it heel to toe initially. When this is easy with a backpack, increase the length of your stride. Try doing this on a hill traverse or on an up or down slope.
- Try Exercises 31, 58–62, 80–82, 84–86 (using a tree to anchor the tubing in 86), 88, and 93. You can try these while standing with one foot on a log or rock, or while standing uphill or downhill. Using hills for balance is particularly useful for climbers, backpackers, scramblers, and snow-sport enthusiasts.
- You may be able to make a balance circuit made up of segments of balance challenges that last 30–120 seconds each.
- Try linking any of the balance challenges in this list.

The important thing is to maintain a stable upright position without straining or hurting your knees or back. Try to simulate the balance and environmental demands of your activity.

Training for sitting balance and abdominal strength is most important for whitewater boating and for mountain bikers. For both sports you can do sitting ball exercises such as Exercises 37–39 and 62 or abdominal challenge exercises such as Exercises 88, 93, and 94. For water sports, train on the water with easy rapids or do agility courses in calmer water. For mountain bikers, the up- and downhill agility cycling drills in chapter 22 are appropriate.

Remember that balance can deteriorate just like strength if you do nothing to exercise it.

Agility

Agility can be described as "moving balance." Training for agility involves setting up obstacle courses in which you have to make quick changes in direction while maintaining your balance. The outdoors is the best setting in which to train for agility. Choose woods, hills, snow slopes, or large open spaces that allow you to move unassisted while adding an element of the unexpected (see chapter 20 for snowboarding and ski agility drills; chapter 21 for water agility drills; and chapter 22 for mountain biking drills).

You can create your own outdoor agility course by using small traffic cones, ropes, ski poles, trees, garden poles, or whatever is handy to set up an obstacle course. The agility course should have at least 10 stations in which you make changes in direction. You could start with a course on level ground, then progress to hills.

Initially, start with fast walking between the stations. Then progress to running. You may progress to adding lunges, jumps, and hops between some stations, depending on the sport you are training for (lunges are most appropriate for cross-country and telemark skiing and for snowshoeing). For downhill skiing and snowboarding, set up your agility course on a hill with mostly jump turns, with an occasional walking lunge on a hillside slope to simulate a traverse. For telemark skiing, set up a combination of running, walking lunges, turn simulations, hops, and jumps. In a good agility circuit workout, you should feel like you are doing body movements similar to those of your activity and at similar speeds.

Precautions: Agility circuits require a high level of aerobic, balance, and strength fitness. You should be able to do basic lunges, hops, and jumps individually and with good form before you do them quickly in a circuit. You should also be able to comfortably do stationary balance exercises from chapter 6. Agility circuits can aggravate any existing lower-body or back problem. Caution should be taken if you are recovering from an injury or have a long-term condition.

Anaerobic Capacity

Some of the best methods of anaerobic training are interval running, cycling, rope skipping, and stair climbing. You can incorporate anaerobic interval training in your outside exercises to make a more complete workout. Do this by doing 1- to 3-minute high-intensity intervals of the above aerobic activities during an outside aerobic workout or in between every 2–3 outdoor exercises to amount to 4–8 intervals per workout.

If you incorporate intervals into your outdoor circuit, you have a few options. You can do an interval training workout before or after your strength, balance, and agility exercises. This would be a 30- to 40-minute block of time that includes an aerobic warm-up. You could mix the interval in with the rest of the circuit, but you would have to warm up, at least for a few minutes, to enable you to safely reach your high-intensity target zone. (See chapter 3 for more details on interval training and precautions.)

TRAINING TIPS FOR OUTDOOR EXERCISES

Hill Running and Sprinting

Running and sprinting uphill are excellent exercises to increase both aerobic and anaerobic conditioning. Hill training interludes between circuit training exercises are excellent for outdoor conditioning. You can use hill running to incorporate an aerobic or anaerobic component into your outdoor program. Exercises on hills can be practiced up slope, down slope, and on the traverse. Slopes can help you to simulate the gravity demands of your activity. Keep these things in mind to gain the most benefit from your efforts:

- Lean into the incline of the hill.
- Emphasize the driving of your arms more than on a flat-surface run. Pump your arms more on steeper hills.
- Focus on the extension of each leg as you push off and the raising of your knee as you bring it forward.
- Look ahead to see where you are going.

A recommended hill-training distance for developing aerobic power is approximately 440–660 yards (400–600 meters). For anaerobic training, use a distance of 220–330 yards (200–300 meters) or 1- to 3-minute interval times. The steeper the slope, the shorter the distance should be.

Stair Running

Stair running and walking are excellent aerobic training for general conditioning as well as for climbing, mountaineering, and backpacking.

Try to find an outside set of connected stairways with at least 5 flights of stairs. You can walk with 1-, 2-, or 3-stair strides. You can run 1 or 2 stairs at a time. You can mix interval sprints of 1–4 minutes during a stair-running aerobic workout. It is better to walk fast or run the stairs in an uphill portion and to walk down the stairs or jog a path to get to the bottom of the stairs. Running down a flight of stairs can lead to knee or ankle problems. See chapter 3 for more information on stair running.

Hops and Jumps

Hop and jump practice can help you to get ready for skiing, snowboarding, snowshoeing, climbing, and glacier mountaineering. It is especially good to do hops and jumps on hills, because this can simulate the demands of your activity. Begin adding these to your program after you have established a good aerobic and strength base and within 4–6 weeks of beginning your activity.

For downhill skiing, a mix of more jumping than hopping is appropriate and should be practiced on a level surface before being done on a downhill slope. For glacier mountaineering, an emphasis on hopping with side-to-side and forward leaping motions is recommended. Try this both up and down a hill. When doing side-to-side hopping, do it on level ground first, then progress to a hill and vary the angle and distances of the hopping. Occasionally try a longer leap if you anticipate having to jump over a crevasse, for example. See Exercises 100 and 101 for technique details.

DESIGNING YOUR OUTDOOR TRAINING PROGRAM

When you design an outdoor training program or try one of the segment circuits at the end of this chapter, choose from exercises in this chapter as well as from chapters 5 and 6; the body region chapters in Part II; and the agility circuits and drills in chapters 20, 21, and 22. Try to have a good mix of lower-body, upper-body, and abdominal exercises that are relevant to your activity. Some of the exercises are very conducive to outdoor training.

For the lower body: Try squats, lunges, step-ups, hops, and jumps (Exercises 95, 97, 98, 100, and 101). Doing them on hills (up, down, and traversing) is helpful for climbers, snowboarders, and skiers.

For the upper body: Try dips, pull-ups, and push-ups in outdoor settings. Exercises 115, 120.2, 120.3, 127, 128, 130, 132, and 136 are all appropriate in outdoor settings.

For the abdominal region: Try Exercises 80–86, and 88–93.

You can do many of the balance exercises in chapter 6 in an outdoor setting. Add additional challenges with logs and rocks.

OUTDOOR EXERCISES

The following exercises are divided into categories for your lower body, torso, and upper body. However, these categories are intended primarily to aid in program design, because the exercises use more of the body than these categories imply. The best exercises for outdoor activities use multiple muscles and joints simultaneously, because we are interested in training the total motion, not simply one section of the body.

Each exercise is adapted to beginning, intermediate, and advanced levels. People with injuries might need to simplify movements to prebeginning levels. Stop any exercise if you feel pain or discomfort.

Everyone, regardless of fitness level, should start at the beginning stage and progress when performance is easy and graceful. Only extremely fit athletes should attempt the advanced versions. Always warm up for at least 10 minutes before starting any exercise program.

LOWER BODY

70 OUTDOOR STEP-UPS

Equipment: Raised platform 1–2 feet high.
Purpose: Develop your quadriceps, gluteals, and hip muscle groups for stepping motions.

Technique: Place one foot on a raised platform 1–2 feet high. Use a step, bleacher seat, park bench, log, or tree stump. Start with low steps and work your way up to higher steps to simulate the highest stepping demands of your activity. Glacier mountaineering will occasionally require step heights that place your knee and hip in a fully flexed position. Weight-shifting (see chapter 25) is quite important for step-up exercises that use the higher step heights found in outdoor settings. It is also important to push off from the back foot once you have weight-shifted onto the step. Once on the step, balance briefly on one leg and then slowly lower yourself down. You may raise your nonstepping knee up into the air and swing your opposite arm with it. See Exercise 98 for details on technique.

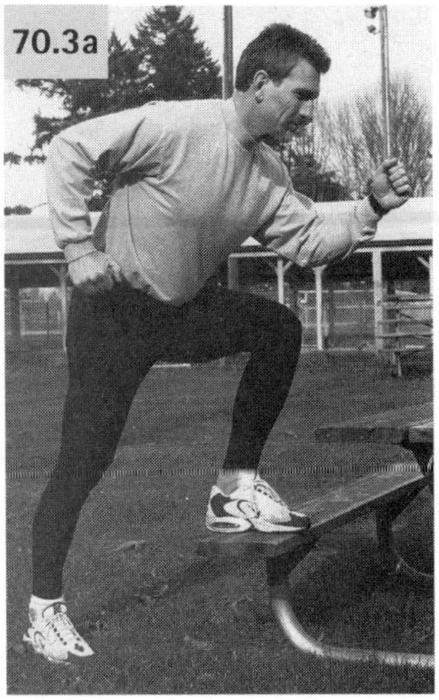
70.3a

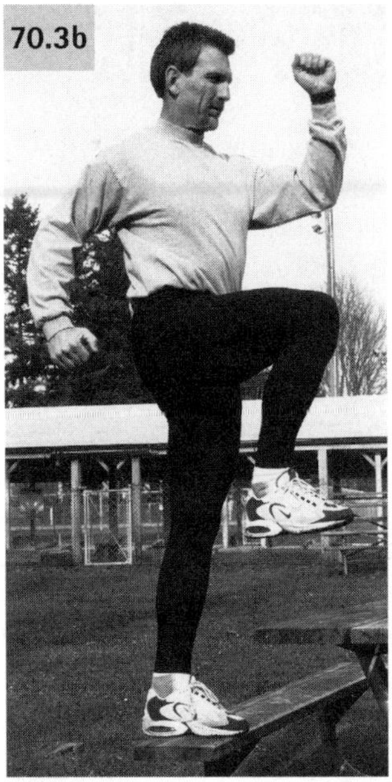
70.3b

Variations: 70.1. Beginning: Use smaller steps. Consider assisting your step with ski poles. **70.2.** Intermediate: Use larger steps such as bleacher steps, rocks, or logs up to a foot high. **70.3.** Advanced: Use very high steps that will bring your leg into a high-step position with your hip almost fully flexed, such as a park bench seat or a foothold on a boulder (70.3a and 70.3b). Because most high stepping is done with some assistance from your arms, you may wish to use ski poles or wooden dowels to assist.

Precautions: Gradually work your way up to a high step, because there is a risk of muscle strains. Do shorter step-ups, lunges, and other exercises as preparation.

71 SQUAT HOPS AND JUMPS

Equipment: None.

Purpose: Develop your quadriceps, hamstrings, gluteals, and torso for snow and climbing activities.

Technique: Warm up by doing 1–2 sets of regular squats, jumps, and hops. See Exercises 95, 100, and 101 for details on technique.

Variations: 71.1. Beginning: In sand, do small continuous hops forward and backward. Do jumps with pauses in between and gentle landings (71.1a, 71.1b, and 71.1c). **71.2.** Intermediate: Do jumps and hops on stadium steps or on a hill; do them uphill, downhill (71.2a, 71.2b, and 71.2c), forward, to the side, and diagonally. Try them over a stretched bungee cord, ball, or log, 6 inches off the ground (71.2d). To increase the difficulty, do them more quickly or raise the bungee cord. **71.3.** Advanced: Add ankle weights and/or speed to the above exercises. Do lateral hops uphill, hopping with your downhill leg. Do quarter turns while jumping uphill. Avoid pauses between hops.

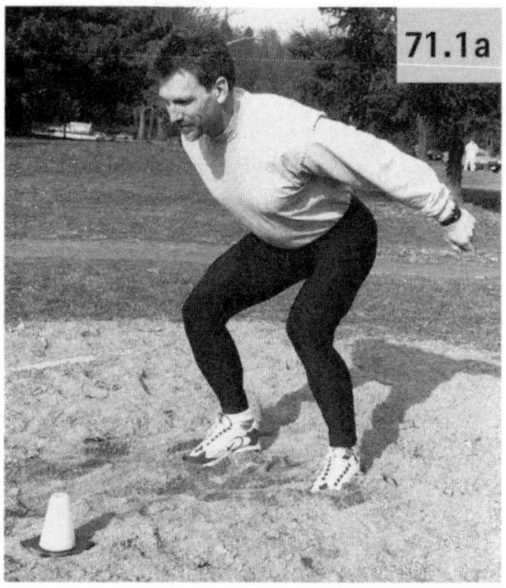
71.1a

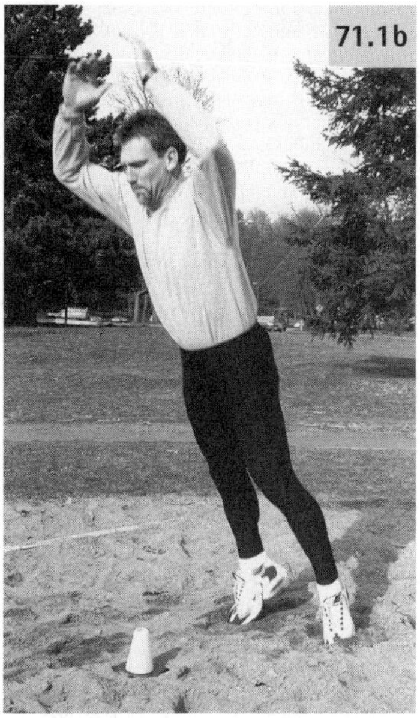
71.1b

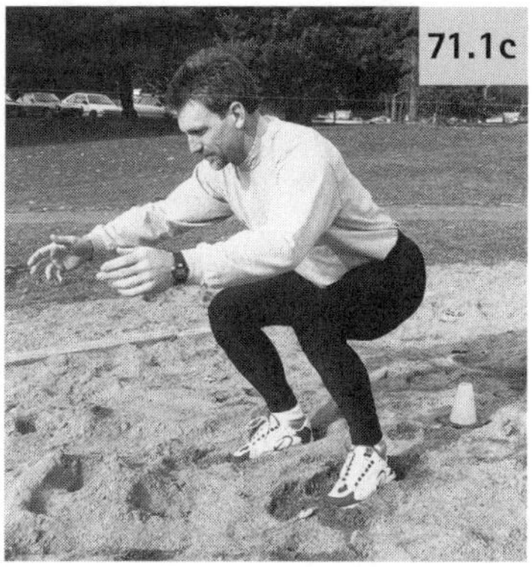
71.1c

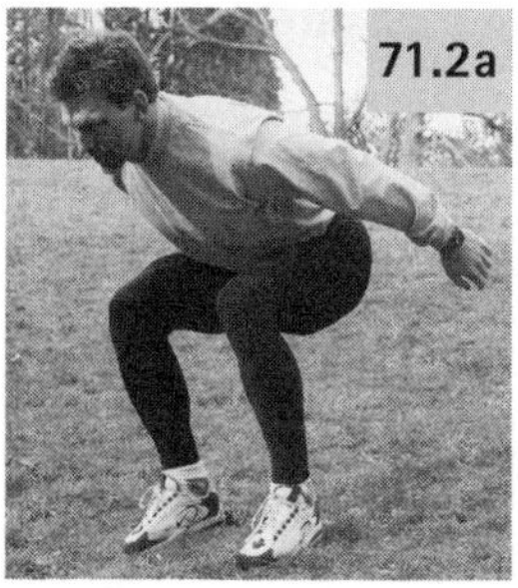
71.2a

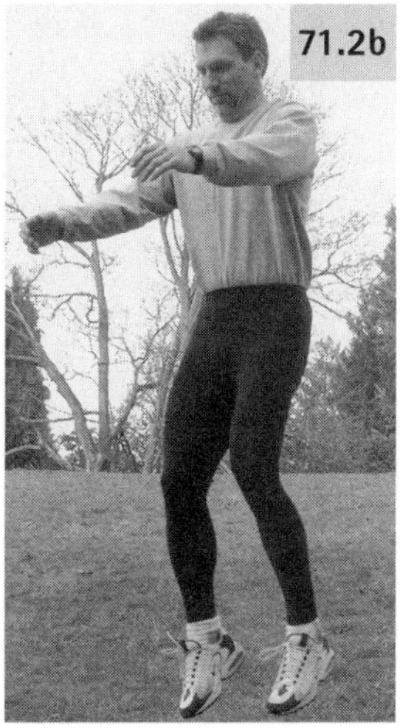
71.2b

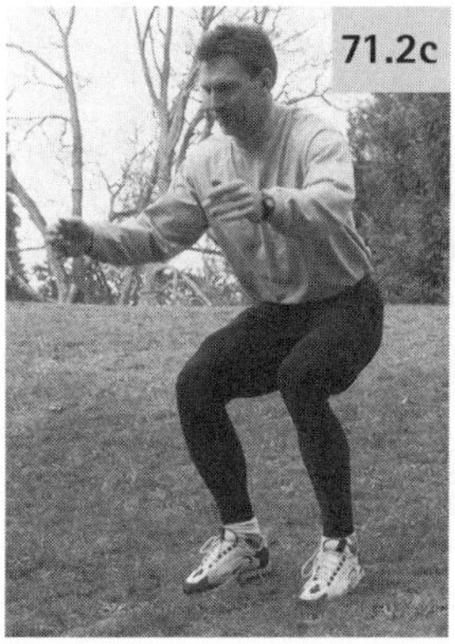
71.2c

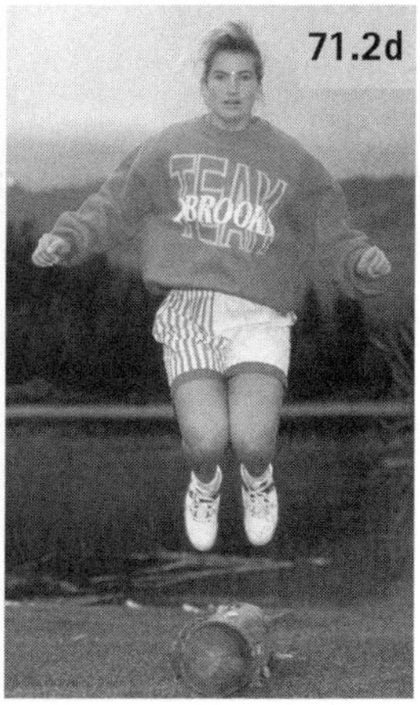
71.2d

TORSO

These exercises are not intended for people with back injuries or low-back pain. No matter what your fitness level, always start with the easiest version to learn the movement and warm up before advancing. Perform torso exercises with great control. Your head should not be pulled forward or allowed to roll back. Find a head and neck position by imagining a string being pulled out the top of your head, not by extending your chin forward. For outdoor circuit training, add any of the functional abdominal exercises from chapter 10 to your torso exercises.

72 SITTING BALL ROTATION

Equipment: Ball.
Purpose: Control rotation forces in a sitting position.

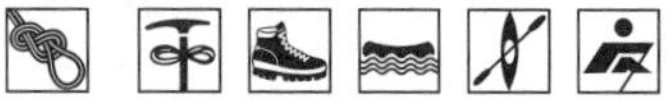

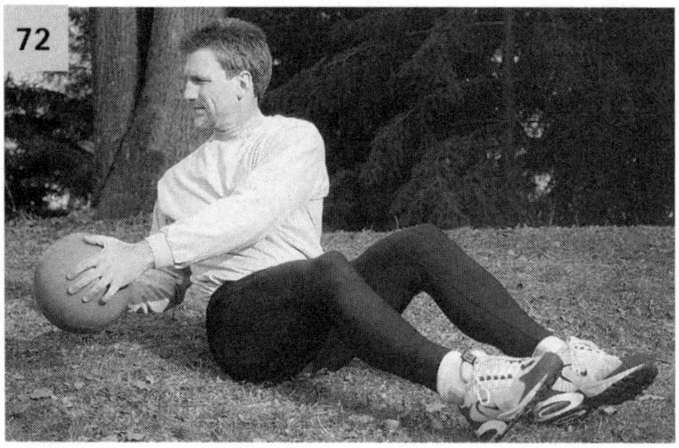

72

Technique: Hold a ball and sit on the ground with your knees slightly bent and your feet touching the ground. Lower yourself backward until you feel your abdominal muscles activating. Rotate your spine and touch the ground with the ball to the right and then the left.

Variations: **72.1.** Beginning: Do the exercise slowly, then increase speed. **72.2.** Intermediate: Hold a weighted ball. **72.3.** Advanced: Perform the movement on an incline, with your feet pointed uphill.

73 OVER AND BACK

Equipment: Ball.
Purpose: Increase the strength of the extensors of your back and gluteals.

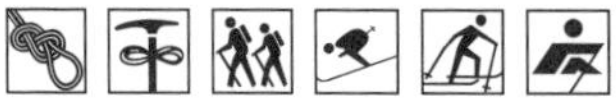

Technique: Lie face-down on the ground. Extend your arms overhead on the ground, keeping them close to your ears. Hold a ball (or imagine holding a basketball) in your hands. Extend your back and raise your shoulders and arms off the ground, moving from side to side as if you were raising the ball over an invisible 6- to 12-inch object (or use a cone or a natural object outdoors). Pause briefly on

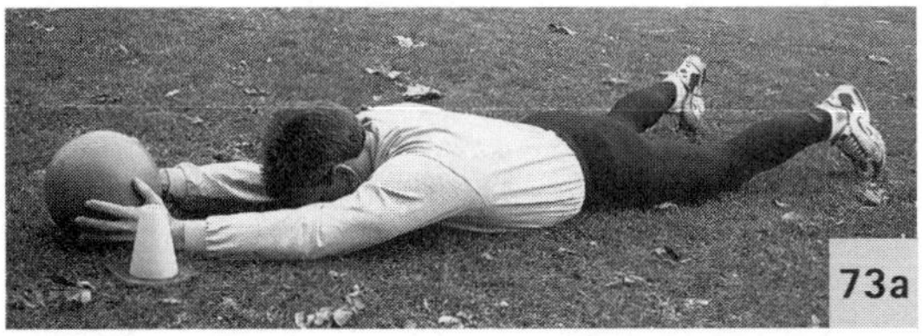
73a

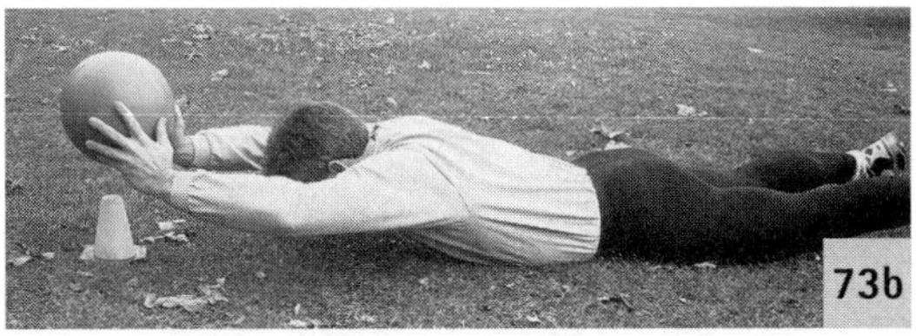
73b

each side. Keep your legs straight and focus on your long, stable spine (73a and 73b).

Variations: 73.1. Intermediate: Hold the ball for 3 seconds without moving side to side. **73.2.** Advanced: Lift a weight ball.

UPPER BODY

For your outdoor circuit, include Exercises 20, 28, 29, 33–35, and any of the exercises in chapter 15 in addition to the following exercises.

74 DIPS

Equipment: Raised surface.

Purpose: Strengthen your chest, anterior shoulders, triceps, and upper back, and improve your ability to push yourself up or away from a surface.

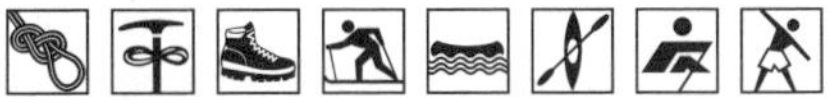

Technique: Dips can be done at different angles, depending on the surfaces you have available. Locate a raised surface that has a height that is between the level of your low back and knee when you are sitting on the ground with your knees in 60 degrees of flexion. You can use the top of a park bench's back or a park bench seat, or a surface on a fallen log or a boulder. It is preferable to have two surfaces within shoulder-width apart. Back up to the raised surface until you are almost touching it. Place the heels of your hands on the top edge of the surface, just outside of hip-width apart, fingers pointing forward. Support your body weight, with your arms straight. Move your feet away from you about 3–4 feet, and keep your knees bent and feet flat. Lower your body by bending your elbows until your upper arms are almost parallel to the ground, then press down against the surface until your arms are straight again.

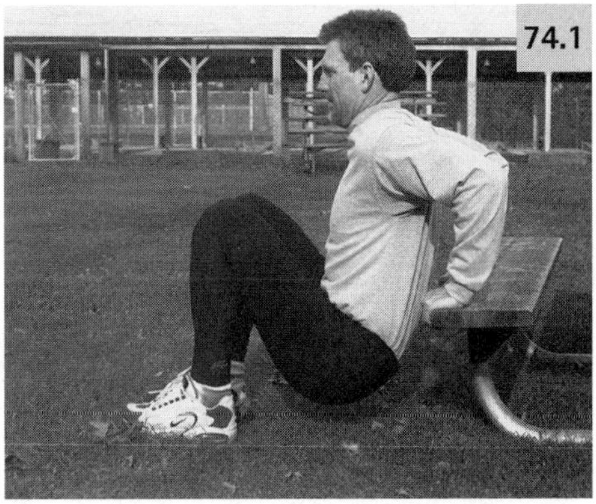
74.1

Variations: 74.1. Beginning: Bend your knees maximally under your body and use your legs to help push

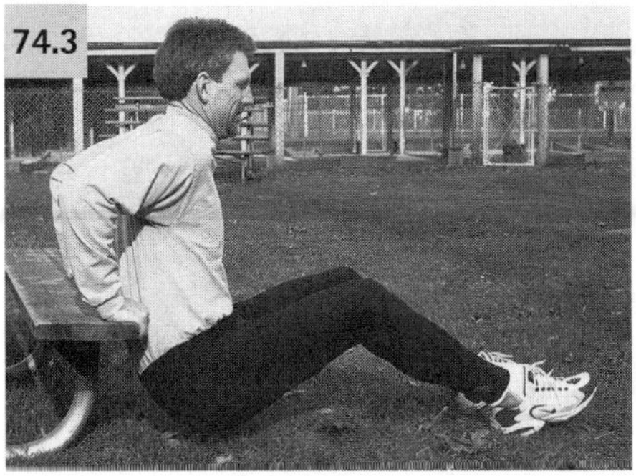

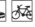
74.3

your body upward to assist your arms, as in a squat-type exercise. **74.2.** Intermediate: Do the movement with your knees less extended. **74.3.** Advanced: Extend your legs straight in front of your body, resting your weight on your heels. The farther your feet are extended, the more difficult the movement.

Precaution: Dips outdoors are potentially stressful to your elbows and shoulders.

75 PULL-UPS

Equipment: Overhead bar.

Purpose: Strengthen your upper back, shoulders, and biceps, and improve your ability to pull up your body weight.

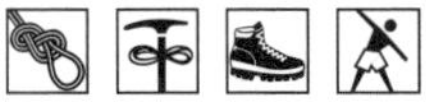

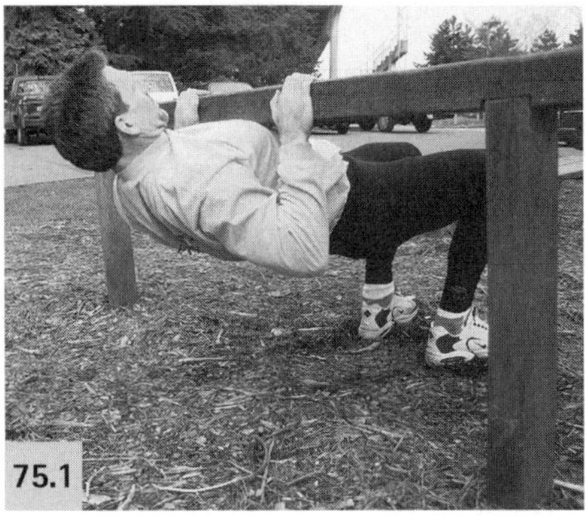
75.1

Technique: Find a jungle gym or some other sturdy overhead bar. Grasp it, palms facing away from your body. Pull your body weight upward until you can see over the bar. Be careful not to reach up with your chin.

Variations: 75.1. Beginning: Do pull-ups on a low bar with part of your weight supported. **75.2.** Intermediate: Do pull-ups with a partner. Have him or her stand behind you. Grasp the bar and bend your knees. Have your partner place his or her hands under the front of your ankles. When you pull up, press down against your partner's hands to relieve some of the effort on your upper body and to unload. **75.3.** Advanced: Do the movements without a partner. When you can do at least 6 pull-ups unsupported, add weight to your body. You can do this with a backpack, ankle weights, and so on.

76 PUSH-UPS

Equipment: None.

Purpose: Strengthen your chest, shoulders, and back to aid in pushing.

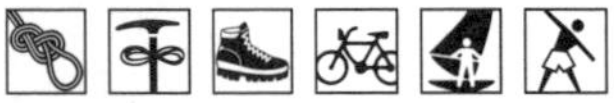

Technique: Identify different surfaces on which you can safely do a push-up in a standing and leaning position as well as on the level ground. Use tree trunks, stairs, boulder faces, and so on. Do the push-up in a slow, controlled manner. See Exercise 115 for technique.

Variations: 76.1. Beginning: Do a push-up while standing and leaning against an inclined surface. Try 10–12 in a set. Next, vary the angle and increase the difficulty until you are doing some on the ground. Have your knees touching the ground. **76.2.** Intermediate: Straighten your knees and have them off the ground; do 8–12 in a set. **76.3.** Advanced: Try plyometric push-ups (see Exercise 77), especially useful for climbers.

77 PLYOMETRIC PUSH-UPS

Equipment: None.
Purpose: Improve your ability to push quickly off a surface, which is helpful for climbers.

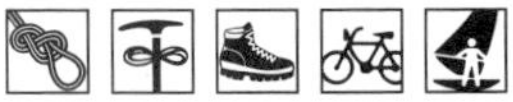

Technique: Start a regular push-up as described in Exercise 115. After lowering your body to the ground, your hands should be placed to the outside of your shoulders and slightly below them. Your spine and body, from the top of your head to your knees, should remain straight, with no swaying or arching of your back. Plyometric (plyo) push-ups are done by quickly pushing your body off the ground explosively from the lowest position, instead of just pushing to the straight-arm position. Your hands will raise off the ground. Start on an inclined hill, and gradually work toward doing these on flat ground. It is tempting to use your back muscles to throw yourself upward, but avoid this. Plyo push-ups are very difficult, so don't expect to do too many.

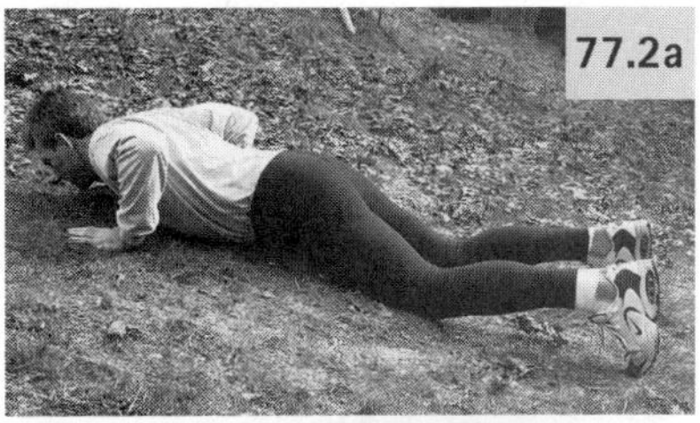

77.2a

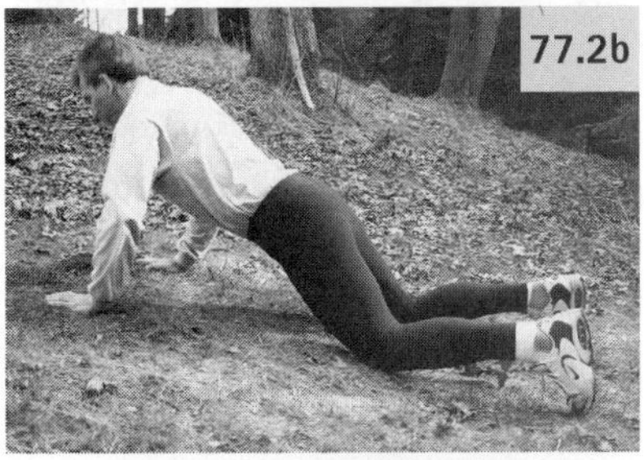

77.2b

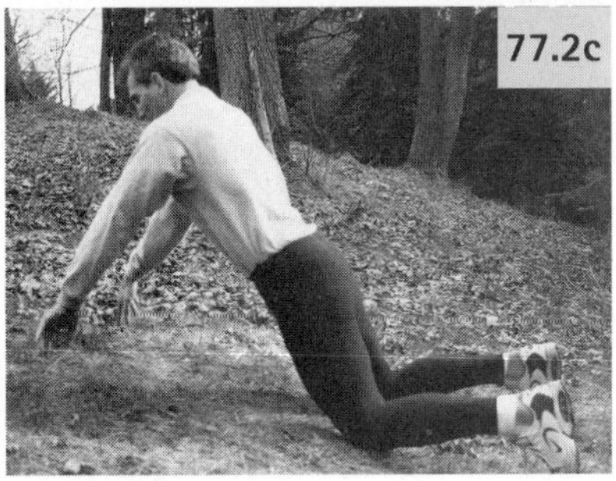

77.2c

Variations: 77.1. Beginning: Try these against a wall or a sloped boulder. Try to do them at angles that will simulate the angles at which you will need to push off during your activity. Try push-ups on an incline (like a grassy hill) with your head uphill and knees downhill. Another way is to stand up, then lean into a park bench or picnic table with your arms straight. Your body will be at an angle to the ground instead of parallel to it, which makes pushing off much easier. **77.2.** Intermediate: Add the plyo push-up on a more level surface. **77.3.** Advanced: Increase speed and repetitions to increase difficulty.
Precautions: Plyo push-ups are a very high-level exercise and are potentially risky to your shoulders and back. Don't do them if you have any active injuries in these regions. Your knees should also touch the ground only minimally or lightly in order to avoid injury.

OUTDOOR "SEGMENT CIRCUIT TRAINING"

This is a more sophisticated method of circuit training most suited for outdoor performance training that increases overall strength within an endurance format. There is greater emphasis on training the torso, and no machines are used.

Design an outdoor circuit of 10–15 stations using exercises from this and other chapters. In most cases, you will alternate between lower-body, upper-body, and torso exercises. Do 1–2 sets at each station, and rest only 30–60 seconds before moving on. You can walk quickly, run, skip, or cycle between stations. This keeps your heart rate at an aerobic level while still providing strength training. You can also incorporate aerobic or anaerobic intervals between stations.

Emphasizing Strength/Endurance

For those activities that require more endurance, follow these general guidelines:

- Do more repetitions (15–20) of each exercise.
- Do longer aerobic intervals between sets (e.g., jog or bike for 3- to 4-minute intervals or 10-minute lower-intensity aerobic sessions).

Emphasizing Speed/Strength

For those sports that are anaerobically oriented, alter the segment circuit training this way:

- Do anaerobic interval training between sets (sprinting, short hill running, or cycling).
- As an alternative to counting repetitions, time some of your sets with a stopwatch or second hand and do as many reps as you can within 30–45 seconds.

Sample Outdoor Workouts

Below are two examples of how to pattern your outdoor workouts using segment circuit training: one an endurance workout (Figure 22) and the other an explosive/anaerobic workout (Figure 23). Guidelines for both are the following:

1. Make sure you do a short warm-up before beginning your outdoor circuit.
2. Fill in the specific exercise that you want to do, choosing from the upper-body, lower-body, and torso exercises in this chapter as well as from other exercises in this book. Try to start with easier exercises that are safe for your spine before

you add variations or advanced levels. If you wish to train for an activity, make your exercises as activity-specific as possible.

3. Try to incorporate some exercises to challenge your balance.
4. Consider adding an agility circuit somewhere in your outdoor circuit.
5. In Figures 22 and 23, numbers in square brackets indicate rest time between sets. You may decide to decrease or eliminate the rest periods as you get more experienced or if you want to get a more aerobic workout.
6. In Figures 22 and 23, each segment of three to five exercises is followed by an aerobic or anaerobic interval. An effort level for each of these intervals is suggested as a percentage, based on resting being 1%, jogging 50%, and maximum output 100%. Pay attention to how you feel and learn how to assign an effort level percentage to that feeling. This takes practice. There is never a need to go beyond 90%. This would increase your chance of injury and require long recovery times.

Endurance Workout with Lower-Body Emphasis

Start with an aerobic warm-up and then move into segments of exercises. Each segment consists of lower-body, upper-body, or torso exercises and is followed by a 5-minute jog/run. Use a stopwatch or second hand to time each exercise set within a segment. Don't count repetitions. The timed sets are followed by short periods of rest. Do exercises at a rhythmic, nonexplosive pace to increase aerobic capacity. See Figure 22.

Explosive/Anaerobic Workout with Lower-Body Emphasis

Start with a warm-up run, jog, or cycle and then start your exercise segments. Each segment consists of lower-body, upper-body, or torso exercises and is followed by a 60- to 90-second sprint, hill run, or hill cycle. Count repetitions instead of timing each set. Exercises are

FIGURE 22. ENDURANCE WORKOUT

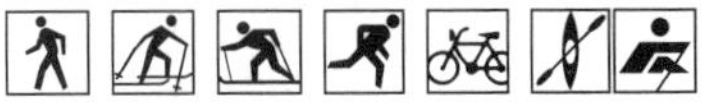

EXERCISE	TIME/INTENSITY	REST PERIOD (SECONDS)
Aerobic warm-up	10 minutes, 70%	
Lower body	30–45 seconds	[30]
Upper body	30–45 seconds	[30]
Lower body	30–45 seconds	[30]
Upper body	30–45 seconds	[30]
Run	5 minutes, 80%	
Lower body	30–45 seconds	[30]
Torso	30–45 seconds	[30]
Lower body	30–45 seconds	[30]
Torso	30–45 seconds	[30]
Run	5 minutes, 85%	
Upper body	30–45 seconds	[30]
Lower body	30–45 seconds	[30]
Upper body	30–45 seconds	[30]
Lower body	30–45 seconds	[30]
Aerobic	5 minutes, 75%	
ADVANCED LEVELS ADD ONE MORE SEGMENT:		
Lower body	30–45 seconds	[30]
Torso	30–45 seconds	[30]
Lower body	30–45 seconds	[30]
Lower body	30–45 seconds	[30]
Aerobic	5 minutes, 70%	Cool down
Flexibility work	5–10 minutes	

FIGURE 23. EXPLOSIVE/ANAEROBIC WORKOUT

EXERCISE	REPS/INTENSITY	REST PERIOD (SECONDS)
Run, jog, or cycle	10 minutes	
Lower body	2 × 8–12 reps (fast)	[60]
Torso	2 × 20 reps	[60]
Lower body (hops and jumps)	3 × 10 reps	[60]
Sprint or hill run	60–90 seconds, 85–90%	[60–90]
Lower body	3 × 8–12 reps (fast)	[60]
Upper body	2 × 8–12 reps (fast)	[60]
Lower body (hops and jumps)	2 × 8–12 reps (fast)	[60]
Sprint or hill run	60–90 seconds, 85–90%	[60–90]
Torso	2 × 12–15	[60]
Upper body	2 × 8–12 (fast)	[60]
Torso	2 × 12–15 (fast)	[60]
Run variations: backward uphill	60–90 seconds	
Lower body	3 × 8–12 (fast)	[60]
Torso	3 × 12–15	[60]
Lower body	3 × 8–12 (fast)	[60]
Jog	5 minutes	Cool down
Flexibility work	10 minutes	

performed with increased speed and intensity (compared to those in the endurance workout in Figure 22), followed by longer rest periods of 60 seconds. This type of training is excellent for sports requiring shorter, more intense workout periods followed by longer rest periods. See Figure 23.

PART II

Body Regions

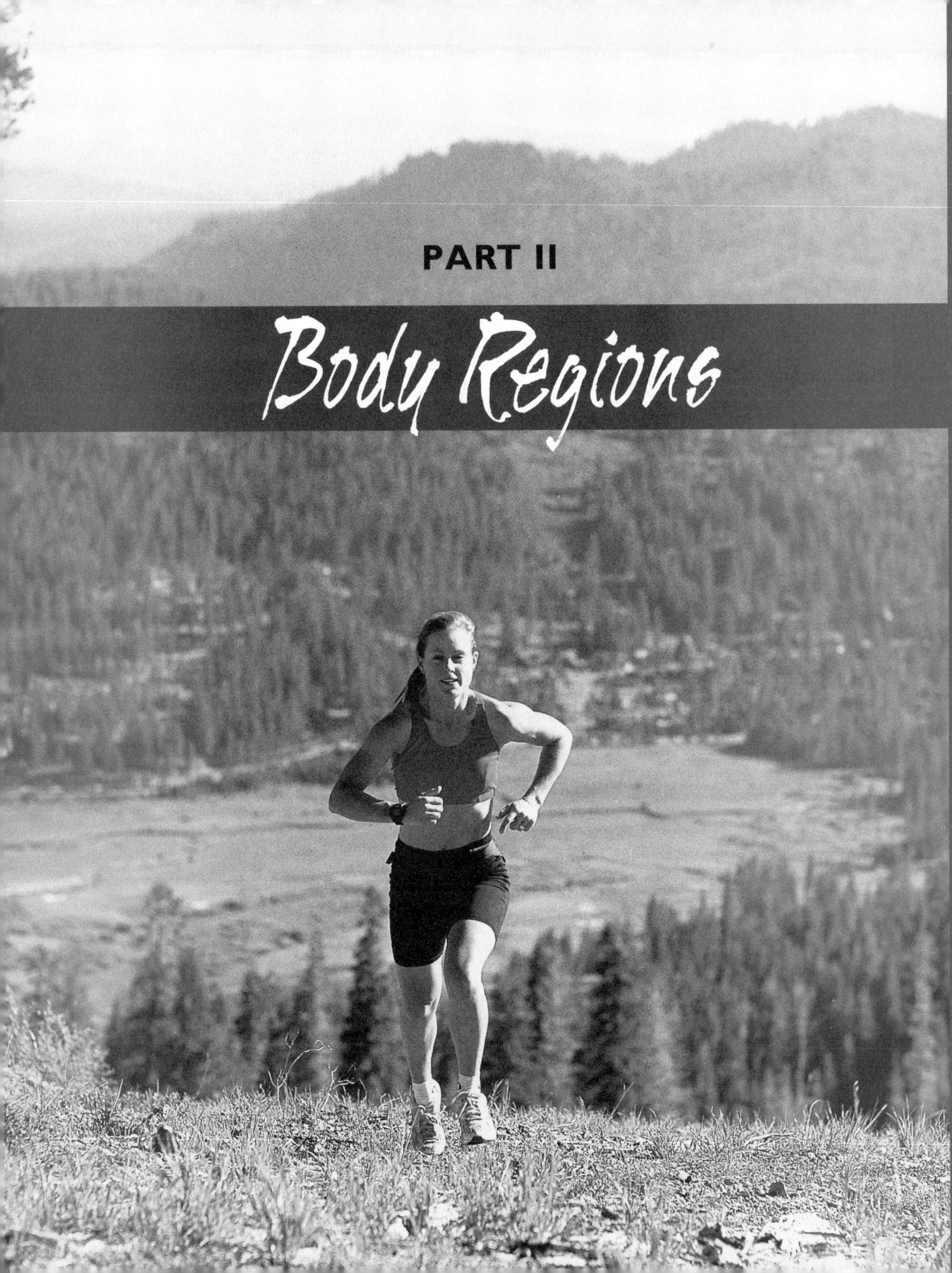

chapter 9 ANATOMY AND MUSCULOSKELETAL INJURY: PREVENTION AND TREATMENT

By David Musnick, M.D., and Mark Pierce, A.T.C.

THIS CHAPTER WILL HELP YOU:

- Understand movement, planes of motion, and anatomy terms used in other chapters in this book.
- Understand why muscles, ligaments, joints, and discs get injured.
- Understand the factors that may predispose you to injury and slow recovery.
- Develop exercise and activity strategies while recovering from an injury.
- Orient yourself to the muscles described in chapters 10–24.

Your musculoskeletal system works as a whole but can be analyzed and exercised in "regions." Learning about your system by using the regions approach can be very helpful in enabling you to analyze and plan a better exercise program. There are many important functional relationships between your body regions. For example, strengthening your shoulder and upper back is critical for arm and hand functional strength. Strengthening your abdominal muscles and balance is important for lower- and upper-body function. Strengthening your shoulder along with your hip and leg is critical for many activities. More examples are discussed in chapters 10–16 and in chapter 25.

The body region chapters are all organized similarly. Each begins with a brief description of the function of the body region and describes functional relationships between the regions. The body region's anatomy, which is presented next, is not comprehensive, as you would find in an anatomy atlas or medical text, but is presented in enough detail to explain its functions without sacrificing accuracy. The anatomy review is followed by a discussion of common muscle imbalances and injury prevention. Exercises and self-tests are then given.

BODY MOVEMENTS

Flexion or *flexing* means to shorten a muscle or set of muscles and bring one part of the body closer to another. *Spine flexion* means rounding your back. Hip and spine flexion will bring your chest closer to your thighs. *Side bending* or *lateral flexion* means bending your back to the side so that your arm and elbow go closer to your buttock if you are sitting, or to your knee if you are standing.

Extension or *extending* means moving a joint from a flexed or neutral position (such as straightening your elbow or knee). In the spine it means the same thing but may also mean arching your back if you are starting upright or neutral.

Neutral is a term usually given to the spine. It indicates a position of spinal alignment in which the joints are positioned to give the spine its normal curves, and is usually near midrange alignment. Details are given in chapters 14 and 25.

Lateral movement (abduction) is away from the midline of your body. *Medial movement* (adduction) is toward the midline of your body. *External* (lateral) *rotation* is a rotation of your feet, knees, hips, and shoulders away from the midline of your body. *Internal* (medial) *rotation* brings these joints toward the midline of your body. *Circumduction* means moving a body area in a circular motion. It can be used in reference to pelvic motion that might occur in a canoe or kayak.

Planes of Motion

Our body movements can be described in three planes of motion. *Sagittal plane motion* is movement in a front-to-back or flexion/extension direction. *Frontal plane motion* is in a side-to-side direction. *Transverse plane motion* is in a rotational direction.

In outdoor and sports activities, demands are placed on your muscles and joints to perform in these combined planes. Many exercises in this book have been chosen or designed to simulate multiplanar demands (see, for example, the balance self-test exercises in chapter 6). This is a major component of functional conditioning.

Pronation/Supination

These terms are usually used to describe motion in the foot and lower extremity (foot, ankle, knee, and hip). When your foot *pronates*, it flattens and rolls inward, and the arch gets slightly closer to the ground. The term *pronation* has been used in relation to the body and may mean a rotating inward of the knee, hip, and shoulder as well as flexing of the spine. *Supination* indicates an outward rolling of the foot and ankle, and an increase in the height of the arch. In relation to the rest of the body, it may indicate external rotation of the knee, hip, and shoulder and an extending of the back. Forces of gravity and the stance phase of gait tend to bring your body into pronation, and ground reaction forces and the push-off phase of walking tend to bring your body more into supination. For more discussion of phases of gait, see chapter 13.

BASIC ANATOMY

The musculoskeletal system includes the bones, tendons, ligaments, joints, cartilage, fascia, and muscles.

A *tendon* is specialized muscle tissue at the end of a muscle that connects the muscle to the bone.

A *ligament* is noncontractile tissue that connects bone to bone. It is a structure that helps to stabilize a joint.

A *joint* is the site of a junction between bones.

Cartilage covers bone surfaces to allow for smooth gliding of joints.

Fascia is a connective tissue.

Muscles that work with opposing forces around a joint or body region are called *agonists* and *antagonists*.

Use the illustrations in this chapter (Figures 24a–c and 25a–c) to identify muscles, bones, and joints discussed in chapters 10–24.

INJURIES

Injuries common to outdoor athletes include tendonitis, muscle strains, ligament sprains, and bursitis.

Tendonitis is inflammation of the tendon, or the structure that connects muscle to bone.

Muscle strains are tears in the muscle belly or tendon, and are also known as pulled muscles.

Ligament sprains are tears to a ligament.

Bursitis is inflammation of the bursa, which is a flat, pancakelike, fluid-filled sac. Bursas are located in places of the body affected by high amounts of movement, in order to help reduce friction and allow the parts to slide and glide more freely. Bursitis commonly occurs in the shoulder, elbow, lateral hip, and kneecap regions.

Predisposing Factors and Prevention

Muscles and ligaments may overstretch and tear when they are subject to excessive mechanical loads that create undue tension. All tissues have a length tension curve of response to loads, which determines whether they will simply lengthen or tear given a certain load. There are many factors that may contribute to whether a sprain, strain, or joint injury will occur. A number of the factors are due to muscle imbalance, which is lack of balance in strength of muscles within a body region or between regions. Specific imbalances are covered in the body region chapters. The following factors may contribute to injury development.

Malalignment. This can be abnormal biomechanics in your feet, legs, knees, hips, pelvis, and low back. Malalignment issues can be discovered by a health-care provider trained to look for biomechanical and structural alignment patterns that can predispose you to injury.

Patterns of tight and weak muscles. Tight muscles usually activate quickly. They may pull joints into misalignment and lead to inhibition of their antagonists. Tight muscles may be a result of pain, joint motion problems (excessive mobility or less-than-normal mobility), or stress and central nervous system issues. Commonly tight muscles are the pectorals, hamstrings, iliotibial band, quadriceps, and the hip flexors. The calf and Achilles tendon are also often tight. See chapter 4 for further discussion of the most common tight and weak muscles.

Inhibited muscles. Inhibited muscles are weaker and activate more slowly. A smaller percentage of a muscle's fibers are recruited when it is inhibited. Such muscles withstand loads less well and are more likely to be strained or to lead to sprains or joint damage due to their inability to control motion. A muscle can be inhibited intermittently or chronically. An inhibited muscle will demonstrate breakaway weakness and will not be able to maintain a sustained contraction during a manual muscle test by a therapist, athletic trainer, or a doctor. If a muscle or muscles are inhibited during your strength training, you may notice that you fatigue more easily or cannot handle increased resistance. If this happens during an activity or a sport, you may feel weaker, have poorer balance and agility, perceive a lower level of performance, and feel more prone to injury.

FIGURE 24a

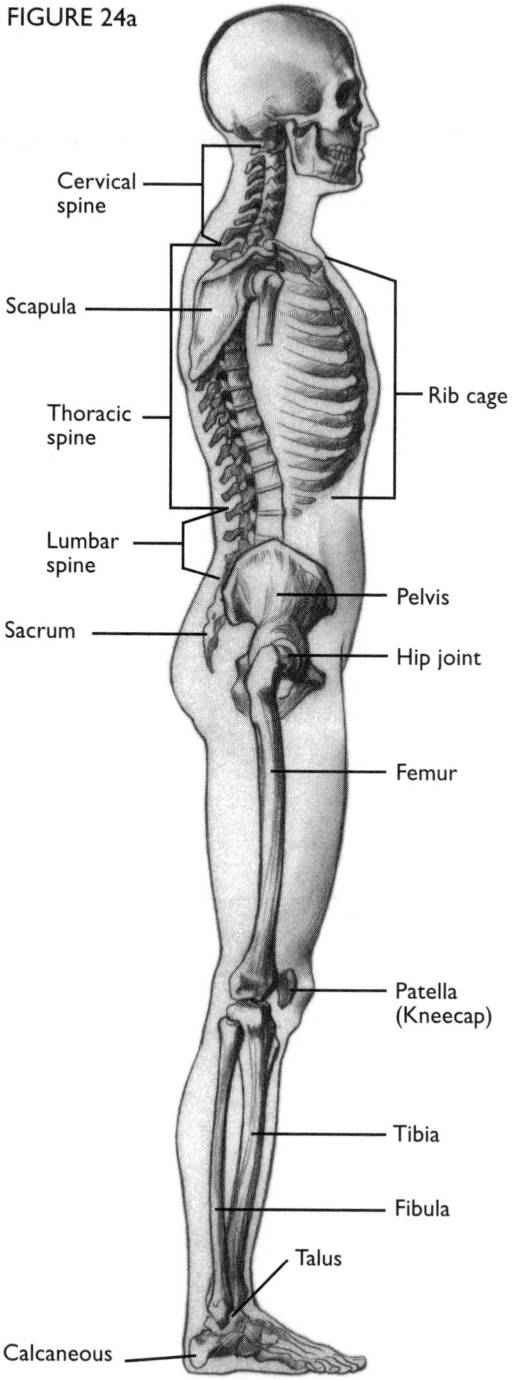

FIGURE 24b

FIGURE 24c

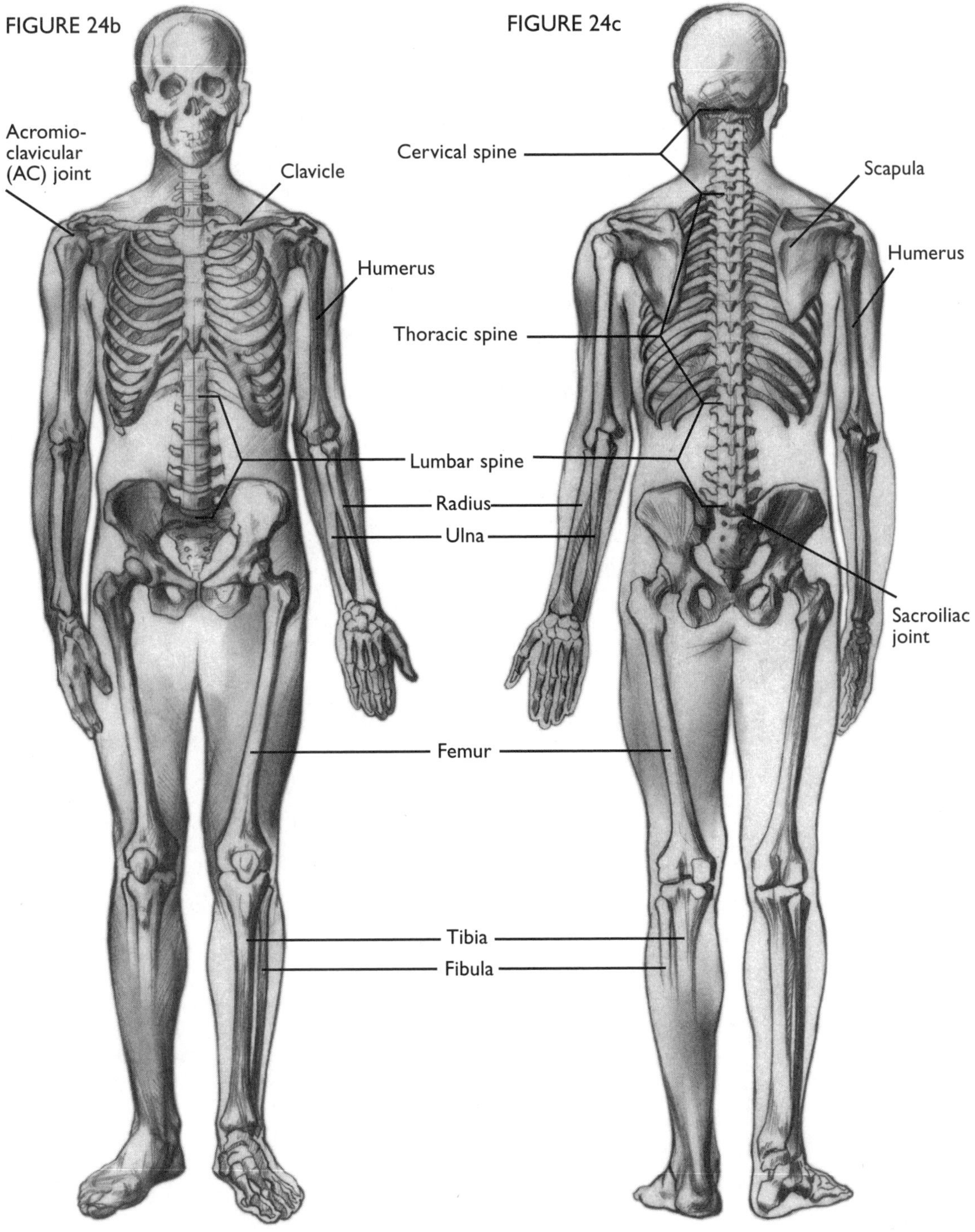

FIGURE 25a

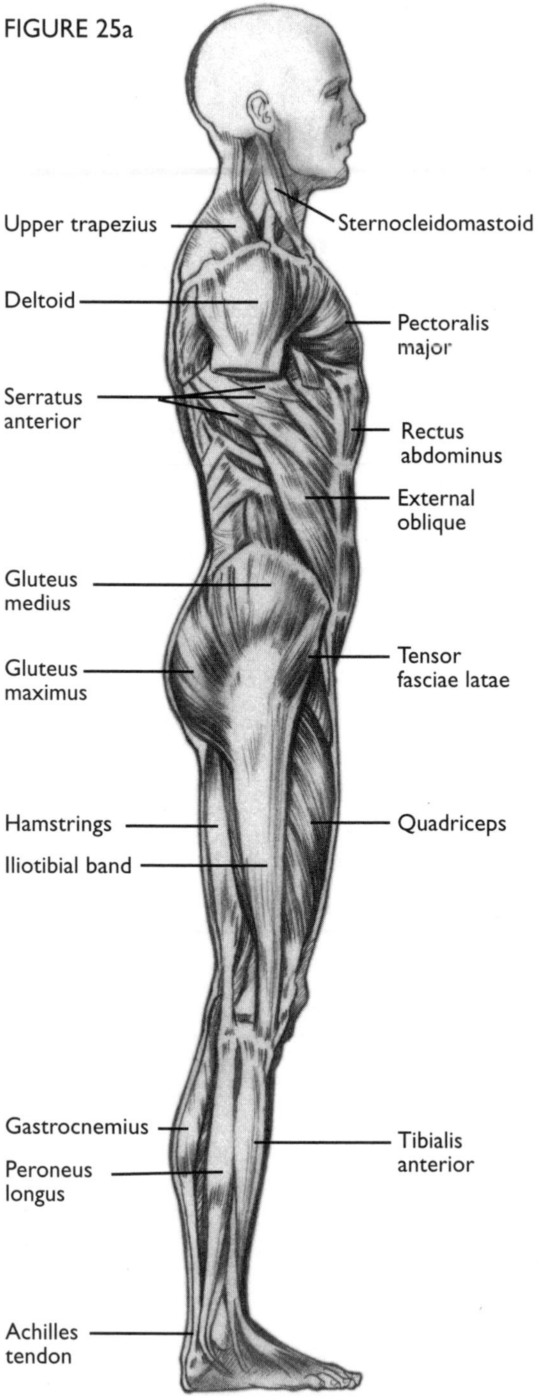
Upper trapezius
Sternocleidomastoid
Deltoid
Pectoralis major
Serratus anterior
Rectus abdominus
External oblique
Gluteus medius
Gluteus maximus
Tensor fasciae latae
Hamstrings
Quadriceps
Iliotibial band
Gastrocnemius
Tibialis anterior
Peroneus longus
Achilles tendon

FIGURE 25b

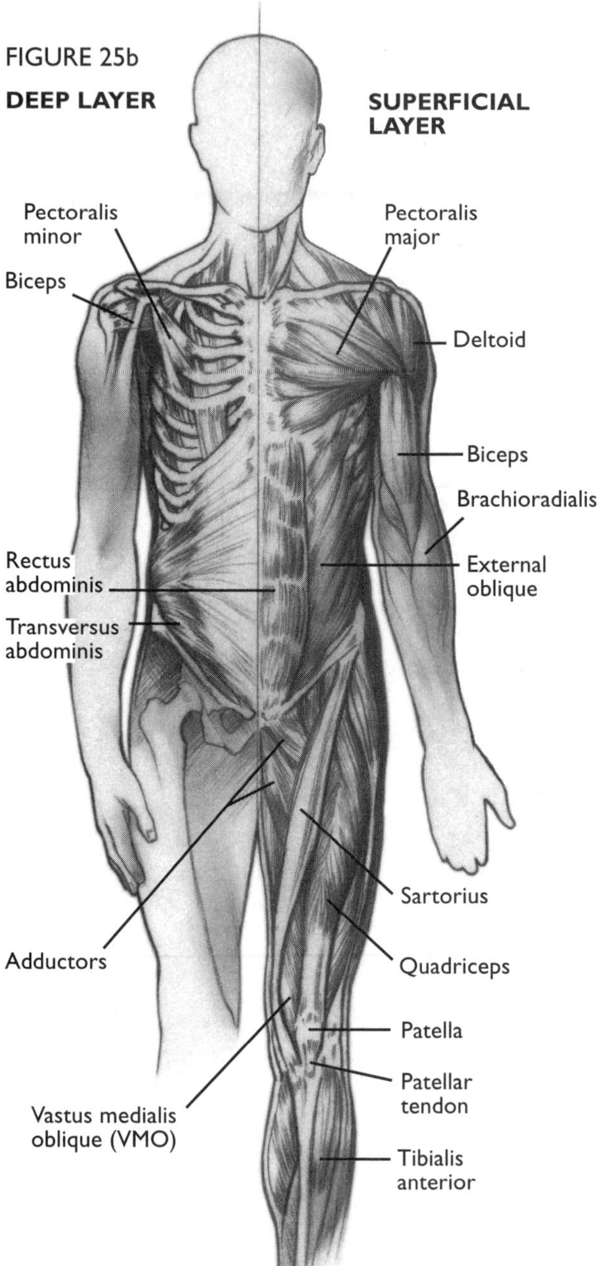
DEEP LAYER
SUPERFICIAL LAYER
Pectoralis minor
Pectoralis major
Biceps
Deltoid
Biceps
Brachioradialis
Rectus abdominis
External oblique
Transversus abdominis
Sartorius
Adductors
Quadriceps
Patella
Patellar tendon
Vastus medialis oblique (VMO)
Tibialis anterior

FIGURE 25c

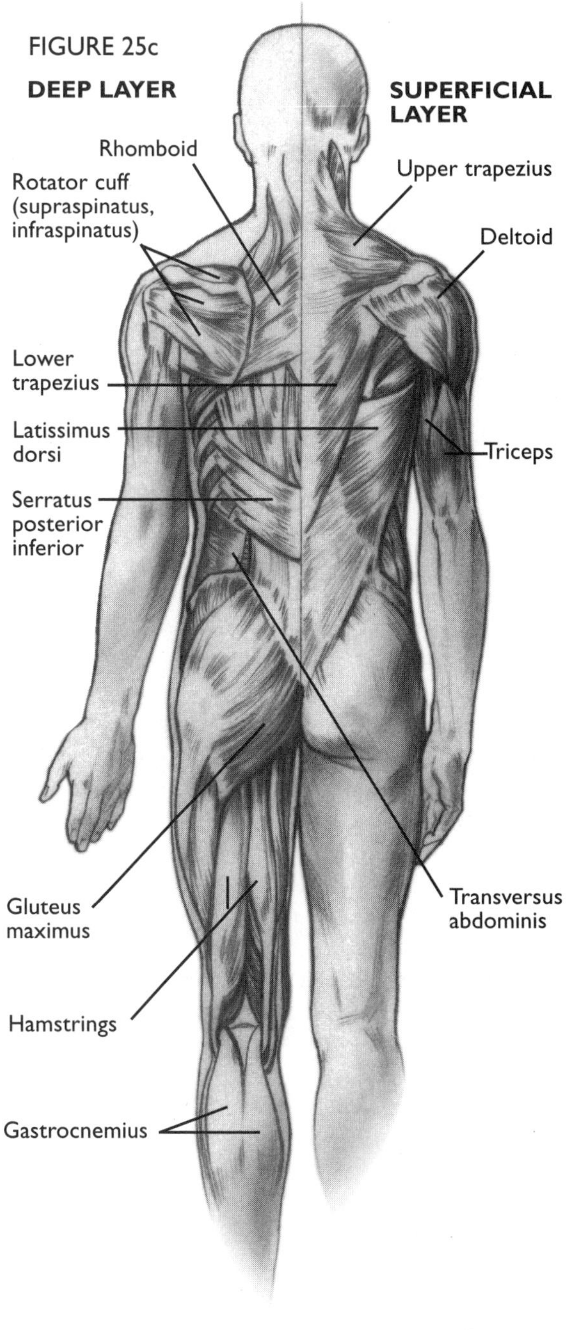

There are many possible reasons that a muscle can be inhibited, including:

- Antagonist (opposing) muscles are tight.
- The muscle is lengthened excessively because of chronic poor posture or excessive stretching.
- Joints are out of alignment.
- A joint is inflamed or has edema (swelling) from injury or arthritis.
- There are loose ligaments in the joint region that relates neurologically to the muscle or is near the muscle.
- Scars from injuries or surgeries can have an effect on muscles near them or, sometimes, on muscles that are on the opposite side of the body or that are far away.
- Internal organ system dysfunction can lead to certain patterns of muscle inhibition via the autonomic nervous system or other mechanisms.
- Certain food and environmental sensitivities can lead to a muscle or groups of muscles being inhibited.
- Cold temperatures may lead to a more generalized pattern of muscle inhibition and an increased risk of injury.

Muscles most prone to being weak or inhibited are the wrist extensors, rotator cuffs, mid and lower trapezius, abdominal obliques, gluteus maximus and gluteus medius, vastus medialis obliques, and the tibialis posterior. Consider spending more time stretching your tight muscles and strengthening your weak muscles. Consider stress reduction techniques if you have chronic neck, shoulder, or upper-back tightness or pain. If you feel generally weak or you injure easily, consider consulting a health-care professional.

Improper recruitment of muscles during joint motions. When body regions move, more than one muscle is usually recruited. If one muscle is not doing its job, another muscle may have to overwork and get strained or develop tendonitis. For example, an inhibited gluteus maximus (buttock) can lead to hamstring problems during hip-extending activities such as climbing, backpacking, and running. Many functional exercises in this book work on recruitment pattern issues.

Ligament laxity and loose joints. Ligament laxity can contribute to a number of musculoskeletal symptoms and signs. If the ligaments are loose around a joint, the muscles that contribute to stabilizing that joint will have to work excessively. They may begin to hurt, have tender points, or eventually have trigger points (firm sensitive areas within the muscle belly). These muscles are also more likely to strain or can lead to joint and ligament injury during activities. Ligaments that are loose may or may not be tender to the touch.

Ligaments can be loose for a number of reasons:

- A prior injury that did not heal completely and healed with a lengthened ligament
- Poor posture
- Genetic reasons, including Marfan Syndrome and Ehlers-Danlos Syndrome
- Constitutional ligament laxity

Constitutional ligament laxity is a condition in which a person has many loose joints and lax ligaments. This is more common in women then men. The most common findings are:

- Hyperextension of the fingers, elbow, and knees
- Multidirectional looseness of the shoulder
- Looseness to inversion of the ankle and frequent ankle sprains
- Flattened arches and pes planus (flat) feet

If you think that you have loose ligaments or are working with a client who has loose ligaments, you will want to emphasize the following:

- Core stability
- Proper movement patterns
- Good posture
- Caution when speeding up an exercise or doing plyometrics
- Balance and agility training
- Exercise of muscles that stabilize the joint area of concern
- Consideration of bracing and taping
- Consideration of referral to a physician who does prolotherapy (ligament stabilizing injections)

Overuse. Excessive use of a muscle or muscles can lead to tendonitis or a strain. This may be from doing an activity or exercise with too much speed, duration, or resistance before your muscles are strong enough to handle the load. Build up gradually in your exercises and activities.

Inadequate equipment can lead to muscles having to work excessively. Footwear must be stable enough to support and control your body's motion. Orthotic supports may be useful in addition to good footwear.

Poor postural habits over prolonged periods may be due to inadequate knowledge of proper posture or to tight or weak muscles or joint misalignment. It can lead to shortened or lengthened muscles as well as joints functioning off their normal axis of motion. See chapter 14 as well as the other body region chapters.

Improper movement patterns during exercise or activities. Form is important in exercise or activities so as to use muscles and joints properly with the least likelihood of injury. Make sure you understand the movement pattern of an exercise or activity before increasing resistance or speed.

Poor balance and agility can lead to injury of the extremities or spine from falling or excessive demands on muscles. Try to incorporate balance and agility exercises (from chapter 6 and the body region and activity chapters) into your program within 6–8 weeks of starting your activity.

Inadequate training and strength to control deceleration. Most musculoskeletal injuries are considered deceleration injuries because your tissues are exposed to quicker and more demanding forces during deceleration than acceleration. The demand for deceleration control is related to the pull of gravity as well as the need to control joint motion while a muscle is lengthening (eccentric contraction). Injuries occur when you cannot slow down and stop motion before failure. Many of the functional exercises address deceleration demands. See chapter 11 for details.

Inadequate strength training at longer muscle length, when muscles are normally weaker. Depending on your activity, you may need to train muscles when they are lengthened. This is especially true in climbing and certain boating activities. See the activity chapters for exercise advice for your activity.

Inadequate muscle training at the highest speeds that will be used during an activity. Do some of your exercises at higher speeds to simulate the speed demands of your activity.

Poor nutrition. Muscles, ligaments, and cartilage require certain nutrients for optimal function as well as for healing after exercise and activities. See chapter 2.

Inadequate attention during a task or activity. Focus your attention on your activity as well as the surface you are on, especially in steep or rough conditions.

Injury Phases and Healing

Different phases of tissue healing occur when you have injured a musculoskeletal structure. If you are doing a strength training program, take these injury phases into account to modify any strength training that involves an injured area.

Acute phase occurs immediately after an injury, lasting 24–72 hours. There may be pain, swelling, limited joint motion, muscle weakness, and muscle spasm. Minimize swelling by using ice or cold water; compression with bandages, braces, or tape; and elevation of a limb above the level of the heart. In addition, protect the joint from further injury by limiting or modifying exercises or activities. Bracing, splinting, crutches, or slings may be used for more severe injuries. As soon as possible, restore pain-free range of motion. On day 2 or 3, pain-free range-of-motion exercises should help reduce swelling and restore tolerance for weight bearing or lifting.

Subacute (fibroblastic/repair) phase may last 14–21 days after onset of the injury. In this phase, there is clearing of swelling and cellular debris, and production of new cells and collagen to strengthen the area. Caution should be taken during this time (and during the remodeling phase, below) to limit exercises and activities so as to prevent worsening the original injury. Remember that the pain will resolve much sooner than it takes to regain full strength and function. An injured tissue may only be 15–20% of its original strength at the end of this phase.

Exercises involving the injured body region should be done in pain-free ranges of motion and with minimal resistance to improve blood flow and decrease swelling. After acute pain and swelling have subsided, an exercise may be done for 2 sets of 12–15 reps. If the injury does not worsen, progress to 3–5 sets of 20–30 reps. If there is pain while exercising or within the following 24 hours, the exercises should be modified to involve decreased resistance. Exercises that involve other body regions away from the injury may be done with less resistance than used prior to the injury. This is important when exercising your arms and shoulders after a neck injury, or your legs after a low-back injury.

Other goals during this phase include regaining full joint motion, muscle length, as well as balance and coordination. Gentle flexibility work can begin in this phase, but remember, injured areas can be injured more from aggressive stretching, so don't hold stretches in painful ranges and limit them to 20–30 seconds. Easy balance exercises can begin early in this phase; you will find many balance exercises in chapters 6, 8, 10, and 11. Functional strength and coordination exercises can begin in the middle of this phase, but should usually be modified to decreased ranges and decreased speeds.

Remodeling phase may begin within 2–3 weeks of the original injury and may last for many months (up to 1 year). In this phase, collagen in the scar tissue is being organized and aligned, and the scar is strengthening, depending upon the exercise and activity stresses. An injured area may only be 40–50% of original strength after 6 weeks, and thus caution should still be used in exercise and activities. Goals during this phase are to develop strong scar tissue and maintain cartilage; increase strength, flexibility, and balance; maintain aerobic capacity; and rehabilitate toward the functional demands of your activity.

In this phase, continue flexibility exercises and gradually increase the resistance of your strength training. Two to 3 sets of 12–15 reps are appropriate. Eight to 12 weeks into this phase, you may add a set of 6–8 reps of higher resistance to develop maximum strength, if you are training for activities that require quick bursts of activity or working against higher loads. Continue your functional exercises in this phase and incorporate more gravity and balance challenges. As you master the movement patterns, you can add speed to these exercises.

Outdoor activities should initially be done with less intensity, distance, and difficulty. Simulate and demonstrate competency in the motion, strength, and balance demands of your activity in a controlled environment before starting your activity. You can start getting back to your activity when you meet the following criteria:

- Injured muscles have returned to normal lengths.
- Injured muscles and ligaments don't hurt when you simulate your activity for short duration.
- You have good balance and coordination.
- You have good muscle strength balance and recruitment in the injured and adjacent areas.
- The joints of your spine have normal motion.
- The joints in the injured or compensating areas have normal motion when compared to the noninjured joint on the opposite side of your body.

chapter 10 THE ABDOMINALS

By Carrie Hall, P.T., and Mark Pierce, A.T.C.

THIS CHAPTER WILL HELP YOU:

- Understand the function of your abdominal muscles.
- Perform a self-assessment of your abdominal strength.
- Learn new exercises that dynamically strengthen your abdominal muscles to meet the challenges of your sport or activity.

Your abdominal muscles are the core stabilizers of your trunk (torso). Essentially, your abdominal muscles are controllers and initiators of motion in rotation, forward and backward bending, and side-to-side movements. Functional abdominal strength provides dynamic control for these movements along with decelerating your body against changes in direction, speed, and surface.

All forms of outdoor activities require your body to be in an erect, semi-erect, or seated position relative to the ground and the forces of gravity. To develop optimal balance, coordination, and total body strength, perform functional abdominal exercises in standing and sitting positions, which are designed for dynamic abdominal function and injury prevention.

Understanding the anatomical and functional roles that your abdominal muscles play during activities will help you make educated exercise choices specific to your sport or activity and enable you to condition your abdominal muscles appropriately to meet those demands.

FUNCTION AND ANATOMY

There are four abdominal muscles positioned in specific layers covering the front, sides, and part of the back of your torso. Along with your back muscles, they form a link between your rib cage, spine, and pelvis. (See chapter 9 for illustrations of the muscles.) As a result, normal abdominal muscle length and strength is critical for proper torso alignment. With their attachments to your rib cage, spine, and pelvis, they provide a solid foundation for movement of your upper and lower extremities.

The first, and deepest, of the abdominal muscles is called the *transversus abdominis*. This muscle has fibers that run horizontally. Therefore, it functions like a girdle to provide support to your abdominal organs and spine.

The next layer is called the *internal oblique*, followed by the *external oblique*. These muscles have fibers that run diagonally to each other and cover primarily the sides and part of the back of your torso. They share the function of providing the primary force to produce torso rotation, but also have very different functions with respect to your pelvis and rib cage, as discussed below. The final layer is called the *rectus abdominis*. This is a muscle that extends from your ribs to your pelvis and is strengthened in the typical "ab" crunch.

The rectus abdominis and the internal oblique curl the rib cage toward the pelvis as in a sit-up. The internal and external obliques, along with the transversus abdominis, provide stability for the spine and pelvis during motions of the extremities.

The terms *upper abdominals* and *lower abdominals* relate to the relative functions of these muscles. The internal oblique and upper rectus abdominis are referred to as the upper abdominals, and the lower external oblique is referred to as the lower abdominals. Upper abdominals play a greater role in controlling movements of your torso on your pelvis (e.g., sit-ups), and lower abdominals play a greater role in controlling the position of your pelvis and spine during leg and arm movements (e.g., lifting your leg to hike up a slope).

ABDOMINAL STRENGTH AND SPINE PROTECTION

Adequate abdominal strength and endurance is critical for spine protection, especially for your low back or lumbar spine. Lower abdominal strength, endurance, and length create a "girdling effect" on your low back and pelvis. This girdling effect protects your spine by decreasing the mechanical stresses on ligaments and discs, thus helping to maintain the integrity of each joint.

Your lower abdominals allow you to position and maintain your lumbar spine in a neutral position while using your arm and legs. Exercising and performing daily activities with a neutral lumbar spine and with your lower abdominals engaged trains your neuromuscular system to recognize this position. The lengths of your lower abdominal muscles adapt and conform to the positions and tensions that they commonly experience. If you consistently train them in an appropriate neutral spine position, they become stronger and gain the endurance to protect your spine for prolonged activities and positions.

COMMON MUSCLE IMBALANCES

It is important to maintain balance in muscle strength and length between all four abdominal muscles, as well as between your abdominal muscles and your back and hip muscles. The most common imbalance is between the rectus abdominis/internal oblique group and between the external oblique/transversus abdominis group. This imbalance also alters the alignment and function of the low back and leaves it vulnerable to numerous injuries.

Most abdominal exercises emphasize strengthening of your rectus abdominis and internal oblique with crunch-type exercises, for example, the bent-knees crunch, oblique curl-up, and feet-in-the-air crunch, as well as the curl-down abdominal machine. Rarely do you see exercises for strengthening your external obliques and transversus abdominis, and if you do see them, the exercises are usually far more advanced than the average person's muscle strength permits (e.g., double leg lifts and leg lowering). Also, rarely do you see exercises to functionally strengthen your abdominal muscles in standing and sitting positions.

Muscle length is rarely discussed with respect to abdominal muscles. The typical postural problem of forward shoulders, increased curve of the upper back, and slumped chest demonstrates shortening of the upper fibers of the rectus abdominis muscle and upper, front fibers of the internal oblique. With this type of posture, it is inappropriate to perform trunk-curl exercises or any variations. These exercises will only further shorten the rectus abdominis and internal oblique and exaggerate the postural problem.

Another common postural problem is a forward-tilted pelvis (excessive lumbar extension curve). This type of posture demonstrates overstretching of the external obliques. Again, trunk-curl exercises will not specifically address this problem. An exercise that promotes a stable neutral pelvic position during progressively more difficult leg motions will more specifically strengthen the external oblique at its optimal length.

INJURY PREVENTION

In order to exercise your abdominal muscles safely, you must not only choose a safe technique, but also be sure you are exercising at the correct level for your strength. It certainly makes sense that you would not lift 30 pounds with your biceps if you could only lift 10 pounds safely and with good technique. Why, then, do we expect all individuals to be able to perform the same abdominal exercises?

Poor abdominal muscle strength, and/or imbalances in strength and length, are risk factors for the development of numerous musculoskeletal injuries and pain syndromes. The most common injury linked to the abdominal muscles involves the low back. Typically, the rectus abdominis and internal obliques become relatively stronger than the external obliques. An injury resulting from trauma, such as a low-back strain resulting from a fall, can be more severe or more difficult to recover from if an individual has poor abdominal strength prior to the injury.

STRATEGIES FOR STRENGTHENING

It is a good idea to plan your abdominal strengthening program to accomplish the following goals: (1) Strengthen your transversus abdominis and your obliques to provide core stability for your back. (2) Learn to use your abdominal muscles in standing or sitting positions (if your sport is a seated one) for dynamic balance. (3) Strengthen your obliques to aid in rotating and decelerating your spine. (4) Do rectus and transversus exercises to improve your abdominal tone and shape.

To prepare for specific activity challenges, you can add any of the other abdominal exercises in this chapter to the basic or intermediate programs that follow.

Basic Abdominal Conditioning Program

To establish a basic abdominal program for the average person desiring good functional abdominal strength and tone, try Exercises 78.3 (2–3 sets of 15 reps), 83, 84, and 92.

Intermediate Abdominal Strengthening Program

Try Exercises 23.1, 78 (progress to 78.5), 83, and 86.

ABDOMINAL EXERCISES

You can begin strength training exercises with 15 reps unless otherwise indicated. Progress your reps and resistance according to the guidelines in chapter 5.

MUSCLE BALANCING EXERCISES

The following exercises provide a foundation for developing muscle balance. It may be advantageous for you to develop competency in the following exercises prior to moving into the functional exercises. This will help you perform the functional exercises with balanced muscle activation patterns while tuning your body's fine motor control.

78 LOWER ABDOMINAL PROGRESSION

Equipment: Firm, comfortable surface.
Purpose: Build the foundation for controlling your lower abdominal muscles and improve the balance between your upper and lower abdominal muscles (external oblique/transversus abdominis).

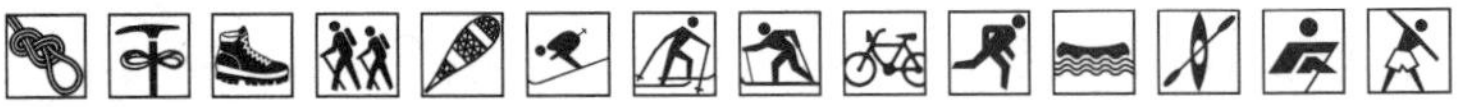

Technique: Once you can perform this exercise, you may progress to variation 78.1 and omit this exercise; continue progressing through the variations in this manner. In order to progress from an easier exercise to the next in this series, you must meet the following criteria: First, the abdominal muscles must be pulled up and in, as if to bring your belly button (umbilicus) toward your spine. This will prevent a "pooched out" abdomen as increased strain is placed on your abdominal muscles from the progressively difficult leg movements. Second, your lumbar spine must remain in a neutral position with a slight extension curve, just enough to fit your hand between your back and the floor, and not move into an exaggerated curve or excessively flatten. The starting position is the same for this exercise and its variations. Lie on your back on a firm surface, such as the floor, with your knees bent and feet flat on the floor, with your shoes off. Place your little fingers on the bony anterior part of your pelvis to monitor pelvic motion. Your goal is to use your abdominal muscles to keep your pelvis from moving. Have your other fingertips on your lower abdominal

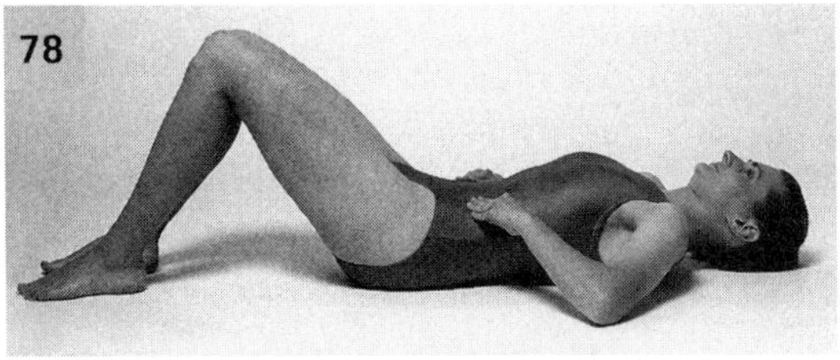
78

muscles. Take a deep breath in, then exhale and pull your belly button toward your spine. Be sure to incorporate breathing to activate the transversus abdominal muscle. Don't concentrate on pushing your back flat but, rather, on lengthening your torso while pulling in your abdominal muscles. Start with 8–10 reps and gradually progress to 15–20 reps, holding each rep for 10 seconds. When you can perform 15–20 reps, without allowing your low back or pelvis to move, you are ready to progress to variation 78.1.

Variations: 78.1. While keeping your abdomen pulled in (this occurs maximally at a full exhalation), slowly lift one leg so that your hip is at a 90-degree angle (78.1a). Breathe in while in the rest position; exhale as you lift your leg. Once you have completed the lift of the first leg, breathe in again, and then exhale while you lift the other leg to the same position (78.1b). Return to the starting position, one limb at a time. A good rule of thumb is to exhale as your legs are moving and inhale while they are resting. Remember that exhalation activates the transversus abdominis, which is required to stabilize your spine as you move your extremities. Alternate the starting leg with each subsequent repetition. Start with 8–10 reps and gradually increase to 15–20 reps with each leg before progressing to variation 78.2.

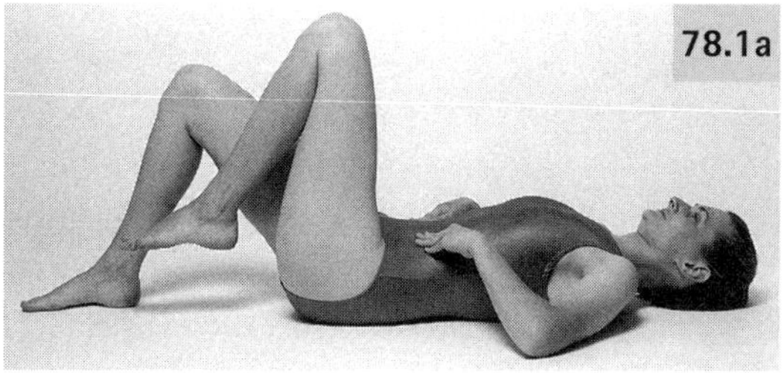
78.1a

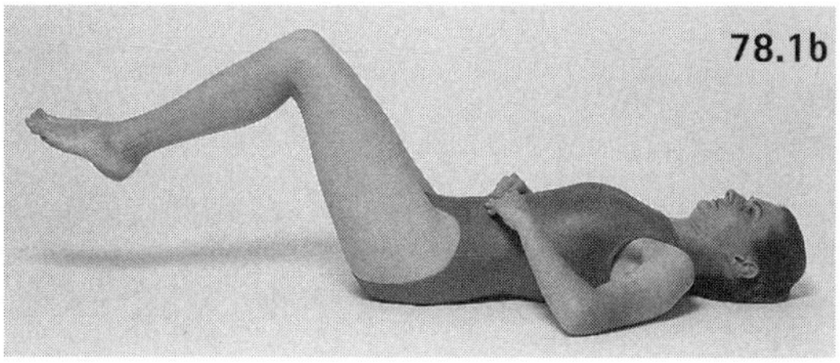
78.1b

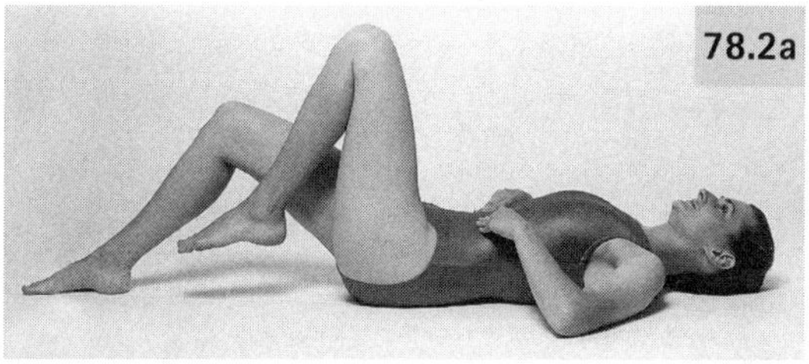
78.2a

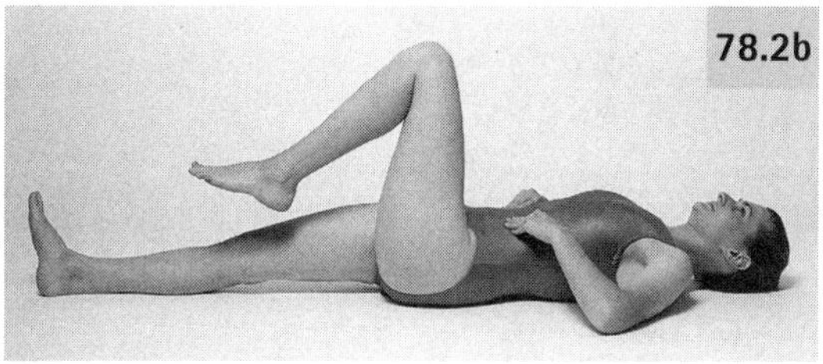
78.2b

78.2. Repeat variation 78.1, but instead of lowering your legs to the starting position, slide one leg down to a fully extended position while keeping the opposite leg elevated off the floor (78.2a and 78.2b). Breathe out as you slide your leg down. Breathe in while your leg is fully extended, and breathe out as you slide your leg back to the same position as your nonmoving limb; repeat with your other leg. As soon as you are unable to stabilize your pelvis and lumbar spine and your abdomen begins to pooch out, stop and rest for a minute before continuing. Start with 8–10 reps and gradually increase to 15–20 reps with each leg before progressing to variation 78.3. **Note:** If your hip flexors (front thigh muscles) are short, you will not be able to fully extend your leg without moving your spine out of neutral. In this case, stop sliding your leg when you notice your back moving from its neutral position. Eventually, your hip flexor muscles will

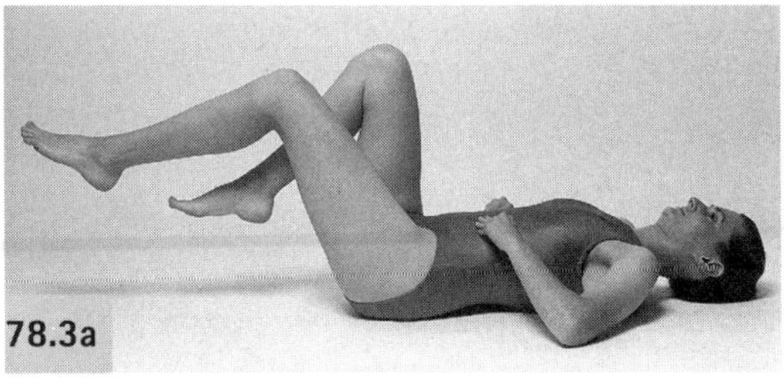
78.3a

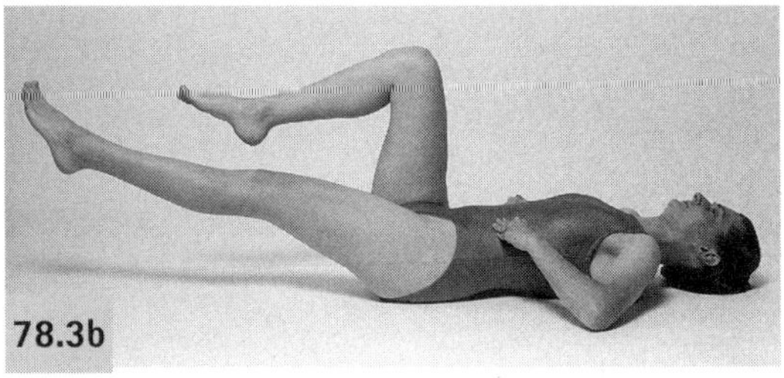
78.3b

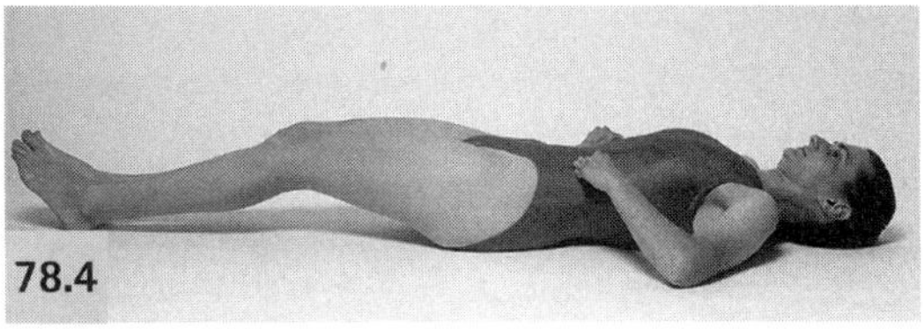
78.4

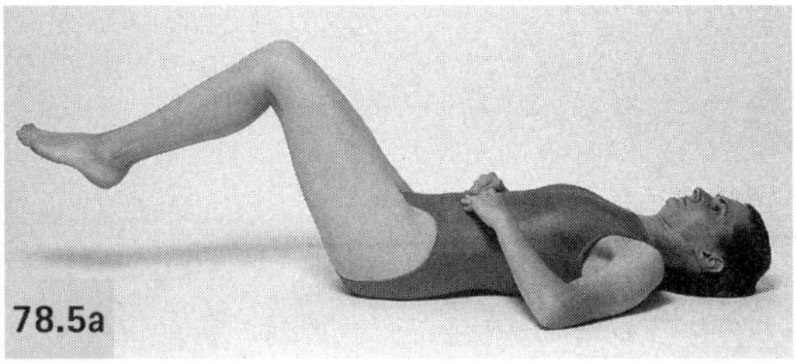
78.5a

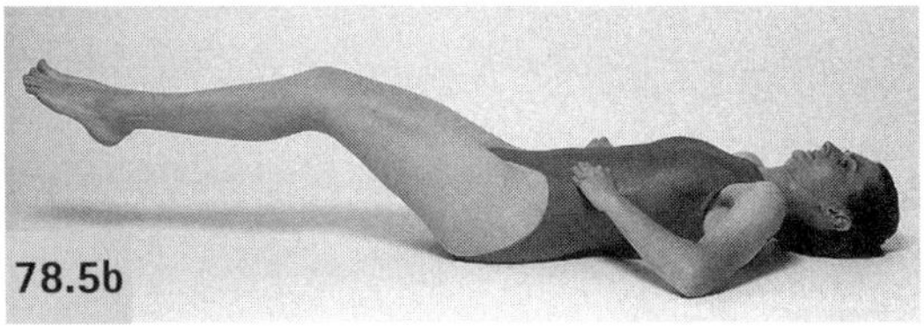
78.5b

lengthen as your abdominal muscles shorten and become stronger. **78.3.** Repeat variation 78.2, but instead of sliding your leg, glide your leg straight to the starting position while keeping your heel 6–12 inches off the floor. Your nonmoving leg should remain in a flexed position off the floor (78.3a and 78.3b). Breathe similarly to variation 78.2. Perform 2–3 sets to develop endurance. In preparation for functional exercises, achieve a minimum of 1 set of 20 reps. **Note:** It is easy to transition from a flat abdomen to a pooched abdomen in this variation. Keep your lower abs tight to avoid this problem. **78.4.** From the starting position, lift both legs off the floor at the same time to the 90-degree position. Breathe in once both legs are elevated. Return to the starting position by lowering both legs at the same time. Breathe out as you move both legs down. Then, slide both legs simultaneously (while maintaining heel contact with the floor) to the fully extended straight-knee position (see photo 78.4), and breathe in as both legs are fully extended. Slide both legs back to the starting position; breathe out as you slide both legs up. Perform 2–3 sets to develop endurance. In preparation for functional exercises, achieve a minimum of 1 set of 20 reps. **Note:** Variations 78.3 and 78.4 are similar in difficulty. You may find that sliding one leg at a time is more difficult than sliding two legs simultaneously, particularly if you have difficulty stabilizing against rotational forces. Choose the variation that is appropriate for you. Variations 78.3 and 78.4 are appropriate goals for the average person. **78.5.** Repeat variation 78.4, but instead of sliding your heels, keep them 6–12 inches above the floor (78.5a and 78.5b). Slowly return both legs to the 90-degree position. Breathe as in variation 78.4. Perform 2–3 sets to develop endurance. In preparation for functional exercises, achieve a minimum of 1 set of 20 reps. **Note:** Only the most fit individuals should try variation 78.5. This is a difficult exercise and takes a high level of strength to perform properly. Don't do this variation if you have an active back problem.

79 UPPER ABDOMINAL STRENGTHENING

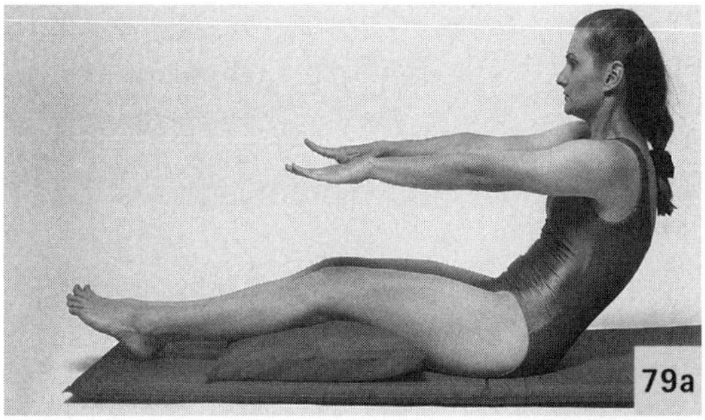
79a

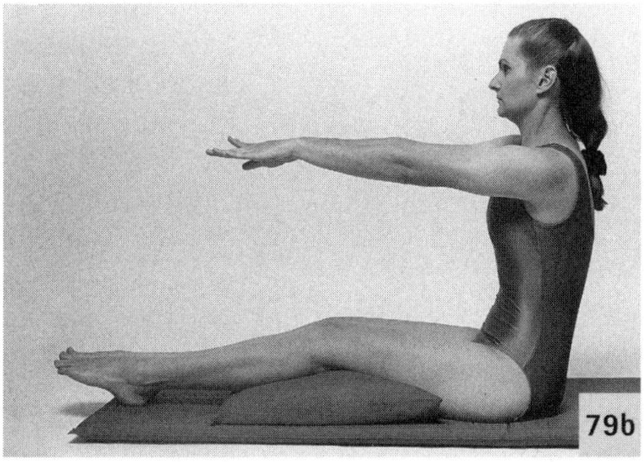
79b

Equipment: Firm, comfortable surface.
Purpose: Strengthen your upper abdominals (internal oblique and rectus abdominis) to flex your torso.

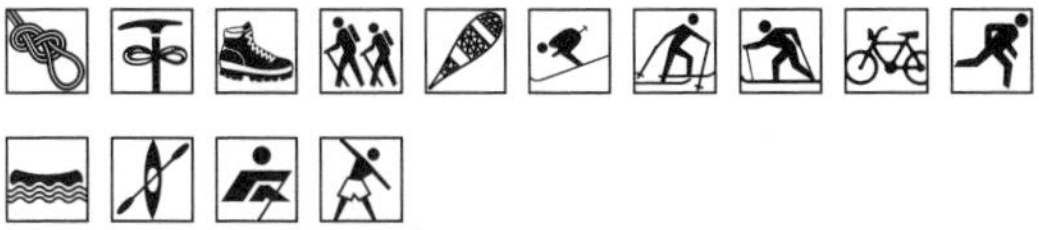

Technique: To determine your start position, which is dependent upon the length of your hip flexors, lie on the floor on your back with your legs out straight. If you can flatten your back against the floor with your legs out straight, this is your start position. If not, place a pillow or pillows under your knees until you can flatten your back against the floor. With your arms straight in front of your body, curl your chin to your chest. Once you have completely curled your chin to your chest, continue to curl your trunk (79a). As you raise your upper body to a sitting position, allow your neck to return to a neutral, relaxed position (79b; note the use of a support under the knees for tight hamstrings). To return to the start position, reverse your movement pattern. The start and finish positions are the same for all variations of this exercise. If your hamstrings are tight, you may need to bend your knees to achieve a full sit-up position. If you are unable to curl upward through a full sit-up, just lift your head and shoulders off the floor. Start with 8–10 reps; achieving 20 reps is an appropriate goal before progressing to variation 79.1.

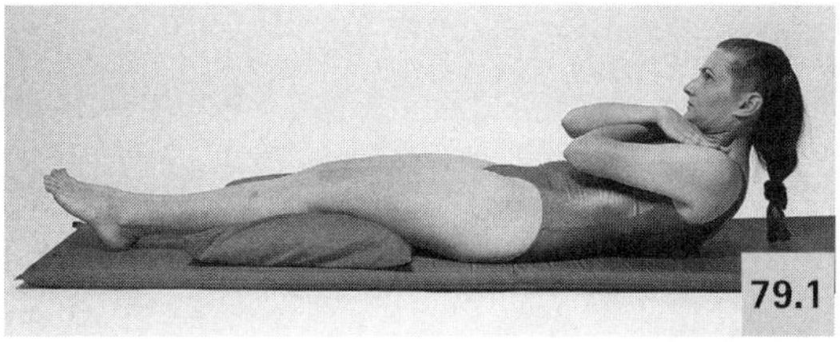
79.1

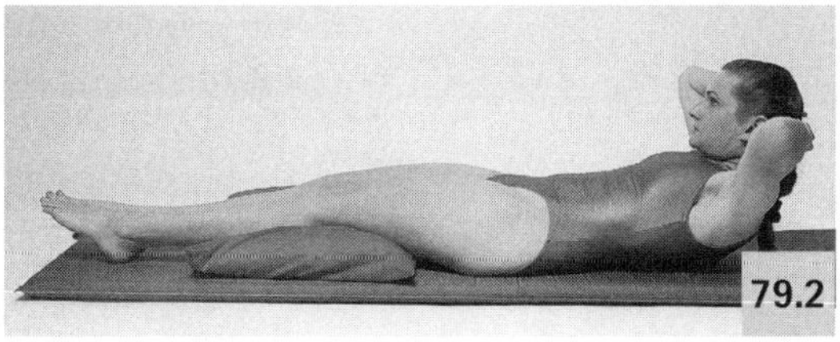
79.2

Variations: 79.1. Arms across chest: With your arms folded across your chest so that your hands are on opposite shoulders, curl your chin toward your chest. Once you have completely curled your chin to your chest, slowly curl your trunk as you come to a sitting position. Maintain the curl throughout the movement. **79.2.** Hands behind neck: With your hands supporting the back of your neck, curl your chin toward your chest.

Once you have completely curled your chin to your chest, slowly curl your trunk as you come to a sitting position. Maintain the curl throughout the movement. Perform 2–3 sets of 20 reps to maintain the endurance of your abdominal muscles and to progress safely to the functional exercises.

Tips and Precautions: You should be able to perform a complete flexing of your torso before you flex (pivot) at your hips. You may notice that once you have completed the curl phase, your feet will want to lift upward. At that point you can secure your feet with a partner, under a couch, or under the bar of a sit-up board. The purpose of securing your feet is to counteract the fact that in order to sit up, you must contract your hip flexors. Without securing your feet, your hip flexors will attempt to lift your legs. If you find the need to secure your feet earlier in the trunk curl phase, it indicates that your abdominal muscles are fatigued and your hip flexors are taking over the motion. Stop and rest at this point. This is your maximum number of repetitions for this set. You must also be able to lift your upper body smoothly, without jerking, to the full sit-up position. Jerking movements indicate that your abdominal muscles either are not strong enough or have fatigued and your hip flexor muscles are trying to take over.

FUNCTIONAL ABDOMINAL EXERCISES

The majority of people continue to exercise their abdominal muscles with crunches, sit-ups, leg raises, and using various machines. This type of training is excellent for developing strength and muscle balance. Unfortunately, these exercises alone don't address all of the real-life functional requirements of the abdominal muscles during activities. To enhance performance in activities, train your abdominal muscles in the same way you wish them to perform. Functional abdominal exercises are designed to dynamically strengthen and challenge your abdominal muscles with movement patterns and balance challenges most commonly encountered during activities. These exercises are appropriate for many outdoor activities (note the activity icons, defined in Figure 1 in the introduction). The exercises are performed in sitting and standing positions and may involve additional equipment.

These exercises are nontraditional and very challenging. Make each exercise safe and pain-free. Start each exercise slowly and in a range of motion that you can control before increasing your speed or range of motion. Most of these exercises should be performed in a neutral zone of low-back alignment to prevent injury. In addition, bring your belly button up and under your rib cage to initially activate your abdominal muscles. Make sure you breathe during the exercises. When you first try an exercise, begin with 8–10 reps in a set for just 1 set, and gradually increase the reps and the number of sets.

If you have a back problem, consult a health-care practitioner skilled in biomechanics and musculoskeletal injuries before starting the following exercises. You should achieve competency in exercises 78.3 and 79.2 before progressing to the functional abdominal exercises.

80 TORSO ROTATIONS: THE TWISTER

Equipment: 3- to 10-pound hand weight (dumbbell)
Purpose: Improve the dynamic strength of your core in the transverse (rotational) plane and improve your ability to react in shortened rotational ranges of motion while engaging your lower body as a stabilizer. Also, condition your neck, abdominals, and hips for rapid changes in direction, and improve your ability to accelerate.

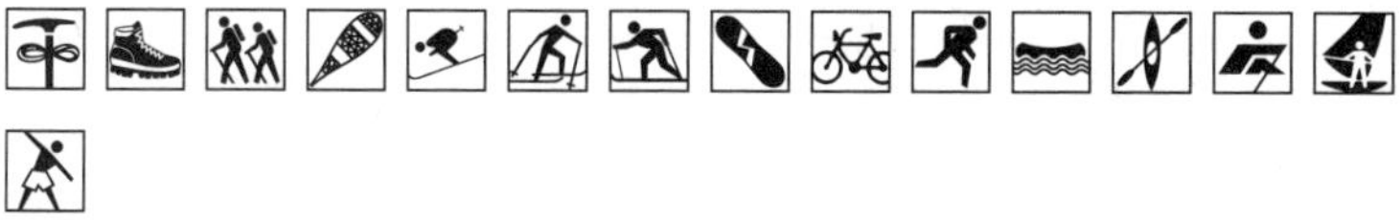

Technique: Grasp the dumbbell handle with both hands and place it firmly in the center of your chest with your elbows at your sides. This will add mass to your core and create resistance for this exercise. Stand with your feet slightly wider than shoulder width apart, maintain a neutral spine and bend slightly at your ankles, knees and hips. Hinge at your hips so that your upper body has a slight forward lean and engage your core (80a). Keep your head and hips still and, without sliding the hand weight across your chest, rotate your shoulders and upper back to the left (80b). Perform the same rotation motion to the right (80c), maintaining a still head and hip position. Do this motion slowly at first to establish your left and right rotational end positions. Once your have performed 5–6 rotations to each side, move faster, rapidly rotating to the left and right in a shorter range without allowing any side-to-side trunk motion. Perform 2–3 sets of 30- to 60-second intervals, resting the equivalent between sets.
Variation: 80.1. Staggered stance twister: Perform this exercise in a staggered stance with your right foot forward for 30–60 seconds and repeat with your left foot forward.
Tips and Precautions: Try to increase the tempo of the exercise before using more weight. Move as quickly as you can, in control. Don't try to overrotate your spine in either direction. Keep your core engaged during the duration of this exercise. Don't perform this exercise if you have an active neck problem.

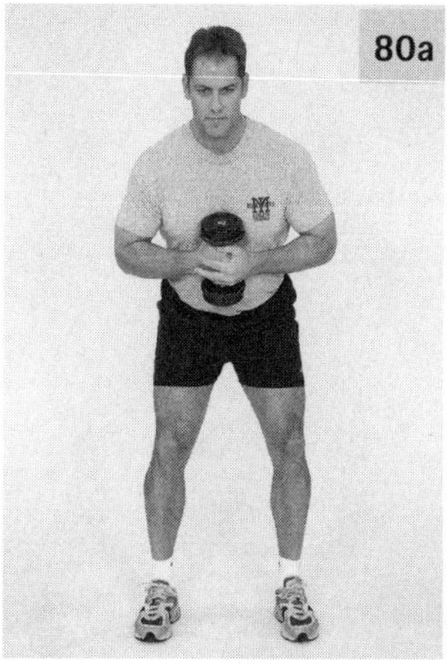
80a

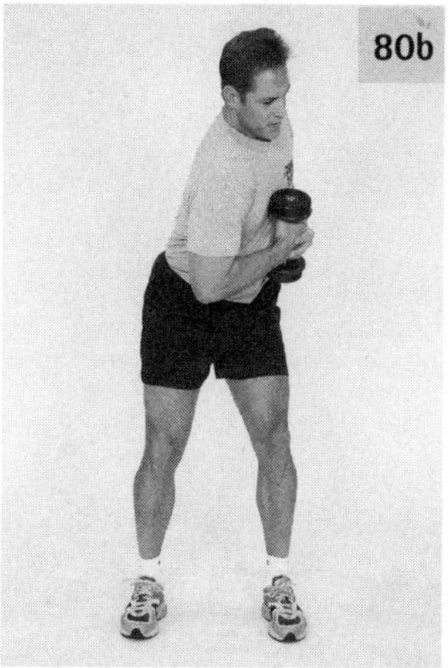
80b

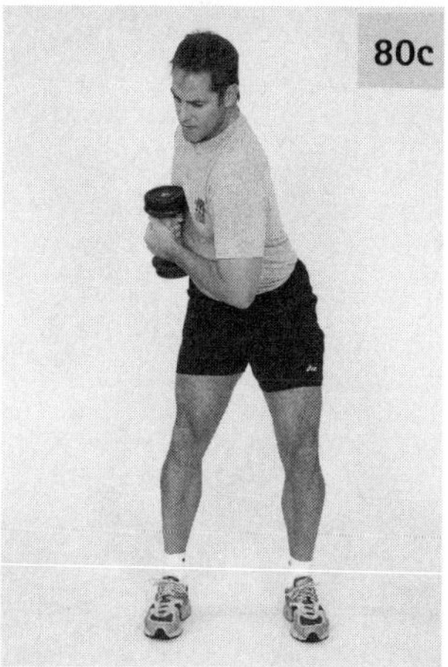
80c

81 SUPINE PHYSIOBALL ALTERNATING PRESS

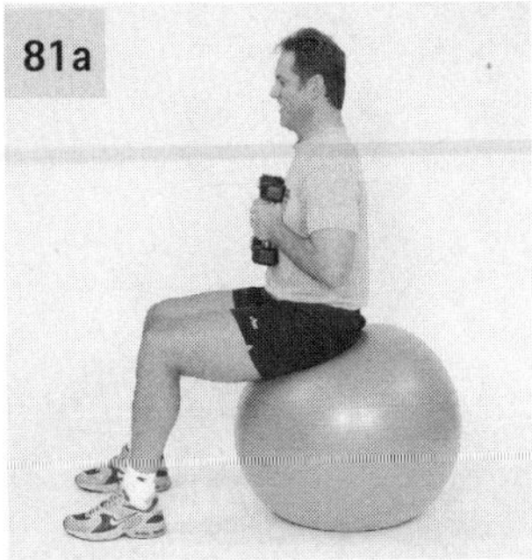
81a

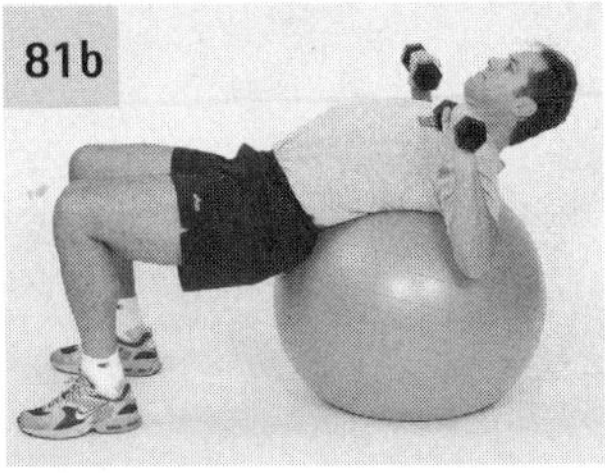
81b

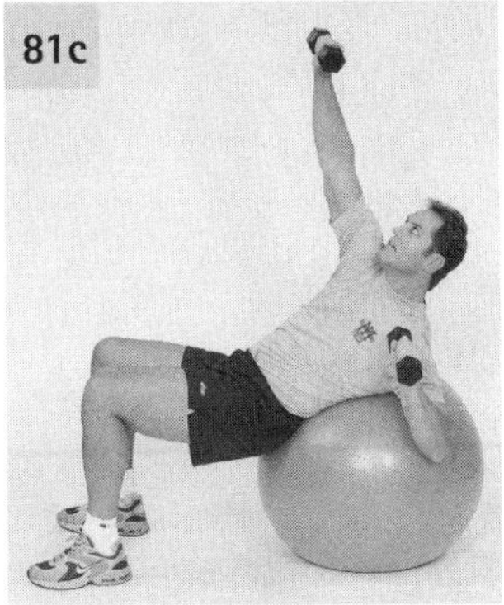
81c

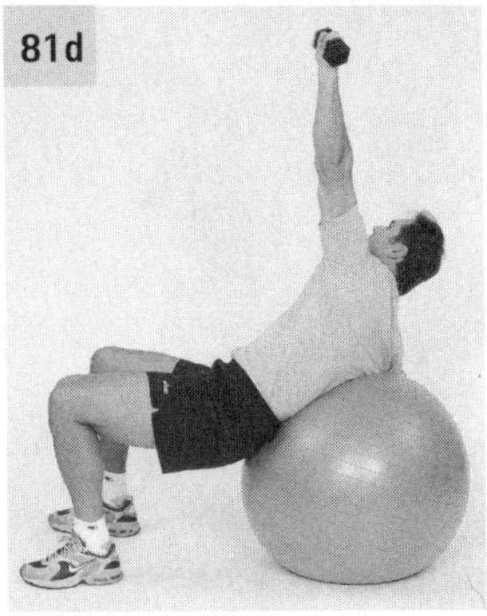
81d

Equipment: A Physioball and 2 hand weights of 2–8 pounds each.
Purpose: Dynamically strengthen your core, shoulders, and arms for rotational challenges. Also, improve your upper thoracic mobility.

Technique: Grasp a hand weight in each hand and hold them close to your chest. Sit on the Physioball and find your balance point (81a). Slowly walk your feet away from the ball until your shoulder blades are on the surface of the ball. Your hips should now be on the ball with your feet flat on the floor and the hand weights resting on your chest. Maintain a neutral spine and engage your core. Next, bring the hand weights slightly outside your shoulders and position your elbows slightly away from your body (81b). Raise one hand weight toward the ceiling while flexing and rotating your upper back and simultaneously allowing your opposite shoulder and dumbbell to drop toward the floor (81c). Slowly, switch arm positions by lowering the weight and returning your upper back to the neutral position, then reach your opposite hand weight toward the ceiling, flexing and rotating your upper back again (81d), completing the cycle. Each time you change arm positions, allow your upper back to flex, extend, and rotate with the motion of your moving arm. Perform 2–3 sets of 15 reps per side.
Precaution: Don't perform this exercise if you have any active neck or shoulder problems.

82 SQUAT TO DOUBLE-ARM OVERHEAD DIAGONAL WALL REACH

Equipment: 3- to 5-pound medicine ball or any soft object weighing 3–5 pounds.

Purpose: Strengthen your abdominal muscles' ability to decelerate your body during backward bending and sideways rotational motions, such as in reaching, moving suddenly in a boat, or pushing off from a rock behind you.

Technique: Stand with your back to a wall and take a step forward about 1 foot from the wall. Place your feet shoulder-width apart. Grasp the medicine ball, with your hands facing each other. Lower the ball down toward the floor and between your feet while bending your hips, knees, and ankles (82a). Squat down to a comfortable level, then return to the standing position while bringing the ball past your chest and raising it over your left shoulder and above your head until the ball touches the wall behind you (82b; note that this exercise should be done near a wall). Once you have touched the ball to the wall, return the ball toward the floor in a squat motion. Then repeat this motion to the right side. Perform 2–3 sets of 15 reps on each side of your body.

Variations: 82.1. Single-leg balance or unstable surface: Try balancing on one leg or changing the surface on which you are standing (e.g., a soft, thick mat). **82.2.** Try the exercise kneeling or half kneeling (one knee and one foot on the floor). Simulate the stance you would normally assume during your sports activity. This is good for boating and cycling activities.

Tips and Precautions: Follow the ball with your eyes through the complete range of motion. This will challenge your neck and upper back as well as your abdominals and legs. Allow your hips to translate forward as you reach overhead to the wall. This will help you maintain balance and add to the demands placed upon your abdominal muscles. Try to reach the ball as high as possible over your shoulder. Maintain your low-back neutral zone while flexing primarily at your hips. This will help limit the flexing of your mid and low back.

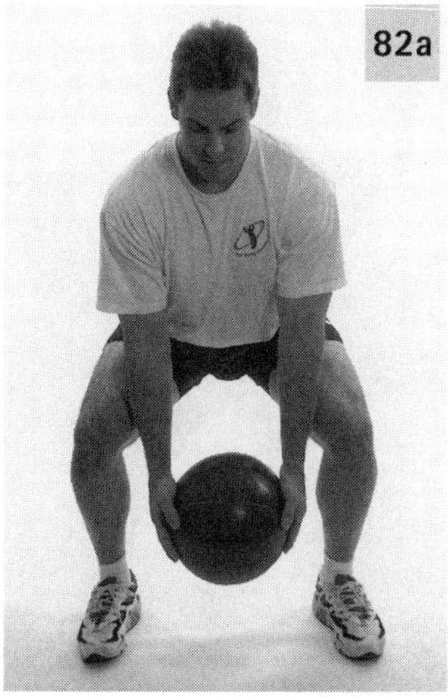
82a

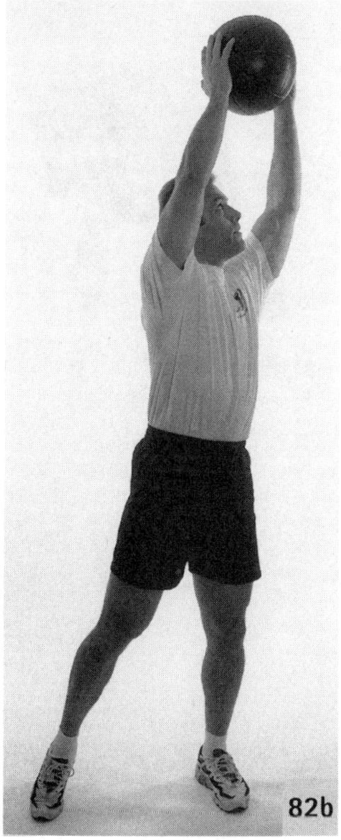
82b

83 STAGGERED STANCE ABDOMINAL CRUNCH WITH ROTATION

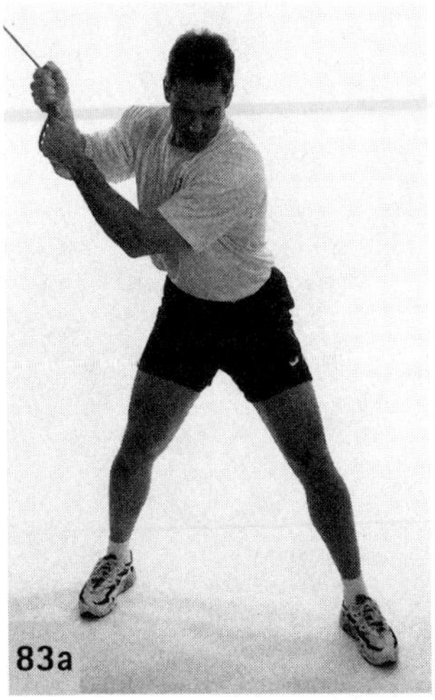
83a

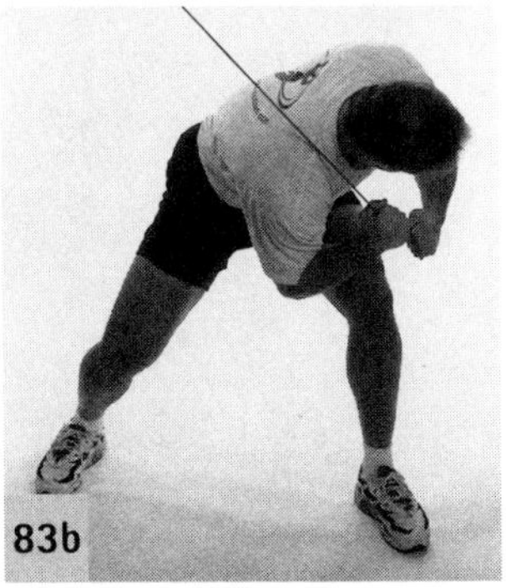
83b

Equipment: 3- to 5-foot piece of medium to heavy tubing and a door or high, immovable object or an adjustable high pulley machine.
Purpose: Increase the functional and dynamic strength of your abdominal muscles in forward and rotational movements. Coordinate this abdominal challenge with your legs to help you develop balance and functional strength for most outdoor activities.

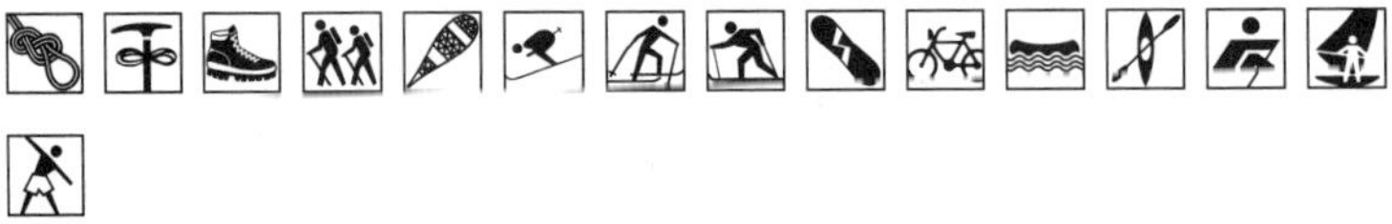

Technique: Attach tubing to a door or immovable object 2 feet above your head. If you are using an adjustable high pulley or FreeMotion machine, set the pulley at a height 2–3 feet over your head. Grasp the tubing or pulley handle with both hands. Stand sideways with your right shoulder facing the door or pulley machine. Step away from the door or the pulley machine until tension is developed in the tubing or the weight stack is off the rack. Stagger your stance so that your left foot is in front of your right foot and your feet are wider than shoulder-width apart. Pull the tubing or handle close to your chest and maintain this hand position during the exercise (83a). Simultaneously flex your hips and knees while rotating your mid back and hips. At the same time, bring your hands and chest down toward your left knee, so that you end within 1 foot above your left knee (83b). Return to the upright start position in a smooth, controlled fashion. Perform the same sequence in the opposite direction. Perform 2–3 sets of 15 reps on each side.
Variations: 83.1. Parallel stance: Use a parallel foot stance, with your feet wider than shoulder-width apart. **83.2.** Hands to knee range: Bring your hands down to touch your knee.
Tips and Precautions: Try to make this exercise smooth and continuous. Coordinate your arm, trunk, and legs through the entire range of motion. Avoid excessive forward positioning of your shoulders. Limit the flexing and rotating of your low back and maintain a low-back neutral-zone posture.

84 SINGLE-LEG STANCE TRUNK SIDE BEND WITH MEDICINE BALL

Equipment: 3- to 5-pound medicine ball or dumbbell.
Purpose: Strengthen your abdominal muscles and improve your ability to function in side-to-side motions while developing balance and coordination.

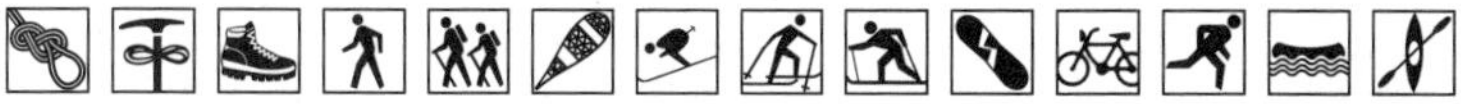

Technique: Grasp the medicine ball or dumbbell with your hands facing each other. Balance on one leg, knee slightly bent, with your toes 8–12 inches from a wall. Reach the medicine ball or dumbbell over your head. In an arc over your head, move the ball or weight toward your right side while bending your trunk to the right; then move the ball or weight to your left side while bending your trunk to the left (see photo 84; note that this exercise should be done near a wall). Try touching the wall with the ball or weight randomly at clock positions of 10:00, 11:00, 1:00, and 2:00. Keep your low back in the neutral zone. Perform 2–3 sets of 30- to 45-second intervals.
Variation: 84.1. Unstable surface: Change the surface you are standing on. Stand on a mat or a half foam roll—start with the roll lengthwise and parallel to your body, with the curved side up. Progress to placing the foam roll perpendicular to your body with the curved side up and then down. Be very careful with the roll in the curved-side-down position.
Tips and Precautions: If you need to assist your balance, touch the floor with your opposite-foot toes. Don't increase your speed or range of motion until you can balance for a full 30 seconds on either foot without assistance from your opposite foot.

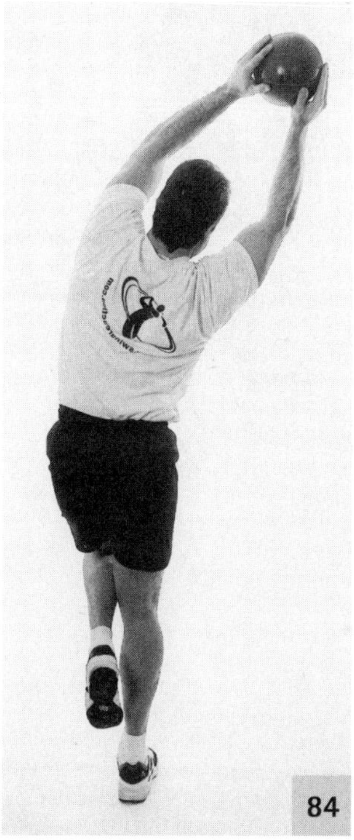

84

85 STANDING SINGLE-LEG ABDOMINAL CHALLENGE WITH DYNAMIC PARTNER RESISTANCE

Equipment: 8-foot belt and a partner.
Purpose: Develop your balance and abdominal strength with a strong base of support against a variety of directional changes experienced during any outdoor activity.

Technique: Both you and your partner should be in the standing position. Place the belt around your waist or chest and under your armpits, running the belt through the buckle but not fastening it. Have your partner take the end of the belt and supply just enough pull on

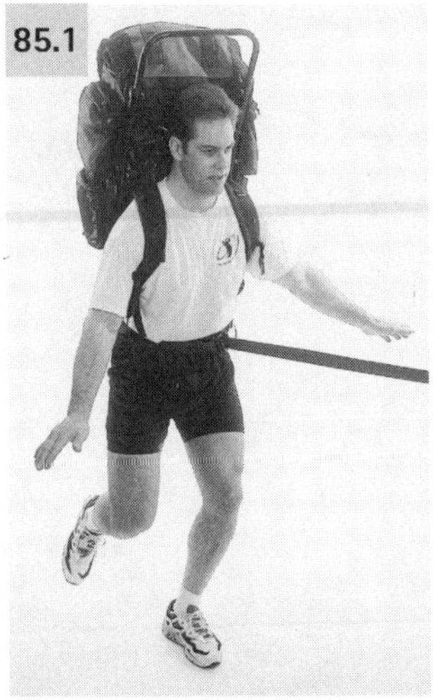
85.1

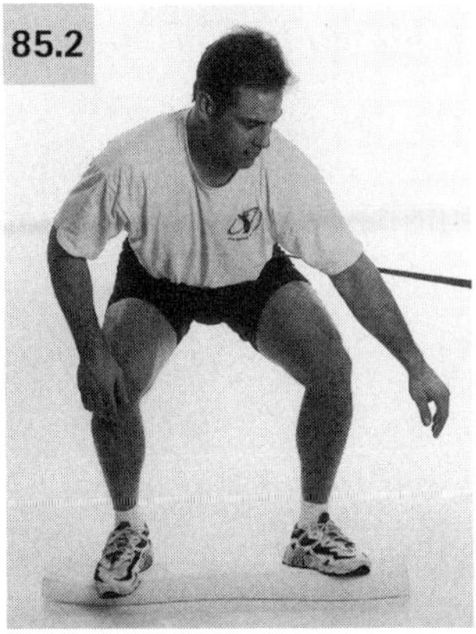
85.2

the belt to challenge your ability to stay rooted to the floor. You will find yourself recruiting your abdominal muscles in order to stay upright. The object is to keep your feet fixed in one place and not let your partner pull you off balance. Also, try this in a stride position, as if you were walking on a log. Have your partner apply tension to the belt for about 3–5 seconds, then change location. Your partner can move around you to various locations, making the tension and location unpredictable. To become successful at this exercise and derive benefit, your partner should not overwhelm you with too much tension or apply the tension too quickly. Each set should focus pulls from quadrants of 10:00–2:00, 2:00–6:00, and 6:00–10:00 around an imaginary clock. Perform 2–3 sets of 15 pulls in each quadrant.

Variations: 85.1. Loaded pack: Try this with a full pack on or while balancing on one foot. Beginning skiers can use ski poles, with their partner using gradual, slower pulls. Intermediate/advanced skiers can have their partners use very quick pulls in variable directions. **85.2.** Do this while standing on a foam roll that is flat side up.

86 SINGLE-LEG BALANCE OVERHEAD DOUBLE-ARM TUBING CHALLENGE

Equipment: 2 pieces of tubing about 3–4 feet long and a door or high, immovable object.

Purpose: Functionally strengthen your abdominals in all three planes of motion, along with developing your abdominal muscles' ability to coordinate trunk stability with your upper and lower extremities.

Technique: Anchor both pieces of tubing to a door or immovable object above your head. Face away from the door. Grasp one piece of tubing in each hand, with your elbows slightly bent and your arms overhead and in eyesight. Step away from the door until a mild amount of tension is developed in the tubing. This is your starting position. Balance on one foot with your knee slightly bent. Alternately, move your hands forward, keeping your elbows still. When one hand moves forward, the other moves backward (86a and 86b). Make sure you use your upper trunk and abdominal muscles to create the motion. Repeat this exercise on the other foot for the same

time interval. Perform 1–2 sets of 30–60 seconds on each foot, moving as quickly as you can.
Variations: 86.1. Arm position challenge: Gradually progress by beginning with your arms in a more overhead position. Once you are experienced with this, do sets with different arm starting positions. **86.2.** Unstable surface challenge: Try balancing on a less stable surface, such as a thick mat.
Tips and Precautions: Perform this exercise on both feet if you are uncomfortable with your balance. Start with short arm and shoulder motions until your strength and coordination develop. If you have a history of shoulder problems, keep the level of your elbows below your eyes during all shoulder movements.

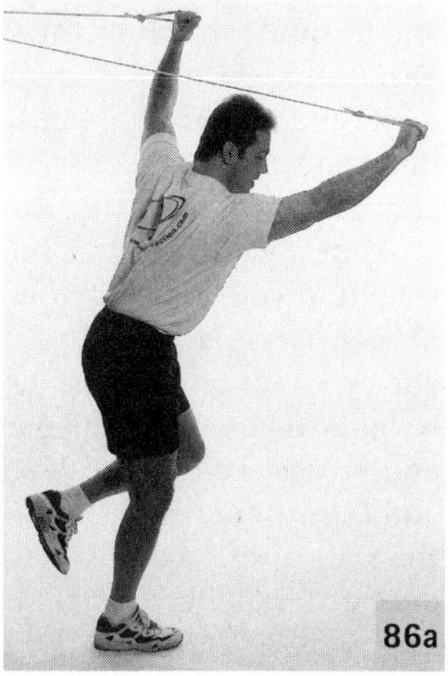
86a

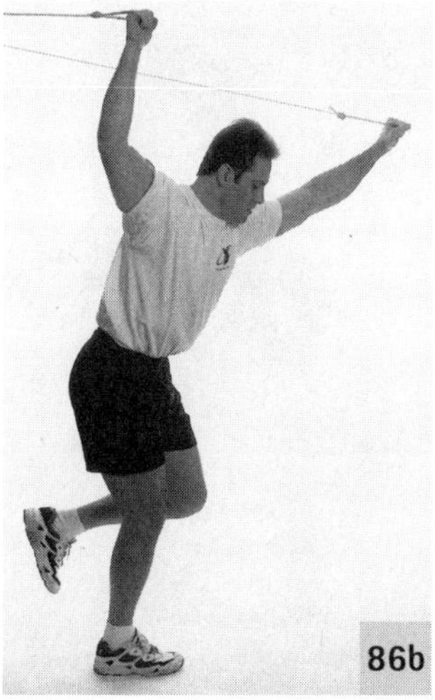
86b

87 BOSU BALL CORE CHALLENGE

Equipment: Bosu ball or disc pillow, a 3- to 8-pound dumbbell or weighted ball.
Purpose: Improve your standing core stability against arm challenges.

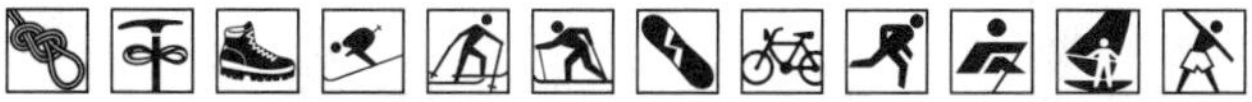

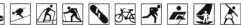

Technique: Grasp both heads of the dumbbell or weighted ball so that your palms are facing each other and position it at your waist. Stand on the Bosu ball or outside perimeter of the disc pillow and balance with your ankles, knees, and hips slightly bent (87a). Maintaining a neutral spine position, engage your core by lifting your tummy inward and tightening your abdominals (especially your lower abdominals). Reach the weight forward at hip height (87b) and return it to the start position at your waist. Do this 5 times slowly (3 counts to reach full extension of your arms

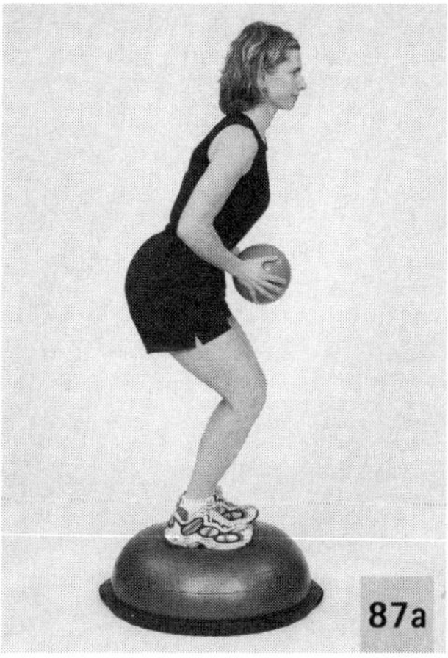
87a

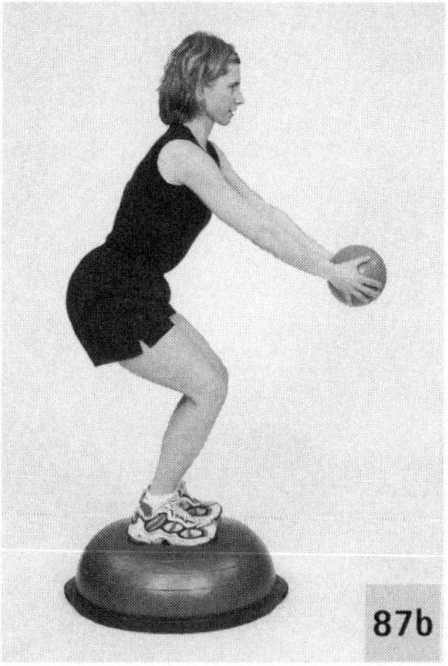
87b

87.1

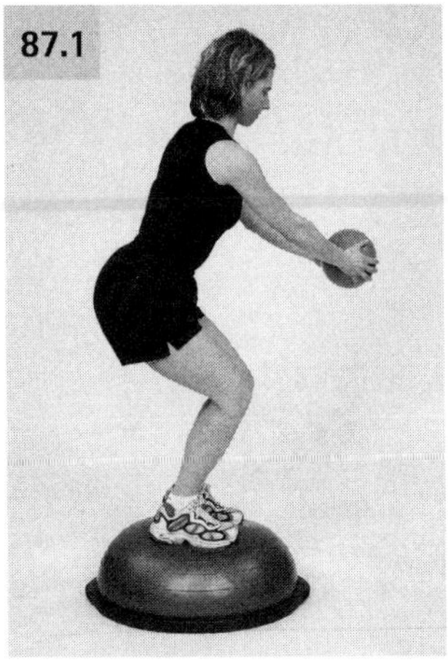

and 3 counts to return the weight to your waist).

Variations: 87.1. 45-degree angle reaches: Do the same hip-height reach and return at a 45-degree angle to the left in front of you 5 times and a 45-degree angle to the right in front of you 5 times. **87.2.** Shoulder-height reaches: Advance this exercise by reaching forward at 45-degree angles to shoulder height, making sure to return the weight to your waist after each repetition. **87.3.** Alternate overhead presses: Grasp a 3- to 8-pound hand weight in each hand and balance yourself on the Bosu ball or disc pillow, positioning your hand weights in contact with your chest (87.3a). Maintain a neutral spine and engage your core. Reach one hand weight toward the ceiling and the other toward the floor (87.3b). Return both hand weights to the start position and switch arm directions while maintaining balance and stability of your core. Perform 2–3 sets of 10–12 reps on each side.

Tips and Precautions: Reach only in a range that allows you to maintain your balance and core stability. If you have any active shoulder problems, don't reach above shoulder height.

87.3a

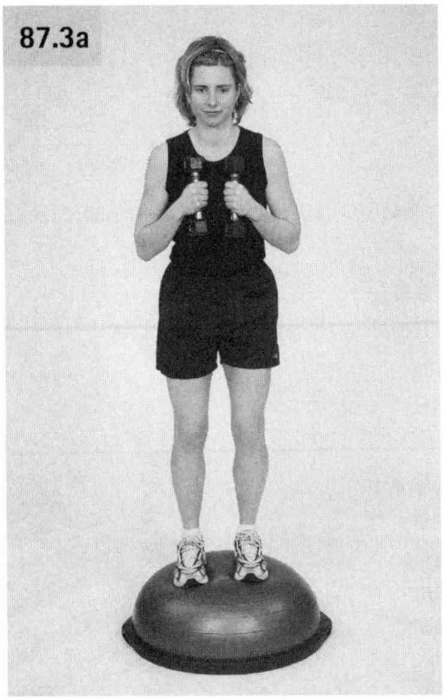

87.3b

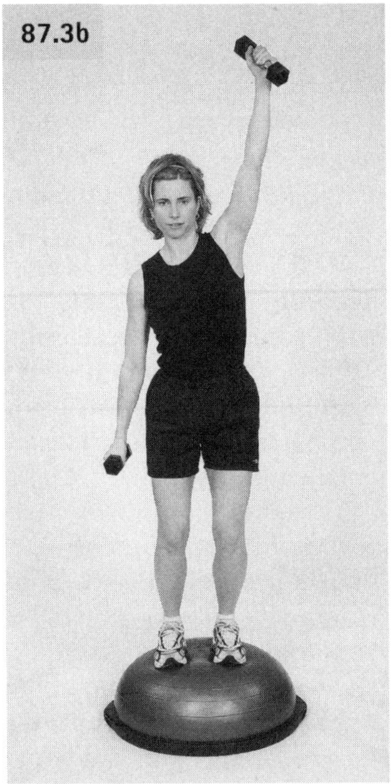

88 KNEELING AB DOLLY/ROLLER CORE CHALLENGE

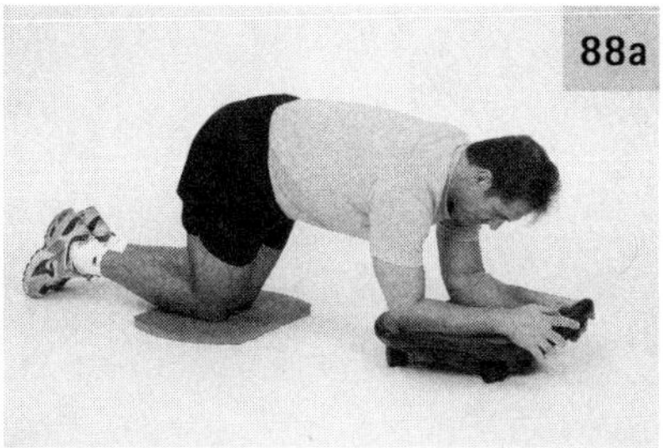

88a

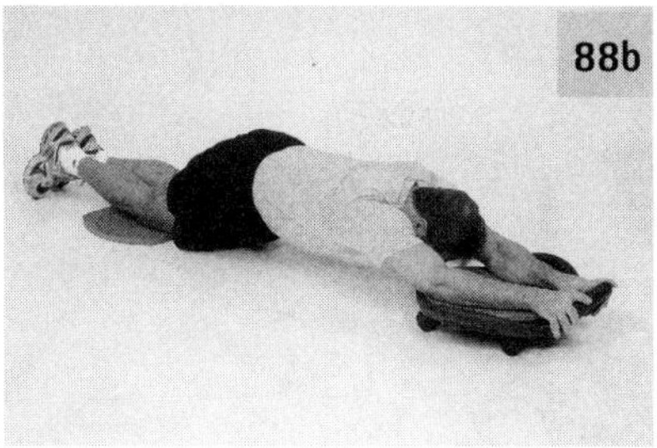

88b

Equipment: Ab Dolly or Ab Roller.
Purpose: Strengthen your core and arm extensors in the sagittal (forward) or frontal (side-to-side) planes in combination with your shoulders and hip flexors.

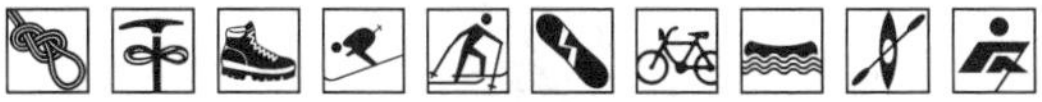

Technique: Basic to intermediate: Kneel on the knee cushion and place your elbows on the Ab Dolly with your hands grasping the top handles. Your hips and shoulders should be in a 90-degree position with your body weight dispersed equally. Maintain a neutral spine position and engage your core (88a). Roll the Ab Dolly forward, allowing your hips to move toward the floor and your arms to reach overhead (88b). Return to the 90-degree start position by pulling with your hips, abdominals, and shoulders, maintaining a neutral spine position.
Variations: 88.1. Advanced: Assume the 90-degree hip and shoulder position kneeling on a pad, with your hands on the outside grips of the Ab Dolly and your arms straight (88.1a). Maintain a neutral spine and engage your core. Keep your arms straight and roll the Ab Dolly forward by hinging at your hips and shoulders (88.1b). Allow your straight arms to reach over your head and at the same pace, reach your hips for the floor. This is an advanced exercise. Start with short ranges, slowly, and get the feel of this exercise before moving in longer ranges. **88.2.** 45-degree angles: Try variation 88.1 moving the Ab Dolly into 45-degree angles to your left and to your right. Always return to the start position before switching sides.
Tip: Try the easier version of all variations first, with your elbows on the dolly, before trying the harder straight-arm position.

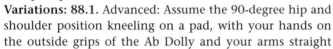

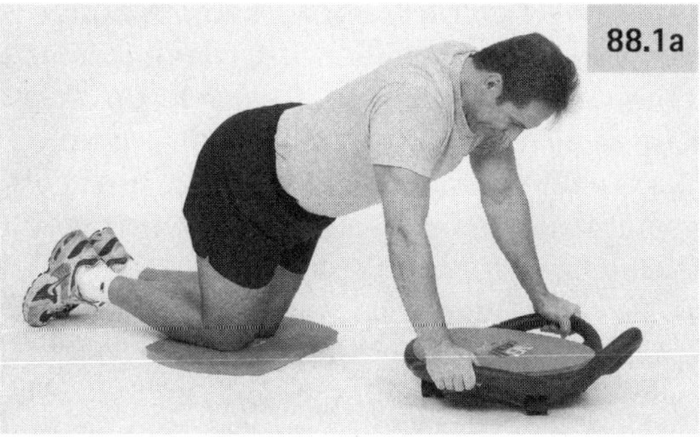

88.1a

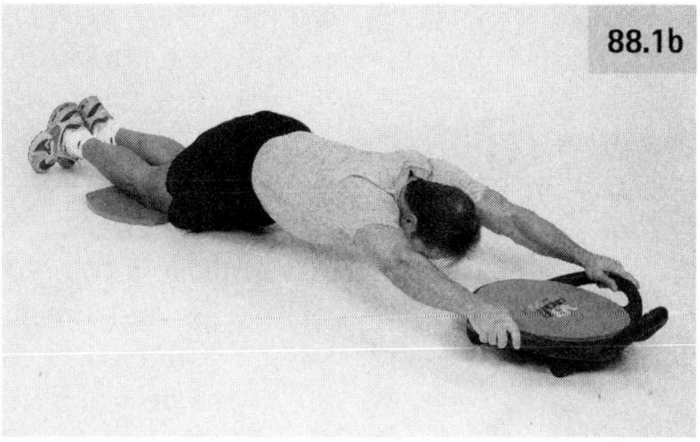

88.1b

89 THE PRAYER

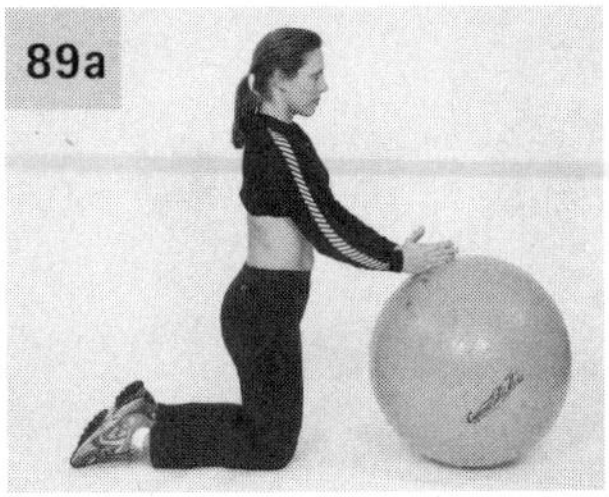
89a

Equipment: Physioball. A mirror is helpful for visual feedback on your mechanics.

Purpose: Strengthen abdominals in an isometric position and help train your abdominals to support neutral spine position.

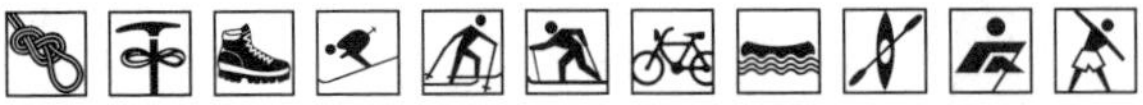

Technique: Kneel in front of a Physioball and rest your forearms on the ball. Clasp your hands, emulating a prayer position (89a). Position your spine in neutral and activate your core muscles. Roll the ball out slowly, allowing your knees to straighten and your arms to move overhead with the ball (89b). Control the descent and keep your spine neutral at all times. Your core should be engaged, with your abdominals working to stabilize this position. Hold this position for a 10 count and return to the start position. Do 3 sets of 10 reps.

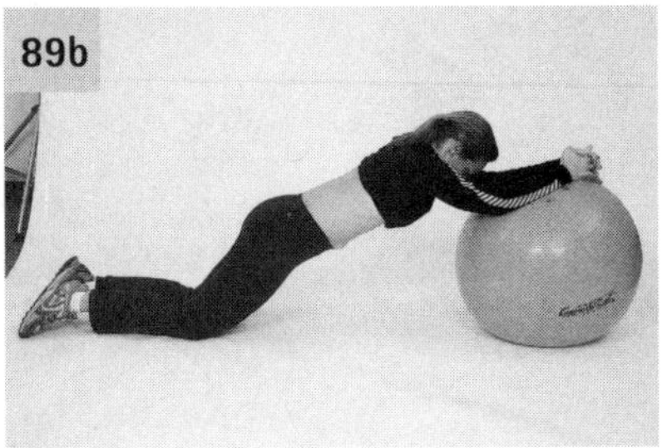
89b

Tips and Precautions: Use something soft under your knees to protect them. Don't allow your back to arch beyond neutral. Don't do this exercise if you have any active neck, shoulder, back, or kneecap problems.

90 THE PLANK

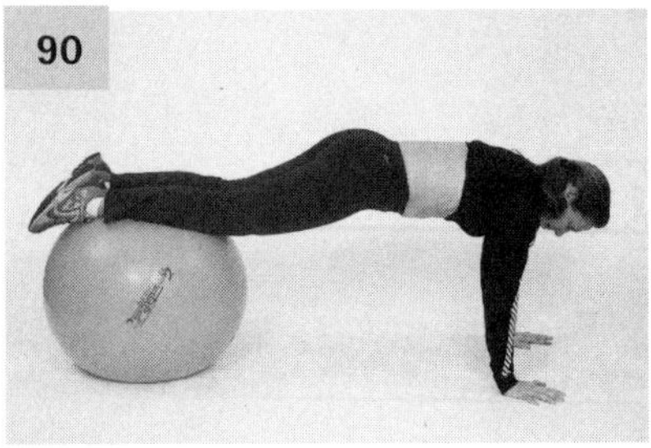
90

Equipment: Physioball. A mirror is helpful for visual feedback on your mechanics.

Purpose: Strengthen abdominals and improve balance while your abdominals and core are engaged.

Technique: Lay over a Physioball face down. Walk out onto your hands until only your shins are supported by the ball and you are in a plank position. Keep your core engaged and your spine in neutral. Don't let your back sag. A mirror is helpful to see if your back is in a neutral position. Use your abdominals to maintain and hold this neutral position for 10 seconds. Do 3 reps. You may eventually want to increase the hold time to 30 seconds.

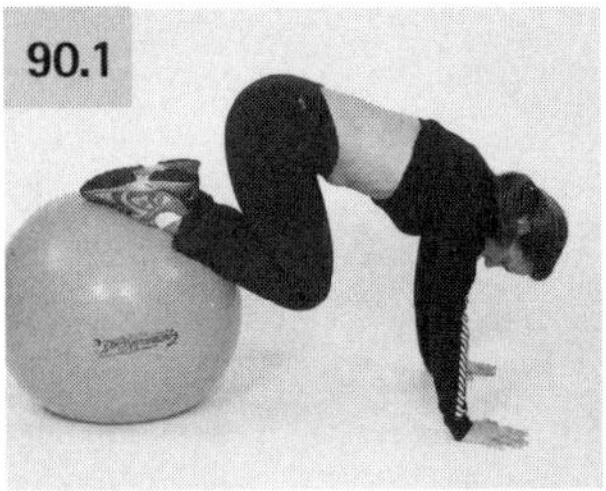
90.1

Variation: 90.1. Plank knee tuck: Position yourself in the hold position of a plank. Bring your knees toward your chest, rolling the ball towards you (90.1). Then return to the start position.

Tips and Precautions: Be careful not to let your back arch beyond neutral toward the floor. If you have sore or weak wrists or shoulders, or a neck or back problem, this exercise is not appropriate for you. The farther you walk your hands, the more difficult the exercise becomes.

91 THE SKIER

Equipment: Physioball. A mirror is helpful for visual feedback on your mechanics.
Purpose: Strengthen your abdominals and prepare your spine for rotational movements.

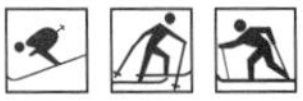

Technique: Lay over a Physioball face down. Walk out onto your hands until only your shins are supported by the ball and you are in a plank position. Pull your knees diagonally toward your left shoulder (91a), then return to a plank. Alternate this rotation to the right (91b). Use your abdominals to pull your knees through. When in a plank, be sure to maintain neutral spine position. A good goal is 2 sets of 10–12 reps.
Tips and Precautions: Your center of gravity will move forward in the direction you travel. This will place a strain on your abdominal muscles, so don't overdo it by moving too far. Maintain your low-back in the neutral zone as much as possible with your core engaged. Try not to let your low back arch.

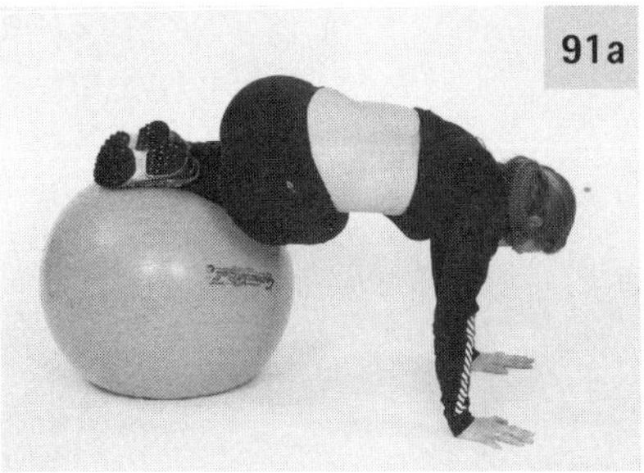

91a

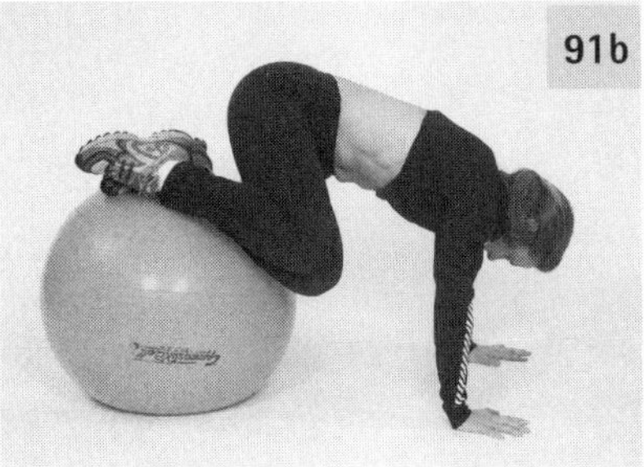

91b

92 SUPINE CRUNCH ON PHYSIOBALL

Equipment: Large Physioball.
Purpose: Strengthen your abdominal muscles in the forward (sagittal) plane of motion and increase your mid to low back's ability to bend and extend. Also challenge your balance in a supine to seated position.

Technique: First, sit on the Physioball and find your balance point. Slowly walk your feet away from the ball until the middle of your back is on the surface of the ball and you are looking at the ceiling. Your hips should now be on the ball and your feet on the floor. Place your arms across your chest and allow your back to slightly extend over the surface of the ball. Curl your chin toward your chest and rise to a semi-upright position, maintaining balance and control over the ball. Perform 12–20 reps for 2–3 sets, resting about a minute between each set.
Variations: 92.1. Hands behind neck: You may wish to bring your hands behind your neck for added resistance and neck support. Don't jerk on your neck or head. Don't rely on your arms to raise your body; use your abdominal muscles. **92.2.** Rotational crunches: For

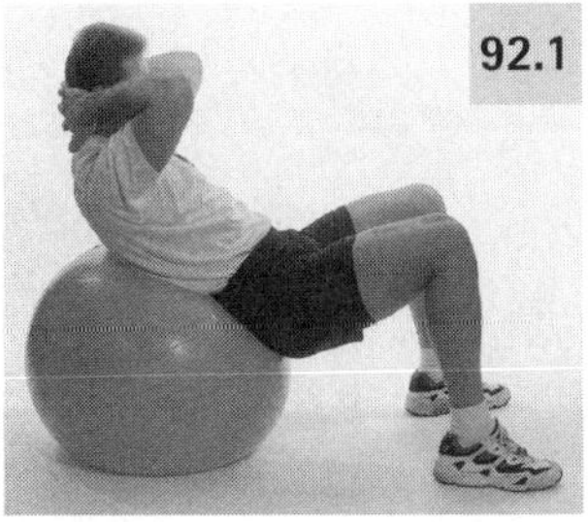

92.1

an additional challenge, add rotation to this exercise by bringing a shoulder toward the opposite knee as you rise to the semi-upright position.

Tips and Precautions: Start slowly! Exercise in a pain-free and successful range of motion. Don't overextend your back. As you reach the top of the crunch, try bringing your hips toward your rib cage. This will mean additional work for your lower abdominal muscles.

93 SUPINE BALL TOSS WITH PARTNER

Equipment: 3- to 5-pound medicine ball and a partner

Purpose: Improve your abdominal muscles' ability to react and to decelerate (slow down), and accelerate (speed up) your trunk against multidirectional external forces.

Technique: Both you and your partner should sit on the floor with your legs straight or knees slightly bent and the soles of your feet facing your partner. With the medicine ball in your hands and your arms overhead (93a), lower yourself, back down, completely to the floor, then sit up and toss the ball at various angles to your partner. Your partner will receive the ball and lower him/herself toward the floor, back down with arms outstretched and overhead (93b). Repeat the motion by having your partner toss the ball back to you; play catch with each other. Toss the ball in different directions to make this exercise challenging in all planes of motion. Perform 2–3 sets of 12–20 reps or until fatigued.

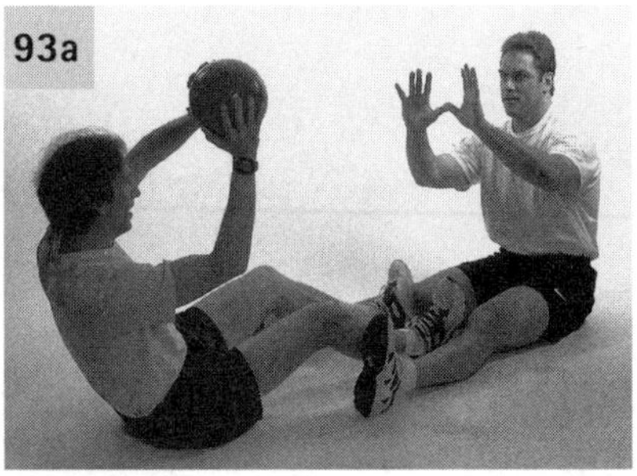

93a

Variation: 93.1. Leg elevation ball toss: Try elevating one foot off the floor, or try bending your knees.

Tips and Precautions: Before attempting this exercise, you should be successful at Exercise 78.2. Keep your feet in contact with the floor at all times. Toss the ball to the left and to the right of your partner. Keep the ball within reach while making it challenging.

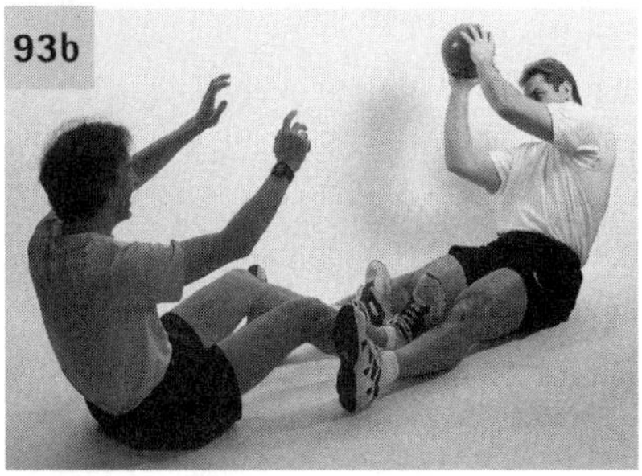

93b

94 SEATED PHYSIOBALL BOATERS/CYCLIST REACTION CHALLENGE

Equipment: Large Physioball, a partner (and 8-foot belt for cyclist variation).
Purpose: Strengthen your abdominal muscles' ability to react to changes of direction in a seated position.

Technique: Sit on a large Physioball with your toes barely touching the ground. Pick one foot up off the ground and try to balance. Work toward balancing with both feet off the ground. Also try pushing off one foot with the other foot on the ground, to challenge your balance. You can use ski poles or dowels as a stabilizing aid. To increase the challenge, perform this exercise with a partner and have him/her push randomly on the ball. Use your poles for safety. This exercise especially benefits boaters. Spend 2–3 minutes on the ball per set, for 3 sets 2 times per week.
Variations: 94.1. Cyclists: The object of this variation is to develop strength and balance control over directional changes. Sitting on the ball, move your feet behind you, making contact with the floor with the balls of your feet in a position similar to how your feet would be placed on your bike pedals. Put your hands on the seat of a chair, bench, or stool, gripping the edges the way that you would grip your bike handlebars. If you have a moving stool, move the stool farther away in front of you and from clock positions of 10:00 to 2:00. Place an 8-foot-long belt around your waist or upper torso and under your armpits, passing the end of the belt through the buckle but not fastening it. Plant your feet firmly on the floor for balance. Have a partner take hold of the end of the belt and try to pull you off balance while changing the pulling direction frequently. Your partner should pull just enough to challenge you, giving tugs in clock quadrants of 10:00–2:00, 2:00–4:00 or 2:00–6:00, and 6:00–10:00 or 8:00–10:00. Perform 2–3 sets of 10–15 pulls in each quadrant. **94.2.** When you become successful at variation 94.1, try it with one foot off the floor. You will need only minimal resistance from your partner.
Tips and Precautions: The partner should not administer an overwhelming force to the exerciser. Allow the exerciser to develop the coordination and strength to meet each challenge.

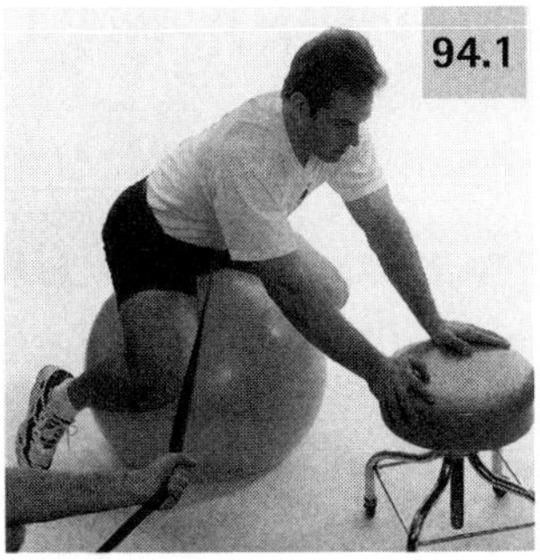

chapter 11 THE KNEE, THIGH, HIP, AND BUTTOCK

By Mark Pierce, A.T.C., Mark Looper, P.T., and David Musnick, M.D.

THIS CHAPTER WILL HELP YOU:

- Understand how this critical body region functions.
- Do basic functional exercises such as squats, lunges, step-ups, hops, and jumps to improve your functional strength.

Your hip, buttock, and knee allow you to position your foot where you want it to go. They allow you to move pedals, run or climb on rocks and trails, and move or stabilize yourself in boats. They also help you to decelerate so that you can control your speed going downhill. They are very important, along with your lower leg and abdominal muscles, in controlling balance.

FUNCTION AND ANATOMY

The muscles described below basically work as movers and decelerators of motion, depending on whether your foot is on or off the ground or how you are using your hip and knee if you are sitting. See chapter 9 for illustrations.

The *psoas muscle* flexes your hip (placing your knee in front of your body and closer to your chest) and works in conjunction with the hip extenders (the gluteus maximus and hamstrings). The hip *abductors* (gluteus medius and minimus buttock muscles) move your foot and knee away from your body when your foot is off the ground. When your foot is on the ground, they slow down side-to-side motion of your pelvis. The abductors work in conjunction with the *adductors* (groin muscles). The adductors are comprised of five muscles on the inner thigh. When your foot is off the ground, they move your leg inward and across the midline of your body. When your foot is on the ground, they assist your hamstrings in decelerating hip flexion and help produce hip extension. They are also responsible for medial hip stability and deceleration during hip abduction. The *iliotibial band* (ITB) on the side of the hip assists the abductors in slowing down your pelvis from moving sideways when your foot is on the ground. When your foot is off the ground, the ITB assists your abductors in moving your leg away from the midline of your body.

The *buttock* region muscle group is the largest and probably the most important for stabilizing us in an upright position and moving us over the ground. It is comprised of the gluteus maximus, medius, and minimus. In addition to the gluteus medius and minimus that comprise the abductor muscles described above, the *gluteus maximus* is a large muscle that is what you sit on. It extends your hip and brings your leg behind you. It also assists external rotation of your hip joint when your foot is off the ground. When your foot contacts the ground, it decelerates hip flexion and internal rotation and sends a powerful muscular extension into the ITB to stabilize the lateral side of your knee. As we propel or push off the ground, the gluteus maximus functions through the ITB to accelerate external rotation of your lower leg. A strong gluteus maximus is important for low-back protection. It aids in decelerating forward (flexing) spine motion (in both the thoracic and low back). It helps to maintain an upright posture along with the spinal erectors and the hamstrings. It is a force coupler between the upper and lower body.

The *quadriceps* (quads), the muscles on the front of your thigh, extend your knee if your foot is off the ground, or decelerate your knee from flexing and collapsing if your foot is on the ground. They work in conjunction with the hamstrings, which flex your knee if your foot is off the ground, or decelerate knee and hip flexion if your foot is on the ground. If you are sitting in a crew boat or on a bicycle, these muscles work more to initiate motion in flexing and extending the knees and hips. If you are walking, especially downhill, these muscles work more to decelerate or control your body and keep you upright. This explains why your quads and kneecaps may hurt more after downhill hiking or running.

The *patellofemoral joint* consists of the *patella* (kneecap), which is imbedded in the center of the quadriceps tendon and slides up and down in the groove on the *femur* (thighbone) as your knee is bent or extended. The knee joint consists of cartilage and many ligaments. When you are bearing weight, tension from the quadriceps muscle group is present in all knee positions, thereby firmly fixing or stabilizing the front of your knee. Knee motion is primarily flexing and extending. The knee joint is much more susceptible to injury than the hip joint. The hip is a very stable joint that can move in many directions. Hips may have tendon problems, but the joint is rarely injured. The hip can become problematic due to adjacent joints, such as the back, that compensate for the lack of hip motion.

Muscle function is often broken down into either open (foot is free to move) or closed (foot is fixed on the ground, a pedal, or a platform, for example) kinetic chains of motion. In order to better understand muscle function in a closed kinetic chain environment, imagine yourself descending fairly steep terrain. When your foot makes contact with the ground, a strong inward rotational force is generated as your foot moves from an arched position (*supination*) and begins to flatten (*pronate*). Your knee and hip then bend to absorb the force of your body weight. This requires muscles that catch you or decelerate your leg's internal rotational force and your hip and knee during flexion. Without proper muscular deceleration, we may overstrain or injure the leg, or accelerate down the hill faster than we can control.

Once we have decelerated, we need our muscles to propel our body over the foot, muscles that externally rotate the hip as well as extend the hip and knee. Thus, the cycle continues, from deceleration to propulsion to deceleration. Exercises in this chapter work on both these functions.

COMMON MUSCLE IMBALANCES

One of the most common muscle imbalances at the hip is weakness of the gluteus maximus (buttock muscle). This often coincides with weaker abdominal muscles. This results in the pelvis being tilted forward, increasing the arch in the low back (*lordosis*). The hip flexes and the thigh rotates inward. Hiking or exercising in this position can stress and strain the low back and lead to hip and knee strains, tendonitis, or bursitis. The gluteus medius can also be weak, especially in people with low-back and sacroiliac problems. This can lead to an excessive shifting of the pelvis and exacerbate low-back problems. It can also cause dysfunction in the knee and kneecap pain syndromes.

The gluteus maximus and *tensor fasciae latae* (lateral hip muscle) both connect to the iliotibial tract. A common imbalance is that the gluteal muscles are underutilized and underdeveloped, and the tensor fasciae latae gets tighter, resulting in shortening of the ITB. This can translate into increased friction over the bony surfaces at the hip and knee, leading to hip and knee bursitis. The hamstrings on many people are tight or weak and thus are prone to "pulling." They can also place more strain on the back or knee. At the knee, a common imbalance is a weaker inner quad muscle (VMO).

STRATEGIES FOR STRENGTHENING

Your exercise program for this body region should address your muscle imbalances and use your muscles in a functional manner. When strengthening your hips, buttocks, and thighs, it is important to do the majority of your exercises in ways that mimic the function of your activity. If you are sitting during your activity, do most of your exercises while sitting as well as some while standing. If you are standing during your activity, do most of your lower-extremity exercises while standing. If you simply would like balanced strength, toning, and would like to stay fit, follow the Basic Strengthening and Toning Program.

Basic Strengthening and Toning Program

This program will give you a basic functional strength foundation, fitness, and toning for this body region. You can add any of the other exercises listed in this chapter to meet specific activity goals.

1. Do stretching Exercises 1, 3, 5, 6, 8, and 9.
2. For the thighs, do Exercises 95.2, 96, and 97.5.
3. For the glutes, do Exercises 102 or 103 and 104 or 105.

Lower-Body Program for High-Level Fitness and Performance

Beginning high-level program:

1. Maintain flexibility in your hip joint, hamstrings, calf, and ITB to lengthen the commonly tight areas. Use stretching Exercises 1–9.
2. Develop strong buttocks, hamstrings, and inner quads to strengthen these commonly weaker areas. Use Exercises 31.1, 35 or 36, 95.2, 97.6, 97.9, 104, and 106.
3. Develop and challenge your balance to improve your muscles to work dynamically. Choose from Exercises 20.1, 32.1, 58–61, 84, and 94 (if you are a sitting athlete).

Advanced high-level program:

Add Exercises 30, 31.2, 34, 75 (with a squat machine), 97.2 (do a deep lunge with weights and progress to a walking deep lunge), 100 and 101 (if you have a need for hopping, jumping, and plyometric moves and power), and 135.

KNEE, THIGH, HIP, AND BUTTOCK EXERCISES

These exercises are basic versions of the squat, lunge, step-up, and jump, and should be practiced before going on to the combination exercises in chapter 5, Functional Core and Strength Training, and the more advanced jumps in chapters 8, Creative Use of the Outdoors in Training, and 20, Conditioning for Snowboarding and Skiing. The exercises in this chapter are considered closed kinetic chain exercises (except for Exercise 96) and are well suited to the outdoor enthusiast. All of the exercises can be done in sets of 15–20 reps except for the hops and jumps; build up your strength and balance before doing hops and jumps.

Note: All of the exercises in this section except Exercise 96 use your hamstrings in a functional manner.

95 SQUAT

Equipment: Level surface to start; may progress to hills or balance equipment (see chapter 6). Variations can be done with free weights or on squat machines.
Purpose: Establish basic buttock, quad, and calf deceleration strength. The squat is also the basis for jumping and plyometrics.

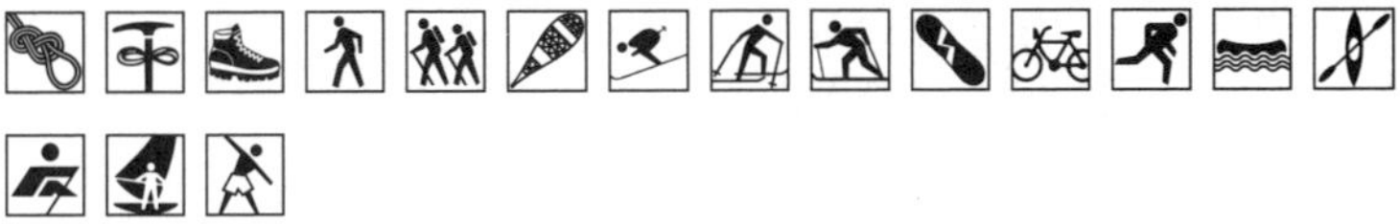

Technique: Beginners should start with mini to half squats. Start with your weight evenly distributed side to side and front to back. Stand with your feet shoulder-width apart. Lower your buttocks until your knees are at an angle of about 60 degrees. Keep your back in a neutral position to avoid excessive flexion. Be sure that your knees are aligned with your first and second toes. It isn't necessary to go lower than having your thighs parallel to the ground. If your knees hurt with a squat, try the unloaded squat (95.1) below. Try 15 reps and do 2–3 sets slowly, then gradually increase speed.
Variations: 95.1. Unloaded squat: Do this if you have knee pain, are working on your balance, or have a neurological condition. Do a squat while holding onto the backs of 2 chairs or while holding 2 ski poles. **95.2.** Add weight: After you have the basic form you can add weights to the squat by holding dumbbells, putting a pack on, or by using a squat machine with a bar (aka Smith machine). If you use dumbbells, try placing them slightly in front of you and place your buttocks slightly back to counter the weight. **95.3.** Squats with biceps

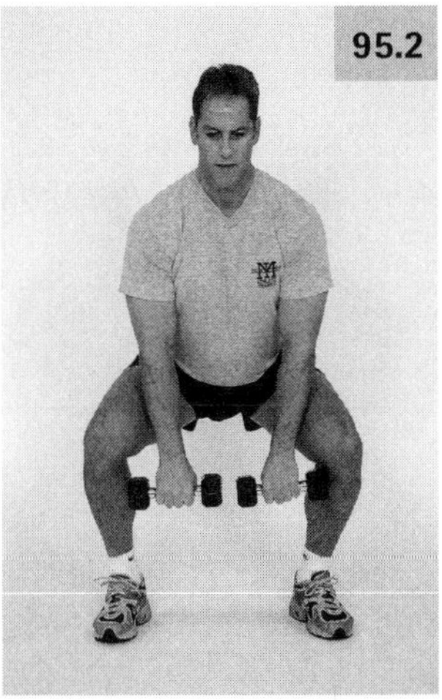

95.2

curl: Start by grabbing 2 dumbbells or hand weights by your side. Activate your core muscles and make sure your back is in a neutral position. Curl the hand weights toward your chest by flexing your elbows. This will be your starting position. As you squat, lower the weights between your knees and allow your buttocks to stick out. Make sure your back stays in good alignment during the whole exercise (see photo 95.2). **95.4.** The Squat and Clean: This exercise is excellent for crew and climbing. It is a difficult lift requiring precise spine positioning and technique. Refer to an Olympic lifting text or have a trainer in a gym demonstrate it to you. Don't do this if you have any active spine problems.

Tips and Precautions: Leg-press machines in recumbent positions are another alternative for building quad, buttock, and hamstring strength. There is no balance challenge with this method, and it is preferable for body builders. You need to maintain a neutral low-back position through the full range of motion in order to be safe in this exercise. A leg-press machine can also possibly overload your knees. Try to avoid excessive weight or knee flexion, which could cause your heels to raise off the platform. For rowing athletes, it makes sense to use a sitting (not recumbent) leg-press machine.

96 HAMSTRING CURLS

Equipment: Ankle weights and vertical surface (such as a wall), or hamstring curl machine (seated).

Purpose: Increase the strength of your hamstrings to flex your knee, especially for cyclists and crew.

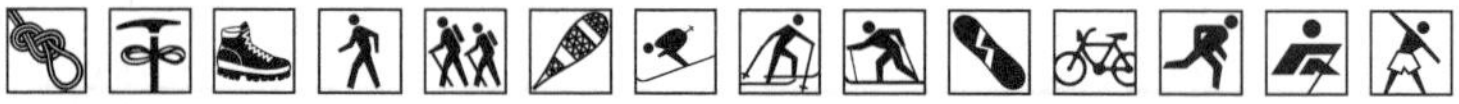

Technique: Standing hamstring curl: Attach an ankle weight to one ankle and stand on the opposite foot with your knee slightly bent. Stabilize yourself by touching a wall. Maintain both thighs in a vertical position while bringing your heel to your buttock. Do 2–3 sets of 15 reps with each leg.

Variations: 96.1. Prone hamstring curl: This type of hamstring exercise can be performed on a typical hamstring curl machine. When using this type of equipment, you may need to adjust the pads for your individual leg length. Adjust the pads so that your knee joint is in line with the pivot point of the lever arm. Lay prone on your stomach with the pads of the lever arm resting just above your heels. Maintain a neutral spine position and try not to arch your back as you bring your heels toward your buttocks. You may need to grip the sides of the machine or the handles for stability. **96.2.** Seated hamstring curl: This machine looks like a seated leg-extension machine

with the lever arm parallel to the floor. Again, adjust the seat position or the pads so that your knee joint is in line with the pivot point of the lever arm. Once you have your adjustments set, sit on the machine with your legs straight and the back of your heels on the pads. Place the restraint across your thighs to stabilize your upper legs and pull or curl the pads and lever arm downward.
Tips and Precautions: Keep your back in a neutral spine position to avoid excessive low-back stress. Try to limit excessive upper-body motion during all of these exercises.

97 LUNGES

Equipment: Level indoor or outdoor surface, hills.
Purpose: Improve your ability to handle your body's weight in a deceleration mode, landing on one foot. Improve your buttock and leg strength. This is an excellent lower-body exercise that is good for thigh and leg strength and balance.

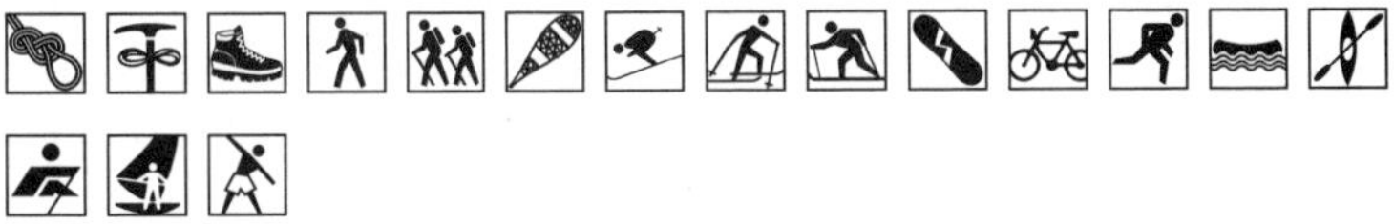

Note on progression: Many lunge variations are described below. If you are rehabbing an injury, are just starting to learn lunges, or are an older person, begin with an unloaded lunge (97.1) and then move to the basic lunge technique. Then go to the Basic Lunge Progression at the end of the lunge descriptions and determine which variation is best suited for your abilities and strength needs. If you are at a higher level of fitness, you may move rapidly through the lunge progression and then pick a lunge variation that you like and that challenges you.
Note on reps: One repetition is counted as a lunge onto that leg. If you are doing a same-leg lunge and do 10 lunges on your left leg, that is a count of 10 reps. If you are doing an alternating lunge and do 10 on the left and 10 on the right, that is a count of a 10 reps. If you are doing a variation that involves a walking lunge, every lunge onto your right leg is one rep—20 total lunges (10 on the right and 10 on the left) count as 10 reps.
Basic Technique: For a forward lunge, start in a standing position with your feet parallel to one another and 1–2 shoe widths apart. Place one foot about 1½–2 feet forward and allow your front knee to bend. The *excursion* of the lunge is the length from where your toe begins in the start position to where your heel makes first contact with the surface after you lunge. If you are shorter than 5 feet, 5 inches, you may want to start with a 1-foot excursion. Progress your

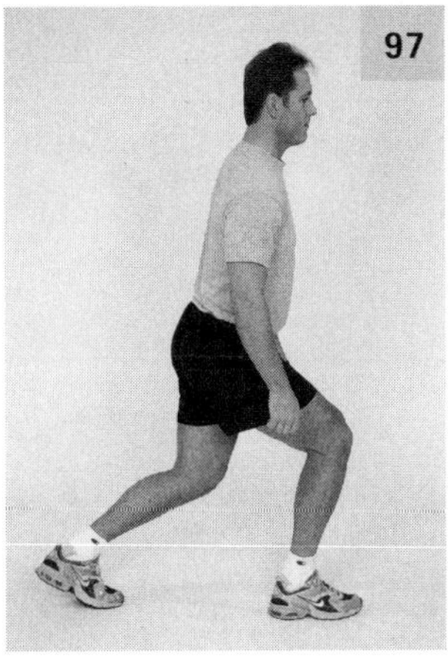

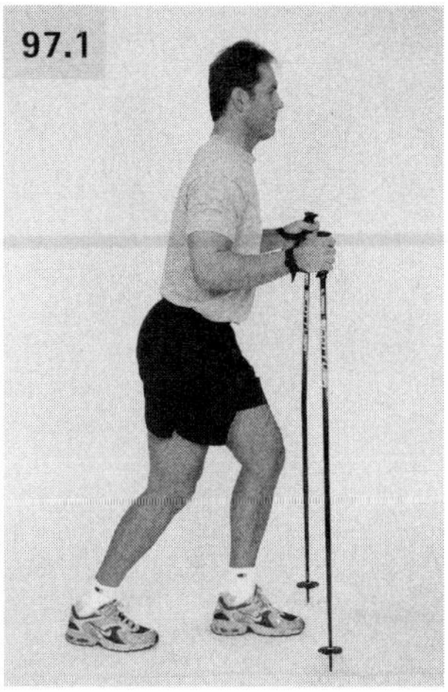

97.1

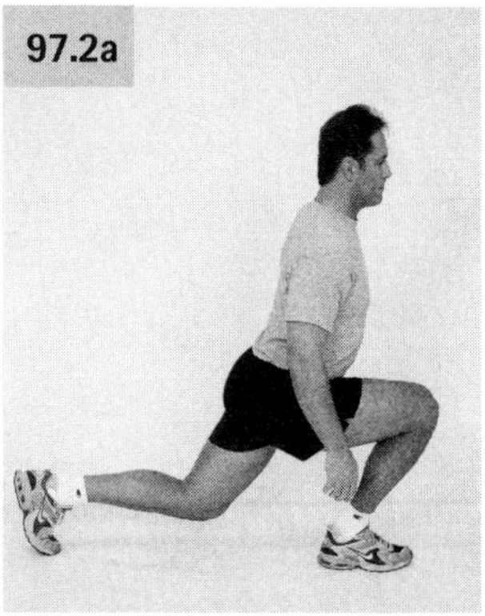

97.2a

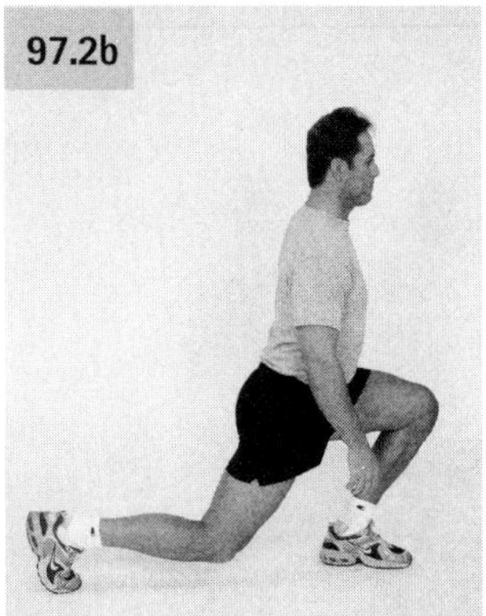

97.2b

lunge excursion gradually. Perform most of your lunges within a $1\frac{1}{2}$-to 2-foot excursion. You may do some of your lunges past this range if your activity requires longer lunge movements. Before progressing to longer lunges, follow these guidelines:

1. The movement should be pain-free.
2. Wobbling or swaying of your knees or torso should be minimal.
3. Keep your low back in a neutral position and allow minimal forward or side-to-side motion of your back during the lunge.
4. Before increasing the excursion of the lunge past 2 feet, try increasing the speed of your lunges while maintaining good control of motion.

Control the speed of knee flexion and stop at about 55–60 degrees. Eventually you may go into a deeper lunge. Allow your back knee to bend and your back foot to lift up at the heel. Try to align your forward knee over your first and second toes (see photo 97). Return to the start position by pushing off your front foot. Initially do your lunge with one foot going forward and back. **Same-side lunges:** Lunge on the right foot for a set of 5–6 reps and then do a set of lunges onto your left foot. **Alternating lunges:** When you have the form and are not wobbling, try alternating the lunge foot that you put forward. Work up to a set with 8–12 lunges to each side. In most workout routines, you'll want to do 2–3 sets of whichever lunge variation you choose. If you are training for an activity that requires speed, try to increase the speed of your lunges to see how many you can do in 30–45 seconds, especially if you are a skier or climber.

Tips and Precautions: If the forward lunge is painful, try decreasing the depth of your knee flexion and add lunges in different directions, especially to the sides. If a lunge is still painful, try unloading it as in variation 97.1. In any lunge, make sure your knee is in line with your foot.

Variations: 97.1. Unloaded lunge ("No Knee Pain Lunge"): Unload a lunge to decrease kneecap pain by using ski poles, dowels, or 2 chair backs to support part of your body weight through your arms as you bend your knee in the basic lunge. Try to support enough weight with your arms so that your knees don't hurt.

97.2. Deep lunge: In this lunge, you take a longer stride with your front foot, bending your back knee so that it almost touches the floor. If you are a telemark skier, increase your lunge excursion as your ability allows, simulating your skiing (97.2a and 97.2b).

97.3. Sidestep (lateral) lunge: Lunge to one side and then the other while keeping your feet facing forward and your back in neutral alignment. Measure your lunge excursion from the inside of your nonlunging foot to the inside of your lunging foot. Perform most of your lunges with an excursion of 1 1/2–2 feet. If you are a telemark or cross-country skier or a mountaineer, some of your lunges should have excursions of 2–2 1/2 feet. You can do lateral lunges with hand weights held at your sides or with ski poles. (A more advanced version of this is a sidestep lunge on stairs. You can do this up 2–3 stairs at a time to simulate sidestepping up a hill in cross-country skiing.)

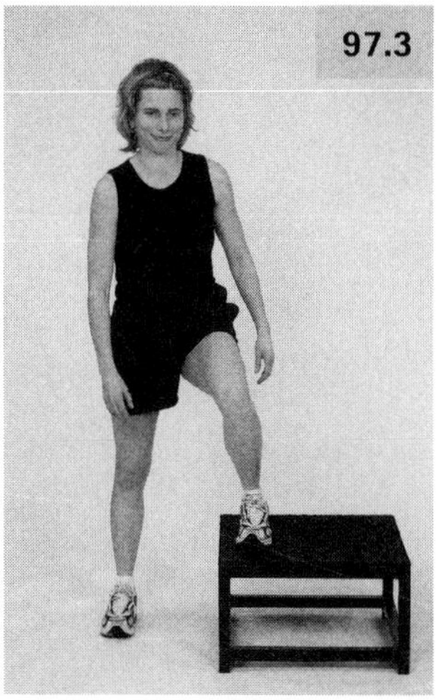
97.3

97.4. Sidestep balance lunge: Perform a sidestep lunge while shaking a partially water-filled beach ball or a Body Blade vigorously side to side. This is excellent training for snowboarders.

97.5. Lunge with hand weights: Do a basic alternating lunge with dumbbells or hand weights that you hold at your side. Start with light weights (3–8 pounds) and work up to as much weight as you can manage pain-free while maintaining good form (97.5a–c).

97.6. Lunge with biceps curl: Doing a lunge with a biceps curl is an excellent way to exercise your arms, back, and legs simultaneously. Hold a pair of 3- to 5-pound dumbbells at your sides (the same position as shown in photo 97.5a). You can start with heavier weights if you already do a biceps curl, but remember that you can't use as much weight as you normally would for an isolated biceps curl. Curl the dumbbells toward your chest as you lunge to a safe range (97.6a), then lower them back to your sides as you return to the upright position. If you don't have back problems you can progress to lunges that start with the dumbbells at your chest (97.6b). This will challenge your back and core stability. Remember to activate your core muscles before doing the lunge. Lower the dumbbells toward your lunge foot (97.6c) as you perform the lunge and return them to your chest as you return to

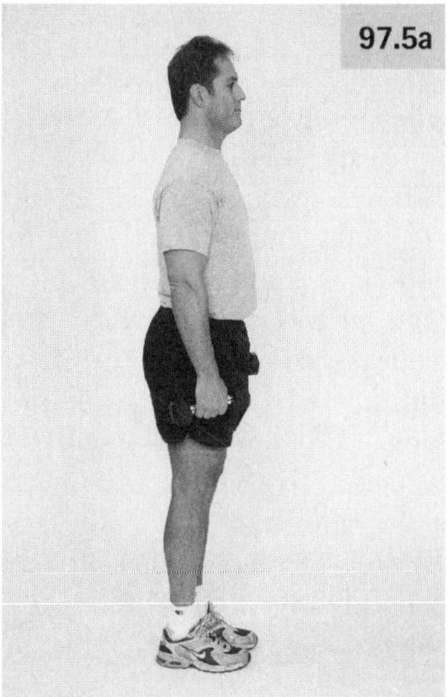
97.5a

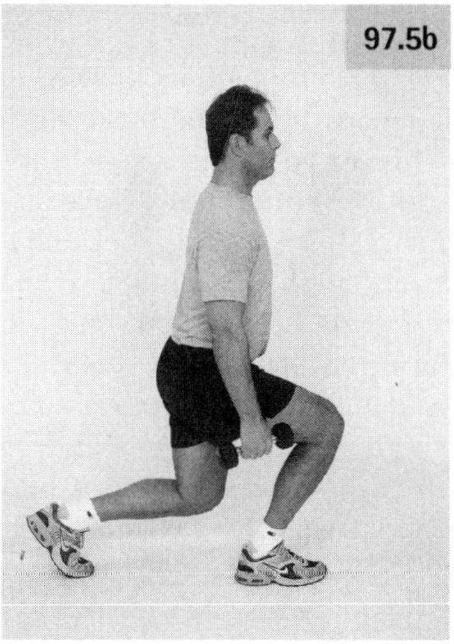
97.5b

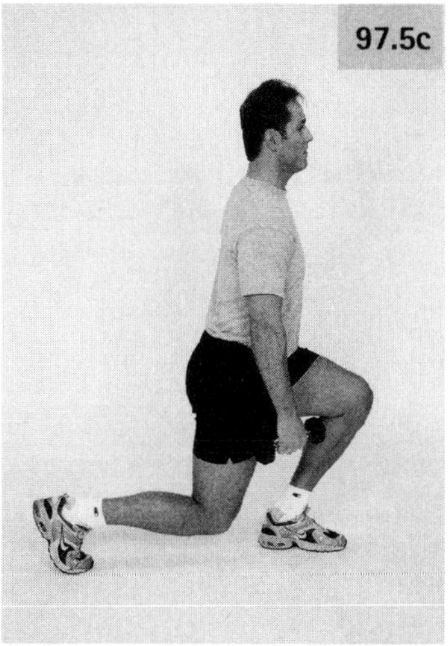
97.5c

97.6a

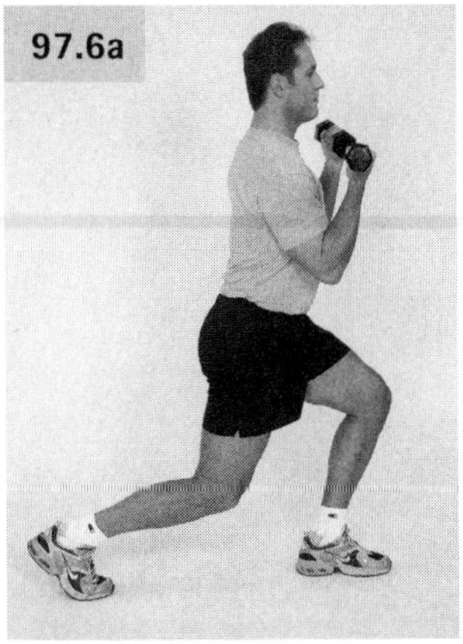

97.6b

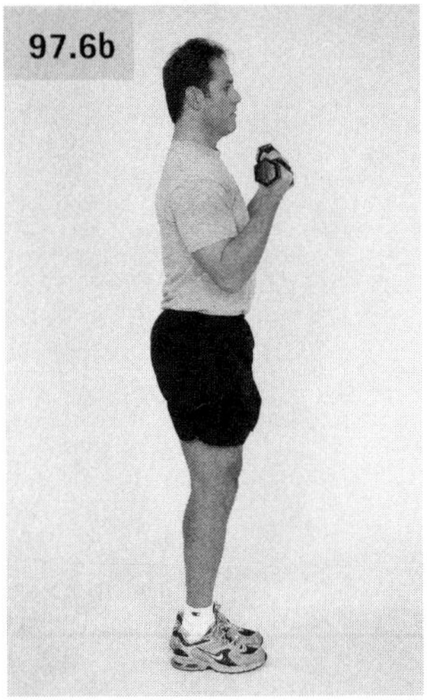

97.6c

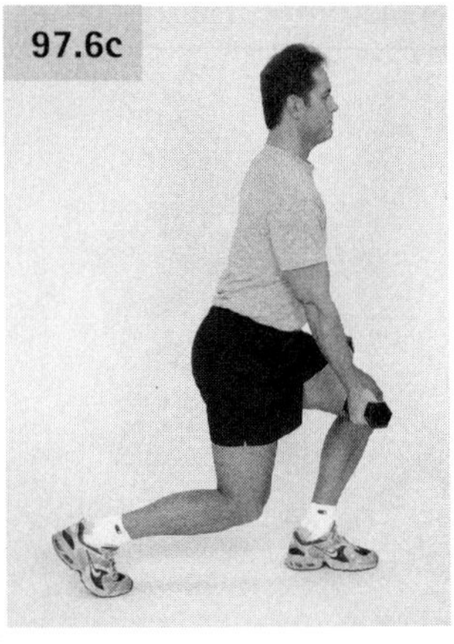

the upright position. This can be done for a same-side or alternate lunge set for 2 sets of 8–12 reps on each leg.

97.7. Lunge with opposite knee reach: Doing a lunge with an opposite knee reach is excellent for telemark skiers (see Exercise 29 in chapter 5).

97.8. Lunge with overhead press: Perform an overhead press with dumbbells while lunging forward with one leg. Remember that you will be able to lift less weight in a lunge than in an isolated overhead shoulder press. This is a good variation for climbers and cyclists.

97.9. Basic walking lunge: Try a walking lunge by stepping forward with each lunge instead of returning to the start position. This helps improve balance during your lunge. Try this lunge initially with 6 lunges forward, turn around and then do 6 lunges to return to your starting position. You can add hand weights or dumbbells to this walking lunge. Initially try a walking lunge with weights at your side and you can progress to doing a biceps curl while lunging. Start with safe successful ranges, making sure you are pain-free and in control without allowing any wobbling at the bottom of the lunge. Once you can perform 2 sets of 8–12 reps, pain-free and in good control, increase the depth, then the length of your walking lunge.

97.10. Walking balance lunge: Do a walking lunge with a partially filled beach ball or a Body Blade. Shake it side to side vigorously, to increase the balance and abdominal challenge.

97.11. Sidestep walking lunge: Do a walking lunge in a sidestepping motion. This is good for cross-country skiers.

97.12. Sidestep walking balance lunge: Do variation 97.11 while shaking a ball or Body Blade.

97.13. Lunge matrix: The lunge matrix is a dynamic advanced whole-body lunge combination exercise (see Exercise 30 in chapter 5). This is a good one for any nonboating athlete to try.

97.14. Rotational (transverse) lunge: Position yourself in the center of an imaginary clock and locate 3:00, 4:00, and 5:00 (to your right and slightly behind you) and 9:00, 8:00, and 7:00 (to your left and slightly behind you). Start by lunging toward 3:00 with your right foot while pointing the toes of your right foot at the 3:00 position. Remember to pivot on your nonlunge foot so that you don't stress your knee. The guidelines for lunge excursion are the same as for the forward lunge. Once you have lunged to a safe range, return to the start position in the center of the imaginary clock and face 12:00. Repeat this lunge maneuver toward 4:00 and 5:00 with your right foot, then switch to your left foot and lunge to 9:00, 8:00, and 7:00. Be very careful with this if you have a knee cartilage, ankle, or back problem.

97.15. Outdoor lunges: Try lunges on outdoor terrain, especially hills (see chapter 8). This will help you better prepare for outdoor activities. Add resistance or balance challenges by holding hand weights or wearing a backpack.

Basic Lunge Progression: This functional progression is designed to safely progress you through various lunges depending on your age, musculoskeletal conditions, and requirements for strength and balance (that can be assisted with lunge exercises). It goes from the easiest to the most difficult lunges. Don't progress to the next level unless you can do at least 2 sets of 6–10 lunges pain-free and in good form. If you don't fit the category named, you can move to a different level. For most people the walking lunge with weights will be the end of the progression. Remember to take at least a 1-minute break in between each lunge set.

1. **Unloaded lunge (97.1):** Do this if you have knee pain or are rehabbing an injured knee, ankle, or hip. Also do this if you are older or have a neurological condition and are trying to improve your balance.
2. **Basic lunge same leg (97):** Perform a set of 8–12 lunges on the same leg then repeat on the opposite side.
3. **Basic alternating lunge (97):** Do alternate lunges in safe ranges on each leg for 8–12 reps on each leg.
4. **Basic deep lunge (97.2):** Do this lunge if your activity requires better buttock strength or deeper lunge motions.
5. **Lunge with hand weights (97.5):** Do this lunge if you require more balance or strength challenge. It is also good for older women who wish to load their arm and leg bones to improve bone density.
6. **Lunge with biceps curl (97.6):** Do this for the following reasons: (a) You are pressed for time and want to exercise your biceps, core, and legs in the same exercise. (b) To improve your balance. (c) As part of a core strengthening program. (d) To incorporate a more challenging lunge. (e) As a biceps exercise. (f) To improve bone density in your arms and legs.
7. **Basic walking lunge (97.9):** Do this for the following reasons: (a) To improve your balance and core stability. (b) To make your lunge more fun and challenging. (c) If you are a mountain climber, runner, snowshoer, or advanced hiker.
8. **Walking lunge with hand weights (97.9):** Do 2 sets of 8–12 reps/steps on each leg. Start with shallow lunging steps in safe, pain-free ranges before progressing to deeper or longer strides. Do this for the same reasons as the basic walking lunge. The added weight will help you build bone density in your arms and legs.

9. **Lunge matrix:** See Exercise 30 in chapter 5. This is the ultimate lunge combination and should not be attempted until you can perform walking lunges with dumbbells for the prescribed number of sets and reps. It is good for any higher-performance athlete in any nonboating sport or activity. Start with the first sequence of lunges for 2 sets of 3 alternate lunges in each of the directions described. When you have mastered this, progress to the second sequence and then the third sequence, doing 2 sets of 3 alternate lunges for each sequence. When you have mastered each sequence of the lunge matrix individually for the prescribed number of sets and reps, put all 3 sequences together for 1 complete set. Start with sequence 1 and complete all 3 alternate lunges on each leg in all 3 directions, then immediately go to the second sequence, then the third, for 1 complete lunge matrix set. If you are looking for advanced conditioning with the exercise, do 3 sets of the complete lunge matrix without stopping.

98 STEP-UPS

Equipment: 4-inch step on a step platform, or stairs or bleachers with a 6- to 8-inch step.

Purpose: Improve your legs' ability to go up steep inclines, steps, rocks, or logs, which is essential to the hiker, climber, or mountaineer.

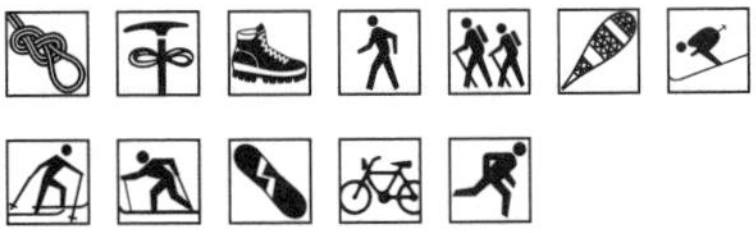

98a

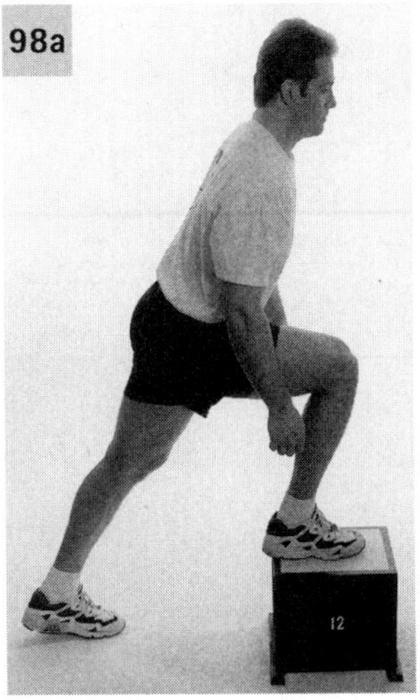

98b

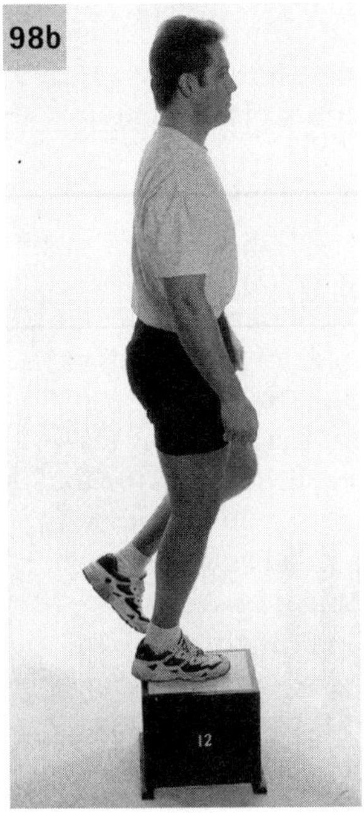

Technique: Start with your feet shoulder-width apart, about 6–12 inches from the step. Lift and place one foot onto the step surface and then shift your weight forward, keeping your back in a neutral position. Shift your weight forward until you feel your back heel lifting off the ground, or until about three-fourths of your weight is on your front foot (98a). Then push off your back foot and straighten your front knee (98b). Place both feet on the step and then return to the start position with your knees slightly bent. You can repeat the step-up with the same knee each time in 1 set, or alternate the stepping-up foot. Increase the height of the step gradually. You can use a staircase and step up 2–3 stairs at a time. Backpackers and climbers should gradually increase step height to simulate the highest step up that you might have to take in the outdoors. This may be as high as 2–3 feet. When doing a high step, weight shifting is very important. You may want to use ski poles to assist you on a high step to simulate a handhold. Do 2 sets of 15 reps. Try to do 1 set of 4–6 high step-ups if you are a scrambler or a climber.

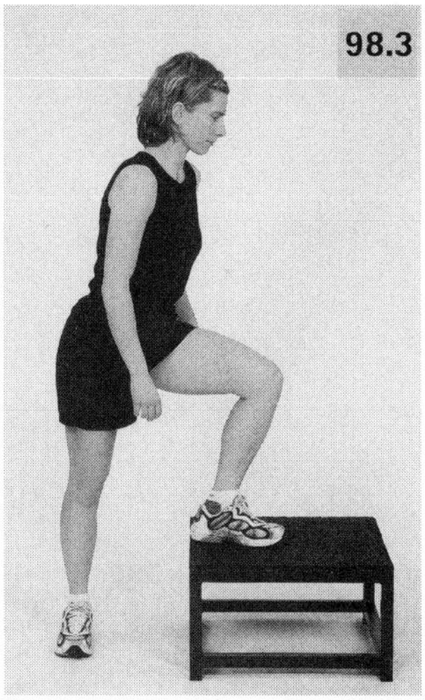
98.3

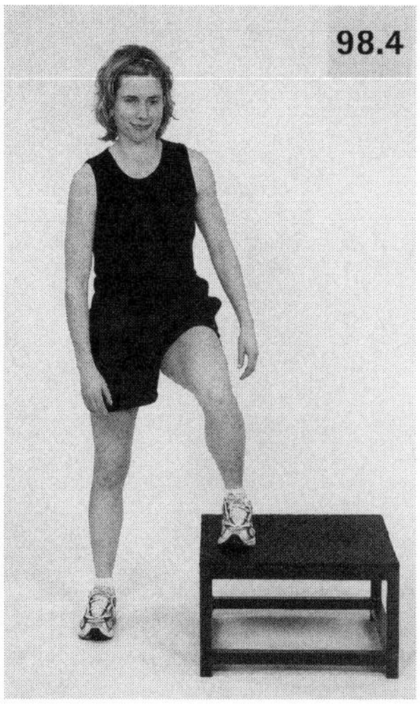
98.4

Variations: 98.1. Do a step-up with an overhead press (see Exercise 35 in chapter 5). **98.2.** Do a step-up with resisted shoulder extension (see Exercise 36). **98.3.** Lateral step-ups: Try standing to the side of the step with your feet parallel and sidestep up onto the step. You can also perform this on a flight of stairs. Try to perform sets of 12–15 reps on each leg. **98.4.** Rotational step-ups: Stand sideways to the step and turn at a 90-degree angle toward the step as you step up. Avoid this exercise if you have a knee meniscus cartilage problem.

99 STEP-DOWNS

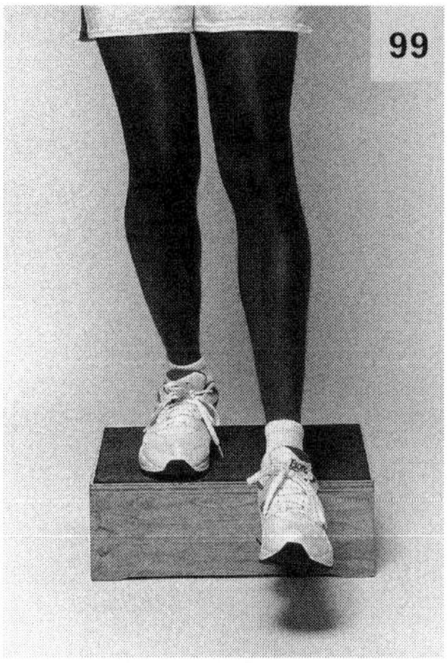
99

Equipment: 4-inch step on a step platform, or stairs or bleachers with a 6- to 8-inch step.
Purpose: Improve your ability to control gravitational forces while moving downhill.

Technique: Stand with both feet on the step, facing "downhill." Balance on one foot and with the other foot reach to the floor in front of you. Allow both knees to bend and try to keep your back in a neutral position. During this initial phase of the step-down, try not to transfer your body weight over the descending foot. Touch your heel to the floor and then return back to the start position. Use the foot and leg on the step to raise yourself back to the start position. Do 2 sets of 15 reps.

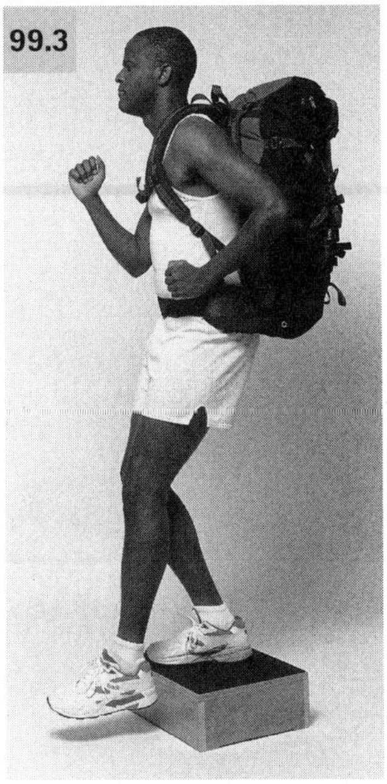
99.3

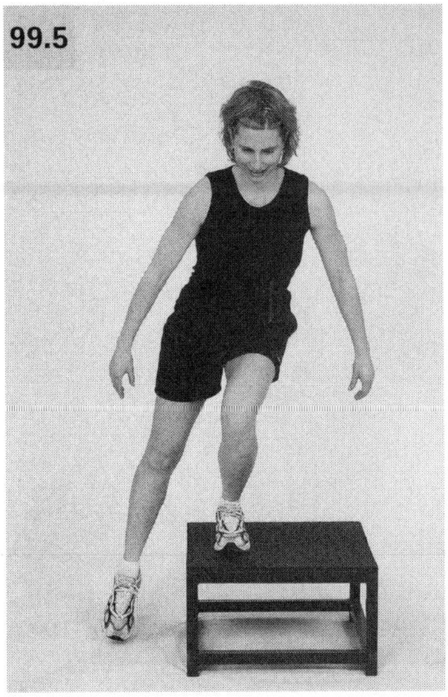
99.5

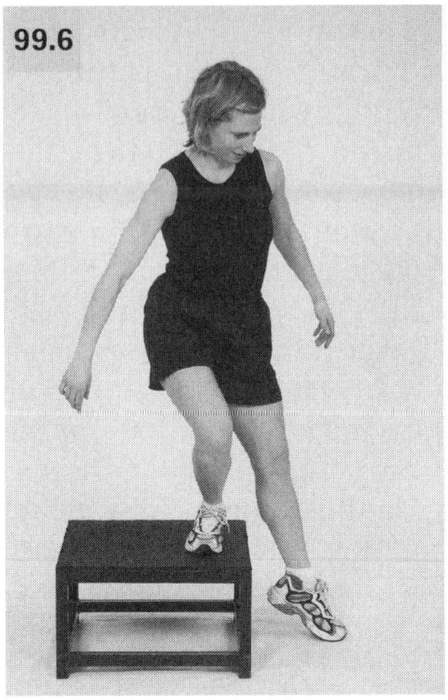
99.6

Variations: 99.1. Variable height: Increase the step height, especially if you are a scrambler or climber. You can use 2–3 stairs. **99.2.** Variable distance: Increase the distance from the step to the ground touch area to 10 inches away, and so on. **99.3.** Loaded step-downs: Add resistance by wearing a backpack or holding hand weights. **99.4.** Continuous step-downs: On stairs, do connected step-downs of 2–3 stairs for 30 seconds to 4 minutes. **99.5.** Lateral step-downs: Try stepping off to the side of the step, keeping your step-off foot parallel to your stance foot. Don't put weight on the step-off foot, just touch the floor with your toe or heel and return it to beside your stance foot. **99.6.** Rotational step-down: Try stepping off the step while turning at a 45- to 50-degree angle. If you are balancing on your left foot, turn and step off at a 45- to 50-degree angle to your right with your right foot pointed in that direction.

Precaution: Avoid lateral and rotational step-downs if you have low-back and especially sacroiliac problems.

JUMPS AND HOPS

You can begin adding jumps and hops to your program after you have established a good aerobic and strength base. You should be able to do Exercises 31, 34, 58, 59.3, 61, and 95–99 before doing hops and jumps. You should not do these if you have any ongoing musculoskeletal injuries.

Vertical jumps are appropriate for rock climbers. Hopping (or leaping) and landing on the opposite foot is more functional for mountaineering and snowshoeing. For glacier mountaineering, emphasize hopping with side-to-side and forward leaping motions. Try this both up and down a hill. Do side-to-side hopping on level ground first, then progress to a hill and vary the angle and distances of the hopping motion. Occasionally try a longer leap if you anticipate having to jump over a crevasse, for example. You may begin with a short run before some of your hops. For downhill skiing and snowboarding, in general, a mix of more jumping than hopping is appropriate and should be practiced on a level surface before doing them on a downhill slope. Jumps are also functional for crew preparation.

A hop is performed by leaping and landing on one foot. Hops can begin and land on the same foot or begin on one foot and land on the opposite foot. In general, a hop requires more balance and strength than a jump. A jump begins and finishes on both feet. Try basic jump exercises prior to hop exercises.

Your hops and jumps can start out small and progress to longer distances to simulate the motions of your activity. You can vary the amplitude, direction, and slope with your jumps. You can do your hops and jumps in sets of 3–8 reps initially in the same direction and distance. As you increase in your general strength, perform your hops and jumps with greater distances and speeds.

Hops and jumps engage your torso and arms to propel weight off the ground, so they are considered total body movements. Do an aerobic warm-up and some lunge or squat exercises before doing hops and jumps. After performing jumping and hopping exercises, cool down with a 5- to 10-minute aerobic period consisting of a brisk walk, cycle, or run.

Proper form is imperative while hopping and jumping. Don't allow your knees to bend more than 90 degrees when you land. Protect your back by doing most of your bending from your hips, knees, and ankles. Hops and jumps should not be done if you have limited motion in your ankle or if you have a knee, back, or foot problem. If you have sore knees or any other problems that make landing from jumps uncomfortable, try the same routine but use water jumps or uphill jumps to soften the impact.

100 THE BASIC JUMP

Equipment: Level floor or ground; progress to using hills, snow, and/or a backpack.
Purpose: Improve your ability to balance while decelerating and propelling your body in an explosive manner, such as in activities on snow, on climbing walls, and in the mountains. Also to improve power in runners.

Technique: Stand with your feet slightly farther than shoulder-width apart, with your arms in a relaxed position at your side. Wind up by bending your knees and hips (100a). Allow your trunk to move forward while you bring your arms behind you. Simultaneously push off with both legs while swinging your arms forward, and let your entire body extend completely to maximize the full power that you are generating (100b). Land on both feet. When landing, think of yourself as a shock absorber as your feet, ankles, knees, and hips share the impact of contact. Your feet must land in the same direction as the start position with no loss of balance (100c). When learning a new jump, practice 2–4 of them and gradually build to 8–12 in a set. The more explosive the jump, the fewer you should do in a set.
Variations: 100.1. Vertical jump: Start with more knee bending and less hip flexing. Thrust your arms overhead and upward. This is good for climbers. **100.2.** Squat jump: This emphasizes the lower body and does not use the arms for momentum. From a half squat, jump straight up for maximum height. Do this as described for variation

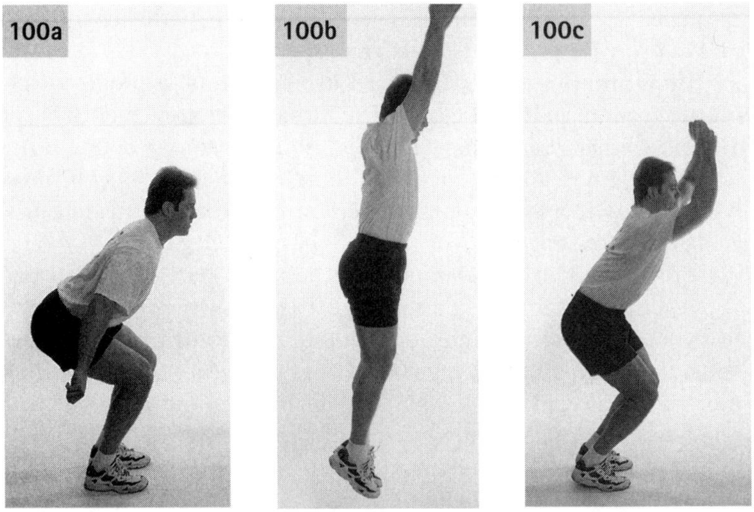

100.1, but place your hands behind your neck. **100.3.** Double-leg forward, uphill, and downhill jump: Jump forward and land on both feet. Going uphill, try for maximum height, land softly, and absorb landing forces with your legs. Try 4–8 reps per set and rest 3 minutes between sets. Try these backward, sideways, and at an angle (100.3a). These are specifically designed for snowboarders. In downhill jumping, be careful and keep your back from flexing excessively. Use your hips, knees, and ankles to absorb the impact rather than your low back. To simulate skiing, alternate turning your body to the left and right with each jump. Try this with lower-amplitude jumps before increasing the height of your jumps (100.3b). **100.4.** Rotational jump: Start with your feet shoulder-width apart, jump, and rotate 90 degrees to your right or to your left. Upon landing, jump and return to your initial starting position. As your balance and strength improve, increase your rotational jump to between 90 and 180 degrees in both directions. As you land your jump, reach across your body with your left hand to hip level. Repeat the same jump-and-reach motion to the opposite side. Perform this motion for 8–12 reps on

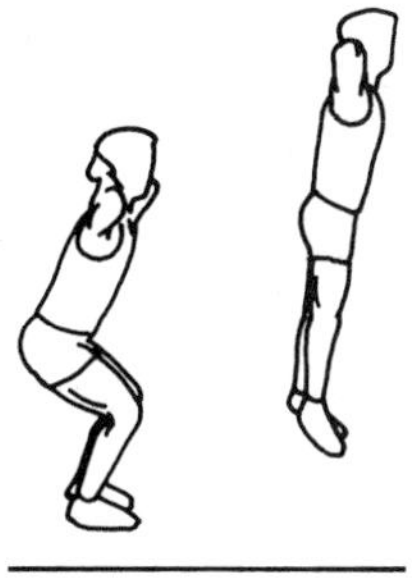

100.2

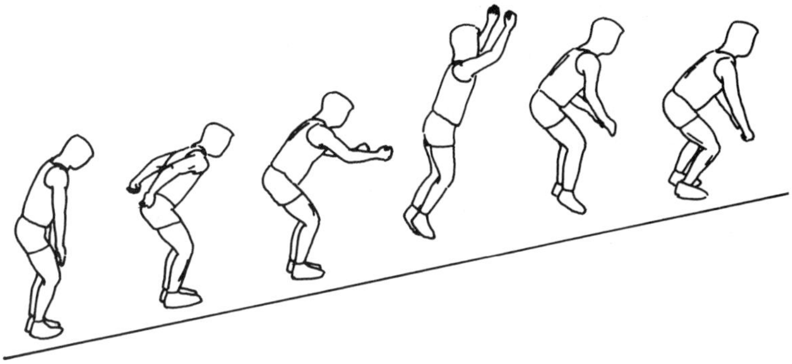

100.3a

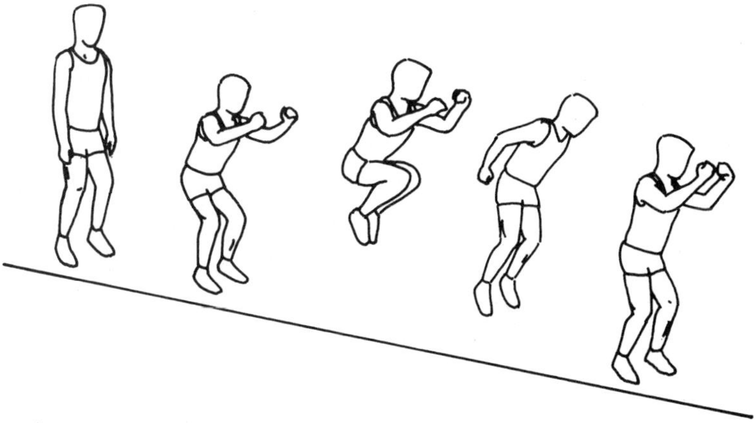

100.3b

each side. For an additional balance and strength challenge, progress your left-hand reach from hip level toward your right foot. Repeat this in the opposite direction. These are excellent for snowboarders. **100.5.** Lateral jump: Follow the directions for exercise 100.2, but take off and land on both feet. You can do this over a step or a log to make it more challenging (see Exercise 71.2d). These are good for snowboarders, windsurfers, and alpine skiers. **100.6.** Lateral jump with ball toss: Do exercise 100.5, and have a partner throw a ball to your side in the direction that you are jumping. These are good for snowboarders, windsurfers, and alpine skiers. **100.7.** Loaded jump: Increase the jump challenge by using ski poles or wearing a loaded backpack while performing the previous jumps. Use your ski poles to help during the push-off phase. Pole-assisted jumps are most appropriate for telemark and downhill skiers. Pack-loaded jumps are most appropriate for backcountry snowshoers, telemark skiers, and mountain climbers.

101 THE BASIC HOP

Equipment: Level floor or ground; progress to using hills, snow, and/or a backpack.

Purpose: Improve your ability to balance while decelerating and propelling your body in an explosive manner, such as in activities on snow, on climbing walls, and in the mountains. Also to improve power in runners.

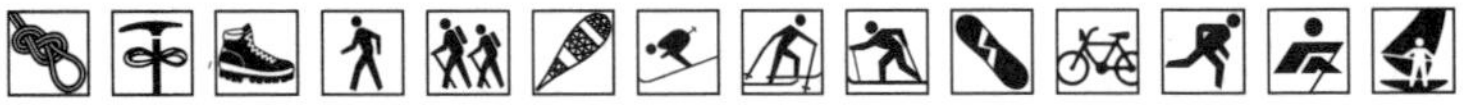

101a

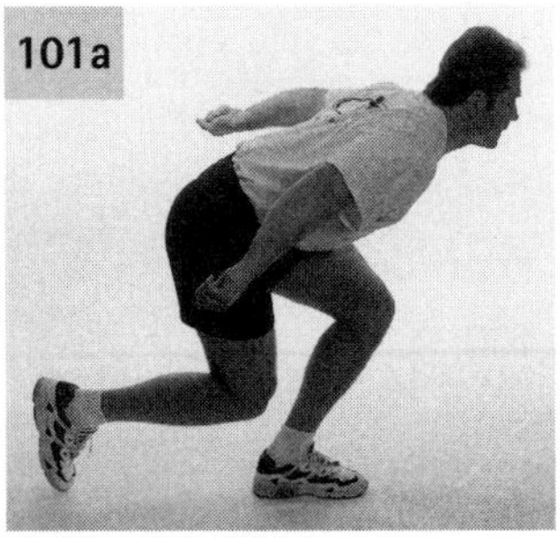

101b

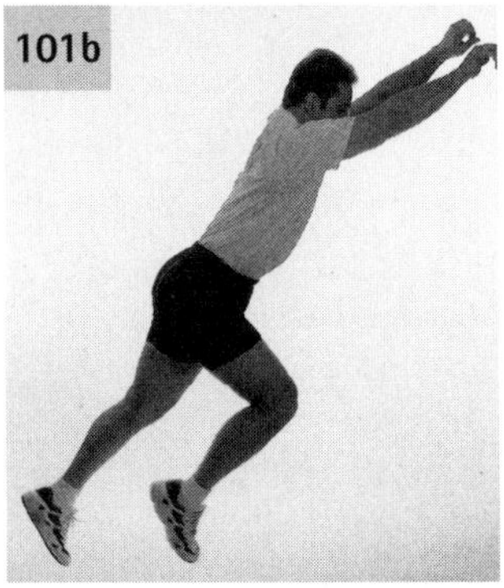

Technique: Balance on one leg with your stance leg slightly bent. Lift your opposite foot off the ground with your knee flexed. Your trunk should be forward and your arms hanging freely by your sides. Wind up by bringing your arms behind you, allow your trunk to flex farther forward, and bend your stance knee farther (101a). Then simultaneously push off your stance foot and bring your arms forward (101b), and land on your opposite foot. You can add resistance or a balance challenge by wearing a backpack.

Variations: 101.1. Vertical hop: Perform Exercise 101, but don't flex your trunk as much in the wind-up phase. Bend your knee farther and propel yourself upward. This is useful for climbers. **101.2.** Lateral hop: Stand on your right foot. Side-bend your torso toward your hop direction (left, in this case) while you move your standing hip to the opposite side (to the right) to load and maintain balance. Wind up your arms to the right in front of your body. Push off from your right foot, swinging your arms to the left, and land on your left foot. This is useful for skiers and snowboarders. **101.3.** Try a very short run and a hop (good for runners, mountain climbers, hikers, and backpackers). **101.4.** Try a forward hop while shaking a partially water-filled beach ball or a Body Blade side to side to increase the balance and abdominal challenge. **101.5.** Hop up or down a hill or incline (good for skiers and climbers).

GLUTEAL AND THIGH EXERCISES

In addition to the exercises below, there are other exercises in this book that are buttock dominant and will train your glute muscles. You can integrate these to get a more diverse buttock workout: Exercises 30–32, 34–36, 97, 100.1–.3, 101, 135.

102 GLUTEUS MEDIUS SIDE LYING

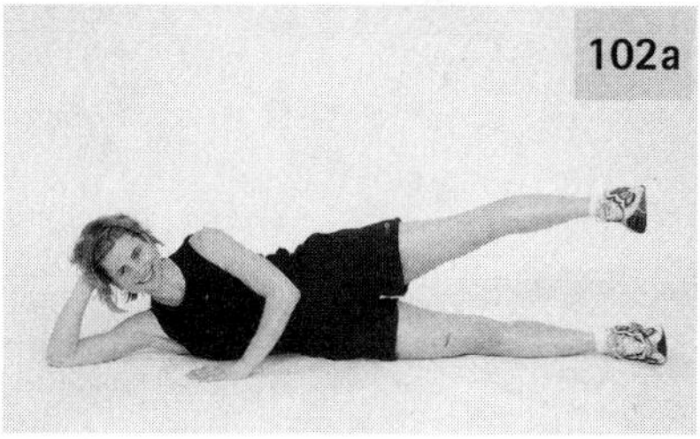
102a

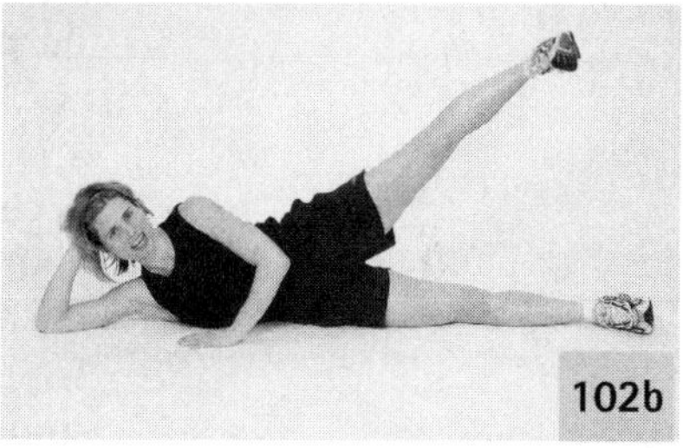
102b

Equipment: Exercise mat, ankle weights.
Purpose: Target the gluteal muscles in an isolated fashion for toning.

Technique: Lay on your right side with your spine in neutral alignment and your head supported on your right hand. Engage your core. Tighten your thigh muscles and maintain a straight right leg as you elevate your right lateral ankle toward the ceiling so that your feet are about 18 inches apart (102a). Pause motion at the end of your range for 1–2 seconds and return your right leg beside your left in a smooth, controlled fashion. Perform 2–3 sets of 12–15 reps on each side. After you have mastered this, increase your range of motion by moving your straight leg about 2–3 feet from the leg resting on the floor (102b). You can add ankle weights after you have mastered the basic form.

103 GLUTEUS MEDIUS STANDING PULLEY

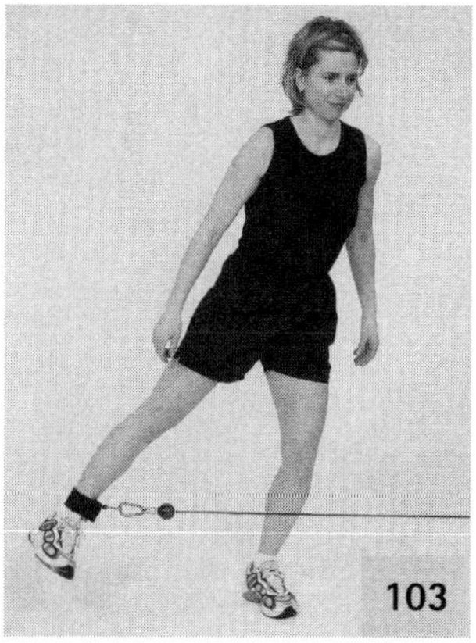
103

Equipment: Low pulley cable machine.
Purpose: Improve your balance and glute tone and strength.

Technique: Attach an ankle cuff to the low pulley cable and then to your ankle. Balance on your free leg and foot, at an angle to the pulley that allows you to move your leg with the resistance outward (abduction). Maintain a neutral spine position with your core engaged and abduct your leg against the resistance in a range that

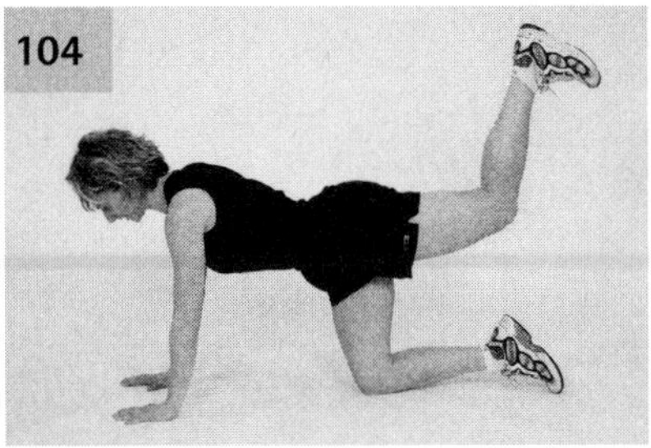
104

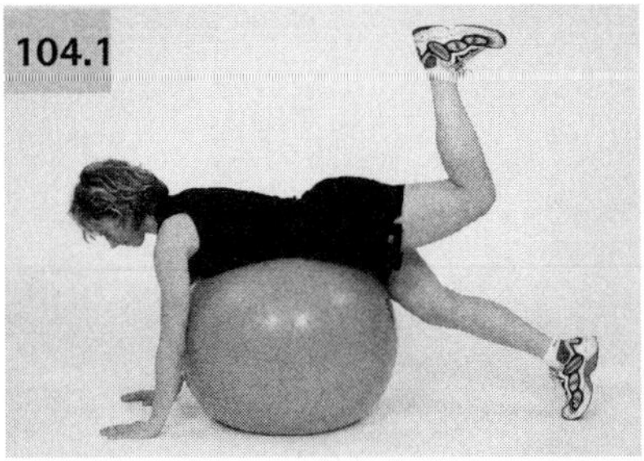
104.1

allows you to keep your hips and spine still. Perform 2–3 sets of 12–15 reps on each leg.

104 QUADRUPED GLUTEUS MAXIMUS

Equipment: None (Physioball for variation).
Purpose: Improve glute tone and strength.

Technique: Start on your hands and knees with a neutral spine and your core engaged. Maintain your right knee in a 90-degree angle and raise your right heel toward the ceiling, pivoting only at your hip joint (photo 104), then return your right knee to the floor. Do 2 sets of 12–15 reps. Perform this again on the opposite side in the same controlled fashion for an equal number of sets and reps.
Variation: 104.1. This same exercise can be done on a Physioball for an additional balance challenge.

105 GLUTEUS MAXIMUS STANDING PULLEY

Equipment: Low pulley cable machine.
Purpose: Improve your balance and glute tone and strength.

Technique: Attach an ankle cuff to the low pulley cable and then to your ankle. Balance on your free leg and foot, at an angle to the pulley that allows you to move your leg with the resistance backwards. Your balance-leg knee should be slightly bent. Maintain a neutral spine with your core engaged and extend your leg against the resistance in a range that allows you to keep your hips and spine still. This may only amount to a 1-foot-length movement behind your stance foot before you feel your low back extend. You may wish to position yourself far enough away from the pulley so that you have continued resistance on your moving leg as it travels in the forward direction.
Precaution: If you have an active back problem, avoid this exercise.

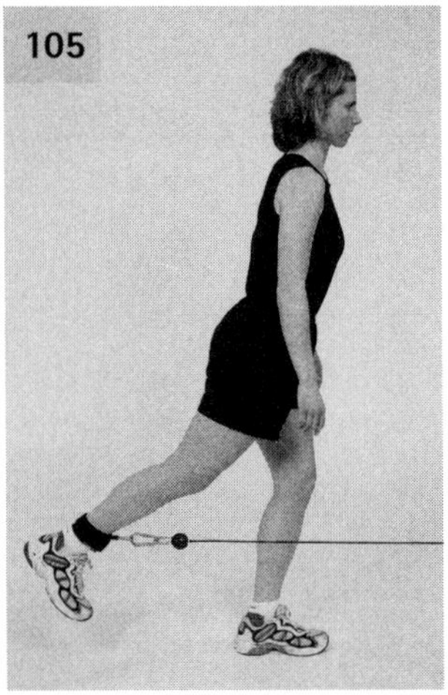
105

106 REVERSE LUNGE

Equipment: Chair.
Purpose: Strengthen your gluteus maximus and work on single-leg balance while lengthening and extending your back muscles with your core engaged.

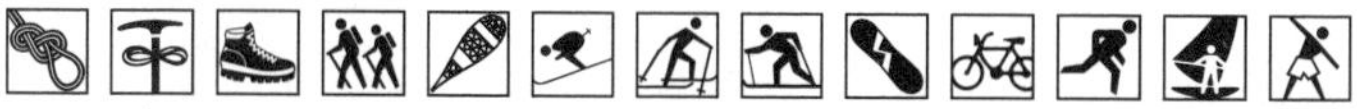

Technique: Stand on one leg with your fingertips lightly touching the back of the chair for balance or support. Be sure your core is engaged and your spine is in your neutral position to optimize your back and buttock muscles. Keep your chest elevated and straighten your opposite knee behind you. There should be a straight line running from your shoulder through your hip and along your elevated leg. Be sure to maintain a slight arch in your back (106a). The weight on your stance leg should be through your heel to keep the muscle focus on your buttock and not your thigh. Reach back at a diagonal with your back foot by bending from your hip joint on your front leg (106b). Hold each lunge for a slow 10-count and return to an upright position. When returning to your start position, focus on your glutes pushing you back up instead of your quads. Initially do a set of 2–3 reps. Progress to holding the reverse lunge position for a maximum of 30 seconds.

Tips and Precautions: Keep your trunk lengthened and arched so as to fully use your back muscles. Don't let your weight-bearing knee travel in front of your toes. Don't let your hips push out to the sides; keep them even and parallel.

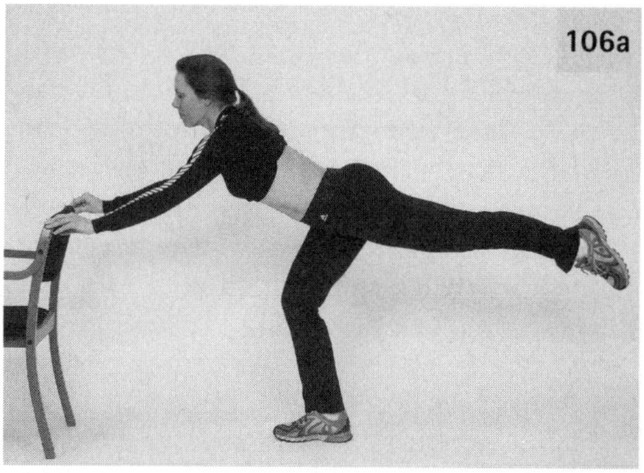
106a

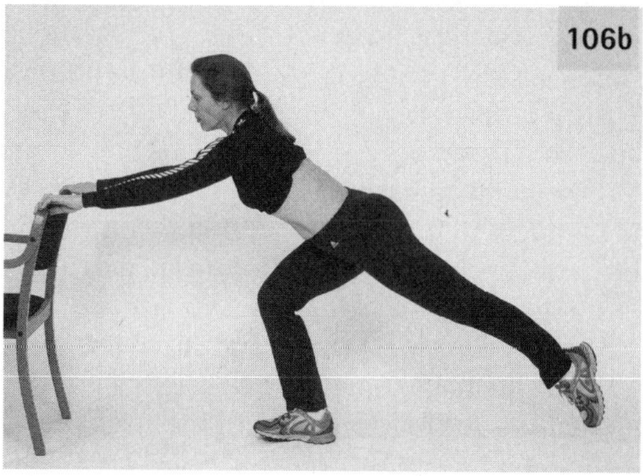
106b

chapter 12 THE ANKLE AND LEG

By John Rumpeltes, P.T.

THIS CHAPTER WILL HELP YOU:

- Understand the function of your ankle/leg and learn what exercises work that region.

Your ankle joint is essentially a hinge joining your foot with your lower leg. Your foot must alternately absorb shock and become a rigid lever to propel your body forward. Your lower leg muscles contribute significantly to balance, as well as propulsion (as in walking uphill) or deceleration (walking downhill or stepping down). Shock absorption requires your muscles to decelerate forces from above in a controlled manner so as to transfer these forces smoothly. With propulsion, the muscles affecting your foot hold it relatively rigid, so there is adequate leverage to push your body forward. The ankle joint moves primarily in *dorsiflexion* (the movement of the ankle that pulls your foot and toes up to your shin) and in *plantar flexion* (the movement of the ankle when standing on your toes or in the push-off phase of walking or running).

Self-Tests

Many activities require advanced balance ability. An ankle injury may contribute to a loss of balance ability. If you have had a serious ankle injury or feel unsure of your balance abilities, try these self-tests and some of the balance exercises in chapter 6.

Note: If you have pain with these self-tests or are not able to increase your motion with the exercises suggested, consult a health-care provider.

1. **Dorsiflexion Tightness.** While standing with your feet parallel and shoulder-width apart, squat slowly, keeping your heels on the ground, until reaching the first barrier to further motion (your back should stay straight). Now look down directly over your kneecaps toward the floor. If mobility is restricted, your toes will be in view under your kneecaps. The farther you can move your knees out over your toes without lifting your heels, the better your mobility is in dorsiflexion. Now repeat this self-test, noting your foot's arch position at the beginning and end range of the squat. If your arch flattens and your knee moves inward, this is a sign of your body compensating for restricted motion. If you are restricted in your motion, do Exercises 9 and 10.
2. **Plantar Flexion Tightness.** Start in a standing position and rise up on your toes. Your heel should rise at least 2–3 inches above the floor and you should bend at least 45 degrees in your first (big) toe joint.
3. **Joint Looseness.** Sit in a chair and cross one leg so that your ankle is on your opposite knee. Hold your heel and gently try to move it upward. If your heel and sole of your foot move upward excessively on one side compared to the other side, you may have loose ligaments. If you have a history of ankle injuries and repeated rolling of your ankle, you also may have loose ligaments. A person with this problem should wear more stable shoes, consider ankle bracing, and do

functional exercises that emphasize balance. (See chapter 6.)

FUNCTION AND ANATOMY

The two bones of the lower leg, the *tibia* and *fibula*, run parallel and contact each other as they sit on and cradle the *talus bone*, thus forming the ankle joint. The muscles of the lower leg play a major role in balance, deceleration, and propulsion, linking the supportive foot to the leg and body above. The muscles can be divided into two groups: the *plantar flexors* (calf, etc.) and the *dorsiflexors* (tibialis anterior, etc.). The dorsiflexors decelerate the toes and foot moving toward the ground just after heel contact. This allows for controlled lowering of the foot. The dorsiflexors also lift the foot and toes as they swing forward, to assure clearance with the ground. The plantar flexors help with balance by maintaining the body's center of gravity over the foot. They also support the arch of the foot. When walking or moving, the plantar flexors propel the body forward or decelerate the body moving forward over the fixed foot. See the illustrations in chapter 9.

COMMON MUSCLE IMBALANCES

Calf muscle shortness or tibialis anterior weakness is common in the lower leg, which alters ankle and foot function. Balance abilities are frequently not very good, resulting from weakness or ligament laxity in the foot, leg, or torso/hip/buttock region. Calf and Achilles stretching should be essential components for the outdoor enthusiasts' fitness program. Entire hip, thigh, lower leg, and ankle muscle training can be incorporated for optimal balance and strength using the balance exercises in chapter 6 and the lower-extremity exercises in chapter 11.

INJURY PREVENTION

Problems in ankle/leg function can lead to inefficient hiking, running, and so on, and can predispose an active individual to injuries. The most common problems in lower leg or ankle function are due to decreased motion in the foot or ankle or increased motion due to foot type or ankle ligament looseness. Tight calf muscles and Achilles tendons (see Self-Test 1, Dorsiflexion Tightness, above) are more common than tight ankle joints, but both may be loosened up with stretching and functional exercises such as a squat or lunge (see chapter 11). These changes can result in compensations that include increased flattening of the foot during movement and/or increased mechanical tension within the muscle-tendon tissue of the calf group and Achilles tendon.

Ankle joints may be loose as a result of bad sprains that did not heal well. With joint looseness, there can be problems in the foot, knee, hip, or back, and balance abilities may be compromised.

ANKLE/LEG EXERCISES

Many of the exercises in chapters 5, 6, 8, and 11 use the muscles of the ankle/leg region for strength and balance. Exercises 9 and 10 are good for flexibility.

chapter 13 THE FOOT

By Katrina Sullivan, D.P.M., and Mark Pierce, A.T.C.

THIS CHAPTER WILL HELP YOU:

- Understand foot function.
- Learn about footwear and orthotics.

Your foot acts as a dynamic foundation for your body during standing and movement. It is helpful to understand what happens to your foot during walking to understand how alterations in foot support can affect the rest of your body.

FUNCTION AND ANATOMY

The walking cycle (the gait cycle) has a few phases. At *heel strike,* the heel of the foot (or shoe) makes initial contact with the ground. During the *stance phase*, the foot is on the ground bearing weight. It must be flexible enough to adapt to various surfaces and be able to *pronate* (flatten) somewhat to accomplish this. The foot has two important roles during contact with the ground: it is a mobile adapter to uneven surfaces and a shock absorber. As we walk or run, we load more weight on the foot until the *toe-off (push-off) phase,* when the foot has to be more stable and *supinate* (go into an arch-up position) to propel the body forward. Those same joints that allowed movement now need to lock tight for proper function.

The foot is comprised of twenty-eight bones and numerous joints, muscles, tendons, and ligaments. The foot is divided into three regions: heel area (*rearfoot*), arch area (*midfoot*), and ball of the foot with toes (*forefoot*). See Figure 26.

COMMON MUSCLE IMBALANCES

Excessive relaxation of the arch and rolling in of the ankle (pronation) during contact with the ground can place the ankle, knee, or leg in a position of internal rotation stress while that structure is trying to accept the body's weight. This contributes to overuse injuries. A tight, high arch can lead to shin splints and stress fractures, since the full impact stress of loading is transmitted directly up the leg. A tight arch may not relax during Self-Test 1, Body Rotation Foot Arch (below).

INJURY PREVENTION

Function of your foot can influence function of your ankle, leg, knee, hip, back, and even upper body. Foot, ankle, knee, hip, or back pain may result from inadequate foot support. Balance and agility may also be compromised by inadequate foot support. This is why proper foot position or posture can be key for exercise and activity participation. How do you tell if your arch is working properly? The inner arch usually maintains a moderate air space between the skin and the ground during standing. There should be minimal callus formation on the bottom of your foot and your toes should remain straight. Hammertoes and bunions are a sign that your arch is not maintaining proper posture during gait. In addition, try Self-Test 1, Body Rotation Foot Arch (below).

Footwear for Active People

There is no one shoe that will fit all people or perform best for all activities. In shoe gear selection, two main categories must be considered: fit and function—the right shoe for the right

FIGURE 26

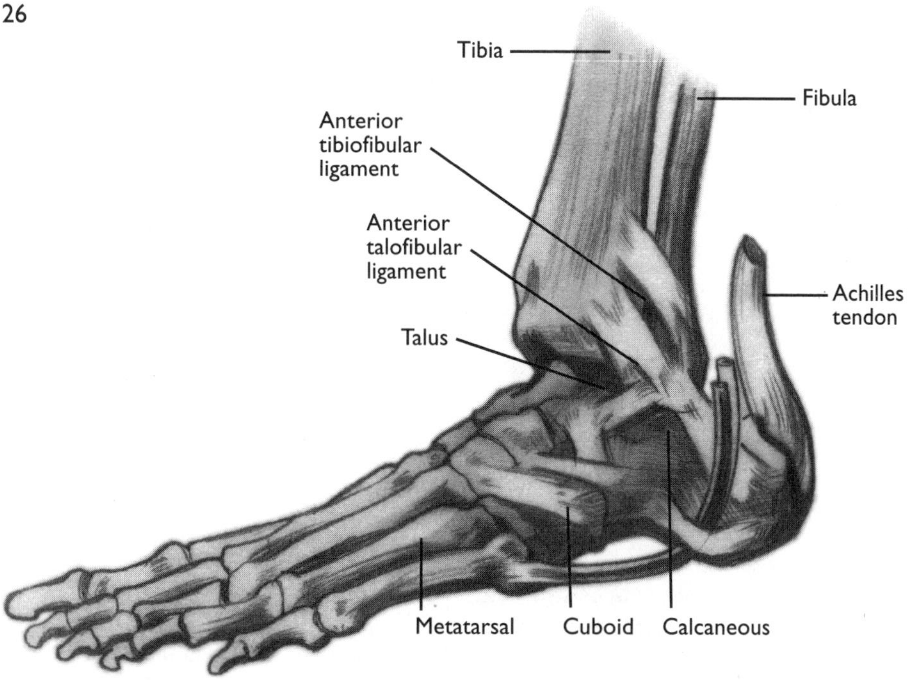

activity, with a proper fit. Today's athletic shoes are designed with particular activities in mind.

Shoe fit takes the primary role in this equation. Adequate width in the ball of the foot and toe region is very important for your foot to function within the shoe properly. The shoe needs to be long enough, a thumb's width from the end of your longest toe. Make sure you have both feet measured for width and length before you buy shoes. If you have orthotics, bring them with you when you try on shoes and make sure the shoes you purchase come with a removable insole. The shoe needs to have a firm heel counter to provide support to your foot. The arch placement or lack of arch is the least important feature, since that is the easiest to modify with ready-made arch supports or custom orthotics.

High-arched individuals do better with a curve-lasted shoe (in-flared near the big toe) as long as they don't overpronate. (The *last* is the shape that the shoe is built around.) People with flat feet and people who are overpronators (the arch sags and the ankle rolls inward) do better with a semicurved- or straight-lasted shoe.

To choose footwear, understand the activity and your needs for stability and support. Learn your foot type: high arch vs. low, narrow vs. wide, good function vs. injury prone, and any abnormal shape or idiosyncrasies. Once you have determined your needs, learn about the current shoes being offered that meet those requirements. Many magazines carry seasonal shoe reviews, and reputable outdoor stores have knowledgeable staff who can teach you about the brands that they carry. Try shoes on after doing an activity on your feet (they will be slightly larger) and wear the same socks that you would use for that sport. If you are unsure about your foot type or needs, seek medical advice prior to shopping. Also try Self-Test 2, Shoe Stability (below), on any new shoe before you purchase it.

For walking, you should have a running or

a walking shoe that is stable in the rearfoot and has a sole that resists torsion. For running, you should have a running shoe. Running shoes vary in stability and vary in regard to medial support. Visit a store that specializes in running shoes and ask for evaluation by a salesperson with some experience in evaluating running shoes while you are running (you'll actually do a test run in the store). For hiking, there are a variety of shoe options in regard to lightness and stability. In general, if you pronate excessively, you likely would benefit from a more stable shoe that has more support in the heel counter and arch. There are many lightweight hiking boots out there, and many of them are not adequate for a full day on a trail or if more stability is needed. For a day trip, a steeper trail, or for hiking on snow or scree slopes, choose a more sturdy and stable hiking boot that is still comfortable. An all-leather shoe with rearfoot support and a sole that resists torsion (twisting) is preferable for such day hikes and for backpacking trips. For scrambling, a stable leather boot is a necessity. For rock climbing, there are special climbing shoes, and you can use stable hiking boots for the hike in. For mountaineering, mountaineering boots can be rented or purchased to provide stability and protection in the snow. You can put a generic orthotic or a custom orthotic in any athletic shoe. Make sure that your athletic shoe has a removable insole so that you can replace it with an orthotic if needed.

Self-Tests

1. **Body Rotation Foot Arch.** Stand with your bare feet flat on the ground. If the inner side of the middle of your foot is almost touching the floor, you likely have pronated (flatter) arches. Next, rotate your upper body to the left as far as you can go while keeping your feet flat on the floor. Your right arch should flatten and your left arch should rise up. If this does not happen, you might have high-arched feet. (See chapter 12, Self-Test 1, Dorsiflexion Tightness.) If your ankle and Achilles tendon are tight, this is very commonly associated with a high-arched foot.
2. **Shoe Stability.** If you have feet that pronate, it is desirable to have a stable shoe or boot to wear. The following method will help you determine if your shoes are unstable. In one hand, hold one of your shoes where the sole material meets the heel, and with your other hand, hold the sole in the widest part of the forefoot (Figure 27a). Attempt to twist the shoe, first from the forefoot and then from the heel. A slight twist is OK, but if you can twist it more than 25 degrees, it is probably not very stable (Figure 27b). Also try pinching

FIGURE 27. Testing shoe stability: (a) Grasp shoe and (b) twist shoe; if it twists more than 25 degrees it is probably not very stable.

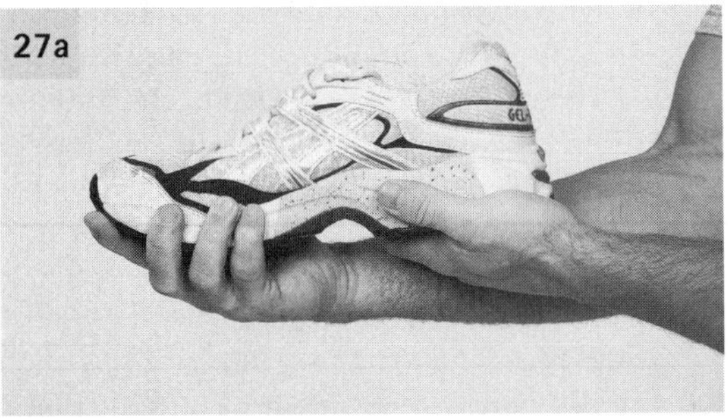

27a

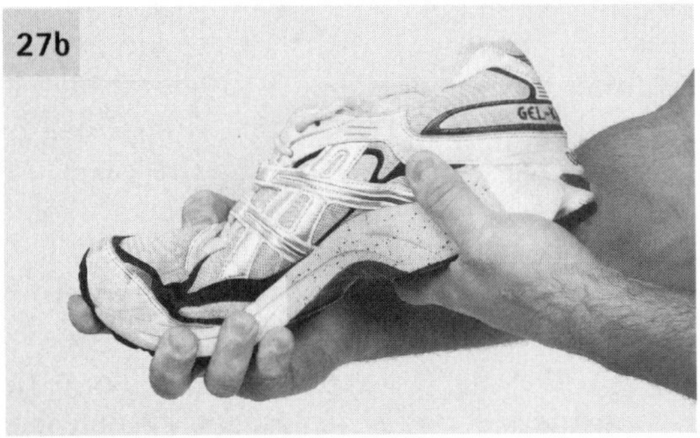

27b

the material 11/2 inches above the superior part of the heel counter. If you can pinch it and touch your thumbs together, it is likely not very supportive. Also try to fold the shoe in half. If you can do this, the sole is not very sturdy. Try to pinch the part of the shoe that contacts your Achilles tendon. If you can fold the rear of the shoe toward the insole, don't buy or continue to wear the shoe.

Orthotic Use and Selection

To understand the indications for when to use an orthotic versus an arch support, it is important to understand the difference between these devices. A functional biomechanical orthoses (corrective orthotic) works by realigning the foot into its ideal mechanical alignment (see Figure 28, below). A corrective orthotic is custom-made for the individual by casting the foot in plaster in a neutral position. Supplemental materials are then added to the orthotic to balance the foot for optimal function. The foot is balanced in relationship to the ground and the leg it supports. The goal is to restore the major joints of the foot to their best position and to control excessive motion during gait. Corrective orthotics can be extremely helpful to support alignment of your feet and lower extremity in all weight-bearing activities, including biking, hiking, running, walking, and skiing.

FIGURE 28. Left, accomodative orthotic; right, corrective orthotic.

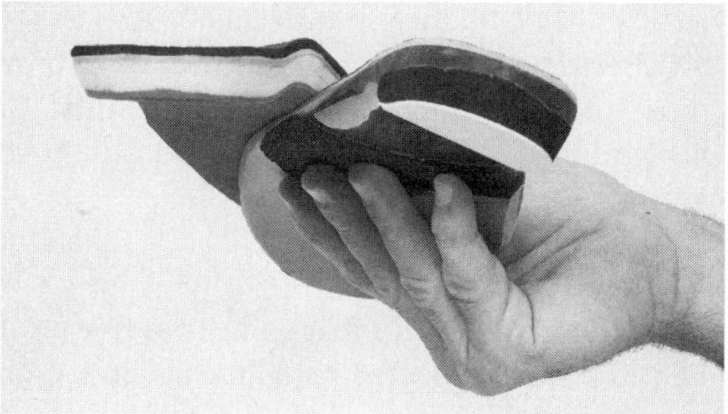

Accommodative orthotics are generic, off-the-shelf insoles that have some plastic stabilizing material that may provide functional support in between a custom orthotic and an arch support (see Figure 28, left). Accommodative orthotics are thinner than corrective orthotics and don't have angulation in the heel. If you have any type of foot pain or slightly flattened arches and are on a tight budget, these generic supports are a good place to start. They may work reasonably well in many walking and athletic shoes. It makes sense to try these on in a store and see if they are comfortable and support your feet.

Generic arch supports are relatively inexpensive inserts that are usually made of foam and simply are a device to fill in the space between your arch and your shoe. They don't provide much, if any, mechanical support. Their primary use is for comfort, especially if you have toe pain, plantar fasciitis, or a heel bursa problem.

If you have foot, ankle, or knee pain, consider consulting a podiatrist or sports medicine specialist to see if orthotics might help you. Investing in an orthotic can often help with foot pain and improve balance and athletic performance.

chapter 14 THE NECK, MID BACK, AND LOW BACK/CORE

By Kim Bennett, P.T., David Musnick, M.D., Anne Marie Trumbold, P.T., and Mark Trumbold, P.T.

THIS CHAPTER WILL HELP YOU:

- Understand the concept of your core.
- Learn neutral spine alignment to be used in many activities.
- Develop protective strategies to observe during exercise and outdoor activity to prevent injury.
- Learn exercises to improve motion and stability while strengthening and protecting your back.

Your spine is a crucial system for you to protect and strengthen. When functioning ideally, it has the ability to perform multiple tasks simultaneously. It protects your spinal cord in your neck and thoracic regions and protects your discs and nerve roots in all spine regions. It allows mobility in many directions. Your neck allows you to move your eyes and it protects your spinal cord and the nerves that go to your shoulders and arms. Your thoracic spine and rib cage protect your chest organs and allow for significant rotation to help you position your arms and hands. Your low back and sacroiliac joint transfer forces and loads from your legs and pelvis. This part of the spine protects the nerves that go to your legs.

Protection and proper positioning of your neck, mid back, and low back are essential for injury-free exercise and outdoor activities. These regions contain discs, bones, joints, and nerve tissue and can be injured or become painful from poor posture, lifting, or motions during activities. Injuries to spinal nerves from disc, joint, or arthritis problems can compromise muscle strength. Muscle strength can also be compromised from problems of the facet and sacroiliac joints. Mobility in your spine can be lost from muscle weakness, from wear and tear arthritis (see chapter 31), or from guarding of loose joints. Pain in any part of your spine can make your activities less enjoyable and decrease your abilities to move quickly, lift or pull, and make appropriate balance adjustments. This chapter is essential reading for any person who wants to ensure the safety, strength, and preservation of one of your most important pieces of equipment, your spine.

FUNCTION AND ANATOMY

Your spine is composed of vertebral bones stacked in a column with discs in between (for whole-body illustrations, see chapter 9). These discs act as shock absorbers and controllers of motion. Nerves exit at openings formed by the facet joints (which join adjacent vertebral levels) between the vertebral bones. Your spine must protect these structures and allow for movement to help you position your head, arms, and legs.

Low Back

Your low back (lumbar spine) has five levels of vertebrae connected to a triangular sacrum bone, which is connected to your pelvis through your sacroiliac joint. See Figure 29 for a picture of low-back detail. Your low back has a normal, slightly arched/extended curve. It contains the nerves that go to your legs. Your low back has limited movement compared to the other spinal areas. If your thoracic spine does not rotate well, your low back (and neck) will be forced to compensate, which can lead to joint pain and eventually arthritis. Your lower-back discs can become painful from prolonged flexed sitting and standing postures as well as from improper lifting.

Sacroiliac Region

Your sacroiliac (SI) joint plays a role in transferring forces from your legs to your upper body. The stability of your SI joint and the strength of surrounding muscles are very important for spine and lower-body function. There are anatomical variations in the structure and ability of the SI joint to fit together in a stable manner. The muscular stabilization of the SI joint is called *force closure*. Certain muscles are involved in stabilizing (or affect) the position of the SI joint. These include the latissimus dorsi (on the opposite side of the joint), spinal muscles (multifidi, quadratus lumborum, erector spinae, and the deep spinal rotators), deep hip rotators (piriformis and deep buttock region muscles), gluteals (gluteus maximus, medius, and minimus), and the hamstring muscles. In this book we refer to these muscles collectively as the *extended core*.

FIGURE 29

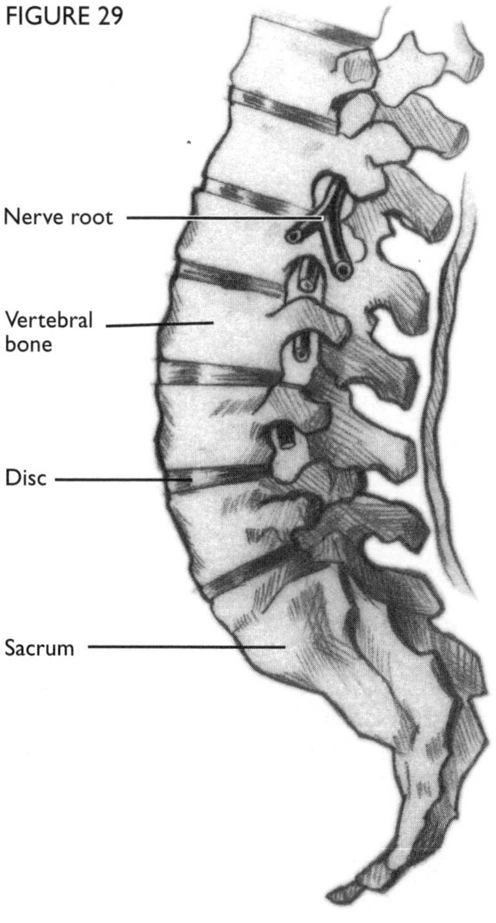

People with less-stable joints or weaker muscles may have problems with the SI joint. Such problems can manifest in any of the following ways: (1) Pain in the SI joint or ligaments on top of the joint (buttock pain). (2) Difficulty walking or running. (3) Weakness or giving way of a leg. (4) Persistent muscle pain, spasm, or trigger points in any of the muscles of the abdomen or extended core. (5) Popping or clicking in the low back. (6) Recurring strains or sprains of the knees, ankles, or feet. If you have persistent SI problems, consult with a manually trained physical therapist along with a physician such as a chiropractor, osteopath, physiatrist, sports medicine specialist, or orthopedic medicine (nonsurgical) specialist. If you are seeing any of the above practitioners and your SI is still not stable, you could try prolotherapy, which involves ligament injections to stabilize the SI area.

If you have sacroiliac or low-back problems or you would like to generally strengthen your back, consider choosing from the following exercises, which can strengthen your abdominals and extended core muscles: 31, 34, 36, 78–80, 83, 84, 86, 88, 92, 93, 95, 96, 98, 102–110, 120, 131, 132, 180, and 182.

If you have low-back and especially SI problems, be especially careful with Exercises 31, 32, 33.1, 34, 36, 102–110, and 131. Consult your physical therapist and health-care provider before doing exercises in this book that note precautions for people with low-back problems.

Your low-back discs, facets, and SI joints are

the most commonly injured from improper lifting and abnormal movement patterns. Consider consulting with a health professional competent in assessing and treating (with exercise and other methods) SI and low-back problems if you have persistent low-back problems.

Mid Back

Your mid back (upper back or thoracic spine) contains ribs, joints, and discs. It must be flexible to rotate and bend in many directions. It has a normal, flexed curve. In some people there is a scoliosis curve and in others there is a lack of the normal flexed curve. These alignment issues can lead to problems with motions or compensations elsewhere in the neck or low back. One of the most common thoracic problems is a lack of normal rotation and extension, which can lead to excessive forces on the joints and discs of the neck and low back. The thorax contains many muscles related to spinal rotation and bending. It is important to do some flexibility work to maintain your mid-back motion. Exercises 17, 18, 19, 23.1, 80, and 83 are good to do on a regular basis for this purpose. A rotary torso machine may be used in a health club or you can do Exercise 109 if you have special needs for enhancing your back rotation.

Cervical Spine

Your neck (cervical spine) encloses your spinal cord and nerve supply to your arms. Its primary function is to position your head and eyes. It moves in many patterns, including flexing, extending, rotating, and combined motions. Neck, shoulder, and arm and hand pain as well as headaches can occur from joint and disc problems. Your neck is closely related to your jaw, shoulders, and your upper thoracic spine. Tight shoulder muscles can pull on your neck. The posture of your low back directly influences your neck and head position. Getting your low back into good alignment can help with alignment of your neck.

In the neck region it is more important to maintain flexibility and to practice good lifting and posture habits than to work on pure strength. It can be important to work on neck muscle strength while moving the head into flexion or extending or while keeping the neck and head in a stable, nonmoving position. For such exercises refer to a physical therapist trained in exercise and manual therapy.

THE CORE

It is difficult to address the back muscles solely as a functional unit because they are so closely integrated with the pelvis. All of the muscles that attach the spine to the pelvis, including the abdominals, back muscles, and pelvic floor muscles, make up the *lumbopelvic complex*.

When stable, the lumbopelvic complex is the link that allows you to generate force through your arms and legs, which is crucial for all sports and for movement in general. In the case of a golfer, volleyball player, kayaker, canoer, or any throwing athlete, the latissimus dorsi on one side of the body and the gluteus maximus on the opposite side work with the trunk muscles to generate the power behind the motion. These muscles link the pelvis and back to the arms to transfer force from the legs through the trunk to the shoulder. The entire system must be strong and stable in order to generate maximum force and to avoid injuries. An important, basic foundation to this lumbopelvic complex is the group of muscles commonly referred to as the core.

Most fitness enthusiasts, athletes, trainers, and physical therapists have heard of or teach the concept of the core. A comprehensive understanding of exactly what the core consists of is crucial. For background on the abdominal muscles involved, see chapter 10. Many people inaccurately believe that contracting the core means solely tightening the lower abdominals or transversus abdominis. This is partially true, but is by no means the whole equation. The core musculature actually consists of muscles above, below, and on all sides of the spine, making up the remainder of the equation. Only when all of these muscles are simultaneously contracted can spine stability be achieved.

A stable spine can be likened to a tent pole. The pole must first be set on a stable base of support, such as solid ground, so that it doesn't sink as soon as weight is placed on it. The pole must then have guide wires on all sides with equal tension to hold the pole erect upon its stable base. Without one or the other, the system will fail. The core muscles accomplish both of these functions, working all day to give local support to the trunk and pelvis.

So what exactly are these core muscles and how do we contract or engage them? As stated before, they surround the spine and abdominal cavity from above, below, and on all sides. From above, we have the *diaphragm*, which, fortunately, most of us don't have to worry about since its function is involuntary.

From below, we have the *pelvic floor muscles*. These are primarily the muscles used to contract the sphincters of the rectum and the urethra for control of bowel and bladder function, again, which most of us are unaware of. Developing awareness and proper use of these muscles can help us improve spine stability. These muscles function as the solid ground in our tent pole analogy. Women who have had children certainly understand the importance of the pelvic floor; however, it is equally as important in men. For both sexes, the pelvic floor musculature can be strengthened by performing the exercise known as the Kegel: Tighten the deep muscles of your pelvis that you would use to stop the flow of urine or to squeeze down on a bowel movement. This contraction can be held for a count of 10 without letting the intensity of the contraction fade. If you lose the full contraction sooner, this lesser time will be your starting point. The goal is 10-second holds for 10 to 15 repetitions. This exercise should be practiced in multiple positions, such as sitting and standing. Try feeling the difference in the support of your trunk when you stand and perform a Kegel with 100% intensity versus fully relaxing your pelvic floor. Holding a 100% intensity Kegel at all times is not realistic, but we can comfortably live with a certain degree of tone in the supportive pelvic floor muscles, which should be a comfortable intensity.

Surrounding the front and sides of the trunk, we have the *transversus abdominis*, which is the deepest of all the abdominal layers. These fibers run horizontally (unlike the vertical alignment of the rectus abdominis or "six-pack" muscle) and attach to the ribs, pelvis, and ultimately to the spine through a thick, fibrous layer of tissue. Due to this horizontal alignment, the transversus abdominis works like a drawstring drawing the abdominals inward and depressing the ribs. You can feel this by laying on your back with one hand over your ribs and the other over your lower abdominals. As you fully and forcefully exhale without lifting your shoulders, your ribs will depress and the lower abdominals will tighten and flatten. However, you must learn how to contract the transversus abdominis while breathing regularly. If your stomach pooches out, you are incorrectly compensating with the rectus abdominis.

From behind, on either side of the spine, we have the muscles known collectively as the *multifidi* (one multifidus on each side of the spine). Each multifidus runs vertebra to vertebra, and from the vertebrae to the pelvis. They provide inner support to the spine as well as allow the spine to arch back and rotate. If you lie down on your back with your knees bent, and then place your fingertips along the thick muscles approximately an inch from either side of your spine at waist level, you will be on the multifidi. Slightly arch your back, at the level of your waist, and feel the multifidi tighten under your fingers. If you flatten your back you will feel the loss of the contraction. Feel the multifidi in a sitting position: arching slightly will activate the multifidi, and going into a flexed or slumped position will turn them off. In essence, the multifidi are engaged in neutral sitting (see definition of neutral spine below) and in standing, but not in slumped sitting or in poor flexed standing posture. The key is to learn to engage the multifidi with as little movement in the spine as possible, working toward a goal of no spine movement at all. This means learning to activate your core muscles simultaneously in many postures and during your movements.

To do this, you must understand the concept of the *neutral spine*. A neutral spine position is simply the comfortable place between too much of a flat-back posture (pelvic tilt backward) and too much of a swaybacked/arched-back posture (pelvic tilt forward). When your back is flattened, it is easy to contract your transversus abdominis, but you cannot easily activate your multifidi. When your back is excessively arched, it is easy to contract your multifidi, but your transversus abdominis is at a disadvantage. The key is to be able to contract your transverse abdominis, multifidi, and pelvic floor simultaneously. This can most efficiently be accomplished in the neutral spine position.

Practice activating your core while standing and sitting so that it becomes second nature. Your core should be engaged during all activities and exercise, perhaps not 100% effort at all times, but you should always aim for a certain amount of tone. Activate your core more strongly with heavy lifting or when you need to generate more force with your body. You will need to be able to activate your core while in neutral positions and while moving in and out of neutral positions. Mastering and applying the concept of engaging your core (and your extended core) and learning to find neutral spine position can help you to prevent spine injuries.

NEUTRAL ALIGNMENT

In addition to understanding the concept of a neutral spine, knowing what overall neutral alignment is, and knowing how to balance the muscles acting around your neck and back, are both important in protecting this vulnerable region.

There are obvious curves in the normally aligned spine when it is viewed from the side. The neck and low back have a slight arch backward and the mid back has a flexed curve. Normal curves indicate correct vertebral stacking designed to protect the component parts of the spinal system.

In adults the normal curves of the spine result in an alignment that, when ideal, brings the ear over the shoulder, the shoulder over the center of the hip joint, and the hip joint slightly in front of the center of the knee and ankle joint. This is called a *neutral alignment*.

Neutral alignment indicates that the individual joints of the spine are in normal alignment with one another, which is necessary for good maintenance of joint structure. When there is good alignment at each vertebral segment, joints are in their most balanced position, with weight distributed over the vertebral bodies and two facet joints. Muscles, ligaments, and bony structures are arranged so motion can occur most freely in each direction the joint moves. Muscles and ligaments are balanced (adapt) in length and strength to allow this to happen, and pairs of adjacent joint surfaces are held parallel and spaced apart, with forces equally distributed across their cartilage liners. See chapter 25 for discussion and illustration of neutral alignment in sitting (Exercise 180) and standing (Exercise 182) postures. It is best to practice first finding neutral in sitting and standing and then to activate your core muscles. Practicing both finding neutral and engaging your core are an important part of keeping your spine safe during exercise and your activities.

Find neutral alignment while sitting, then activate your core: Do Exercise 180 to find neutral while sitting. Once in neutral you should be able to feel your multifidi in your low back. Next do a Kegel and then find a comfortable level of resting tone in your pelvic floor muscles. Next activate your transversus abdominis muscle by minimally exhaling and tightening your lower abdominals so that your belly button moves toward your back. You should then be able to breath comfortably in this position.

Find neutral alignment while standing, then activate your core: Do Exercise 182 to find neutral while standing. Once in a neutral position, do a Kegel and then activate your transversus abdominis muscles.

Applying the Concept of Neutral in Exercises and Activities

The following examples give you an idea of what to look for in achieving neutral alignment and what to avoid. Once you have the idea, apply this to other settings and activities.

When you are ready to lift, stop and take a minute to find neutral back and neck alignment, then activate your core muscles enough to provide support for this alignment but not to pull you out of it. Then lift the weight, trying to maintain a neutral spine alignment. Note that in some of the functional exercises in this book, you may be moving in and out of a neutral alignment. When moving in and out of neutral alignment, move slowly at first to get your movement pattern down and to prevent injuries.

Bending your neck forward under pressure stresses the facet (intervertebral) joint and places ligaments and the back wall of the disc at risk. You might see this happening to someone who is doing abdominal crunches and beginning to pull himself up using his head as a handle as he fatigues, rather than lifting his upper body with his upper abdominal muscles. Use your hands behind your neck to support it in crunch exercises. Doing squats with a bar across the shoulders with the neck held flexed will result in muscle contraction across these flexed segments, compressing them out of alignment. Latissimus pull-downs are frequently done with excessive forward neck posture and low-back flexing. See Exercise 120 for pictures of good and improper neck positioning during this exercise.

These examples illustrate cases where the stack of vertebrae in poor alignment is subject to brief episodes of fairly high levels of pressure, sometimes with quick thrusting motions. Because of poor alignment, joint structures are not protected, placing disc, ligaments, muscles, and joint surfaces, including their cartilage linings, at risk.

In exercise during which joint loading may be less but forces are constant for prolonged periods, static poor alignment can lead to similar joint irritation and discomfort and may ultimately lead to injury. In the case of biking, for example, in an attempt to create less wind resistance, riders often bend forward in the mid back and round their shoulders forward. This creates a sharp, extended angle in the neck and forward head and compresses the space into which the lungs should be expanding. Bending at the hips, keeping the back flat (chest slightly raised), and keeping shoulders and neck tucked slightly back creates less stress on the back of the neck and the mid back as well as opening up the area of the chest cavity.

Another example of static loading out of alignment occurs while hiking with a top-heavy backpack. A backpack loaded so a bulky object is perched at the top, forcing the head forward, will result in compression at the back of the vertebral segments. Reloading the pack so there is room for the neck to move back into its neutral alignment and making sure that weight is distributed to the hip strap reduces these forces.

COMMON MUSCLE IMBALANCES

The most common muscle imbalances in the spine are due to tightened or weakened muscles. Tight hamstrings can cause excessive flexing and more stress on the discs of the low back. Very tight quadriceps can cause excessive arching of the spine and more stress on the joints. Tight abdominal and chest muscles affect mid-back position. Tight and/or weakened upper neck and shoulder muscles can lead to poor neck alignment.

Weaker gluteal and abdominal muscles can contribute to low-back problems. Weaker neck flexors can contribute to neck problems.
Many conditioning programs concentrate on or emphasize abdominal strength and neglect strengthening the upper and lower back muscles and the buttocks. The key to functioning your best and avoiding injuries is to balance all of these muscle groups.

INJURY PREVENTION

Problems in one area of the spine can lead to problems in another area. Problems can be due to acute injuries or to wear and tear from poor posture over many years. It is important to be aware of good posture while you are exercising and while you are engaging in your outdoor activities. Back and neck problems are more likely when you are subjecting your spine to lifting, prolonged sitting, and carrying packs. Injuries can occur during lifting, falling, and abrupt shifts in a boat.

The postural deviations most people have include a head too far forward of the shoulders, the shoulders slumped forward and turned in, the back of the skull resting too close to the back of the spine, and the mid and low back excessively rounded. Postural patterns such as those can lead to disc or joint problems and shortened muscles.

POSTURE AND LIFTING

Certain postures and motion patterns are likely to lead to spine pain and injury. In general, it is safer when lifting to be close to the object that you are lifting and do most of your lifting with your legs and buttocks.

Low Back (Lumbar Spine)

Posture: In general, sitting or carrying things with a flexed, slumped low back can put excessive pressure on your discs. It is best to sit with a neutral posture.

Lifting: Try to avoid lifting with your back flexed and rotated when your knees are relatively straight (see incorrect lifting posture in Figure 30). Many people pick up their dumbbells, packs, skis, or even boats in this position. You should position yourself and lift with your hips and knees flexed (bent) and your back in a neutral position, with your core engaged. It is important to face the object and position yourself close to it. Then move it close to your center of gravity (torso area); Figure 31 shows correct lifting posture. Once you have the object positioned, use your legs and buttock muscles to stand up and try to keep your back in neutral alignment. Avoid extending your back too much during the lifting. Your thigh and buttock muscles are much stronger than your back muscles. Your joints and discs are also safer using this positioning. (See chapter 17 for details on lifting packs.) Remember that proper positioning and lifting is important no matter how light something looks.

Mid Back (Thoracic Spine)

Posture: Good thoracic posture in neutral is with a normal flexed curve and avoids excessive flexing, extending, rotating, or side bending.

Lifting: Avoid lifting while reaching behind you, or while you are extending and rotating your thoracic and lumbar spine. This can injure your neck, shoulders, ribs, or thoracic joints.

FIGURE 30.
Incorrect posture.

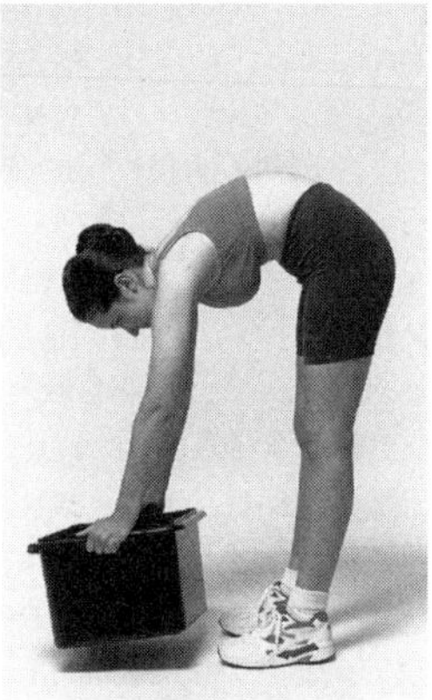

FIGURE 31.
Correct posture.

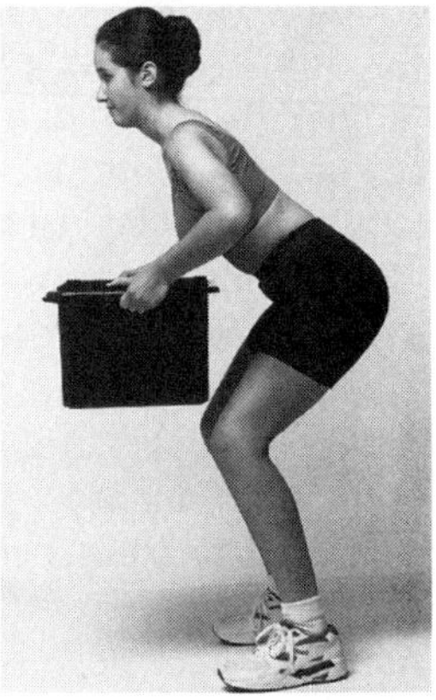

Neck (Cervical Spine)

Posture: Neck pain and problems are most likely to occur in a forward head position. When sitting, standing, or carrying a pack, try to position your neck in a neutral position. Avoid having something on your back that pushes your head forward.

Lifting: Your neck muscles are involved with lifting. Avoid excessive head and neck flexing with lifting. Be careful when you are lifting an object with an elevated arm that is away from your body. If you feel pain in your neck with weight lifting, decrease your resistance and make sure your form is good.

STRATEGIES FOR SPINE EXERCISE PROGRAMS

There are many schools of thought regarding what spine exercises each individual should do. You can go on from the basics to exercise your extended core muscles, which will provide a program for spine and sacroiliac stability.

Basics: Start by learning how to activate your core muscles, as described above. Then proceed to Exercises 180 and 182 to learn how to get into a neutral spine position while sitting and standing. Then combine activating your core muscles with neutral spine postures. Finally, practice safe lifting techniques. Once all of these have been mastered, you can decide to do particular spine exercises depending on your particular spine problems and the demands of your work and activities.

Extended core exercises: 31, 34–36, 55, 70, 117, and 120.

Static and Dynamic Exercises

The spine can be exercised statically (tonically) or dynamically (phasically). In static-type exercises certain muscles are activated to provide stability and protection for your spine. These will usually be your core muscles, along with spinal extensors and rotators that are very close to the spinal bones as well as your abdominal and buttock muscles. There are many exercises in chapters 5, 6, 8, and 10 that will accomplish this. Dynamic exercises are used to increase the motion and strength of your spine. This can be done with exercises that work directly on spinal rotation.

Static, stabilizing exercises: 21.1, 22, 25, 27, 57, 69, 88, 108, 109, and 115, and BST Exercises 42–47.

Dynamic spine exercises: 23, 24, 38, 60, 72, 73, 82–84, 86, 93, 110, 131, 133.

Choose a few exercises from each group and vary them in order to develop a complete and diverse spine exercise program. Remember to always start with the easier exercises that have fewer spine precautions before you proceed to the more difficult exercises. The basic and intermediate spine exercise programs below are examples of how to put some of these exercises together.

Basic Spine Exercise Program

1. Learn neutral spine in sitting and standing: Exercises 180 and 182.
2. Learn to engage your core muscles as described in this chapter.
3. Try practicing engaging your core while in neutral postures.
4. Develop static strength of your core: Exercises 78, 84, 107 (Skydiver), and 108.1 and BST Exercises 42 and 45.
5. Maintain or improve spine/torso rotation: Exercises 19, 23.1, and 24.
6. Develop basic strength of your extended core muscles: Exercises 23.1, 92, 97.10, 98, 99.5, 104, 105, and 120.

Intermediate Spine Exercise Program

1. Perfect steps 1–3 of the basic program.
2. Intermediate static exercises: 107 (Superman), 108.2, 108.3 or 108.4, and 109.1.
3. Intermediate dynamic exercises: 25 and 83.
4. Intermediate extended core: 24.1, 31.1, 34, 80, 109, and 135.

SPINE EXERCISES

You can begin strength training exercises for the spine with 3–5 reps, in order to get your form and posture correct, and gradually progress to 10–15 reps after you have gained strength and are sure of your form. Progress your reps and resistance according to the guidelines in chapter 5. Use special precautions if you have a problem in your neck, mid back, or low back. If you are currently being treated by a health-care provider familiar with spinal problems and exercise, please consult that person before doing these exercises.

Note: In addition to the exercises below, spine rotation exercises can also be useful. They can help to maintain or increase your thoracic spine rotation, which is especially important for your thoracic and lumbar spine function. They can improve the strength of your abdominals. They can also facilitate health of the facet joints and discs in your spine. Such exercises include Exercises 19, 23, 24, 72, 80, and 83. Finding a neutral spine is described in Exercises 180 and 182.

107 SPINE EXTENSION SERIES

Equipment: Mat.
Purpose: Strengthen your spine extensor and buttock muscles and improve stability in extension positions.

Technique: Prone extension (Skydiver): Lie on your stomach with your arms at your sides. Activate your core and tighten your buttocks. Lift your chest and thighs off the floor, keeping your knees straight. Draw your shoulder blades down and in toward your spine as you rotate your arms outward until your thumbs are facing up to the ceiling squeezing your shoulder blades together. Try to arch throughout your entire spine equally, not just in your low back (107a). Work up to 10-second holds for 10 reps. **Prone extension with side bending (Superman):** *Starting position:* Lie on your stomach with your arms overhead. Activate your core and tighten your buttocks. Lift your arms, chest, and thighs off the floor allowing your entire spine to arch (107b). Hold this position for 2 seconds. *Side-bend left:* Keeping the arched position and your core engaged, reach back with your left arm as you side-bend your body to the left. Place your left hand on the back of your left thigh.

107a

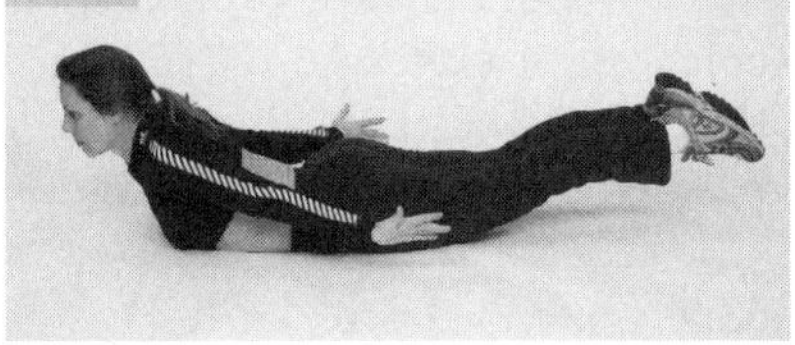

Turn and look at your thigh to maximize your side-bend position (107c). Hold this position for 4 seconds, then return to the starting position, remaining in the arch. *Side-bend right:* Reach back with your right arm as you side-bend your body to the right. Place your right hand on the back of your right thigh. Turn and look at your right thigh to maximize your side-bend position. Hold this position for 4 seconds then return to the starting position. Rest if needed. This sequence equals 1 rep. The goal is 10 reps.

Precaution: Avoid this series if you have spinal stenosis, spondylolisthesis, or facet degeneration.

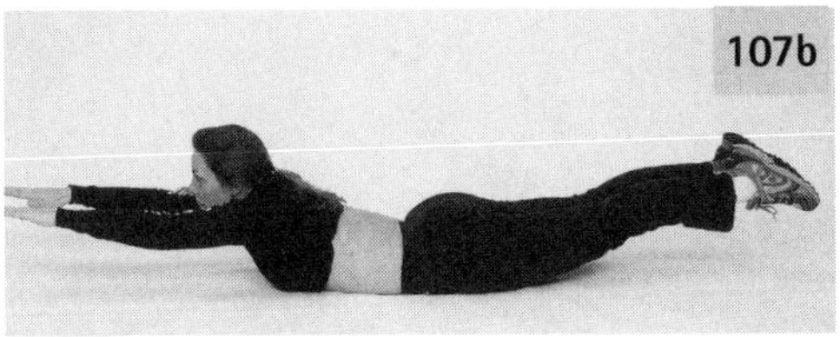
107b

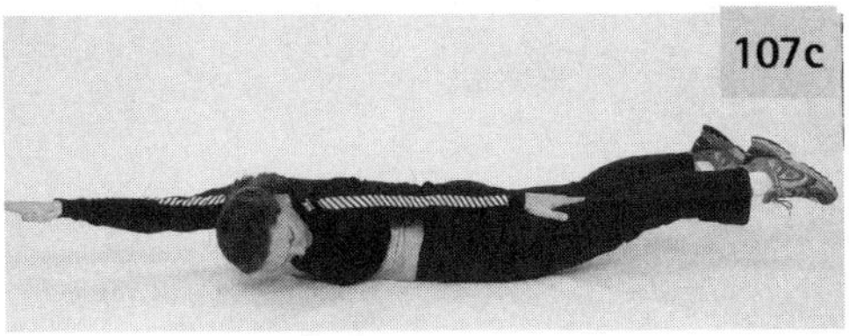
107c

108 SUSPENSION BRIDGE

Equipment: Physioball and padded bench, or 2 padded chairs (pulleys, tubing, or weighted ball for variations).

Purpose: Strengthen and improve the dynamic control of your back extensors.

Technique: Carefully position yourself with your shoulder blades resting on a Physioball or padded chair. Place your heels on a bench or a second chair so as to suspend yourself between the two. Arms are relaxed out to the side. Be sure your core is activated. Lift your hips until you just feel your low-back muscles tighten, but don't excessively arch. Start with 10–15 seconds, with a goal of 30–40 seconds.

Variations: 108.1. Physioball bridge: Make a bridge of your body by bending your knees 90 degrees and placing your feet on the floor (108.1a). Once you can maintain control in this basic position, try straightening one of your knees and raising one of your feet off the ground (108.1b). **108.2.** Single-leg suspension: Suspend yourself as in the main version of 108 and raise one leg toward the ceiling. **108.3.** Straight or diagonal pullovers with tubing: Position yourself as in the main version of 108, but do so in front of a pulley or in front of tubing with handles anchored appropriately. Get into a stable and balanced position and move your arms so that they are over your head. Have a partner give you the handles of the pulleys or of the tubing. Pull them in front of you toward your waist while maintaining

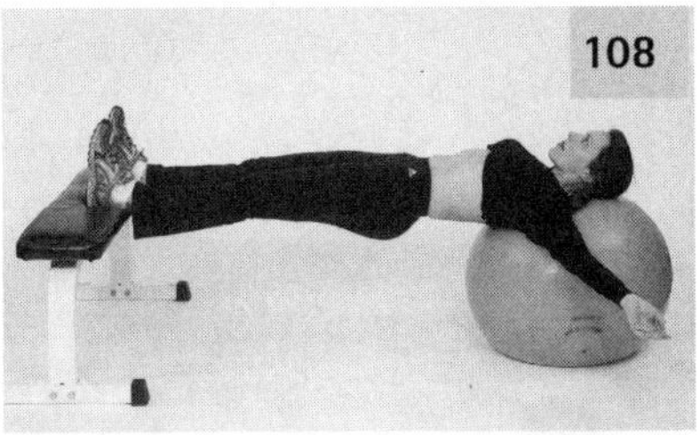
108

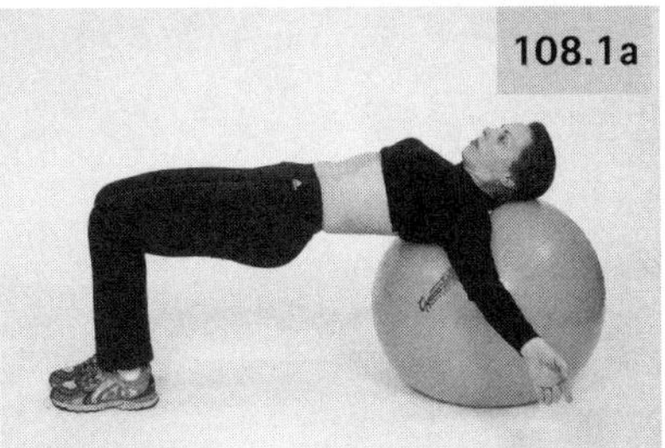
108.1a

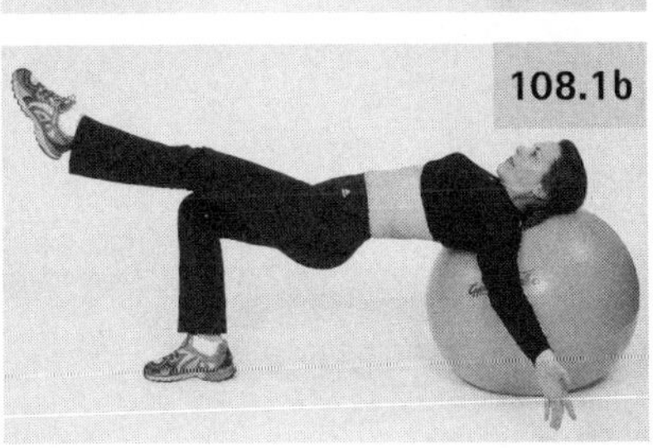
108.1b

EXERCISE 109 110

108.2

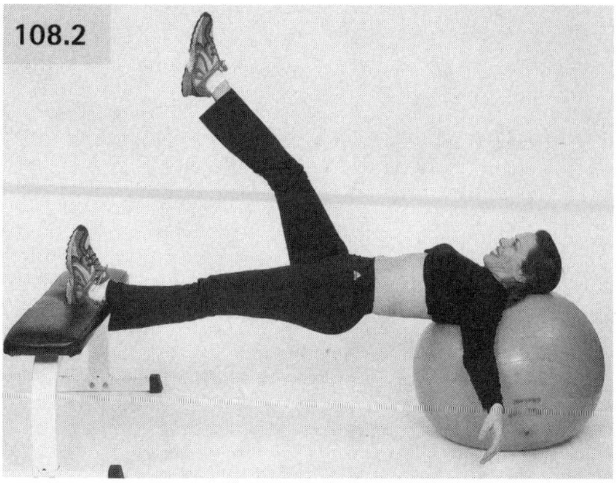

108.3

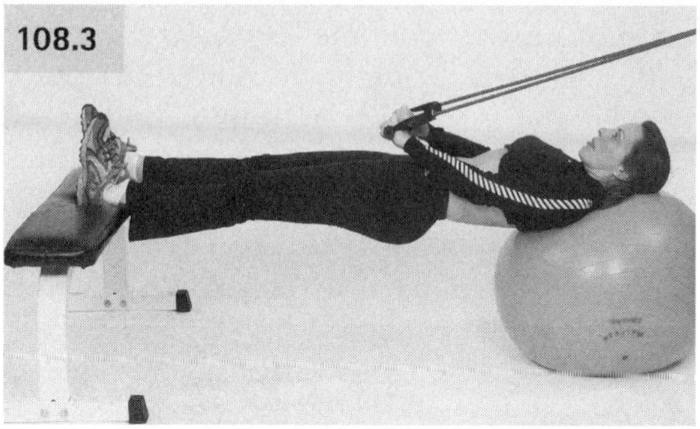

108.4a

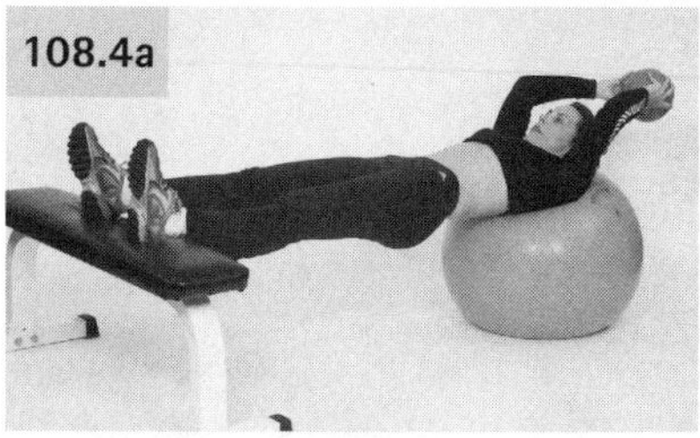

108.4b

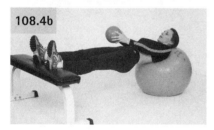

a straight-arm position. **108.4.** Straight or diagonal pull-overs with a ball: Position yourself as in 108.3. Instead of grabbing onto the handles of pulleys or tubing, you will be holding a weighted ball. Start by holding the ball over your head (108.4a) and carefully bring it to your waist (108.4b). The arm motions in 108.3 and 108.4 can also be done in diagonal patterns. Diagonal patterns will challenge your frontal and transverse planes of balance.

Precaution: Avoid this exercise if you have any active neck, mid-back, or low-back problems.

109 T-POSE

Equipment: A stable chair with a high back.

Purpose: Improve static strength of your core, spine extensors, and extended core muscles, and improve your balance. This exercise is also a very good buttock exercise.

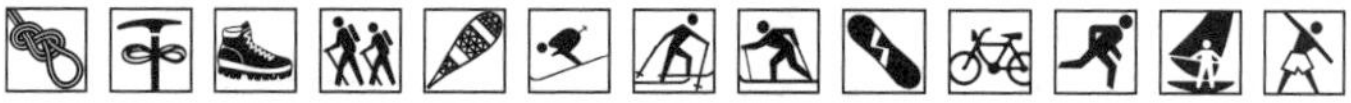

Technique: T-Pose with assistance: Stand on one leg with your hands on the back of a chair for support. You should stand far enough back so that you have to slightly reach for the chair. Your stance leg should be slightly bent with your knee behind your toes and your weight over your heel (109a). With your core engaged, lift your opposite leg and pivot your body forward from your hip until your body is parallel to the floor (109b). Your spine should remain neutral. You should be able to draw a straight line from your shoulders through your hip, knee, and ankle. In this position, shift your weight farther onto your heel to maximize the contraction of the

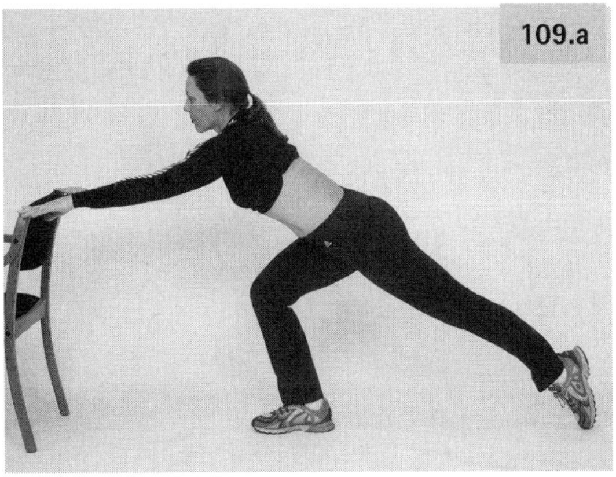
109.a

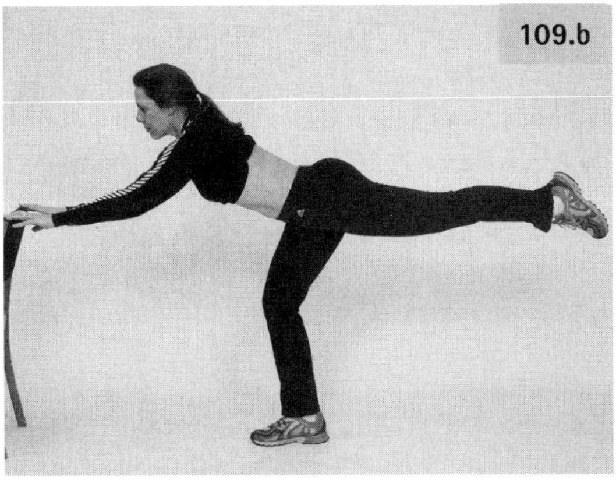
109.b

buttocks. Work up to holding for 60–90 seconds.
Variations: 109.1. T-Pose without assistance: Use the same technique as above, except balance without holding on to the chair. Work up to a 60-second hold. **109.2.** T-Pose with a squat: Use the same technique as above while performing small squats on your stance leg. The goal is 2–3 sets of 10–15 reps on each leg.
Precaution: Avoid this exercise if you have an active sacroiliac or hip problem.

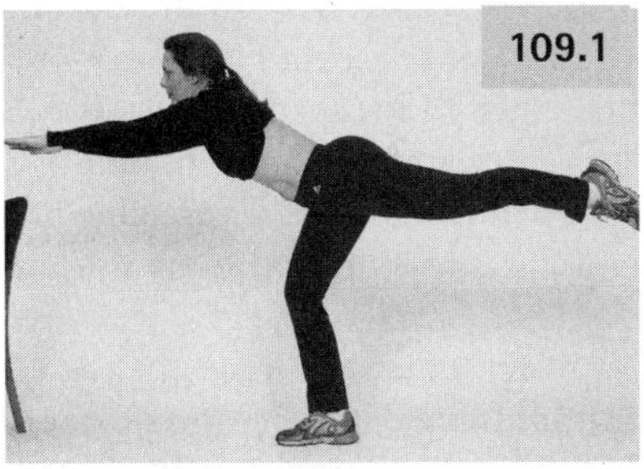
109.1

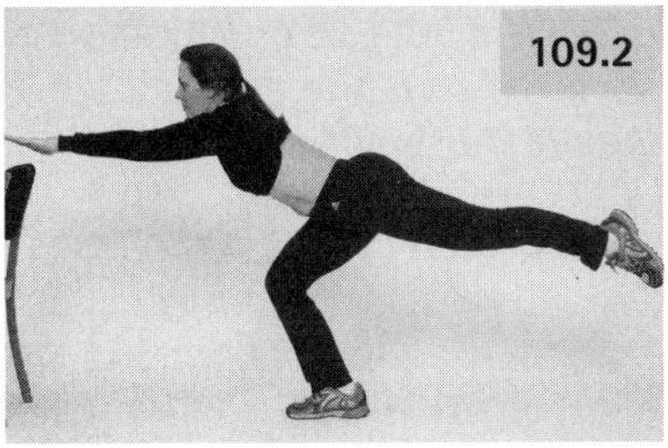
109.2

110 WAITER'S BOW

Equipment: None.
Purpose: Improve your ability to bend at your hips while maintaining your spine in good alignment.

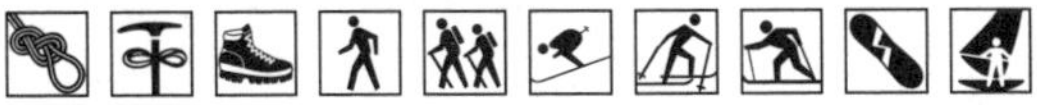

Technique: Stand with your knees slightly bent with your low back in neutral and your head held level (110a). While maintaining a neutral spine, flex at your hips until your hips and low back are at a 45- to 60-degree angle with the floor, or you feel the pull of your hamstrings. Allow your hips and buttocks to translate backward as you flex your hips. Keep your chest up and mid back extended. Maintain your neck in a neutral position and avoid hyperextending your neck. Do this 6–8 times slowly until you have the motion pattern down, then progress to bending your knees while you are bending at your hips (110b). Do this with progressively deeper knee bending to simulate positions that you will have to lift in.
Precaution: This exercise can aggravate an active back problem and should be stopped immediately if you have any back pain.

chapter 15 THE SHOULDER, UPPER TORSO, AND ARM

By Mark Pierce, A.T.C., Carrie Hall, P.T., and Sarah Meeker, P.T.

THIS CHAPTER WILL HELP YOU:

- Understand the function and anatomy of your shoulder, upper torso, and arm region.
- Learn exercises to functionally strengthen and provide balance to this region.

Your shoulder is a highly mobile joint, which allows you to move your arm and position your hand. This joint has the largest range of motion of any joint in your body and must be a stable structure that can provide a base from which your arm and hand can function. This versatility of function is made possible by a balance in muscle forces around your shoulder joint and shoulder blade.

Each muscular force that acts to move the arm must be countered by another force, which keeps the ball stable in the socket. Common overuse injuries are usually a result of an imbalance between the dynamic muscular forces around the shoulder joint.

FUNCTION AND ANATOMY

The shoulder joint is a "ball and socket" joint. (For illustrations, see chapter 9.) The socket component is a part of the shoulder blade (*scapula*) and the ball is the top end of the arm bone (*humerus*). There are a number of key ligaments in the shoulder that help to stabilize it. These include the ligaments that stabilize the AC joint and the ligaments that compose the anterior and posterior capsule of the shoulder. If these ligaments are loose (from injury or in an individual with generalized ligament laxity), muscles that make up the shoulder region (especially the rotator cuff muscles) will have to work excessively to stabilize the shoulder. The muscles can be tender, be in spasm, or might not function properly. The telltale signs of this might be tendonitis, muscle pain, clunks, clicks, or shoulder subluxation (partial dislocation). Working on muscle balance and strength is extremely important, but if a problem persists despite this, you should consider consulting a physician who can evaluate and treat ligament laxity with injections (prolotherapy) and, if necessary, surgery.

It is important to note that the shoulder region is very related to the neck region. Shoulder muscles may not function well if there is a disc or a joint problem in the neck. This should always be investigated in any case in which shoulder muscles are not able to work properly.

Muscles around the shoulder girdle have a number of different functions. They may primarily act as decelerators, stabilizers, and movers. Muscles often play multiple functional roles, depending on the activity and motion patterns of the shoulder. Scapular muscles move the shoulder blade upward and downward to coordinate the motion of the blade with your arm. They also act to track the shoulder blade over your posterior upper rib cage to provide a mobile base of support for arm and hand activities.

The rotator cuff (also called simply "cuff") muscles primarily stabilize the ball in the socket against excessive upward and forward migration during arm movements powered by your deltoid and other larger mover muscles. The cuff muscles also help to rotate your arm inward (internal rotation) and outward (external rotation).

The shoulder blade muscles include the *upper*, *middle*, and *lower trapezius* (traps), *rhomboid major* and *minor*, and *serratus anterior*. Their functional role involves keeping your shoulder blade in proper relationship to your upper back during arm motions. Since the shoulder blade creates the socket half of the shoulder joint, your shoulder blade must rotate upward as your arm rises, in order to maintain the relationship of the socket to the ball. These muscles must also control blade position on your upper back while the arm is lowered. A weakness or lack of coordination of the scapular muscles may lead to altered shoulder joint function and could lead to excessive use of your cuff muscles and possibly strains and tendonitis. The scapular muscles are often overlooked in strength training but their function is paramount. These muscles should be exercised with some sets using lower weights and many repetitions due to their endurance role. Exercises 111–115, 117–120, 122–124, and 128–134 strengthen the scapular muscles.

Several muscles cross the shoulder joint and connect the arm bone (humerus) to the shoulder blade (scapula), collar bone (*clavicle*), or trunk. They generally fall into two groups. The first group is deep and close to the joint, and travels a short distance. It creates a cufflike structure that acts to keep the ball pulled into the socket and helps to stabilize the joint. These muscles include the *supraspinatus*, *infraspinatus*, *teres minor*, and *subscapularis*. They have some mover function in that they can rotate the ball in the socket and thus are strengthened with internal and external rotation motions. Most people don't specifically and functionally exercise the cuff muscles. Use Exercises 31.1, 121, 121.1, 131, and 131.1 to strengthen your cuff.

The second set of muscles that cross the shoulder joint is more superficial. These are the ones that you can see on body builders. Their primary function is to move the arm. They tend to be longer muscles than the rotator cuff and attach lower on your arm bone. Because they attach farther from the shoulder joint, they have a good mechanical advantage to move your arm but are not good at stabilizing the ball in the socket. They work with your cuff and scapular muscles to raise and lower your arm. These include the *deltoid*, *pectoralis major* (pecs), *latissimus dorsi* (lats), *triceps*, and *biceps*. The deltoid, along with the biceps, helps to move your arm in front or to the side and over your head. The lats and pectorals help to bring your arm closer to your body.

Strengthening of the elbow flexors (biceps, *brachioradialis*, and *brachialis*) and extensors (triceps) is important, because they are both movers and stabilizers. A primary role of the elbow flexors and extensors is to move objects. Examples include lifting a pack, putting an ice ax in the snow or ice, paddling a kayak, and so on. Training for this function is important if you frequently will be lifting heavy or lighter objects. Exercises to train for this function are dynamic exercises, including biceps curls, triceps extensions, and rows with free weights, pulleys, or tubing. This can also be done with machines, but there is less coordination training accomplished.

Shoulder muscles also can work to control movement of all or part of your body's weight through space as in pulling, lowering, and pushing. Examples include climbing on rock walls, boulders, or ice; paddling or rolling a kayak; and so on. You may train for this function by doing pull-ups, dips, or push-ups. Free-weight biceps elbow flexion exercises (curls) and triceps elbow extension exercises are useful for building a strength base for these functions.

When your hand is performing strong resisted tasks, your elbow works as a "brace" to transfer the forces from your hand to your shoulder girdle and torso. Your arm and hand are then used in weight-bearing positions. Four examples of this dynamic are isometric hanging by your fingertips from a ledge or bar, keeping bicycle handlebars steady on a long ride, holding an ice ax in an arrest position, and bracing a paddle in whitewater kayaking. Exercises that train for this type of function are push-ups (including use of an isometric hold at various elbow ranges), dips in a gym or outdoors, or using climbing walls. Exercises 88, 94, 115, 127.1, and 130 work on this function.

The shoulder region frequently functions with the abdominal, hip, and leg regions. See the activity chapters for training programs that incorporate these concepts. Some of the most important functional relationships and applicable activities follow:

- Arm elevation related to hip, low-, and upper-back extension: mountaineering, backpacking, kayaking, snowboarding, snowshoeing, scrambling, gym or rock climbing
- Same-side hip extension/flexion with internal rotation related to external shoulder rotation, while the opposite hip relates to internal shoulder rotation: mountaineering, gym or rock climbing, downhill skiing, snowboarding, scrambling
- Hip extension related to arm push-off or pull-down: mountaineering, gym or rock climbing, scrambling
- Elbow and shoulder extension with hip flexion and extension, during any activity using poles, especially uphill: downhill skiing, telemark skiing, cross-country skiing, snowshoeing
- Right shoulder/arm, left hip (gluteal area), spinal extensors, and rotators, along with oblique abdominals, in deceleration of torso flexion and rotation: windsurfing, telemark skiing, cross-country skiing, snowboarding, snowshoeing, canoeing, kayaking

COMMON MUSCLE IMBALANCES

Since the shoulder joint depends so heavily on muscles to maintain its integrity and proper joint mechanics, it is particularly vulnerable to injuries resulting from muscle imbalances. An imbalance between the superficial and deep muscle groups that surround the shoulder joint, or an imbalance within a group, are common causes of shoulder injury.

Muscles that commonly become tight, strong, and overused are the latissimus dorsi, upper trapezius, pectoralis major, and rhomboid major and minor. Muscles that tend to be weak or underused are the rotator cuff and the middle and lower trapezius. When performing exercises to strengthen the weak muscles (cuff and lower traps), some attention should be paid to exercises that isolate the muscles in less functional positions (Exercises 117 and 121, this chapter). If you were to load up the weights in an attempt to strengthen the subscapularis (internal rotation), you could expect to recruit pectoralis major, latissimus dorsi, and teres major. The goal of the exercise is to find and work at the threshold where subscapularis can internally rotate your shoulder alone without the help of the bigger, stronger muscles. This may mean that you are working with much smaller amounts of weight. Since the weak, underused muscles tend to be stabilizers, they must not only be strong, they must be resistant to fatigue. Thus, endurance training with higher reps and lower weights is an important component of the strengthening program of the cuff and traps (Exercises 117, 121, 123, and 124, this chapter).

The shoulder and upper back work functionally together with the buttock, hip, and leg region during many sitting and standing activities. Performing some exercises that functionally integrate these regions can improve your ability to lift, reach, pull, push, and maintain your balance.

INJURY PREVENTION

Injuries of the shoulder are quite common and usually involve the rotator cuff (supraspinatus and infraspinatus) and the long head of the biceps. These are prone to injury, including strains and tendonitis, because they are frequently loaded excessively and subjected to friction. The injuries in this region may also heal slowly because of poor blood supply and associated neck problems. Motions that may load them excessively are straight-arm elevations to your front or to your side. Exercises 123 and 124 and other arm elevations should be done with much less weight than biceps curls (start with one-fifth the weight and gradually work your way up). Be careful to keep heavier loads (packs, boats, windsurfing boards, climbing gear, etc.) closer to your body and lift them in front or to your side.

Balance and agility are important in preventing shoulder sprains and bruises due to falling. If you work on balance and perform some of your shoulder training in unison with your abdominal, hip, and leg regions, you can decrease your risk of shoulder injuries.

STRATEGIES FOR STRENGTHENING

A well-rounded shoulder region program is designed to maintain balance between all of your shoulder muscle groups. It includes exercises for the rotator cuff and shoulder blade upward rotators (mid and lower trapezius and serratus anterior) that typical upper-body programs don't include. It should include exercises for your upper back, biceps, and triceps. Many of the functional exercises in this chapter include shoulder, torso, and hip combinations. Careful attention to form is also critical to promote muscle balance and optimal joint motions.

Basic Shoulder/Upper-Back Program

The following exercises are recommended for establishing a basic strength program for this body region. You can add exercises to this program according to your physical and activity goals.

Use this progression: Exercise 117 (mid and lower trapezius), 121.1 and 121.2 (rotator cuff), 115 (serratus anterior), 122 (deltoid and upper trapezius), 125 (biceps), 126 or 126.1 (triceps), 111 or 114.1 and 127 (chest), 120 and 118 or 131 (upper and mid back).

All exercises can be done in 2–3 sets of 15 reps. You might finish the sets for one exercise before moving to the next. In doing this you will need to take a minute break between each set. Another way to more efficiently do the above exercises is to do a set of one exercise followed by one set of another without taking a break (i.e., chest then back, biceps then triceps, finishing with deltoids and upper trapezius). You can also do these in a circuit fashion without a break between sets.

SHOULDER, UPPER-TORSO, AND ARM EXERCISES

The exercises in this chapter are described in two sections: first are the isolated and more conventional exercises for specific muscle areas and second are the more functional exercises that work the entire region.

For Exercises 111–128, pictures are included only for a few exercises that are less commonly known. The other exercises are commonly done in health clubs and are well known to most trainers. The terms *hand weights* and *dumbbells* refer to free weights and are used interchangeably. You can begin strength training exercises with 15 reps unless otherwise indicated. Progress your reps and resistance according to the guidelines in chapter 5.

CHEST

The various bench presses are done to strengthen your chest, shoulders, and triceps, which will increase your ability to push. For these press exercises, start with 12–15 reps in a set. Progress to 1–2 sets of 6–8 reps to work toward maximum strength.

111 DUMBBELL FLAT BENCH PRESS

Equipment: Bench and dumbbells.
Purpose: Challenge your ability to coordinate your arm motions while gaining strength in your chest, shoulders, and triceps. By using a pair of dumbbells instead of a regular barbell, the challenge of balance and coordination increases. Target muscles: middle pectorals, serratus anterior, anterior deltoid, and triceps.

Technique: Grasp a pair of dumbbells and lie back on a bench with your knees bent and feet resting on the bench. Pull your abdomen up and in to ensure your back remains stable throughout this exercise. Extend your arms so they are perpendicular to the ceiling, with the dumbbells directly over your shoulders and palms facing your feet. Lower the dumbbells, while allowing your elbows to bend, until the dumbbells meet the level of your chest. Return the dumbbells to the start position while lifting them in the same path. Perform 2–3 sets of 15 reps.

112 DUMBBELL INCLINE BENCH PRESS

Equipment: Incline bench and dumbbells.
Purpose: Put more emphasis on your upper chest and anterior shoulder. As you change the angle of the bench to an incline, the workload is placed on different parts of the target muscles: middle pectorals, serratus anterior, anterior deltoid, and triceps; emphasis on the upper pectorals.

Technique: Hold a pair of dumbbells with your palms facing forward. Lie back on an incline bench with your knees bent and feet resting on the floor. Pull your abdomen up and in to ensure your back remains stable throughout this exercise. Extend your arms vertically toward the ceiling while positioning the dumbbells directly above your shoulders. Lower the dumbbells with an outward semicircular motion while allowing your elbows to bend until the dumbbells meet the level of your chest. Return the dumbbells to the start position in the same path. Start with 2–3 sets of 15 reps.

113 DUMBBELL DECLINE BENCH PRESS

Equipment: Decline bench and dumbbells.
Purpose: Increase your strength and ability to push your body in an upward direction. Target muscles: middle pectorals, serratus anterior, anterior deltoid, and triceps; emphasis on the lower pectorals.

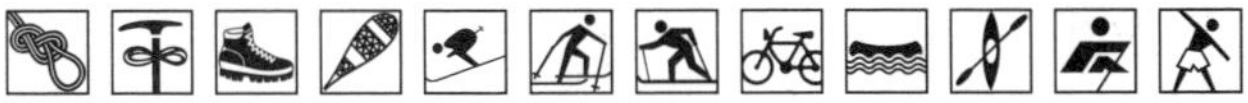

Technique: Lie face up on a decline bench and grasp a pair of dumbbells with your palms facing forward. Lower the dumbbells in an outward semicircular motion while allowing your elbows to bend, until the dumbbells meet the level of your chest. Return the dumbbells to the start position while lifting them in the same path. Start with 2–3 sets of 15 reps.

114 FLAT, INCLINE, OR DECLINE BENCH PRESS

Equipment: Bench and barbell.
Purpose: Develop sheer power and strength for pushing; however, the limitations on versatility and range of motion inherent with barbells make them a second choice after dumbbells. Target muscles: pectorals, serratus anterior, anterior deltoid, and triceps.

Technique: Use a spotter if possible. Lie face up on a flat, incline, or decline bench, with your knees bent and feet resting on the bench or floor. Pull your abdomen up and in to ensure your back remains stable throughout this exercise. Extend your arms so they are perpendicular to the ceiling, with the barbell directly over your shoulders. Grip the barbell with both hands and lower the barbell to your chest. Push the barbell straight above your chest to a point of balance. Perform 2–3 sets of 15 reps.
Variation: 114.1. Seated chest press machine: Some health clubs offer a seated chest press machine. Adjust the vertical seat position so that the handles are at chest height and the horizontal seat position so that it provides you with a mild stretch across the chest when the weight stack is at rest. Grasp the handles with your palms down and your wrists in neutral (not bent into flexion or extension). Press the weight forward, keeping your back against the seat, and in a controlled fashion return to the start position. Perform 2–3 sets of 12–15 reps.

115 PUSH-UP

Equipment: None.
Purpose: Develop upper-body strength and coordination. Improve your ability to push while using your entire body. Target muscles: serratus anterior, pectorals, anterior deltoid, triceps, and abdominals.

Technique: Lower yourself to the floor and position yourself on your hands and knees. Place your hands a little wider than shoulder-width apart, with your elbows straight. Next, move your feet backward until you are balanced on your hands and the balls of your feet. Your body, arms, and legs should be relatively straight and your abdominals tight. You are now in position and ready to perform a push-up; remember to keep your back straight during the entire exercise. Start by bending your elbows, in control, and lower your chest toward the floor until your elbows reach a 90-degree angle. Once you have lowered yourself to this position, immediately extend your arms and raise yourself back to the start position. Do 2 sets of 5–15 reps.

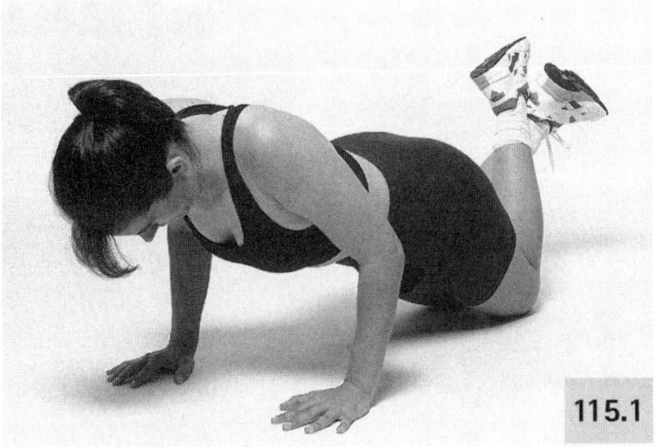

115.1

Variations: 115.1. Knee push-up: This is a good place to start if you have any doubts about your ability to perform regular push-ups. Kneel on your hands and knees with your hip angle halfway between 90 degrees and lying on the floor. Position your hands so that they are under your shoulders, with your fingers facing forward. Lower yourself toward the floor and try to touch your chest to the floor, then push up to a straight-elbow position. Do a set with your hands in this position, then do another set with your hands wider than shoulder-width apart and with your shoulders and hands rotated inward. **115.2.** Wall push-ups: You can strengthen your ability to push from standing and angled standing positions by standing near a wall and doing a regular push-up, leaning and pushing at various angles. This is a good osteoporosis prevention exercise. **115.3.** Plyometric push-ups can be done if you need speed and explosive strength. See Exercise 77 for details.

Tips: A good rule of thumb is that if you cannot perform 5 regular push-ups in a row with good form and back positioning, start with knee push-ups (115.1). When you can perform 10 knee push-ups in a row, advance to regular push-ups.

116 FLAT BENCH DUMBBELL FLIES

Equipment: Bench and a pair of 5- to 20-pound hand weights.

Purpose: Enhance your strength for motions that involve moving your arms inward. Target muscles: pectorals, anterior deltoid, biceps, and triceps.

Technique: Grasp a pair of hand weights with your palms facing each other and lie face up on a bench with your feet resting on the bench. Extend your arms completely so that the hand weights are positioned directly over your chest and touching each other, with your palms facing inward. This is your starting position. Next, lower the hand weights in an arc and out to your sides, while allowing your elbows to bend. When the hand weights reach the level of your shoulders, return them in an arc to the starting position directly over your chest. Start with 2–3 sets of 15 reps.

UPPER BACK/SCAPULA

117 STOMACH-LYING ELBOW LIFT

Equipment: Pillow, 2 towels (dumbbells and bench for some variations).

Purpose: Strengthen the different parts of your trapezius and provide balance for your shoulder blade. Target muscles: middle and lower trapezius, posterior deltoid.

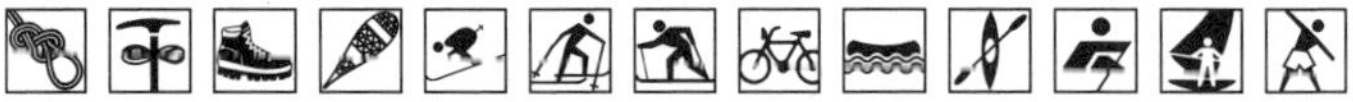

Note: Begin with the standard exercise and progressively build to variation 117.6. Don't progress to the next variation until you are able to complete 15 reps of the current level with correct technique. When learning the exercise motion pattern, don't use any weights. Gradually advance to using a light weight (2–5 pounds).

Technique: Lie on your stomach with a pillow under your abdomen and chest. Roll up two towels lengthwise and place one (or a face cushion) under your chin and one under your forehead to support your head. Place your hands on the back of your head. Barely lift your elbows. Keep your neck muscles (upper trapezius) relaxed, and contract the region between your shoulder blades (lower trapezius). Keep the contraction just enough to lift your elbows so as not to use your rhomboids to excessively squeeze your shoulder blades together. Hold the contraction for 5 seconds. Lower your elbows and repeat up to 20 times. Stop when your neck muscles become tense.

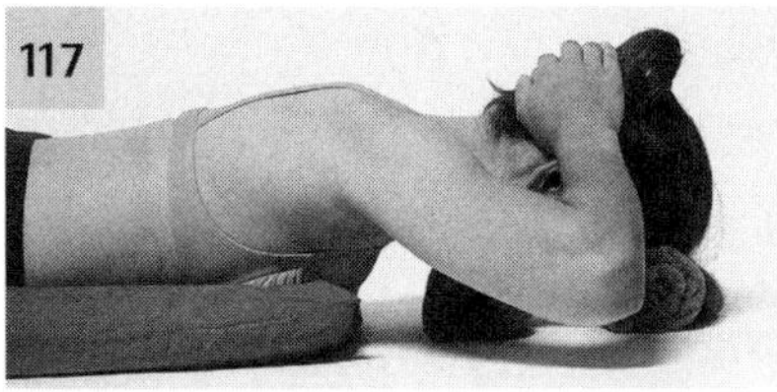

117

Variations: 117.1. With arms extended: Start as above. Slowly extend your elbows so that your arms are straight and reaching overhead. Don't move your shoulders during this exercise. Bend your elbows so that your hands return to the position behind your head. Lower your elbows to the floor. Repeat 15 times. Stop when your neck muscles become tense, as this is an indication that the middle and lower trapezius are fatigued. **117.2.** With arm extension overhead: Start as in Exercise 117, above. Straighten your elbows while extending your arms to meet over your head. Be sure not to tense your neck muscles (upper trapezius) during this variation. If you are unable to keep your neck muscles relatively relaxed, you are not ready for this level

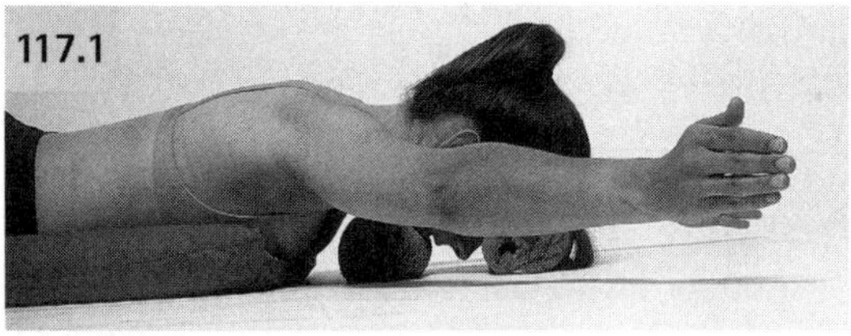

117.1

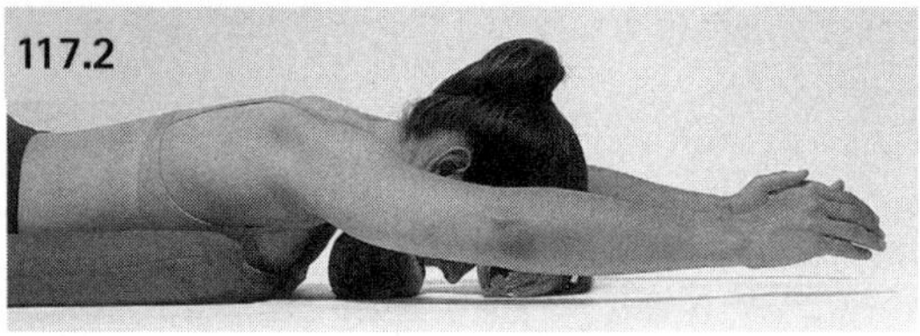

117.2

of exercise. Return your hands to your head, then lower your elbows and relax. Repeat 15 times. **117.3.** Horizontal arm lifts: This isolation exercise strengthens your middle trapezius muscle. Set up the pillow (or cushion) and towels as in Exercise 117, above. Position your arms straight out from your sides at slightly more than a 90-degree shoulder angle. Rotate your forearms so that your thumbs face upward and front elbow crease faces forward. Barely lift your arms off the floor. Hold your arms up for 3 seconds. Lower your arms and then relax. Repeat for 15 reps. **117.4.** Diagonal arm lifts: This isolation exercise strengthens your lower trapezius muscle. Set up the pillow (or cushion) and towels as in Exercise 117, above. Position your arms midway between straight out from your sides and straight up in front of your head. Bend your elbows slightly. Rotate your arms so that your thumbs face upward. Barely lift your arms off the floor. Be sure to lift your entire arm, not just your elbow. Hold your arms off the floor for 3 seconds. Lower your arms and then relax. Repeat for 15 reps. (The end position is the same as in variation 117.1.) **117.5.** Reverse horizontal fly: This isolation exercise strengthens your middle trapezius and posterior deltoid muscles. Lie on your stomach on a weight bench. Bend your knees if they extend too far off the bench. Pull your abdomen up and in. Your head should be slightly off the bench and in line with your spine with your chin tucked. Hold a pair of dumbbells with your palms facing forward and thumbs up. Your arms should be relaxed at chest level and resting on the floor, or against the bench if the bench is tall. Keep your elbows slightly bent (117.5a). Raise the dumbbells in a semicircular motion directly out from your sides, with your thumbs pointing up toward the ceiling; raise your arms to just below chest height (117.5b). Don't lift beyond chest level. Lower to the start position using the same path. Exhale in the up position and inhale in the down position. Do sets of 15 reps. **117.6.** Diagonal reverse fly: This isolation exercise strengthens your lower trapezius muscles. Lie on your stomach on a weight bench. Bend your knees if they extend too far off the bench. Pull your abdomen up and in. Your head should be slightly off the bench and in line with your spine. Hold a pair of dumbbells with your palms facing inward and thumbs up. Your arms should be resting on the floor, or against the bench if the bench is tall. Keep your elbows slightly bent (117.6a). Raise your elbows in a semicircular motion diagonally upward toward your head to just below the level of your head. Your shoulders and arms should be at approximately a 135-degree angle. (117.6b). Don't lift your elbows above the level of your head. Lower to the start position using the same path. Do sets of 15 reps.

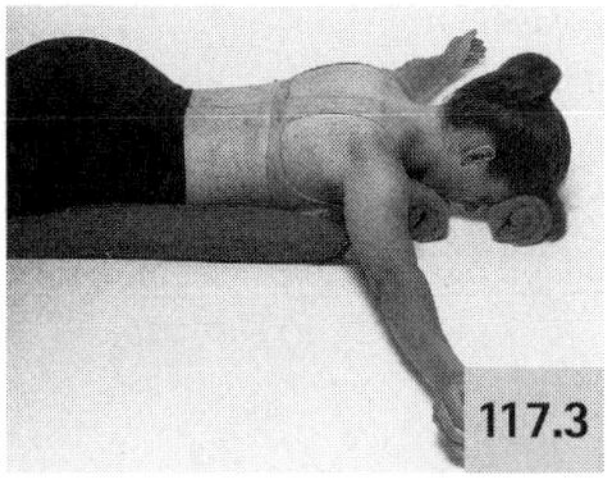
117.3

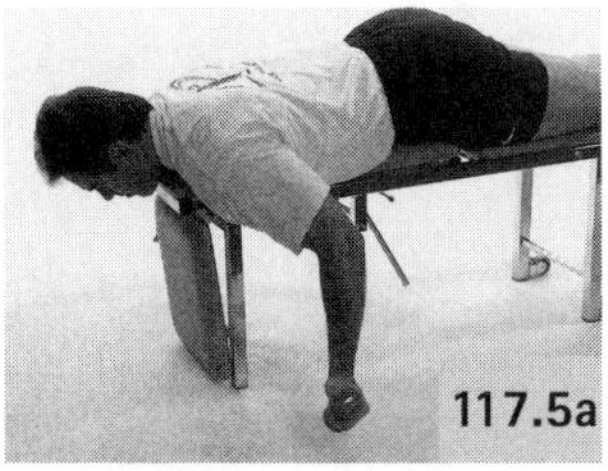
117.5a

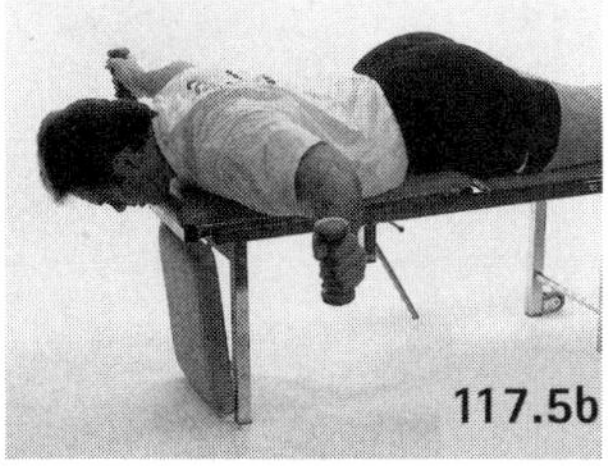
117.5b

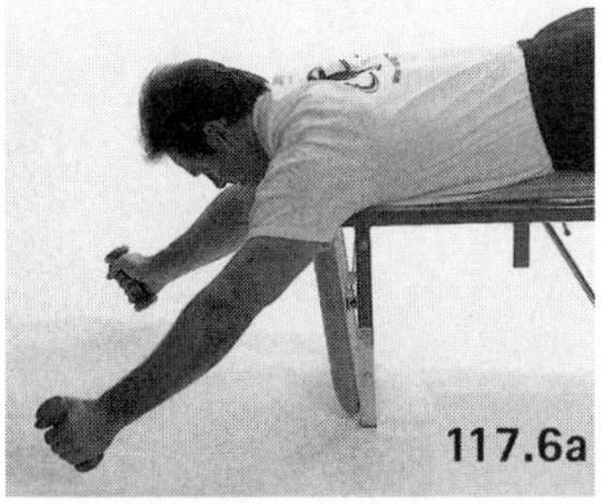
117.6a

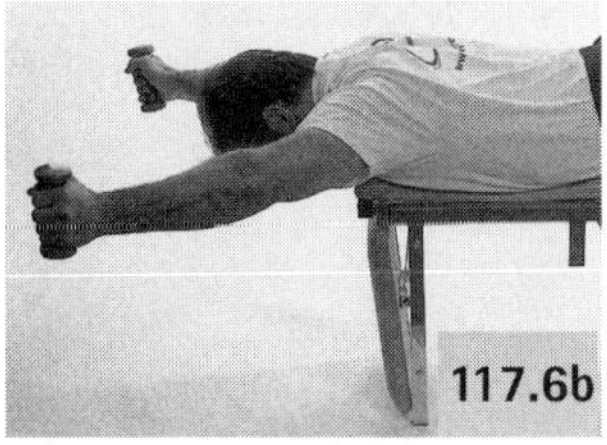
117.6b

118 PULLEY/CABLE ROW

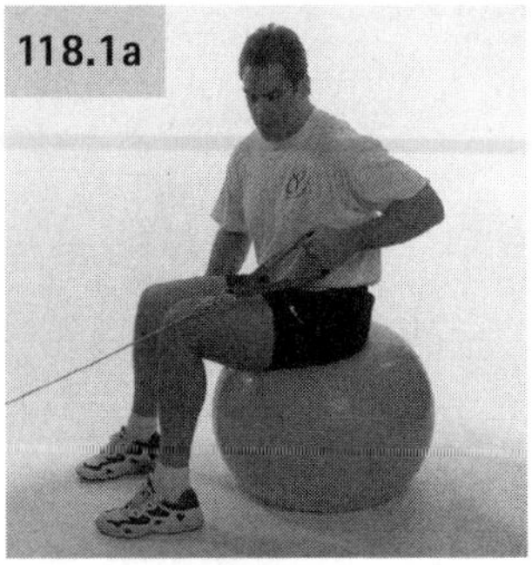
118.1a

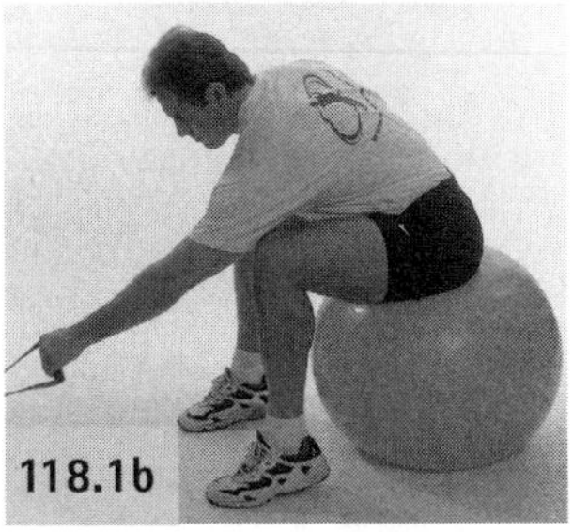
118.1b

Equipment: Pulley cable row machine (Physioball or bench for variation).

Purpose: Strengthen your upper back for rowing and pulling activities. Target muscles: rhomboids, trapezius, latissimus, erector spinae, biceps, and posterior deltoid.

Technique: Grasp the handles of the low pulley with your palms facing inward while maintaining a neutral low-back position. Straighten your knees until they are slightly flexed and bring your back to an upright position with your arms extended. Keeping your back straight, bend at your hips and reach the handle toward the pulley. When your hands are just past your knees, return your back to the upright position and pull the handle to your ribcage. Make sure you end the pull with your chest up and your elbows slightly behind you and to your sides. Do 2 sets of 15 reps.

Variations: 118.1. Seated one-arm rows: Do the above exercise with a pulley or tubing and one arm while sitting on a bench or a ball. Position your knees so that your feet are flat on the floor. **118.2.** Cross-body row/arm extension: Use less weight for this variation than you would use for a standard row. Position the left side of your body so that you are standing perpendicular to a high pulley. Grasp the handle with your right hand so that your arm is across your face, and bear most of your weight on your right leg with your knee bent. Simultaneously pull the handle toward and past your right hip while pushing off your right leg and transferring your weight to your left leg. Then let the pulley go back to the starting position, transferring your weight to your right leg.

119 BENT BARBELL ROW

Equipment: Barbell and bench.

Purpose: Gain balance while strengthening your entire back, rear shoulders, and biceps. Some outdoor activities require your upper body to be in a bent-over posture while pulling with either one or both arms. This exercise will benefit your balance and strength to meet those requirements. Target muscles: posterior deltoids; upper, mid, and low back; trapezius; and biceps.

Technique: Squat and grasp a barbell with your palms facing toward your body and slightly wider than shoulder-width apart (119a). Once

you take hold of the barbell, stand up straight and place your feet shoulder-width apart. Next, bend your hips and knees and assume a position in which your back is parallel to the floor with your low back in a neutral position. At the same time you are getting into position, lower the barbell toward the floor. Keep your back straight and stable, and row the barbell to your chest, allowing your knees and hips to flex slightly to assist your back during loading (119b).
Precaution: Don't attempt this exercise if you have a history of low-back problems unless you are supervised. Try Exercise 118 or 131 instead.

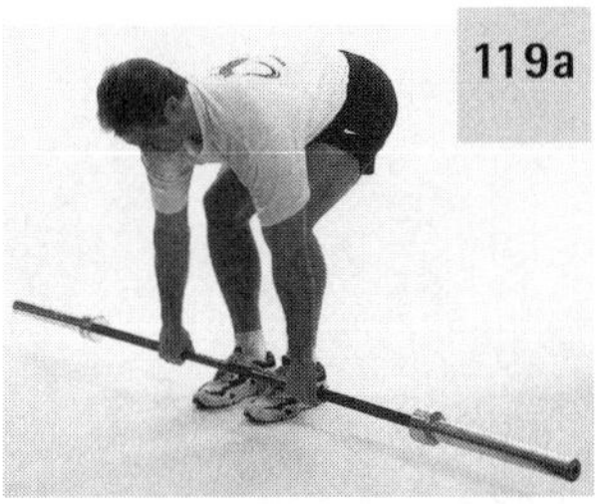
119a

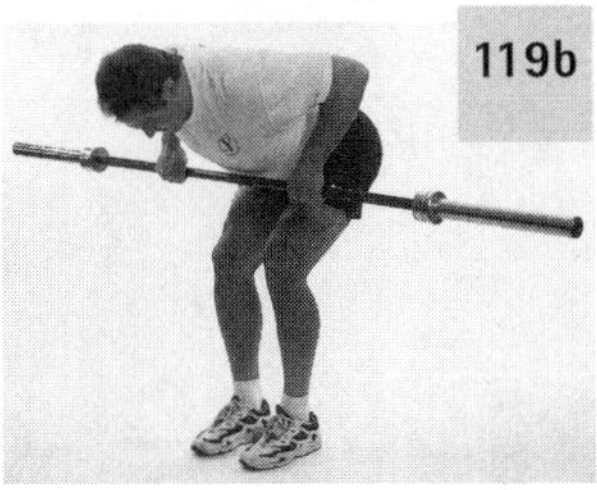
119b

120 LATISSIMUS (LAT) PULL-DOWNS TO THE FRONT AND REAR

Equipment: Lat pull-down machine.
Purpose: Strengthen your arms, shoulders, and upper back for pulling and climbing activities. Target muscles: latissimus, teres major, and biceps.

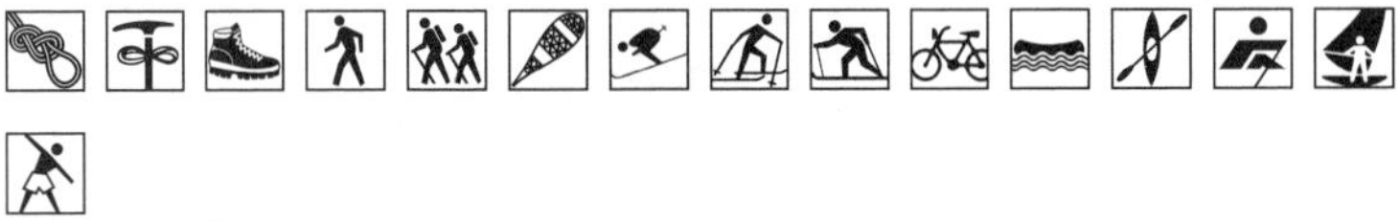

Technique: Select a comfortable weight and start by gripping the bar with your hands apart a distance about 6–10 inches wider than your shoulders. Sit on the bench and allow your arms to extend over your head. Maintain a safe posture in your neck and low back. Once you are seated and gripping the bar, keep your head level and pivot backward at your hips until you have the overhead pulley in sight. You should now be in a semireclined position. Pull the bar to your upper chest. Return the bar to the starting position with your arms in front of you and overhead. You may allow a small amount of forward and backward motion to occur with your upper body during this exercise. Don't bend forward while pulling down. Perform 2–3 sets of 15 reps.
Variations: 120.1. Pull-down to the rear: Assume the same starting position as a pull-down to the front. Maintain a safe posture throughout the exercise by keeping your head level, stomach tight, and your low back in the neutral zone. Pull the bar down to meet the top of your shoulders (120.1a), without bending forward with your neck or upper back (120.1b, poor neck posture). Return to the starting position in control of the weight and allow your arms to extend overhead.
The following variations are good for boating, climbing, and mountaineering activities. **120.2.** Single straight arm lat pull: You will need a high pulley and a handle for this variation. Tubing can be substituted for the cable if pulleys are unavailable. Attach a single handle

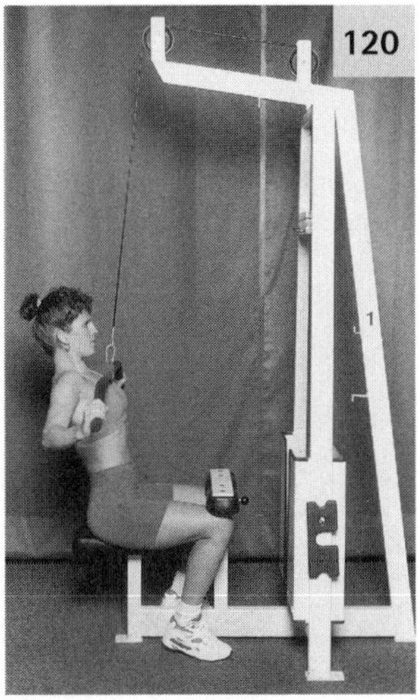
120

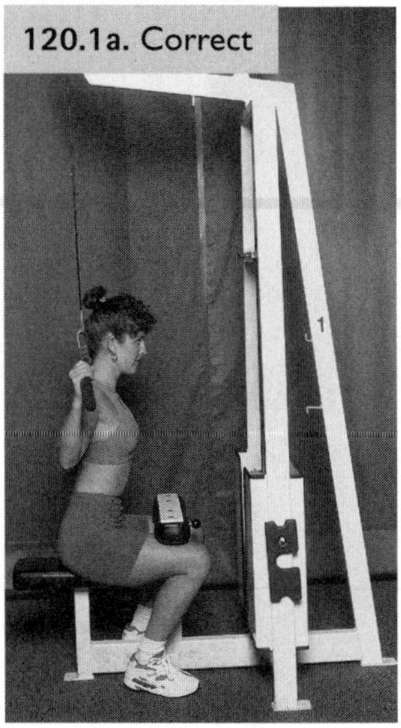
120.1a. Correct

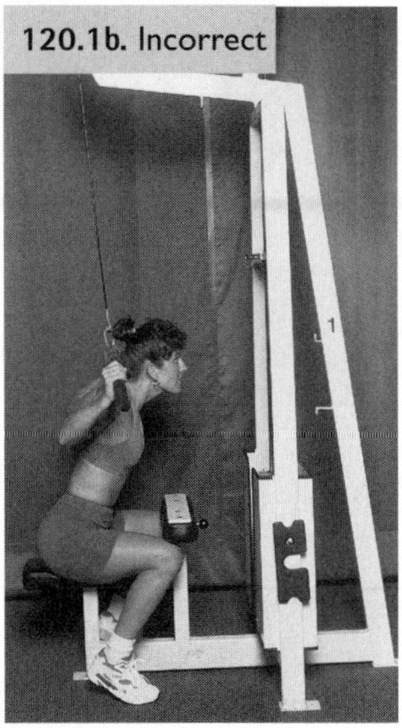
120.1b. Incorrect

to the cable and stand so your body faces sideways to the cable. Position your arm so that it is halfway between parallel to the floor and overhead, and slightly forward from the side plane of your body. Once your arm is at the top of the motion, return your straight arm to your side. This can also be done with both arms simultaneously. **120.3.** Start in the same position as variation 120.2, but position your arm halfway between straight ahead and directly out to your side. Pull the cable down across your body to your opposite leg. **120.4.** Do variation 120.3 with a bent elbow so that the ending position is with your elbow at your side and your palm facing outward. **120.5.** Do Exercise 34, the standing lat pull-down, which uses your legs and shoulders simultaneously.

Tips and Precautions: For the front pull-down, pull the bar down toward the top of your chest and at the same time exhale and raise your chest up to meet the bar. This will create a slight amount of extension in your upper and mid back during the pull-down portion of this exercise. This will also prohibit you from rounding your upper back and overextending your neck. If you need to translate your body forward during the pull-down, pivot from your hips. Try not to bend forward with your upper back and neck.

SHOULDERS

121 ROTATOR CUFF ROTATIONS

Equipment: Bench and 1- to 5-pound dumbbell (pulley for variations).

Purpose: Provide balance for your shoulder and strengthen the usually weak rotator cuff muscles. Target muscles: supraspinatus, infraspinatus, teres minor, subscapularis, and posterior deltoid.

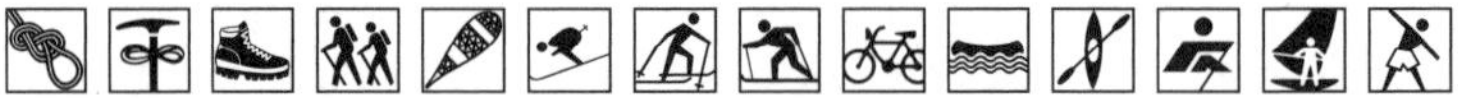

Technique: Kneel and position your upper body lengthwise alongside a bench with your shoulder and upper arm supported on the bench. Position your arm to extend out from your side, with your elbow bent down at 90 degrees. Your arm should hang from your elbow down, not from your shoulder. (You can also do this lying on your stomach on a bed, adjacent to the edge of the bed.) Place one or two rolled towels beneath the front of your shoulder. Keep as much of your shoulder supported on the bench as you need. Grasp a light dumbbell in your hand. Slowly rotate your shoulder externally so that your forearm is raised parallel to the floor, and the back of your hand faces the ceiling (121a). Then rotate your shoulder in the opposite direction (internally) so that your palm is facing the ceiling (121b). Don't let your shoulder displace into the towel roll. Think of keeping your shoulder pulled "away" from the towel roll. Your range of motion will be more limited in internal rotation versus external rotation (possibly only about 10–20 degrees' difference). Do 2–3 sets of 15 reps.

Variations: 121.1. Standing external rotations: Stand sideways next to a pulley that is at armpit level, grasping the pulley with one hand so that it crosses your torso, with your elbow flexed to 90 degrees (121.1a). Rotate your arm externally and weight-shift in the same direction as your hand is moving. Allow your torso rotation to occur naturally (121.1b). Do a set of 15 reps. **121.2.** Standing internal rotations: Turn your body 180 degrees (121.2a) so that you are rotating the pulley toward your chest (internally); weight-shift in your legs in the same direction as your hand is moving. Allow your torso rotation to occur naturally (121.2b). This can also be done with pulleys at different heights.

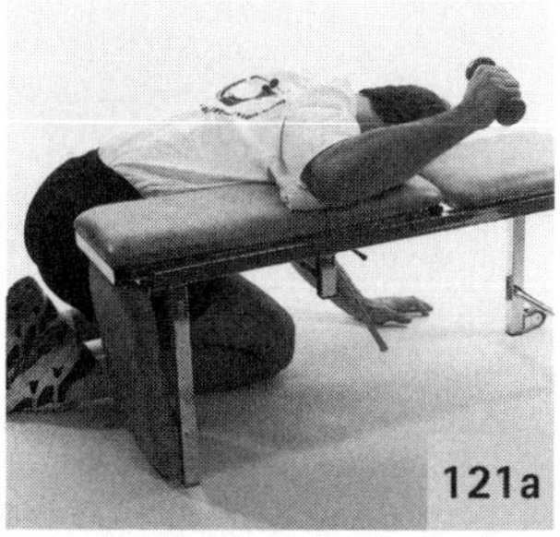
121a

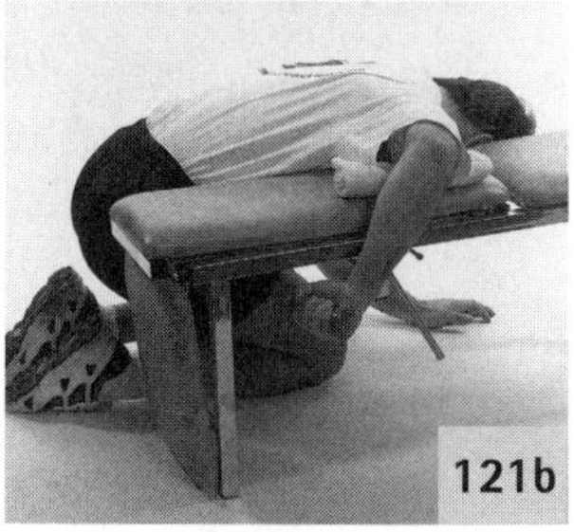
121b

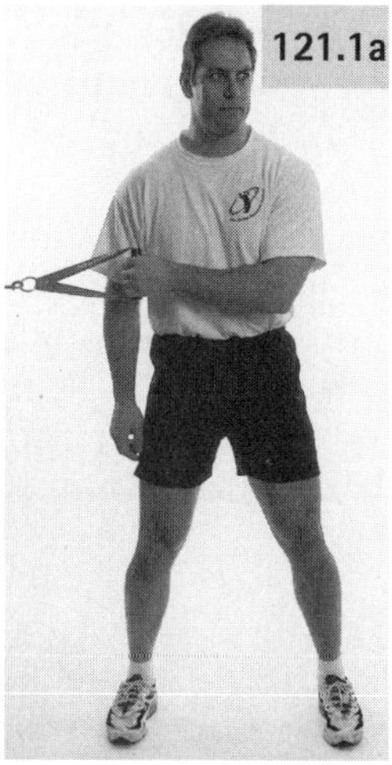
121.1a

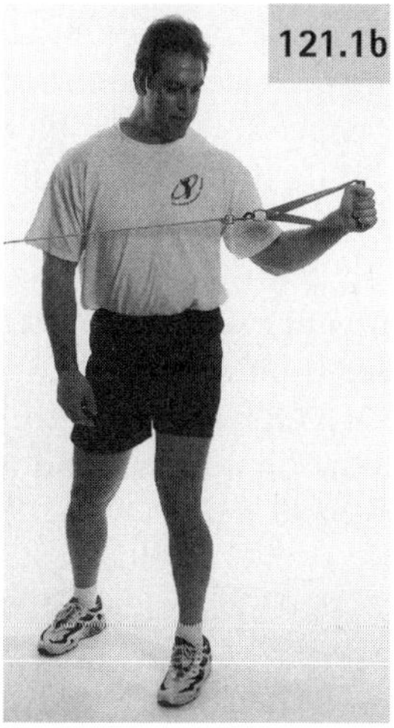
121.1b

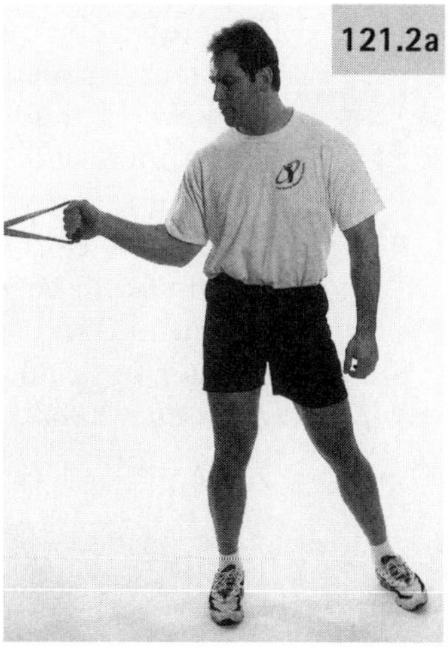
121.2a

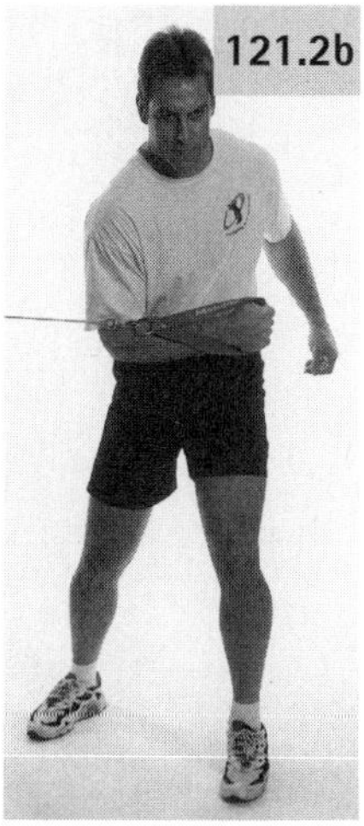
121.2b

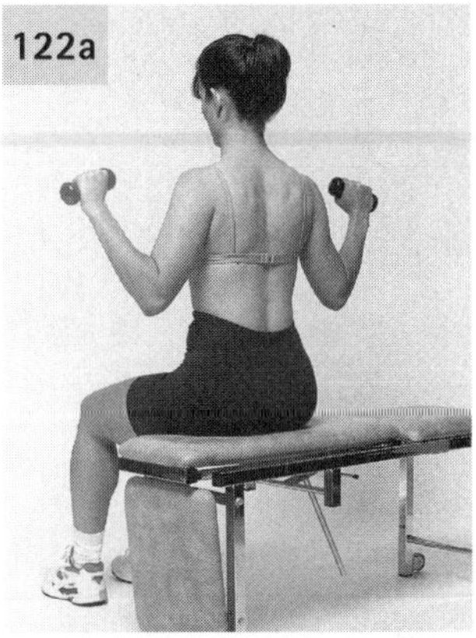

122a

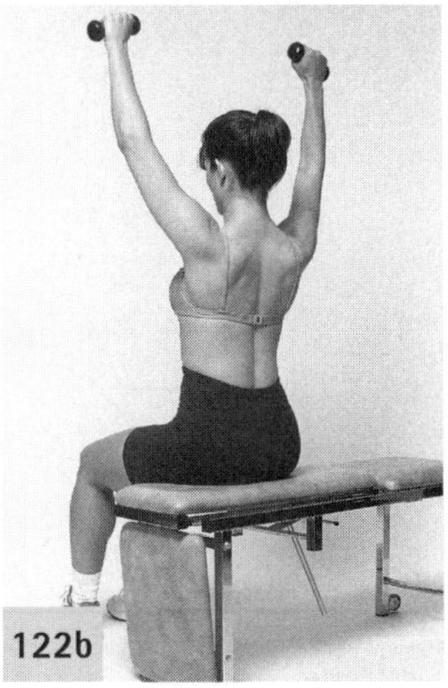

122b

122 DUMBBELL OVERHEAD PRESS

Equipment: Bench, mirror, and dumbbell.
Purpose: Improve your ability to press objects overhead. Target muscles: deltoid, supraspinatus, triceps, and trapezius.

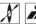

Technique: Sit at the edge of a flat bench (or stand up), facing a mirror if possible. Hold a dumbbell in each hand. Place your feet hip-width apart and sit with your back erect, looking directly into the mirror. (If standing, be sure your pelvis and spine are in neutral.) Hold the dumbbells at shoulder height, palms facing forward (122a). Extend your arms upward until your arms are fully extended (122b). As you extend your arms, be sure your upper trapezius relaxes after the halfway point and you squeeze your lower trapezius to finish the motion. At the end of the motion, your shoulders should not be up around your ears, but relaxed, with your elbows fully extended above your head. Your arms, however, should be in line with your ears, not in front of your head. Exhale in the up position and inhale in the down position. Perform 2–3 sets of 15 reps.

123 LATERAL DUMBBELL RAISE

Equipment: 1 pair of 3- to 8-pound dumbbells.
Purpose: Strengthen your rotator cuff and provide more balance to your traps. Target muscles: deltoid, supraspinatus, and trapezius.

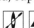

Technique: You can perform this exercise standing or sitting. Standing is more challenging to balance, and therefore requires more core and lower-extremity control. Grasp a pair of light- to moderate-weight dumbbells, holding them with your palms facing each other. Bend slightly at your hips, maintaining a neutral spine, and allow the dumbbells to hang below your shoulders by your waist. Raise the dumbbells to your sides so that your elbows and hands form a straight line with your shoulders. Slowly return the dumbbells to the start position in a controlled fashion with your hands facing each other. Exhale in the up position and inhale in the down position. Perform 2–3 sets of 15 reps.

122
123
124
125
EXERCISE

124 FRONT DUMBBELL RAISE

Equipment: 1 pair of 3- to 10-pound hand weights.
Purpose: Improve your ability to elevate your arm over your head and provide more balance to your traps. Target muscles: deltoid, supraspinatus, trapezius, and serratus anterior.

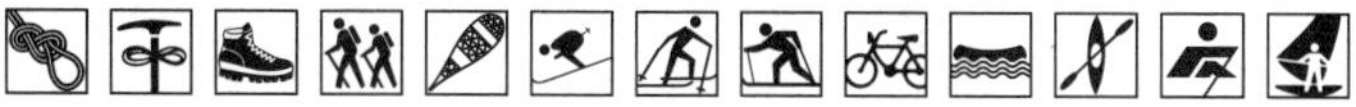

Technique: This exercise may be more beneficial when done with your back against a wall to monitor the position of your shoulder blades. Grasp a dumbbell in each hand. Hold the dumbbells so that your thumbs face upward. Have your abdomen pulled up and in. With your elbows slightly bent, raise the dumbbells, one at a time, in a semicircular motion to arm's length overhead. As you raise your arms overhead, relax your upper trapezius at the halfway point and squeeze your lower trapezius to complete the motion. Return to the start position, maintaining your shoulder blades against the wall while you lower your arms. Exhale in the up position and inhale in the down position. Perform 2–3 sets of 15 reps.

BICEPS

125 DUMBBELL AND BARBELL CURLS

Equipment: 1 pair of 3- to 20-pound hand weights.
Purpose: Strengthen your arm flexors. Strong biceps are helpful for pulling, lifting, and climbing activities. Target muscles: biceps, brachialis, and forearm flexors.

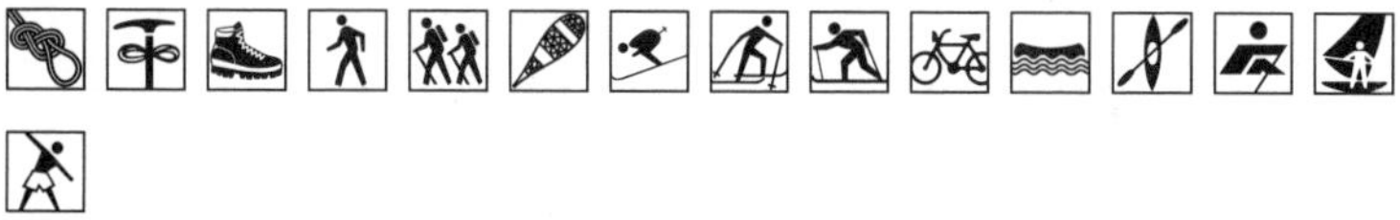

Technique: Stand holding the dumbbells at your side, with your knees slightly bent. Have your palms facing inward at the start. Curl the dumbbells by bending (flexing) your elbows and lift the weight toward your chest. Do 2–3 sets of 8–10 reps with each arm.
Variations: 125.1 Concentration curl: Hold a dumbbell in your hand, palm forward with a straight arm, and brace your elbow against your knee (125.1a). Keeping your elbow against your knee, curl the dumbbell toward your shoulder (125.1b), then lower it in a controlled fashion. Perform 2–3 sets of 10–12 reps for each arm. **125.2.** Squat curl: Stand upright and hold a straight bar in both hands with your palms forward, or a pair of dumbbells about shoulder-width apart. Curl the weight to your shoulders with your upper arms close to your sides

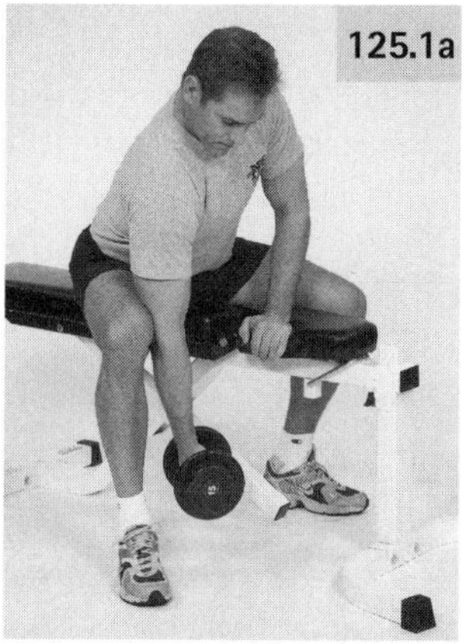

125.1a

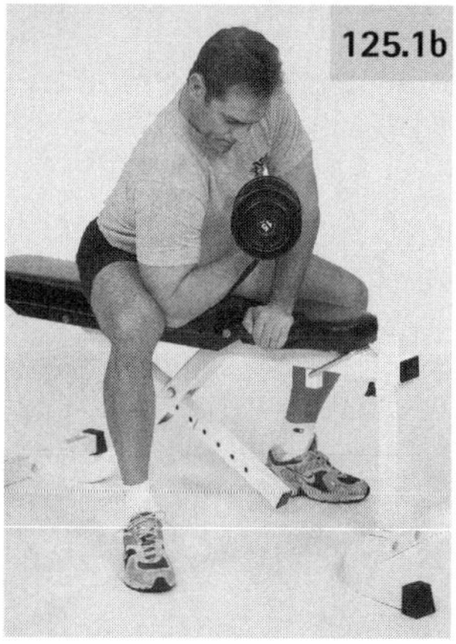

125.1b

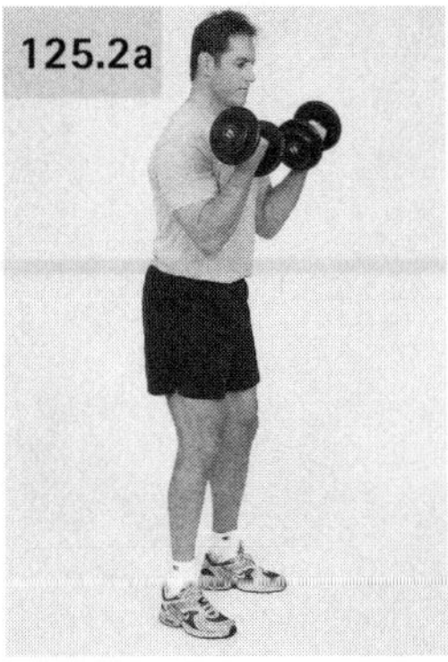
125.2a

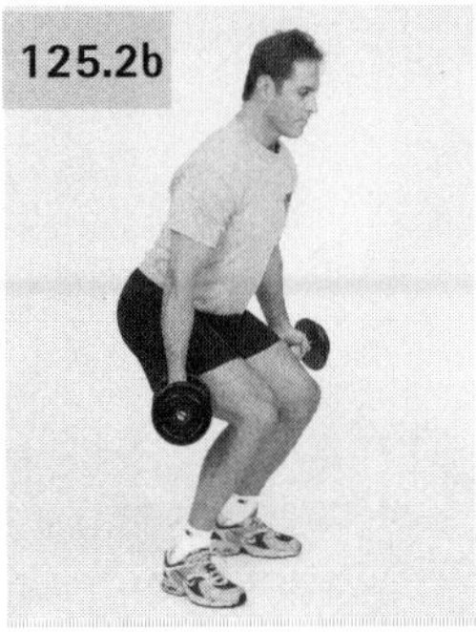
125.2b

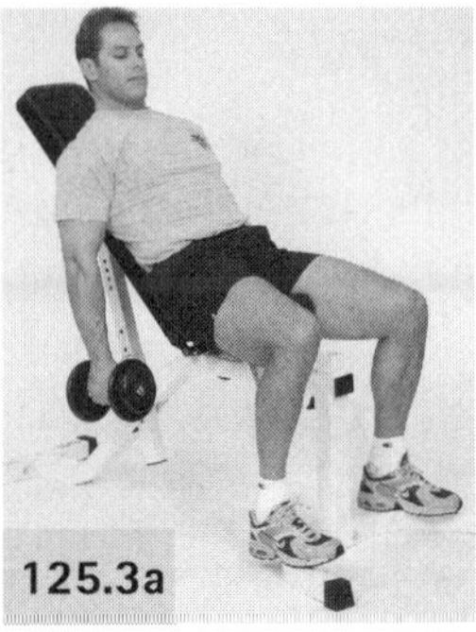
125.3a

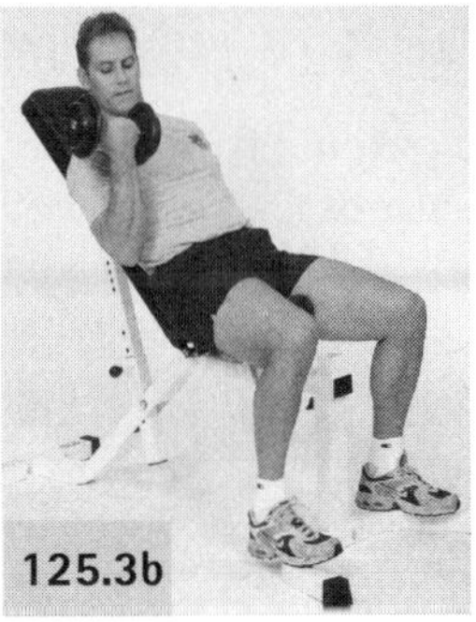
125.3b

(125.2a). As you lower the weight, perform a half or mini squat, then return to the upright position, curling the weight toward your shoulders (125.2b). **125.3.** Incline dumbbell curls: Grasp a pair of dumbbells and sit with your back on a 45-degree incline bench with your arm extended and perpendicular to the floor (125.3a). Alternately (125.3b) or simultaneously, curl the weights toward your shoulders. Perform 2–3 sets of 8–12 reps for each arm. **125.4.** Straight bar curl: Grasp a straight bar with your palms facing forward about shoulder-width apart and arms straight. Stand with your knees slightly bent, assume a neutral spine position, and engage your core (tight stomach, shoulder blades close together, and head positioned with your ears over your shoulders). Curl the bar toward your shoulders keeping your upper arms by your sides. Return the bar to the start position without allowing your elbows to go behind the midline of your body. Try to minimize any body swaying or hip thrusting while lifting the weight, and don't hold your breath. Breathe in on the way up and out on the way down. Perform 2–3 sets of 10–12 reps. **125.5.** Hammer curl: Grasp a pair of dumbbells and assume a standing position with your arms at your sides and palms facing inward (125.5a). Bend your knees slightly and engage your core with your spine in the neutral position. Maintain your wrist in neutral with your palm facing inward; curl one of the dumbbells toward your chin. At the top position (125.5b) pause motion, and then return the weight to your side. Perform the same motion on the opposite side and do 2–3 sets of 15 reps.

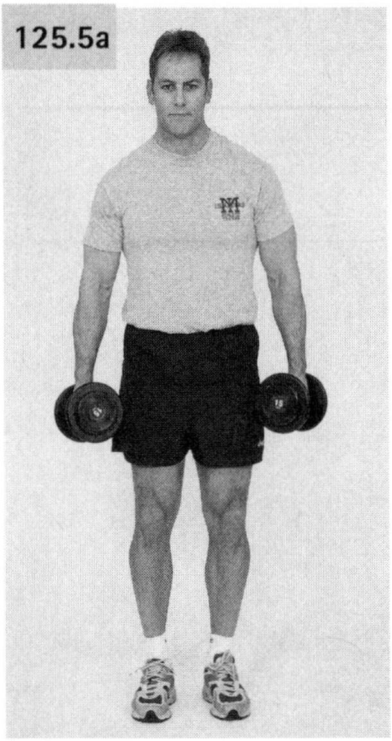
125.5a

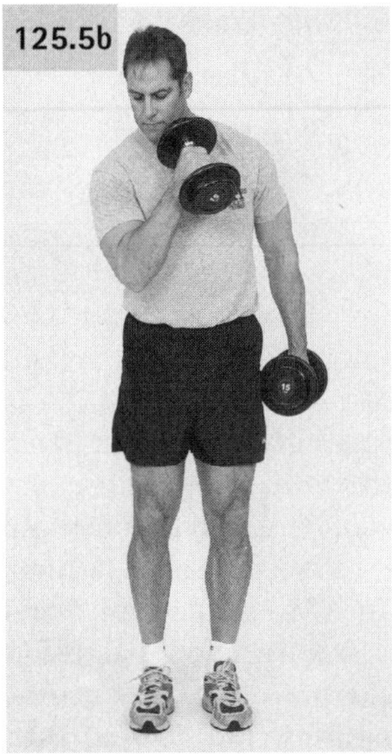
125.5b

TRICEPS

126 TRICEPS EXTENSIONS

Equipment: Barbell, dumbbells, or a high pulley weight machine.
Purpose: Isolate the triceps muscles and develop strength for arm extension and shoulder-arm stability. Target muscles: triceps and serratus anterior.

Technique: This exercise can be performed with free weights or various machines. If you choose free weights, lie face-up on a bench and place your feet on the bench. Grasp the dumbbells and position them over your chest with your arms straight, hands about 10 inches apart (palms facing each other). Once you feel balanced and in control of the weights, slowly bend your elbows and lower the dumbbells toward, then past, your forehead; then return the weights to the starting position keeping your upper arms stable and still. Perform 2–3 sets of 15 reps.
Variations: 126.1. High pulley: Try this variation on a high pulley machine. Either attach a straight bar, cambered bar, or rope to the cable using a carabiner. If you are using a straight or cambered bar, place your hands palms down about shoulder-width apart on the bar and pull it down so that your elbows are directly below your shoulders. Slightly bend your knees and position your upper body in a forward lean (126.1a). Maintain a neutral spine and engage your core. Keeping your upper arms still, extend your elbows and press the bar toward the floor until your arms are straight (126.1b). Pause a second and return the bar to the start position. **126.2.** Low pulley: Adjust the pulley machine so that the pulley arm is close to the floor and place a bench or seat about 2–3 feet from the low pulley. The best handle device to use with this exercise is a short rope that is attached to a carabiner and knotted on the ends. This exercise is the safest when you use a spotter. Sit on the bench and grasp the rope ends in each hand. Pull the weights off the rack and turn, facing away from the weight stack and pulley. Sit facing away from the low pulley with your elbows pointing toward the ceiling and your hands behind your head. If you have a spotter, have him or her pull the rope up to your hands and grasp the rope in each hand. Maintain a neutral spine position and keep your elbows still while pressing the resistance overhead. Return to the bent-arm position while stabilizing your core and upper arms. Only move at the elbow joint. This is a great isolation exercise for the triceps. Have your spotter assist by returning the weight to the stack. Precaution: If you are limited in

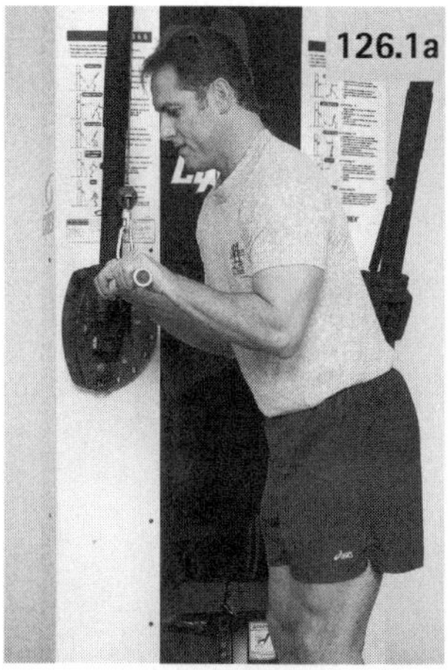

126.1a

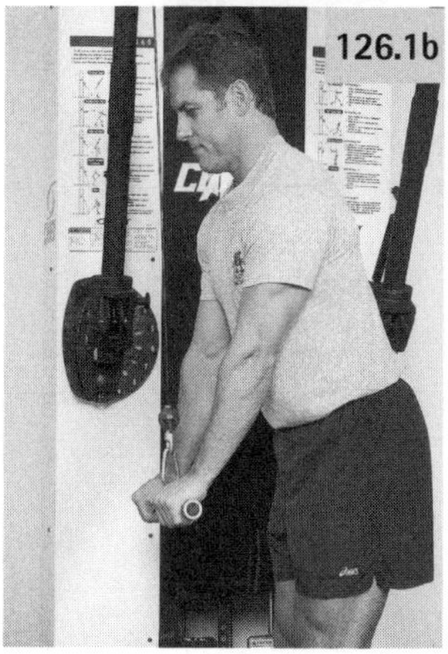

126.1b

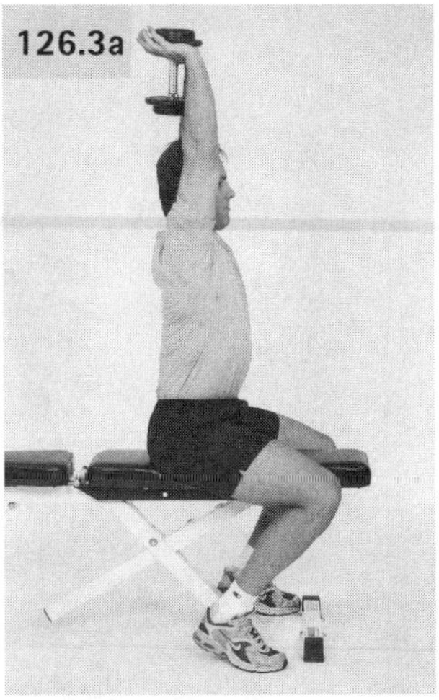
126.3a

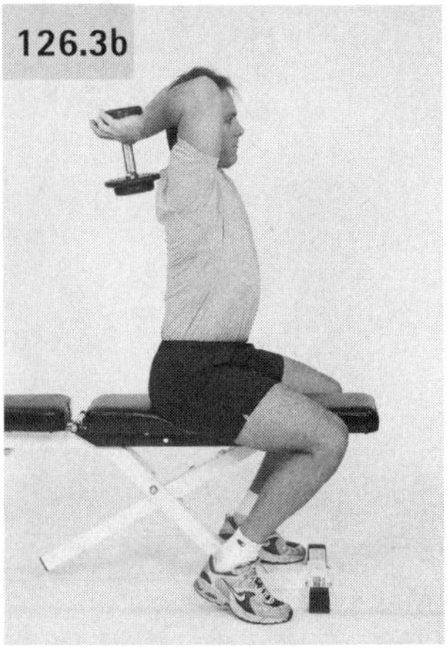
126.3b

shoulder flexion or have an active shoulder or neck problem, don't do this variation. **126.3.** Seated French triceps press: This variation is similar to variation 126.2. Instead of using a pulley and weight stack system for resistance, use a single dumbbell. Grasp a dumbbell with both hands so that your fingers overlap and contact the inside surface of the dumbbell head. The easier way to do this is to place the dumbbell on your lap in a vertical position and place your handhold on the bottom head of the dumbbell. Sit in on a chair or bench in neutral spine position and raise the dumbbell over your head into a straight arm position (126.3a). Maintaining a neutral spine with your core engaged, lower the dumbbell behind your head, keeping your elbows pointed toward the ceiling and your upper arms close to your ears (126.3b). Return to the start position by extending your elbows while keeping your upper arms close to your ears. Perform 2–3 sets of 10–12 reps. Precaution: If you are limited in shoulder flexion or have shoulder or neck problems, don't do this variation. **126.4.** Reverse triceps extensions: The body positioning for this exercise is the same as for variation 126.1, with the exception of the hand positions. Assume the same start position, but with your palms up, and extend your elbows to a straight-arm position. Perform 2–3 sets of 12–15 reps. **126.5.** Triceps press: Again a similar body position to that in variation 126.1, using a straight bar. The difference with this variation is the addition of shoulder motion with the movement. Place your hands about 6 inches apart with your palms facing down on the bar. Allow your elbows to point outward and your shoulders to abduct (upper arm moves outward), and bring the bar to your chest. You should be feeling weight resistance at this point. Assume a slight forward lean position with your spine in neutral and your core engaged. Extend your elbows and press the bar directly toward the floor. Return to the start position by bending your elbows while allowing them to move outward, bringing the bar back to your chest. You may need to move your head to one side of the cable. Perform 2–3 sets of 10–15 reps. If performing multiple sets, change sides after each set.

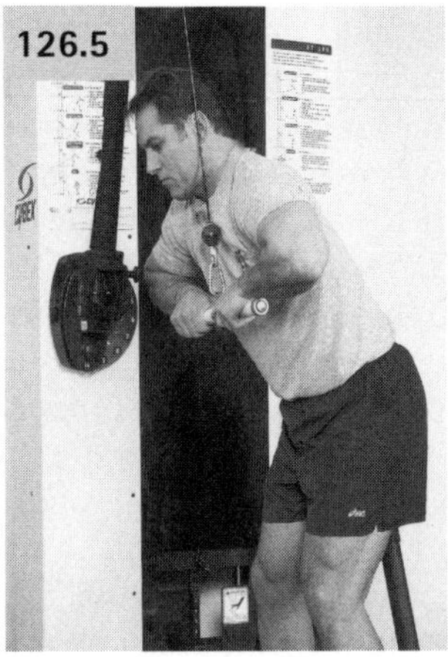
126.5

127 DIPS

Equipment: Dip machine that will unload body weight, or 2 chairs.
Purpose: Improve your ability to push your body vertically and push yourself with poles. Target muscles: triceps and pectorals.

Technique: Use a setting on the dip machine that will unload about half of your body weight. Lower yourself and then raise yourself up with your chest and arms. Do 12–15 dips in a set and decrease the amount of weight assist if you are not fatiguing by the end of the set. To do a dip with chairs, place them facing away from each other and start by balancing on your toes, holding onto the backs of the chairs while in a semi-upright position (127a). Lower yourself between the chairs until your chest meets the level of your hands (127b). You can assist with your legs to make this easier. Perform 2–3 sets of 15 reps.
Variations: 127.1. Angle isolations: Try isometric holds of 3–5 seconds at various locations during the dip. This is a good exercise for climbers. **127.2.** See chapter 8 for outdoor and reverse dip variations.
Tips and Precautions: Using machines (e.g., Gravitron, Cybex) to unload part of your weight during dips (and chin-ups) allows you to reduce the workload of the exercise until you are able to perform the exercise safely.

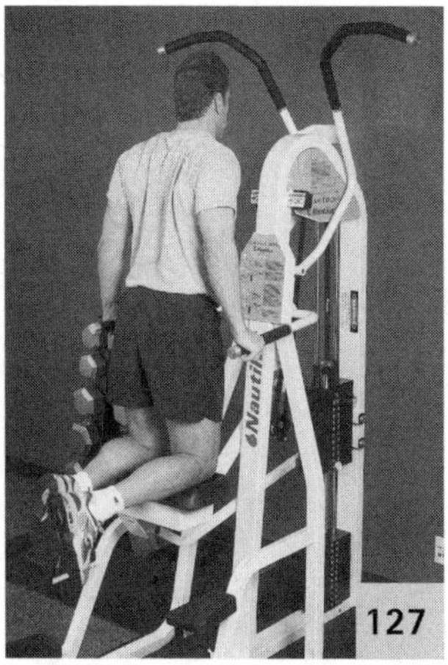

127

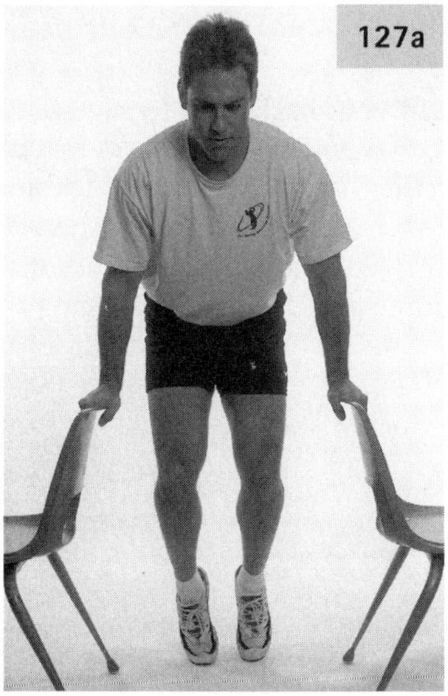

127a

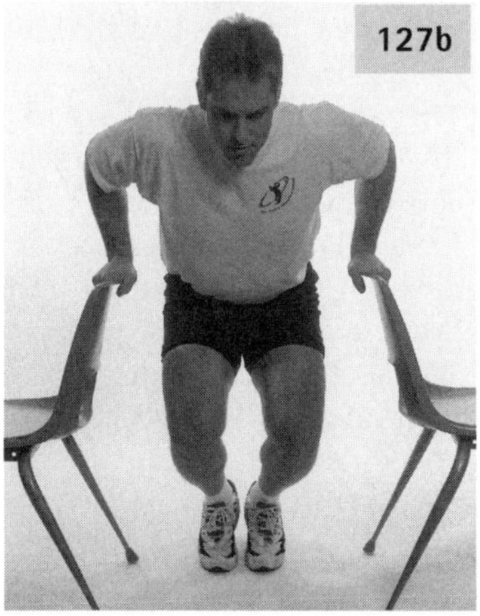

127b

128 CHIN-UPS

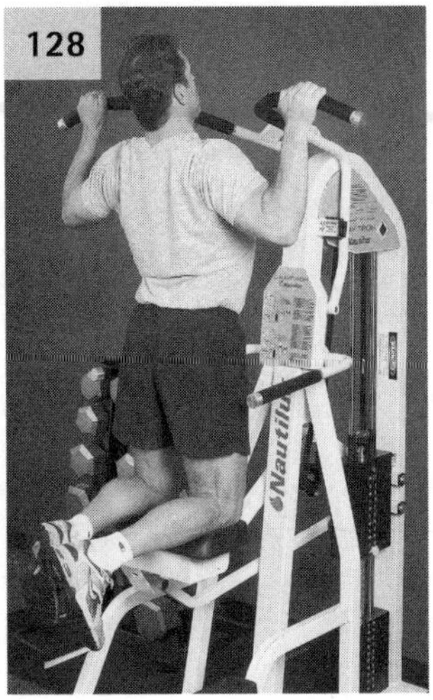

Equipment: Assisted chin-up machine or chin-up bar.
Purpose: Develop the strength and muscular endurance required to pull yourself up on climbs. Target muscles: posterior deltoid, biceps, trapezius, rhomboids, and serratus anterior.

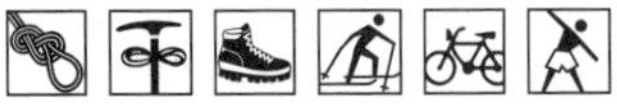

Technique: With an assisted chin-up machine, unload about half of your body weight and place your feet or knees on the platform. Use a handhold of palms forward and facing each other. Raise yourself up until your hands are at the level of your chin. Lower yourself to the start position. If you can do a chin-up with your full body weight, you can use a chin-up bar about 6 inches higher off the floor than you can reach with arms extended overhead. Jump up or climb onto a stool and hold the bar with your hands slightly more than shoulder-width apart, with your hands facing forward. Pull up and try to touch your chin to the bar. After you have pulled yourself to the top, lower yourself slowly and return to the start position. Perform 2–3 sets of 15 reps. Gradually work up to a set of less weight unloading at 6–8 reps.
Variations: 128.1. Variable grip pull-ups: Try changing your grip width or the position of your hands. Occasionally grip the bar with your palms facing you, or use an alternate grip. **128.2.** Prone grip pull-ups: Climbers and scramblers should do this exercise with palms facing away.
Tips and Precautions: Try to prevent your back from hyperextending by keeping your abdomen pulled up and in. Tighten your stomach muscles throughout this exercise. Try not to swing back and forth. Make sure to exhale on the way up, and inhale on the way down. If you are having trouble completing a full chin-up, have an exercise partner assist you. For example, while you are hanging on the bar, bend your knees and allow your partner to grip the front of your ankles. This will give you a foundation from which to push. You may then govern the amount of assistance suitable for your needs, without having your partner lift you.

FUNCTIONAL SHOULDER, UPPER-TORSO, AND ARM EXERCISES

Chapter 5 contains numerous functional shoulder exercises that integrate the upper- and lower-body regions. (See Exercises 20–22, 28–31, and 33–39).

The following exercises are functional exercises that focus primarily on the upper-body region. Not well known in health clubs or discussed in other texts, they are described in detail here.

Target muscles are not listed for these exercises because these exercises integrate multiple muscle groups and body regions. Some of the exercises are better simulations of certain activities but still have applicability for the others listed. See how you feel in relation to your activity after you have given an exercise a few weeks of practice.

129 SINGLE-ARM DUMBBELL PRESS

Equipment: Bench and a 5- to 20-pound hand weight.
Purpose: Improve the dynamic strength and function of the muscles surrounding your chest, shoulders, arms, neck, and anterior torso.

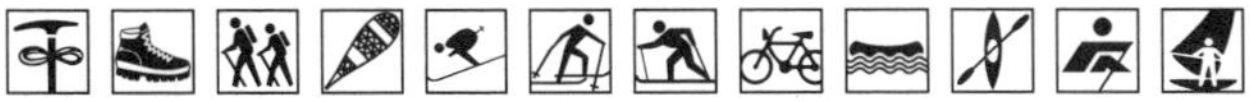

Technique: Hold the hand weight in your right hand and lie face up on the bench. Next, slide your body to the right, so that your right shoulder blade and right buttock are off the bench. Your right foot and leg will need an adequate purchase on the floor to help support your body from falling off the bench. Your left hand may grasp its same side of the bench for additional support. Press or push the dumbbell in your right hand directly over your chest and reach it toward the ceiling (129a). Next, bring the hand weight down toward your right armpit and allow your upper body and neck to slightly rotate to the right. Follow the hand weight through its path with your eyes and head (129b). This will enable your upper body and neck to move in coordination with your arm. Repeat this motion with the other side. Start with 1–2 sets of 12–15 reps, then move up to 2–3 sets of 15–20 reps.
Tips and Precautions: Follow the motion of the hand weight with your head and eyes. Move slowly at first and develop your most efficient path in which to move the hand weight from over your chest, then toward the floor. Allow gravity to assist you during the downward phase, and try not to let the hand weight drift outside the plane of your shoulder. Move quickly and in control through the full range of motion.

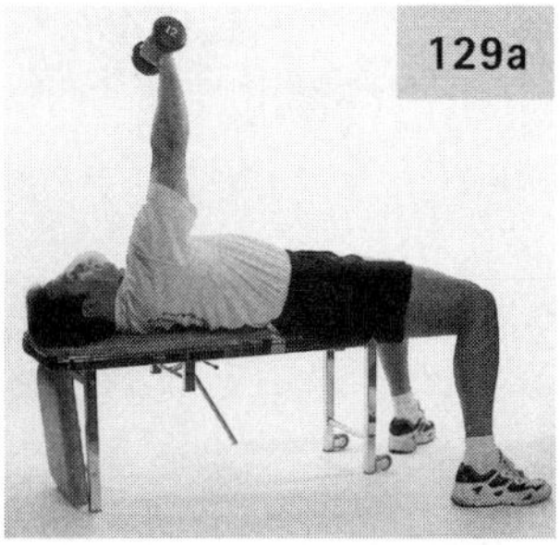
129a

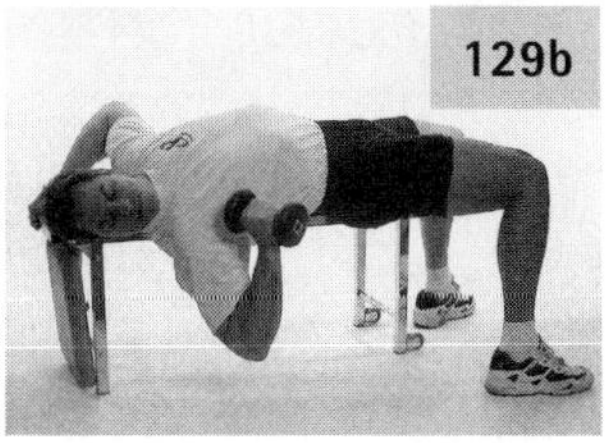
129b

130 VARIABLE-LEVEL PUSH-UPS

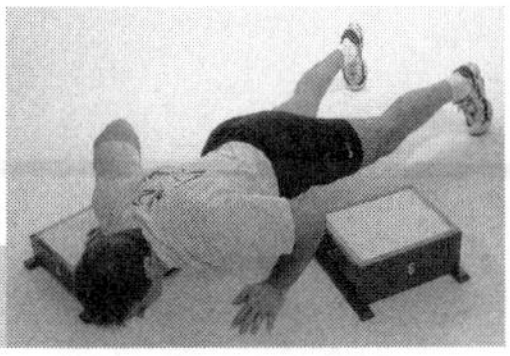
130a

Equipment: Staircase (or any other series of multilevel steps).
Purpose: Increase the synergistic and functional strength of your chest, shoulders, abdominals, and arms. Improve coordination between your upper and lower body by varying the style of a push-up.

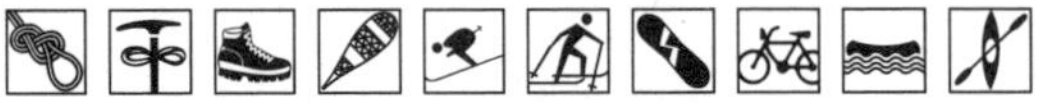

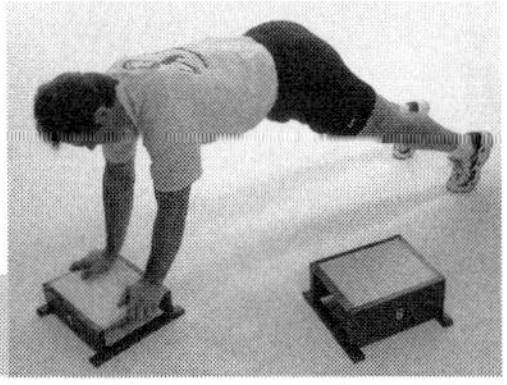
130b

Technique: Once you have mastered the push-up (see Exercise 115), make it more challenging by placing your right hand on an elevated surface, such as a 4- to 8-inch step, while keeping the other hand on the floor. Now, perform a push-up (130a). While you are in the "up" position, with your arms straight, step the left hand up from the floor to the same level as the right hand (130b). Again, perform another push-up, then step the right hand down to the floor while the left hand remains on the step, and perform another push-up (130c). Finally, bring the left hand down to the floor to match the level of the right hand and perform a push-up (130d). Repeat this sequence by leading with your left hand and traveling to your left. Each time you relocate your hand, perform a push-up. Perform 2–3 sets of 15 reps with any combination of surface or elevation challenges.

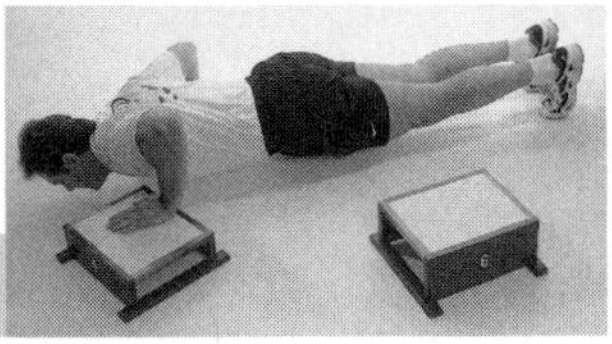
130c

Variations: 130.1. Push-ups against a bench or boulder: Push-ups can also be performed by leaning against a bench or boulder at various angles (130.1a and 130.1b). This is good for climbers (who should wear a pack) as well as for individuals wishing to prevent osteoporosis. **130.2.** Elevated push-ups: Try elevating your feet on a 2- to 4-inch step, then proceed with the push-up sequence from left to right and from right to left.

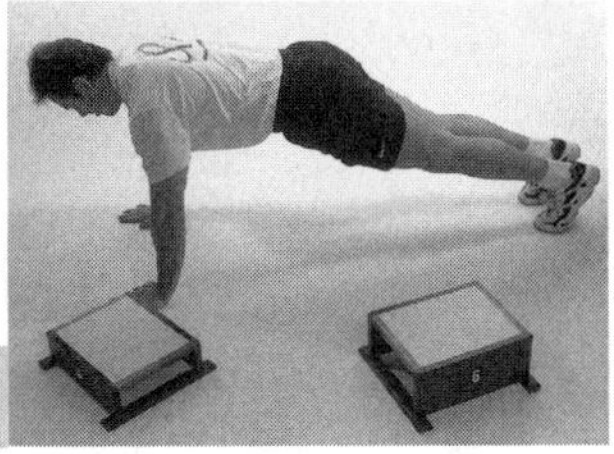
130d

Tips and Precautions: When attempting this exercise for the first time, limit your hand positions to a shoulder-width apart, and lower yourself only as far as you feel comfortable. If you have any recent history of shoulder or neck problems, this exercise could aggravate it. Always exercise in a pain-free range of motion. Be careful and move slowly at first, then increase your speed while maintaining your control.

130.1a
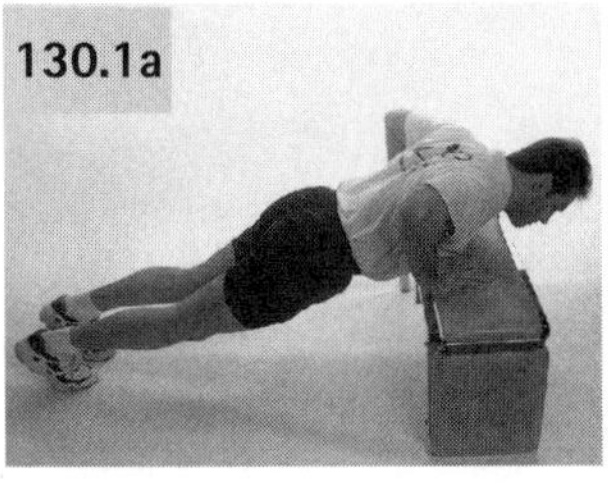

130.1b
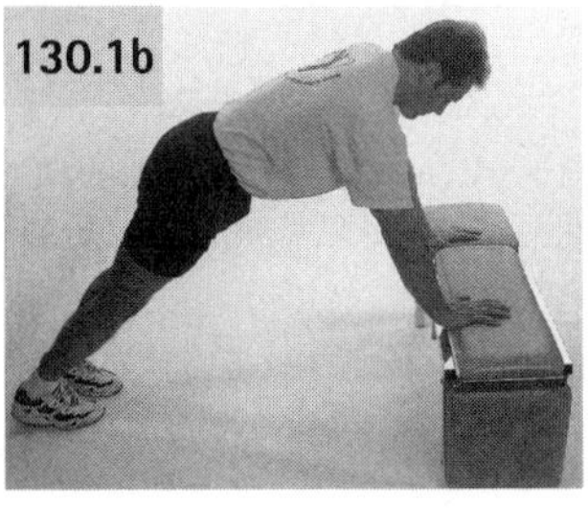

131 SINGLE-ARM DUMBBELL ROW

Equipment: Bench and a 5- to 30-pound hand weight.
Purpose: Increase your strength, flexibility, and muscular coordination of your back, posterior shoulder girdle, arm flexors, and abdominals. Combine complementary body regions with respect to their functional unity.

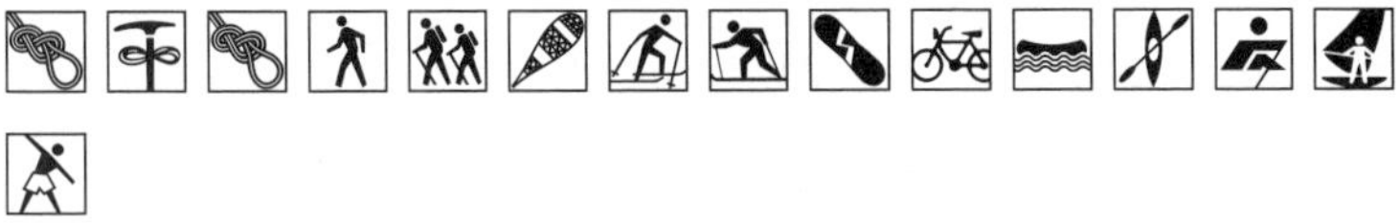

Technique: While holding the hand weight in your left hand, step to the left side of the bench. Place your right hand and right knee on the bench so that your right shoulder is over your right hand and your right hip is over your right knee. Your left foot remains on the floor for support and balance. Now you are in position and ready to start. Reach the hand weight in your left hand toward the floor while turning your hand so that your palm faces outward when you have reached the bottom. Make sure you follow the hand weight with your head and eyes, and allow your upper body to rotate in unison with your left arm (131a). Next, pull the hand weight toward your left rib cage while rotating the hand weight so that your palm is facing inward when you have reached the top. Again, make sure you follow the hand weight with your head and eyes, and allow your upper body to rotate in unison with your arm (131b). Repeat this sequence on the opposite side by bracing yourself on the bench with your left hand and left knee. Perform 2–3 sets of 15 reps on each side.
Variations: 131.1. Row with external rotation: To strengthen your shoulders' external rotators, use a lighter weight and rotate your shoulder at the top of the row portion of this exercise. Make sure that your elbow is close to your side when executing the external rotation. **131.2.** Incline/decline rows: Try this exercise with one end of the bench elevated 2–4 inches. This will create either an incline or a decline, depending on which side you are facing.
Tips and Precautions: If you have a history of neck or low-back problems, find a comfortable start position and move only in a pain-free range of motion.

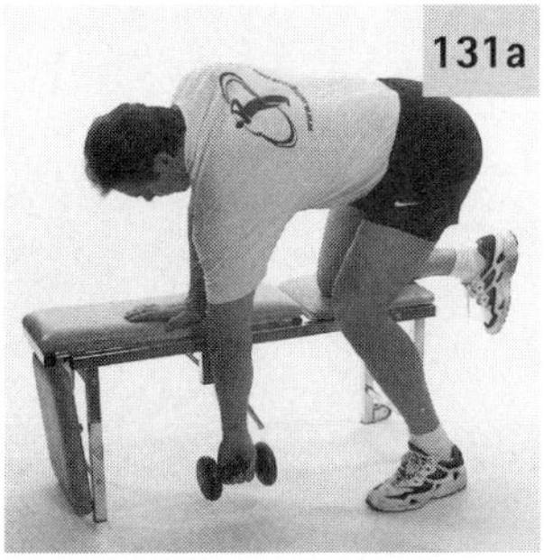

131a

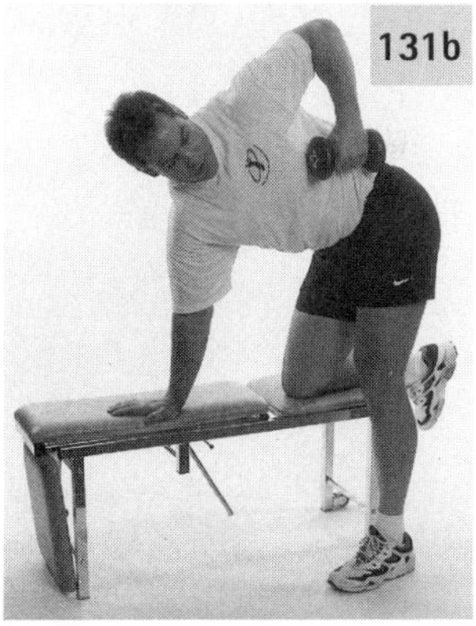

131b

132 SINGLE-LEG HIP, KNEE EXTENSION/PULL-DOWN

Equipment: High pulley machine or 4-foot length of tubing.
Purpose: Challenge your balance and strength, as well as coordinate the muscles that are responsible for pulling you up a hill or climbing a rock face.

Technique: Stand tall with your right arm extended overhead. Balance on your left leg with your knee bent, and touch the floor with your right forefoot for a balance assist. While pulling the pulley handle or tubing to your chest, push off with your left leg and buttock and come to a balanced stance with your left leg straight. After you have completed a set balancing on your left leg, repeat the same maneuver while balancing on your right leg. Perform 2–3 sets of 15 reps on each leg, 2–3 times a week.
Variation: 132.1. Unstable surface and grip change: Try the pull-down while balancing on a thick foam pad, or change your grip on the bar or tubing; for example, use an underhand grip or a grip that allows your palms to face each other. This changes the loads on various muscle groups responsible for pulling and rowing.
Tips and Precautions: If you have a history of knee or neck pain, reduce the depth of the squat portion of this exercise. Make sure that you don't extend your neck too far, and remember to move in a pain-free range of motion and only as far as you can balance. Keep your assist foot directly next to the balancing leg throughout the entire motion of this exercise. When your balance has improved, keep your assist foot up in the air until you can complete a full set without touching your assist foot to the floor.

133 STAGGERED STANCE CROSS DIAGONAL ROW WITH DUMBBELLS

Equipment: 3- to 20-pound hand weight.
Purpose: Increase the strength and coordination of your shoulders, arms, back, and legs in unison and in all directions of motion.

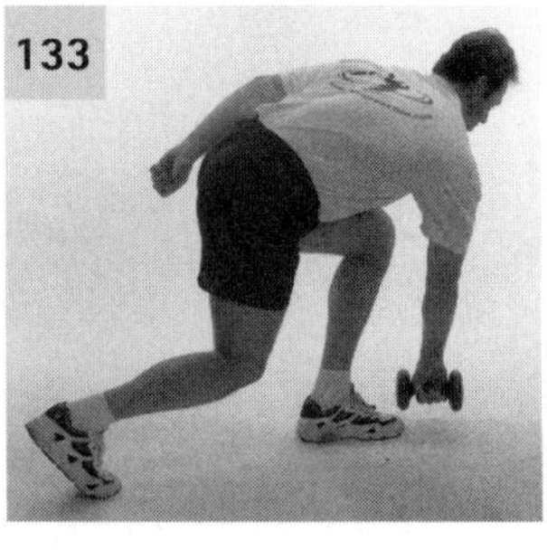

133

Technique: Hold the hand weight in your right hand and stand with your left foot one stride length ahead of your right foot. While bending your knees, hips, and low back, reach the hand weight toward the left foot and twist your right hand inward. Once you have reached as far as you feel comfortable, stand back up while "rowing" the hand weight toward your right hip. You may wish to transfer your balance onto the right leg at this point and prepare yourself for

the next repetition. Perform 2–3 sets of 15 reps on each side.
Variations: 133.1. Wide stance diagonal row: Try moving your feet farther apart or into a wide parallel stance. **133.2.** Unstable surface row challenge: Try balancing on a foam roll with the curved side down and your feet perpendicular to the long axis of the roll. When beginning this variation, start without hand weights and reach only to waist height and across your body while maintaining your balance on the foam roll. When this becomes easier, perform the cross-body reaches toward the floor while holding your hand weights.
Tips and Precautions: Make sure to use your legs and hips during this exercise. Follow the hand weight with your head and eyes through your full range of motion. Avoid this exercise if you have a recent history of low-back problems.

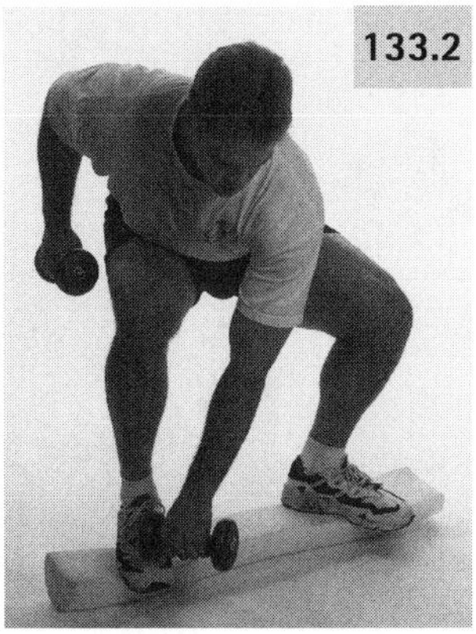
133.2

134 PRONE REACH/ROW/KICK-BACK

Equipment: A flat bench and a pair of 1- to 8-pound hand weights.
Purpose: Strengthen your back extensors, lats, shoulders, and triceps, and improve thoracic mobility into extension.

Technique: Place the hand weights at the head of the bench. Lay face down on the bench lengthwise with your head and chest off the edge of the bench. Grasp the hand weights with your palms down, assume a neutral spine position with your core engaged, and extend your arms fully, overhead (134a). The weights should be off the floor, with your upper arms close to your ears and your upper back slightly flexed at this point. Maintaining a neutral spine, simultaneously pull your upper arms to your sides, squeeze your shoulder blades together, and extend your mid back (134b). Stabilize yourself in this position, keeping your upper arms at your sides, and extend your elbows with your palms facing inward (134c). Return to the start position by reversing this sequence in a smooth and controlled fashion. Perform 2–3 sets of 8–12 reps.
Variation: 134.1. Reach/row/kick-back with a static straight-leg raise: Try this same exercise while elevating and maintaining a straight leg raise. Perform 1–2 sets of 8–12 reps for each leg.

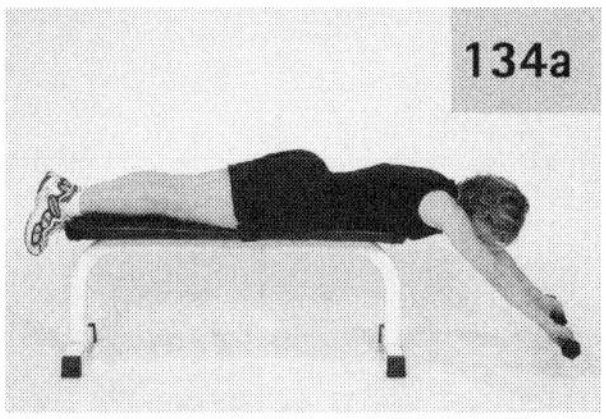
134a

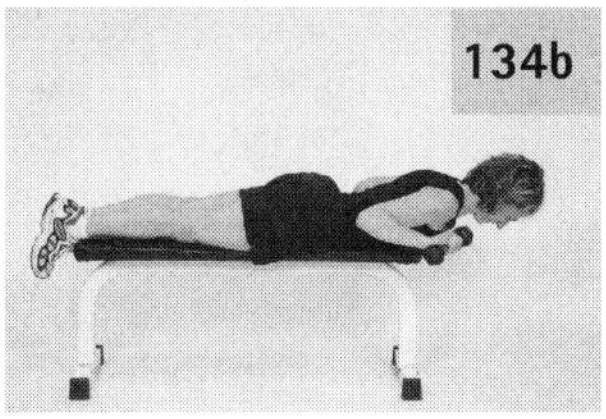
134b

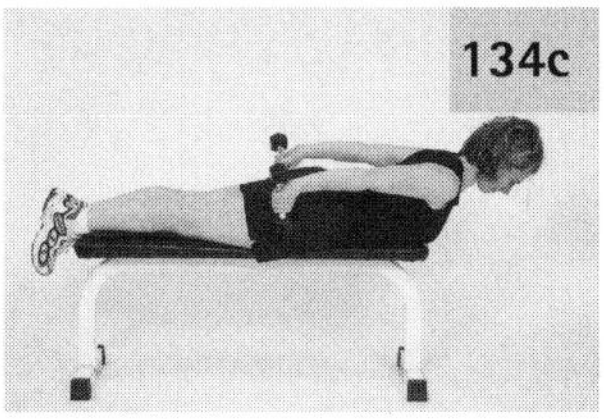
134c

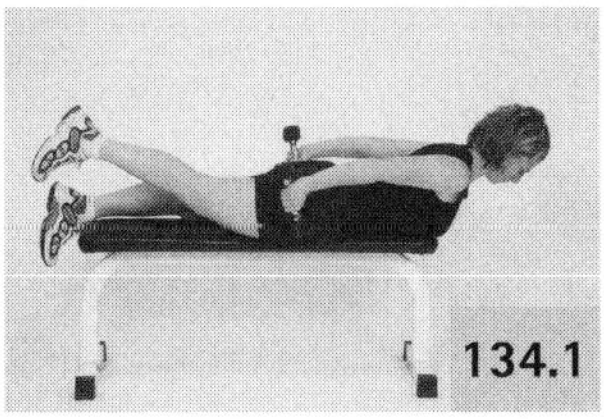
134.1

135 SHOULDER BUTT BURNER COMBO

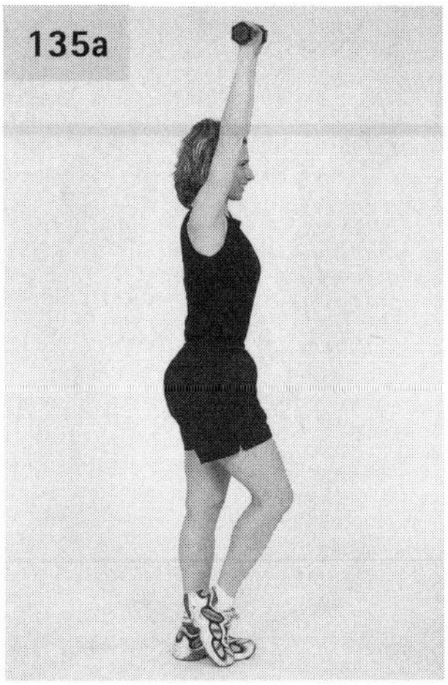
135a

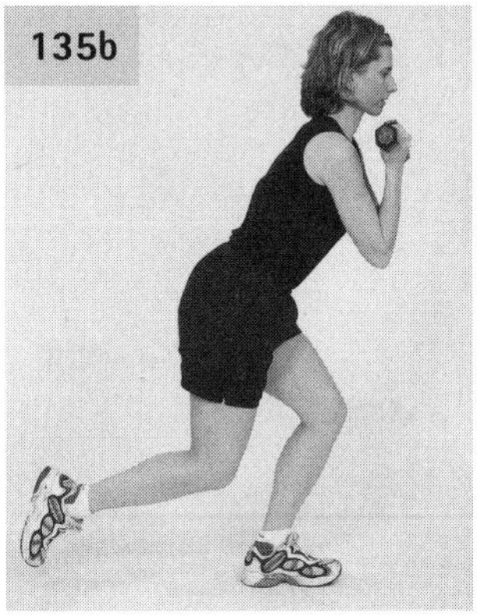
135b

Equipment: A pair of 3- to 8-pound hand weights.
Purpose: Challenge your balance while increasing the strength and coordination of your upper and lower body to function as a unit. Develop strength and balance to move objects from your chest to an overhead position. Combined shoulder, glute, and balance conditioning.

Technique: Hold the hand weights close to your chest, under your chin with your palms facing inward. Balance on your left leg, with the toes of your right foot touching the floor next to the heel of your left foot with your arms straight overhead (135a). Keep an upright spine position and lower yourself in a safe range by bending your left ankle, knee, and hip. Allow your right foot to slide across on the floor, directly behind you or to your left while lowering the hand weights to under your chin (135b). This will aid your balance and control while maintaining most of the work on your left leg. Lower yourself in a safe, pain-free range with your core engaged. Raise yourself to the start position and press and turn the hand weights over your head with your palms facing forward while maintaining your balance through the full range of motion. The motion should be fluid, combining your arms and legs. After you have performed a set while balancing on your left foot, repeat the same coordinated motion while balancing on your right foot. Perform 2–3 sets of 15 reps on each leg.
Variations: 135.1. Alternate direction reach: Try varying the direction you move your assist foot (the nonbalance foot) every repetition. This changes the load and activity of your balance leg and trains your muscles to adjust to various directional challenges. This will change the dynamics of the exercise considerably. **135.2.** Lateral reach: Instead of sliding your assist foot behind and left, slide or reach it sideways in the frontal plane. (See chapter 6 for further description of the frontal plane). Return to the upright position with your hand weight overhead and your assist foot next to your balance foot. **135.3.** Alternating dumbbell presses: The difference in this variation is the alternating arm motions. Start by assuming the single-leg balance position with one hand weight reaching for the ceiling and the other reaching for the floor (135.3a). The palm of the up hand should be facing forward and the palm of the down hand should be facing backward. As you lower yourself, bring both hand weights under your chin, close to the top of your chest with both

palms facing inward. Keep the hand weights close to your chin as you lower yourself. This will help keep your back more upright and help with balance. Slide and reach your assist foot behind you (135.3b). As you raise yourself to the upright position, switch arm positions (135.3c).

Tips and Precautions: When first starting this exercise, make sure to use your assist leg as much as you need. Allow it to slide across the floor or assist you in regaining your balance. Use your knees and hips as much as possible to minimize the involvement of your low back. Try this exercise first without hand weights. When you can complete a full set of 12 reps without hand weights, then add weights.

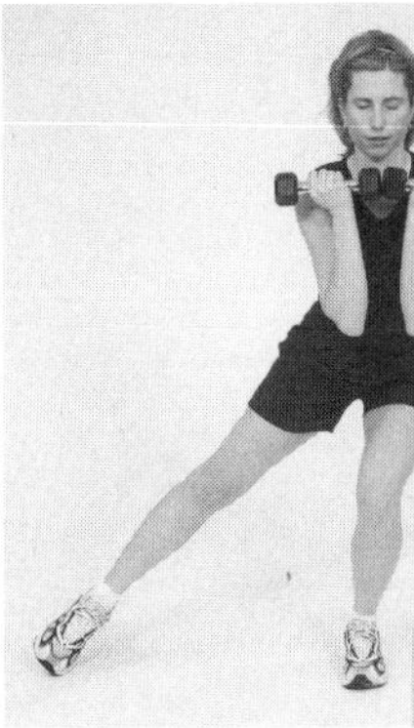
135.2

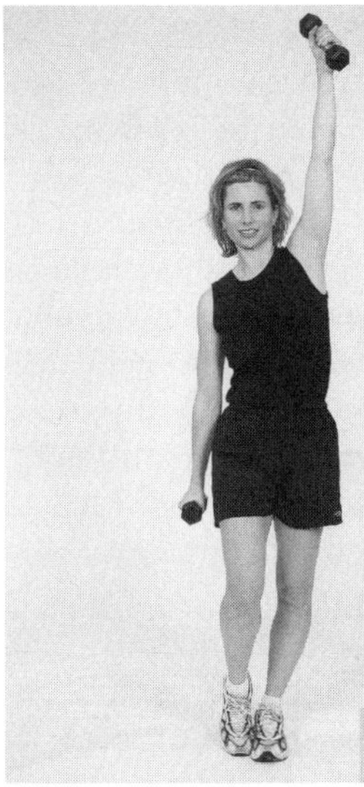
135.3a

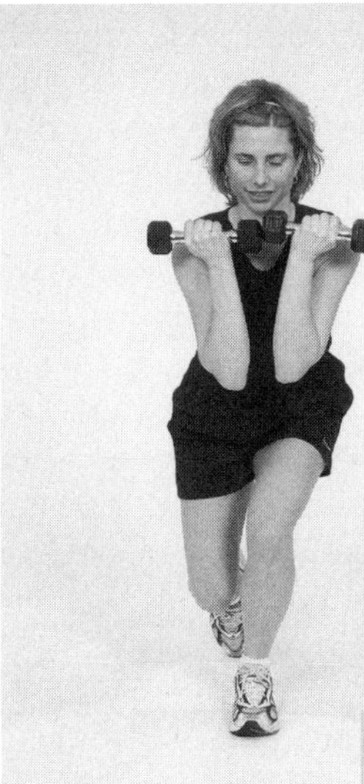
135.3b

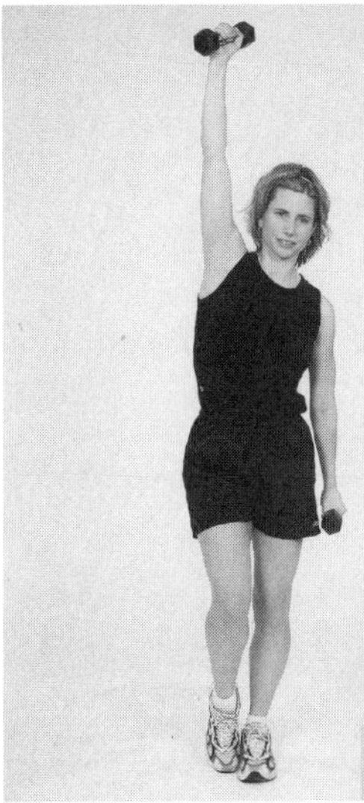
135.3c

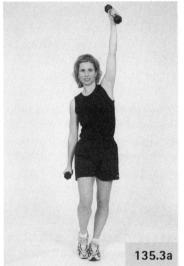

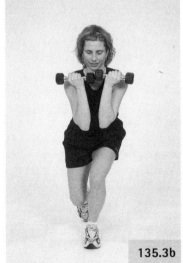

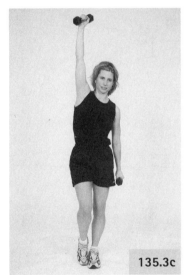

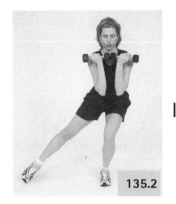

136 STANDING-WEIGHT SHIFT TRICEPS PRESS

Equipment: 5- to 25-pound hand weight.
Purpose: Enhance the coordination of your arms and improve their ability to work together as a unit during elbow extension and side-to-side motions. Stress your triceps, shoulders, and thighs.

Technique: Hold the hand weight overhead with your fingers laced together and your arms extended. Place your feet shoulder-width apart, with your knees slightly bent. Start by squatting to a shallow depth and lowering the hand weight behind your neck. Your elbows should now be pointing toward the ceiling. Next, shift your body weight onto your right leg, then simultaneously straighten your right leg and extend your arms, raising the hand weight above your head. Allow your left foot to rise off the floor so that you are balancing on your right leg when your arms are fully extended over your head. Return to the start position by lowering the hand weight behind your head and repositioning your balance over both feet, with your knees slightly bent. Now, shift your weight onto your left leg and simultaneously straighten your left leg while raising the hand weight over your head by extending your arms. Repeat this motion, shifting your body weight from side to side and keeping your elbows pointing toward the ceiling while extending your arms overhead. Perform 2–3 sets of 15 reps. Try to achieve 15 reps over each side during a 30- to 45-second interval.
Variation: 136.1. Triceps presses with heel rise: Rise up on the balancing foot's toes while you are extending the hand weight overhead. This incorporates your calves into the exercise and increases the balance challenge.
Tips and Precautions: Try to make the transitions from left to right smooth and congruous, and be sure to include your squat in the middle of the transition with your hand weight behind your neck. When you have shifted your body weight, you should be balancing on that foot while extending your arms overhead. Don't hit the back of your head with the hand weight.

chapter 16 THE FOREARM AND HAND

By Craig London, P.T., David Musnick, M.D., and Mark Pierce, A.T.C.

THIS CHAPTER WILL HELP YOU:

- Learn strengthening exercises for your wrists and fingers.
- Learn measures to prevent injuries, including taping.

Your elbow, wrist, and hand contain structures that are relatively small that may be subjected to repetitive or very high loads. Fingers are very susceptible to injury, especially in climbers.

FUNCTION AND ANATOMY

The movements of the forearm are pronation and supination; that is, movement of the forearm from a palm-up position to a palm-down position (pronation) and vice versa (supination). The most powerful supinator muscle is the biceps. The pronator muscles are less powerful than the supinators. Exercises that are effective for these muscles consist of rotating weights in a controlled manner. One effective drill is to hold a hammer (or a light weight) at one end and rotate your forearm from palm up to palm down.

The wrist moves in controlled patterns that allow your hand to achieve the optimal position for fine movements. The movements of flexion and extension are each about 85 degrees. There are also movements of radial and ulnar deviation: movement of your wrist toward the side of your little finger is ulnar deviation, while movement toward your thumb is radial deviation. For anatomy illustrations, see chapter 9 and also the hand detail in Figure 32 this chapter.

There are five *metacarpal* bones in the palm of the hand, and the fingers each have small finger bones (*phalanges*) with many muscles attached. Several muscles originate from the common *flexor tendon*, a site of frequent injury. The muscles quickly form into tendons that travel great lengths to their attachments. This enables a large and effective concentration of forces to produce movement in a very compact manner.

The tendons and a nerve pass through a bony arch and tunnel at the wrist (the *carpal tunnel*). The *carpal bones* in the wrist are small bones that connect the forearm to the fingers. These carpal bones are bound together by numerous ligaments. In a fall on the outstretched hand or in other wrist sprains, these carpal bones can be sprained and the ligaments can loosen. In caring for a wrist sprain it is important to return the carpal bones to good alignment. If after a sprain you experience persistent pain, clunking, or loss of range of motion, seek the attention of a physician and a hand therapist. Carpal bones can stay in dysfunctional positions because of ligament laxity. If this is the case, specialized injections (prolotherapy) may be helpful to stabilize a wrist that is not supporting the activities of the arm and hand muscles.

There are several fibrous sheaths (*pulleys*) that keep the tendons coursing in their proper tracks. These sheaths are a site of injury from overuse and trauma. If the muscle contractions are very strenuous for prolonged periods, the tensile strength of the fibrous bands can be overwhelmed, creating irritation and fraying of fibers. This can also happen if the lines of force

FIGURE 32

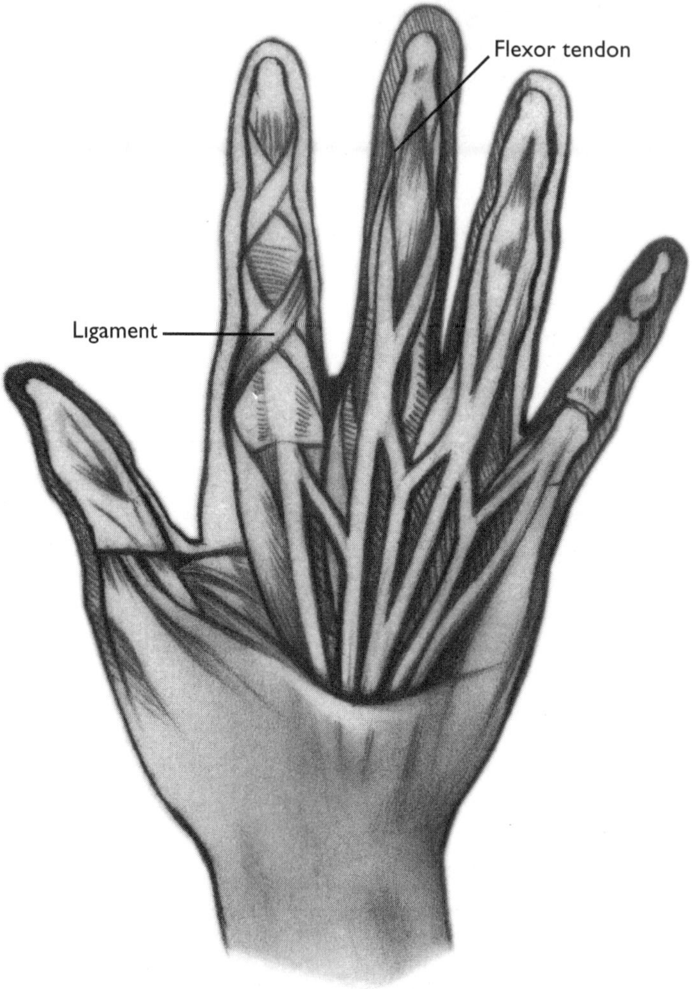

are altered when the fingers are twisted or laterally deviated. This places extra pressure on the ability of the fibrous bands to keep the tendons in place. Rock climbing often places both of these types of pressure on the hand and fingers. To avoid flexor tendon injuries, it is important to use good technique as well as to strengthen your flexor and extensor tendons and the muscles of your shoulder and upper back.

Many of the extensor muscles of the wrist and fingers originate from the same region on the outside of the elbow. Often these muscles are not strong enough in comparison to the overused flexors. To avoid injuries it is important to strengthen these extensors.

There are many muscles and tendons that move the fingers. The pulleys and the tendons are often injured with repetitive fingertip holds, especially if only one or two fingers are used with body-weight resistance.

COMMON MUSCLE IMBALANCES

The most common imbalance in this region is strong wrist and finger flexors combined with extensors that are relatively weak. This can lead to muscle tightness, pain, and overuse injuries. Another common weakness is the inability to lift our body weight, as in pull-up and triceps dip movements.

When considering the function of the hand, wrist, and elbow, vital regions to exercise include the upper back, shoulder, chest, and upper arm because they are important in positioning and stabilization of the arm and hand (see chapter 15). A healthy neck is also important for proper muscle function of the arm, wrist, and hand region, as the nerves to this area exit from the neck. Overuse injuries of the arm, wrist, and hand are very common due to the repetitive uses of the fingers and wrist.

INJURY PREVENTION

Wrist splints and taping can be helpful in prevention and treatment of wrist and hand injuries. Proper taping can add to the load tolerance of your fingers and wrists. The following techniques can be learned quickly and are often used by serious rock climbers.

Wrist taping: The goal of strapping your wrist is to help limit extension of your wrist joint. Excessive extension, especially while weight bearing, can sprain the two rows of carpal bones and the small cartilaginous disc in your wrist. Use 1 1/2-inch-wide tape, and position your wrist in mid range with your fingers spread apart. Start taping on the back of the wrist where your wrist meets your hand. Wrap 2–3 times around your wrist, with appropriate tightness around the creases of your wrist. After taping, make sure that you can extend your wrist just slightly less than your range before you were taped.

Finger taping: If you have had a prior injury, tape a finger joint to support the sheaths and divert some of the forces from your flexor tendons. Use 1/2- or 1/4-inch-wide tape. Tape a figure-eight pattern by starting the first piece on the palm side of the joint just below the joint crease. Tape a diagonal to the superior side of the joint. Continue the tape horizontally around once, and then cross over the joint to the inferior side. Make sure that the crossing occurs on the palm side of the joint. Tape 2–3 times around the joint. Make sure the joint can bend, that the skin is a normal color, and that you can feel the skin on your finger past where you have taped.

FOREARM AND HAND EXERCISES

You can begin strength training exercises with 15 reps unless otherwise indicated. Progress your reps and resistance according to the guidelines in chapter 5.

137 FINGER FLEXOR GRIP

Equipment: Spring-loaded grips, hand and finger putties and balls, elastic bands, and elastic sheets.
Purpose: Strengthen your fingers for better gripping.

Technique: Select one of the several tools available for finger drills, which come in various pressures, and squeeze it briefly for 15 reps in a set. Try a few out and see what feels best for you. Gradually increase the resistance on your fingers with more challenging putties and hand grips.

138 WEIGHT ROLL-UP

Equipment: A rope of shoulder height attached to a 1-foot-long, $1\frac{1}{2}$-inch-diameter dowel on one end and to a weight on the other end.
Purpose: Strengthen and balance your wrist extensors.

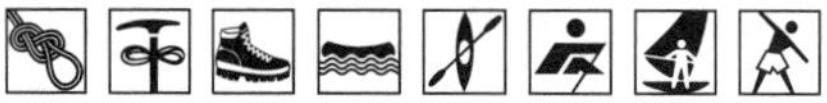

Technique: With your arms in front of you and lower than parallel to the floor, and with your elbows bent, grasp the dowel on either side of the rope and slowly wind the rope up and down. Alternate the hand you are using to wind it up. The intensity of the drill is increased by the amount of weight attached to the rope and by the time it takes to complete. Start with 1 pound and roll at a comfortable pace. Progress from there by doing 4–5 reps and gradually increasing the weight. This exercise can quickly lead to forearm fatigue, so try not to overdo it.

138

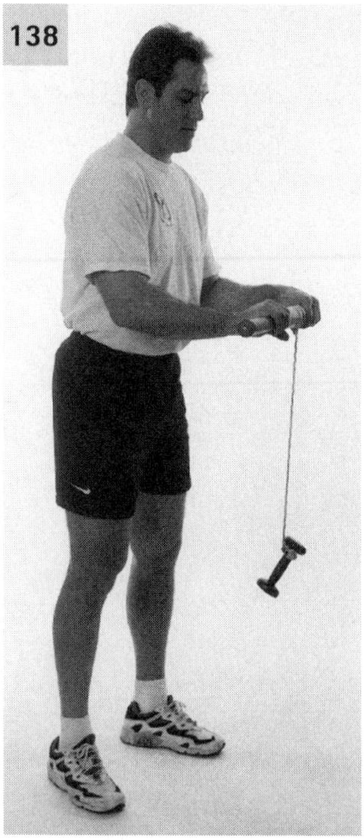

139 DUMBBELL PALMS-UP WRIST CURL

Equipment: A pair of 1- to 10-pound free weights and bench.
Purpose: Strengthen your wrist flexors.

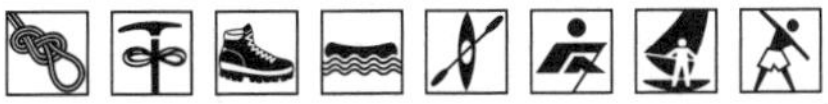

Technique: Grasp a pair of dumbbells and sit on a seat or a bench with your forearms resting on your thighs. Hold the dumbbells palms up. Lower the dumbbells as far as possible (139a), and then curl them up as high as possible (139b). Don't let your forearms raise off your thighs. Do 2–3 sets of 15 reps.

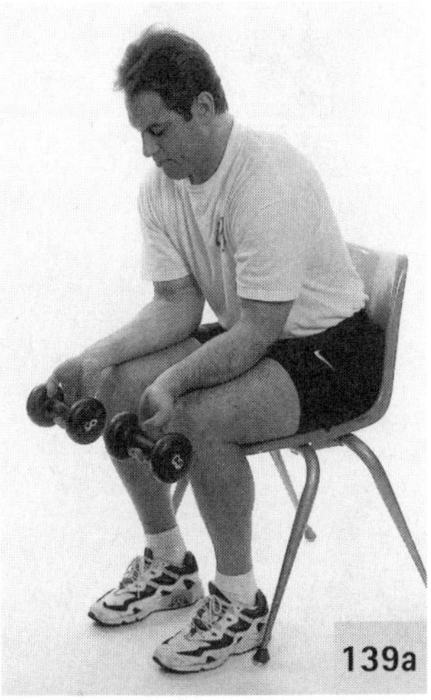

139a

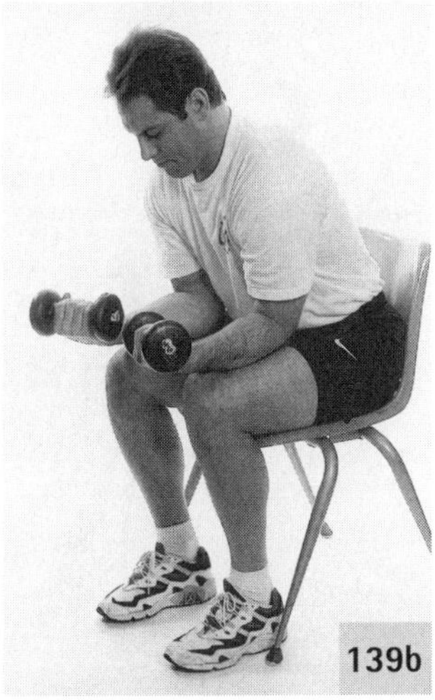

139b

140 DUMBBELL PALMS-DOWN WRIST CURL

Equipment: A pair of 1- to 10-pound free weights and bench.
Purpose: Strengthen your wrist extensors.

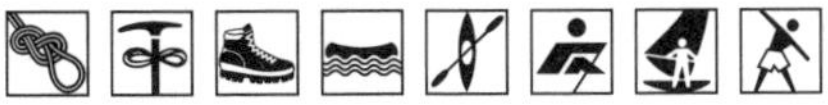

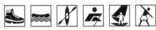

Technique: Begin as in Exercise 139. Hold the dumbbells with your palms down. Lower the dumbbells as far as possible. Don't keep a tight grip with your fingers. Curl the dumbbells upward as far as possible. Don't let your forearms raise off your thighs. Do 2–3 sets of 15 reps.

EXERCISE 141

141 SITTING OLYMPIC PLATE HAND SQUEEZE

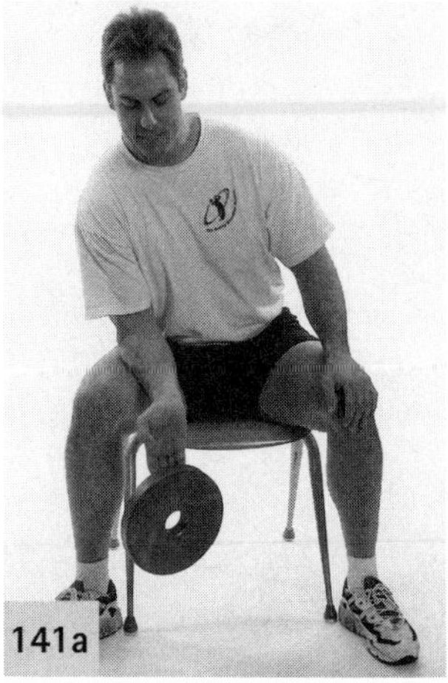
141a

Equipment: 5- to 25-pound Olympic weight plate (one with a ridge).
Purpose: Strengthen your finger flexors and the intrinsic hand muscles. This technique is most useful for climbing athletes.

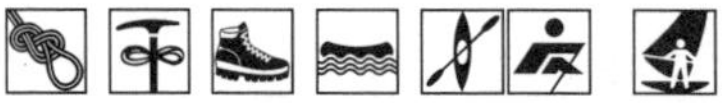

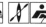

Technique: Sit down with your feet spread apart; with one hand, hold an Olympic plate by the ridge. Lower the plate until your fingers are nearly extended (141a). Curl your fingers upward, raising the plate a few inches (141b). Continue raising and lowering the weight for 15 reps or until you fatigue.

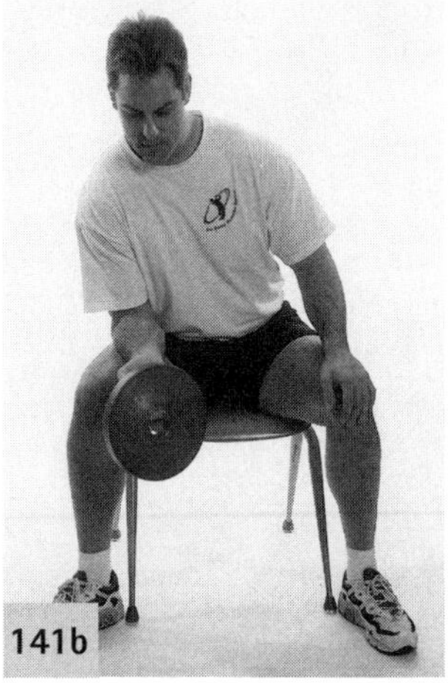
141b

PART III

Conditioning for Outdoor Activities

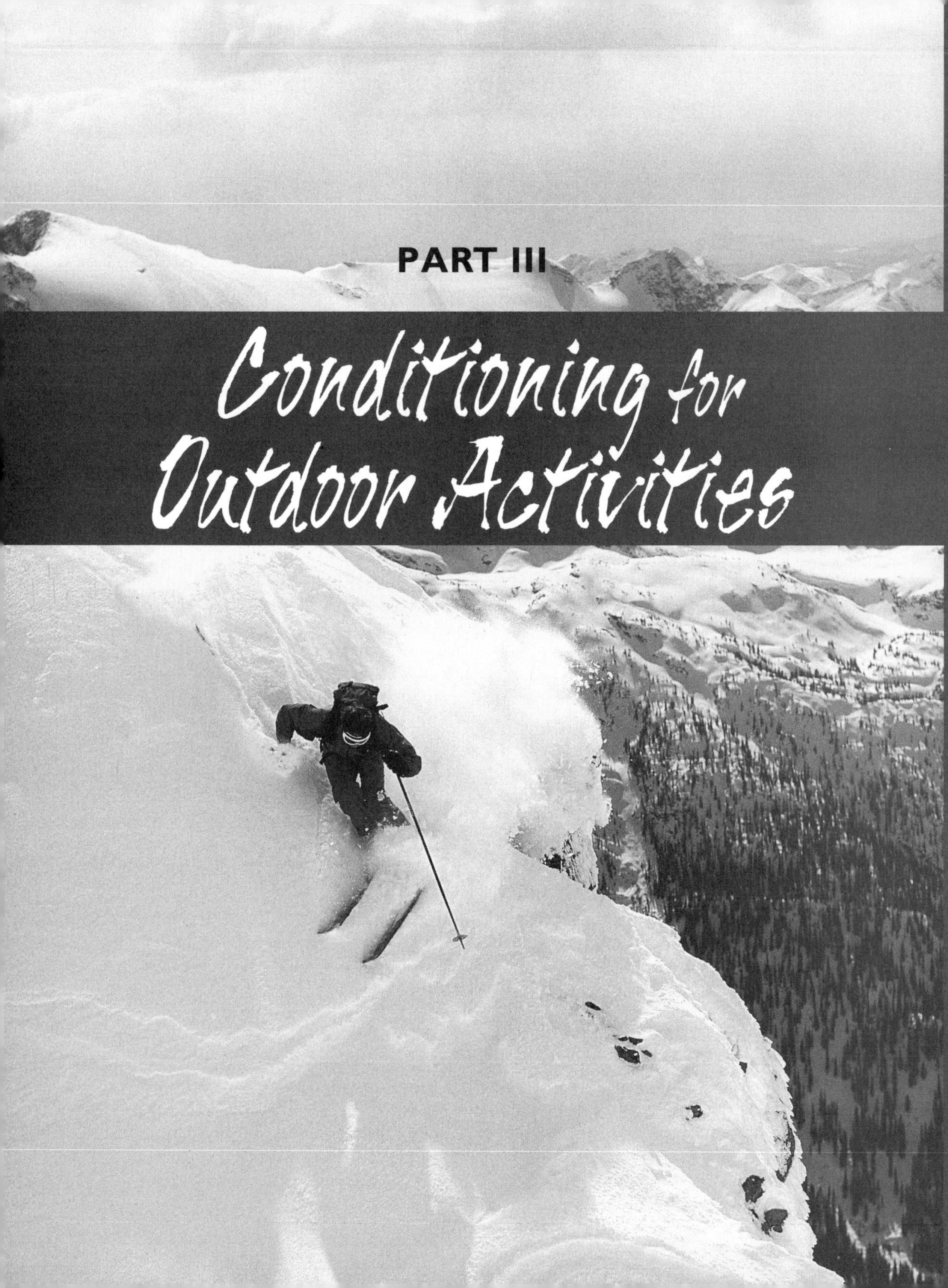

chapter 17 CONDITIONING FOR HIKING, BACKPACKING, AND SNOWSHOEING

By David Musnick, M.D.

THIS CHAPTER WILL HELP YOU:

- Understand the aerobic, balance, and strength demands of hiking, backpacking, and snowshoeing.
- Understand how to avoid common injuries from these activities.
- Develop a basic conditioning program to achieve the goal of a full day of strenuous hiking, backpacking, or snowshoeing.

Getting in shape for hiking, backpacking, and snowshoeing consists primarily of improving your aerobic fitness both in town and on outdoor training days. Some basic strength and balance exercises can help, especially if you are doing steeper trails requiring handholds, areas with river or boulder crossings, or deep snow with uneven terrain. Common problems associated with inadequate conditioning are feeling easily winded, muscle soreness, kneecap area pain (especially with downhill grades), shoulder area discomfort, and falling. Occasionally, back and neck problems can develop if packs are lifted or loaded improperly or during a fall while snowshoeing. If you are in good condition, you reduce the likelihood of developing these problems and you enhance the possibility of enjoying your outdoor activity.

MUSCULOSKELETAL DEMANDS

Hiking and backpacking primarily involve your lower extremity from your hips to your feet. The demands on your knees are greatest in downhill hiking and in large uphill steps. Dynamic balance is important for river crossings. Adding a heavy pack can stress your shoulders, hips, neck, and back. The majority of people with mild back problems can tolerate a pack very well but have to be careful about how they lift the pack on and off their backs, as well as how they position it for good neutral neck and low-back positioning (see chapters 14 and 25 for full discussions on neutral alignment).

Snowshoeing places similar demands on your knees but even greater demands on your ankles because of uneven snow surfaces. The muscles in your buttock, in your inner thigh, and all around your hips are used quite a bit and benefit from strength training. Snowshoeing challenges your balance more frequently than does hiking. But hiking on uneven terrain can put even more stress on your back. Strength training for snowshoers is similar to that for backpackers, but should have more balance, abdominal, buttock, and hip exercises.

MUSCLE IMBALANCES

Common muscle imbalances for hiking, backpacking, and snowshoeing are inadequate strength in the quadriceps and lower legs in controlling downhill motion. The hamstrings may also be somewhat weak in comparison to their much stronger quadriceps counterparts. The hip and buttock muscles are often not strong enough, especially the hip muscles on the front and inner groin in snowshoers.

WARM-UP

Warming up for these activities can be as simple as taking a brisk 5-minute walk around the parking lot before doing some stretches. To prepare for backpacking over river crossings or for snowshoeing, add a short walking lunge and Exercises 59.1 and 61 (for the latter, use your car keys if you don't have a ball available).

STRETCHING

Do some stretching after you have warmed up during your midweek workouts and before you leave the trailhead (if it is not too cold).

Do Exercises 1, 3.1, 5.2, 7–9, and 19.

AEROBIC CONDITIONING

Hiking, backpacking, and snowshoeing are highly aerobic activities that are usually done for many hours at lower intensities, generally at 50–65% maximum heart rate (max HR). They are often done on slopes of varying grades, on boulder fields or scree slopes, or off-trail, which can temporarily increase the aerobic demands to a higher level (often to interval levels). Snowshoeing in deep powder, in very cold weather, or on uneven snow increases the aerobic demands.

The minimum aerobic program (see chapter 3) should be modified in a number of ways to allow your body to more easily meet the aerobic demands of hiking, backpacking, and snowshoeing.

Do 4–5 short aerobic sessions each week at 70–85% max HR.

Within 4–8 weeks of your first moderate hike or snowshoeing trip, begin increasing the duration of the aerobic period of all of your exercise periods to 35–40 minutes, not including warm-up and cooldown. Increases should be gradual, no greater than 10–15% per week.

Six weeks before your first long hike or snowshoe trip, begin one low-intensity, longer-duration (LILD) activity per week at one-third to one-half your expected distance and elevation gain. Gradually increase the elevation gain, distance, and degree of difficulty every week.

In general, in your aerobic program it is good to achieve distance and elevation gains that are within about 60–75% of those expected during your planned outdoor activity. If you are not able to gradually work up to this amount of elevation gain or distance, you may still be able to do the hike or snowshoe trip. You might need to take more frequent breaks or go slower, and you might have more muscle soreness afterward. To preserve your knees, take adequate time and frequent breaks when hiking downhill.

Hiking/Backpacking/Snowshoeing

Inside: Taking step classes, stair climbing on machines (the rotating stair machines are best) or actual stairs, using treadmills, and using EFX cross trainers (this and slide boards are excellent for snowshoers).

Outside: Cross-country skiing, walking, jogging, climbing stairs, and snowshoeing. Stair climbing with single, double, and triple stairs is some of the best in-city training (see stair-climbing options 1–4 in the Modes of Aerobic Conditioning section in chapter 3).

STRENGTH TRAINING

For the most part, you can hike, backpack, and snowshoe without a rigorous strength training program. The program below, a basic one that can be done in a short period of time, can help keep you well toned and make your outdoor activity more enjoyable with less effort, less muscle soreness, and a lower likelihood of overuse injuries. You can do your exercises in 2–3 sets of 15–20 reps because you are working on the endurance aspect of your strength.

Upper-body strength of your shoulder girdle and your posterior back is useful for lifting your pack and for using handholds and ski poles. Strengthening your lower body is important for longer and more challenging trips and to be able to handle steep trails, uneven terrain, or deep snow.

Hiking/Backpacking

The strength training program outlined below is the maximum suggested. You may want to start with a few exercises from each category and build up gradually to doing the entire group. Exercises that involve hops need only be added if you will be crossing rivers or boulder fields. Make sure you do squats and lunges for 4 weeks before adding hops. It is a good idea to vary the lunges you do at each workout.

Lower body: Exercises 70, 95, 97, 97.3, 97.5, 98, 99, 99.3, 99.4, 101, and 101.3.

Abdominals: Exercises 78 (or variations 78.1, 78.2, or 78.3), 82, 84, and 92.

Upper body: Exercises 117.4, 120, 121.1, 123, 124, 125–127, and 131.

Upper/lower body: Exercises 28 and 36 (optional).

Snowshoeing

Do the strength exercises for hiking and backpacking, above, with the following modifications:

Lower body: Add Exercise 97.11.

Abdominals: Add Exercise 86.

Upper body: Add Exercise 127.

Upper/lower body: Add Exercises 31, 34.1, 35.1.

BALANCE AND AGILITY

Consider doing balance exercises within 4–6 weeks of beginning your outdoor activity, to improve your stability on boulder fields, logs, slopes, snow, and river crossings. You can do them twice a week for 5–10 minutes and make them part of your strength workout. Try doing them with a backpack after you have mastered them. If you have kneecap problems and you experience pain with balance exercises, try doing them with ski poles to decrease the weight on your knees.

Hiking/Backpacking

Do BST Exercises 49 and 53, and Exercises 58.1, 58.2, 59.1, 59.3, and 61.

Snowshoeing

Do the above plus Exercise 60.1.

Weight-Shifting Exercises

Weight-shifting awareness and movement are useful techniques for backpackers and snowshoers, especially on river crossings or on steep or unsteady terrain while using high stepping motions (see chapter 25 for a discussion of weight-shifting). Get an idea of how you can move your torso and body weight with more weight on the forward foot so there is optimum weight balance between your feet (and your hands, if there is a handhold or you are using ski poles or a walking stick), so that you can extend your forward knee and move onto that foot in the most stable way possible.

Experiment with weight-shifting while doing step-up Exercises 70.1, 70.2, 70.3, and 98 to find the amount of weight-shifting to your forward foot that gives you the optimum combination of momentum and balance. You can do this outdoors while stepping onto a rock or log or a high step on a trail. Too much weight-shifting forward can lead you to fall forward or cause too much flexing of your low back. In town, try this with a backpack to really notice the importance of weight-shifting. If you are a snowshoer you can use poles during the exercise.

PACK POSTURE

Many people with heavy packs overcompensate in their posture and get into positions of excessive flexion of their back, shoulders, and neck. This can lead to pain. It is more likely to happen when you are tired and on steep hills. It can also happen if the top of the pack or equipment is pushing your neck forward.

Intermittently check your body to see that you are in a reasonable pack-carrying posture.

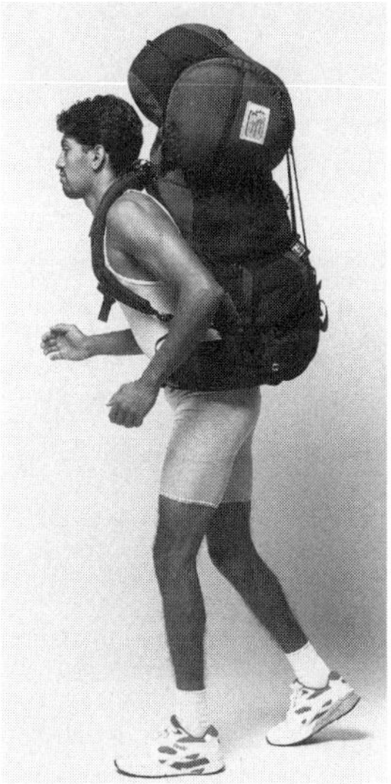

FIGURE 33.
Poor posture.

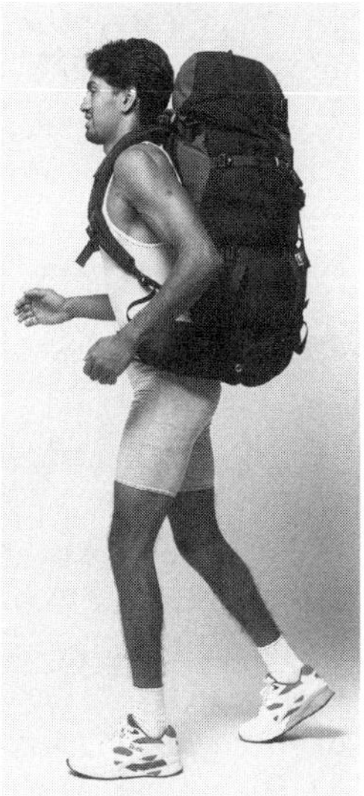

FIGURE 34.
Good posture.

Good pack posture means having your head aligned over your shoulders and looking out onto the terrain or out at the scenery. Have your low back in a neutral position and not slumped forward. Practice Exercise 182 without a pack. Then practice it with a pack or using only low back movement in a much more limited motion (avoid excessive flexing).

It is also important to have well-padded hip straps and secure them on the crest of your pelvic bone so that you carry most of the weight there and not on your shoulders. Carrying excessive weight on your shoulders can lead to shoulder and neck pain, or tingling in the fingers.

In Figure 33, notice the forward head and excessively flexed posture. In Figure 34, the neck and low back are in a more neutral position.

Pack Types and Fit

A pack should be large enough to carry your gear in a comfortable and balanced way. There should be enough room so you don't have to stuff gear in the top in such a manner that your neck is pushed forward. The pack should not sway very much from side to side when you bend slightly to the right or left; this will challenge your back and legs excessively. The waist belt should be very well padded and rest comfortably on the crest of your hips.

Packs: Getting Them Safely On and Off

It is important to use proper body mechanics when lifting your pack. This is a time of increased risk for a back injury. Always bend with your knees rather than your back. When putting a heavy pack on, try squatting down in front of the right-hand pack strap, with your right knee in front of the left. Your right knee can either be on the ground or within $1^{1}/_{2}$ feet of the ground, but should be close to the pack. Your back should be relatively straight.

Raise the pack up to rest on your right thigh, then put your right arm in the strap (see Figure 35a). Stand up carefully using both legs, and minimize any extending in your back (see Figure 35b). If you have back problems, place the pack on one knee and lean it against a tree trunk or a boulder to make it easier to get it on. Removing and lowering your pack requires care and is basically the reverse of this.

Avoid picking up your pack by bending forward and rotating at your low back and then

FIGURE 35a

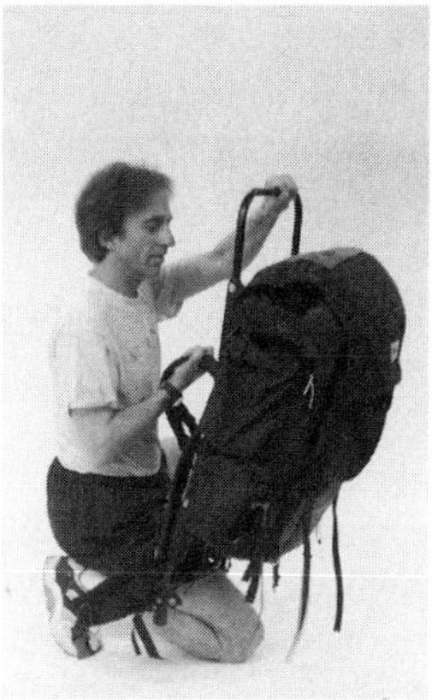

FIGURE 35b

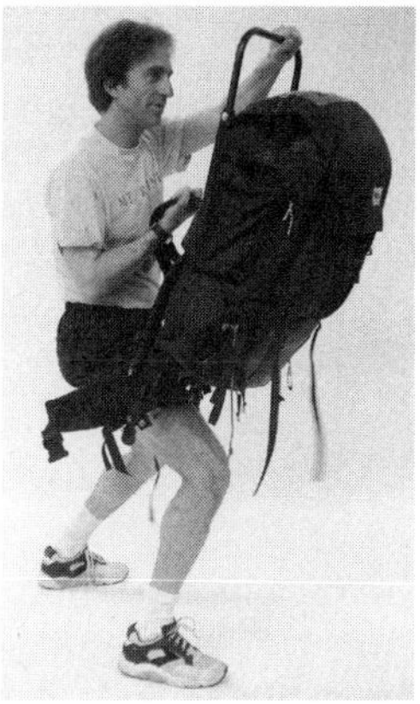

extending your back. These are the positions most likely to lead to injury. A back injury is more likely with a heavy pack, but it can happen while lifting even a light pack improperly, so always use good lifting principles (see chapter 14 for further lifting details).

BOOTS AND STABILITY

The boots you wear can influence how stable you feel on a hike or a snowshoe trip. If you plan on crossing rivers, logs, scree slopes, or boulder fields, you need a full leather boot or a leather combination boot with reinforcement in the heel area. The sole should resist excessive twisting. If you can twist your boot more than 25 degrees (with the top of the boot as 0 degrees, use one hand to twist where the heel meets the sole and keep the other hand on the forefoot), your boot may not be stable enough for any significant backpacking. Try out a boot by doing this twisting test as well as by standing and balancing on one leg and moving your arms in different directions to see how stable you feel. Boots can be too stiff or heavy if you are planning on light day hiking with few balance challenges. For snowshoeing, choose boots that are stable as well as warm. Refer to chapter 13 for further information on shoe fit.

Walking Uphill

Try to avoid excessively long strides or high footholds when hiking uphill. If you have kneecap pain going uphill, focus more attention on step-up exercises, such as Exercises 70 and 98, and practice weight-shifting with a step height of 6 inches or less. Gradually increase the step height to approximate the step reach you want to be able to do in the outdoors.

Walking Downhill

Walking downhill demands lower-extremity deceleration to counter the forces of gravity. The muscles that are most important are the quads, hamstrings, buttock/hip girdle, and calf muscles.

> **PRACTICAL POINT**
>
> It is very important to take breaks and not go too fast when you are walking downhill, even though it may feel less taxing aerobically. There are a lot of forces on your kneecaps when you walk downhill. You can decrease the likelihood of kneecap or thigh muscle pain by taking breaks every 1–1 1/2 hours, by using trekking poles, and by doing Exercises 99, 99.3, and 99.4.

GOAL PROGRAMS

Hiking/backpacking. A 16-mile, 2- to 3-day backpacking trip, or a day hike of 8–10 miles, each with 4,000 feet elevation gain.

In general, 8 weeks of preparation should be adequate. Do the aerobic program listed earlier in this chapter. Include the strength training program listed earlier in this chapter 2 days a week with 2 sets of 15–20 reps. You can add a lower-repetition (8–12), higher-resistance set if you wish to build more strength. Try to incorporate some balance activities into your program during the last month. When you have achieved a 6-mile, 2,500-foot-elevation-gain hike, you will be ready for a longer day hike or backpacking trip. If you are already doing a minimum aerobic and strength program, preparation may take less than 6 weeks.

Snowshoeing. A whole day of moderate snowshoeing, approximately 6 miles with a 2,000- to 3,000-foot elevation gain.

Proceed as in the hiking/backpacking example above, but do more lower-body strengthening and balance work earlier. Use hikes, cross-country skiing, jogging, stair climbing, or snowshoeing for your lower-intensity, longer-duration (LILD) activity. If you use aerobic modes other than snowshoeing, begin shorter snowshoe training activities before your first long trip because of the unique hip and buttock demands of snowshoeing. When you are able to do 4 miles with 1,500–2,000 feet of elevation gain, you should be ready for your longer trip. Give this at least 8 weeks of preparation time.

chapter 18 CONDITIONING FOR SCRAMBLING AND ROCK CLIMBING

By Dan Cauthorn

THIS CHAPTER WILL HELP YOU:

- Understand the special muscle, joint, and movement demands unique to technical climbing.
- Do a dynamic strength training program designed to prepare you for a full day of climbing.
- Create a flexible, 4- to 6-month periodization planning program to develop specific climbing strength, endurance, and technique to achieve these specific goals:
    1. A 10-mile-round-trip, strenuous Class 3 rock scramble.
    2. A multipitch (6–8 pitches) technical Class 5 rock climb.
    3. Thirty minutes of steep (vertical to overhanging) sport/gym climbing.

Scrambling and rock and sport climbing have unique and exacting strength, endurance, coordination, balance, and psychological demands. Overall strength, with special attention to your upper body, and especially your fingers, is a prerequisite to any climbing endeavor. In standard climbing classification, scrambling is basically an aerobic activity of off-trail hiking and mountain peak ascents that involves use of your hands and legs with nontechnical climbing. A scrambling ascent is rated Class 2 or 3 (see Cox and Fulsaas, *Freedom of the Hills*).

Layered onto the physical demands are the complex movements and problem solving skills required for success on steep and exposed terrain. Improving your functional strength and balance can help decrease injuries and enhance performance, and can help you achieve your climbing goals whatever your climbing level.

MUSCULOSKELETAL DEMANDS

In climbers, muscles increase in lactic acid, cramping, and swelling. Many climbers call this "getting pumped." Sport climbers often fail because their arms get pumped and they can no longer hold on. Improving lower-body strength and endurance, often overlooked by new climbers, can help you climb more efficiently and provide rest for your upper body. The muscles in your hand and forearm, along with the supporting muscles of your shoulder and back, also can be strengthened so that you are less likely to get pumped and more able to continue climbing.

Lower Body

Your buttocks, hamstrings, quads, and calves all play significant roles while climbing. Training for strength and muscle balance in your legs is important. Good climbers raise their bodies with their powerful leg and buttock muscles, carefully conserving the strength in their arms. Your lower body also must perform extreme ranges of motion, especially in the flexing of your hips and knees in high stepping on trails, snow, or walls with high footholds (see Figure 36). The climber attempts to rise up from that position using muscles that are in a most disadvantageous position.

Hip and thigh strains can be minimized with

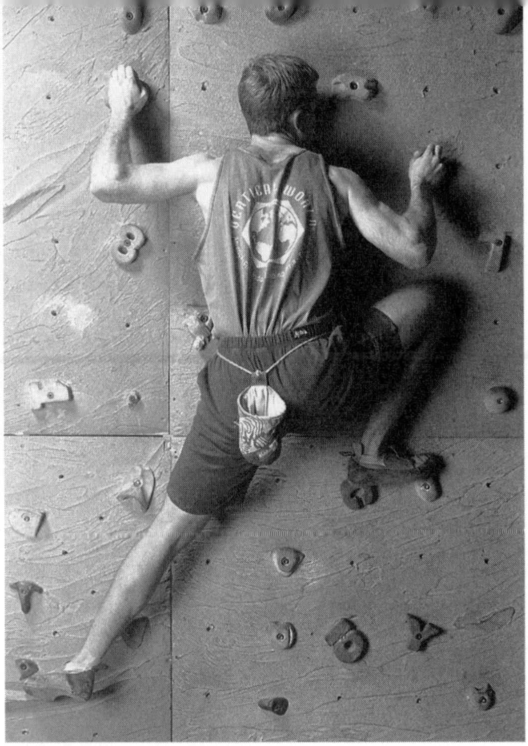

FIGURE 36. High stepping.

proper training during a gradual progression of strengthening exercises to simulate using higher and higher footholds or step heights (if you are training for snow or nonwall terrain). Principles of weight shifting are important to optimize your body position to make these moves more efficient and easier on your body. (See chapter 25 for information on weight shifting.)

Practice stepping exercises (Exercises 70 and 98) using weight-shifting techniques.

Core/Back

Your back is involved in just about every climbing motion. Moves are performed in positions in which your neck and back are very extended, bent, or rotated. Then a climbing move is attempted while your core is twisted at the end of its motion range. Injuries to your back can occur, which may be quite debilitating and even dangerous if you are in the middle of a long climb. Tips to prevent such injuries include:

- Avoid lifting heavy gear with your back; instead, lift with your legs and buttocks (see chapters 14 and 17).
- Train your abdominal muscles.
- Practice some weight-shifting climbing techniques so you move your core (torso, back, and abdomen) and center of gravity well, to preserve your strength. Avoid quick extending motions while hyperextending, as well as quick flexed, rotated positions, especially with a loaded pack.

Upper Body

Climbing activities vary in their requirement for upper-body strength. Generally, the demand increases as the angle of the climb gets steeper and the holds get smaller and farther apart. Scrambling involves a lot of pushing, dipping, rowing, and pull-up maneuvers at different angles but with large hand- and footholds. Technical climbing exerts similar demands on your upper body but usually on steeper pitches with smaller holds. There are more significant demands for strength in your shoulder, upper back, forearm, and fingers. The joints and muscles of these regions are often stressed at various lengths and disadvantageous angles.

Most climbing is done in the forearm pronated position, when your palm is facing the wall. Climbers should do most of their pull-ups in this position.

Movement Demands

Perhaps the most important element concerning the demands of climbing is the actual movement patterns. The ability to move your center of gravity and core in good coordination with your arms and legs is very important and can decrease the strength demands on certain muscles. Training, through climbing-movement drills and exercises to memorize movement patterns (or develop "engrams"), is important. (Refer to Goddard and Neumann, *Performance Rock Climbing* for more details on engrams.)

There are many movement patterns or "moves" that can be practiced on boulders, on rock walls, or on indoor walls. These moves can be practiced by experimenting with hand, feet, and body positioning, and with weight shifting, to find the technique that seems to be most efficient and requires the least effort. It is better to move in ways that don't require putting joints in the end of their range, if possible. Practicing a move with efficient technique can help you integrate moves into a repertoire that you can use when you encounter similar climbing challenges, thus climbing more efficiently and quickly. Good technique and accompanying strength gains are fostered by training specifically to develop balance, weight-shifting skills, and efficient and relaxed moves.

MUSCLE IMBALANCES

Muscle imbalances are common among climbers. The climbing muscles like your chest, lats, biceps, and forearm and finger flexors tend to get strong fast. Muscles that tend to be underdeveloped are your finger/wrist extensors, triceps, rotator cuff, and your lower to mid trapezius. Balancing these muscle groups with training can be important for avoiding injury.

WARM-UP

Try the dynamic warm-up drills in chapter 4. Do all of them, or at least the aerobic and stretching components.

STRETCHING

Scramblers and climbers should do Exercises 1, 3.1, 3.3, 5, 7–9, 11, 13, 16, and 19.

AEROBIC CONDITIONING

The aerobic demands of climbing can be graded from the higher demands of scrambling to the lower demands of multipitch climbing to sport climbing. Aerobic training that is more specific for climbing includes running, hiking, using a treadmill, stair climbing and using stair-climber machines, using rotating climbing walls, using rowing machines, step or high-impact aerobics classes, and using cross-country ski machines. Other aerobic activities can be done intermittently, but are not well suited for training the climbing muscles.

Scrambling

This type of climbing is primarily aerobic. The moves are lower strength, but must be sustained over a long period of time. Most scrambles are 8–12 miles with 3,500–5,000 feet elevation gain. The scrambler should follow and make modifications to the aerobic program for hiking and backpacking in chapter 17. Start increasing your aerobic training within 3 months of your first scramble climb.

Do 4–5 short aerobic sessions per week with sport-specific activities (at least two of these sessions should be 40–50 minutes in length; the others could be 30 minutes). You can do a few aerobic activities in one session to add up to 50 minutes. Nonmachine stair climbing is excellent aerobic training and should be done 1–2 times per week within 6 weeks of your first scramble. Vary your activity with running or fast-walking single, double, or triple stairs.

Start a low-intensity, longer-duration (LILD) activity within 6–8 weeks of your first scramble (this could be a hike or a snowshoe or cross-country ski trip). Each week increase the duration and elevation of your LILD trip until you have reached approximately three-fourths of the mileage and elevation of your first planned scramble. If you anticipate a scramble on snow, make sure some of your training trips involve some snow hiking.

Consider some Fartlek-type interval training 1–2 times per week within 6 weeks of your first scramble. Doing intervals of 30–120 seconds while on a training hike or on aerobic equipment could more quickly improve your aerobic fitness. (See chapter 3 for information on Fartlek interval training.)

Multipitch Climbing

Follow the aerobic training schedule for scramblers, above, but your LILD trips can be shorter to simulate the distances of your approach to your climb. A climber should do training hikes or scrambles, beginning within 6 weeks of the first climb, with a climbing pack of similar weight as would be carried on the approach to the climb. It is important to have enough muscular endurance so that carrying a heavy pack does not drain you before the climb actually begins.

The activity of climbing on a moderate (up to 5.8) multipitch climb can be aerobic if there are long, easy stretches on which a climber can move relatively quickly, and the climbing moves don't seem very difficult to the endurance- and strength-trained climber. On more difficult terrain, the climber moves much more slowly, and strength and power are very important.

Don't forget how strenuous a descent can be in terms of aerobic, strength, and balance demands. Descending even simple terrain can be aerobically strenuous for a tired climber after a long, multipitch climb. Take it slowly and take intermittent breaks for rest, fluid, and food.

Sport Climbing

Sport climbing is characterized by being steep, powerful, and short, and is not usually aerobic but is primarily anaerobic. Much sport climbing is done in climbing clubs and requires only minimum aerobic conditioning. The approaches and descents from the climbing area itself present the aerobic challenges. These can vary greatly according to the climbing area.

Do the minimum aerobic program outlined in chapter 3, with climbing-specific modes of exercise.

Add a LILD activity 1 time per week if your climbs involve a long approach hike.

STRENGTH TRAINING

The following exercises to help you develop strength can be done in conjunction with the climbing-specific exercises at the end of this chapter.

If you are short on time, you can do 1 set each of the abdominal (ab) exercises. Do 2 sets of the other exercises. Do them 2–3 times per week. Climbers and scramblers should start 8–12 weeks before their season. You can do all of your strength exercises on 1 day (2 longer strength exercise sessions per week) or do split sessions (4 shorter sessions per week).

Scramblers

Lower body: Exercises 34, 36, 70, 95.2, 95.4, 97.3, 99, and 120. Alternate Exercise 36 with 70 and Exercise 34 with 120. Focus on Exercise 70 for your step-ups. Add Exercises 30, 106, and 101.3 after 1 1/2 months of strength training.

Abdominals: Exercises 72, 78.1–78.3, 79, 83–85, 86 (with both feet on the floor), 87, and 92.

Upper body: Exercises 34, 115 (or 130.1), 117 (all variations), 120, 120.3, 121, 123, 127, 128.2 (gradually work up to a less assisted dip and chin-up), and 131. Spend more time on your dips than on push-ups.

Forearm and hand (start within 4 weeks of your first scramble): Exercises 137 and 138.

Level I Climbers

Lower body: Do the first exercises listed in the scrambling program above, and add Exercise 35. Alternate Exercise 35 or 36 with 48 and Exercise 34 with 120.

Abdominals: Do the scrambling program above, but omit Exercise 87.

Upper body: Do the scrambling program above, omitting the Exercise 130.1 option.

Forearm and hand: Exercises 137–141.

Level 2 Climbers

These exercises are recommended for sport and more advanced outdoor climbing. Do the Level 1 program with the following modifications.

Lower body: Add Exercises 30 or 31, and also 35.1, 35.3, 95.1, 95.2, 100.1, 101.1, and 106. Do your step-ups with high steps, working up to a step on a chair, a step over 3 steps, or a high step onto a boulder or bleacher, or other similar object.

Abdominals: Add Exercises 78.4, 82, 85 (with a pack on), 86 (balancing on one foot), and 93.

Upper body: Work up to fully unassisted dips and pull-ups. In some of your workouts, substitute Exercises 77 or 130 for 115, 132 for 120, and 133 for 131. Add Exercises 20, 112, 113, 120.2, 120.3, 122, 135, and 136.

Forearm and hand: Add fingerboard exercises (Exercise 147) after 6 weeks of a basic upper-body program.

Timing and Periodization

In general, begin a climbing-specific conditioning program at least 8 weeks prior to your first scramble or climb. If your first climb requires a great deal of finger, forearm, and general strength training, it is better to start 10–12 weeks before your climbing season.

For serious climbers, a year-round strategy is ultimately the best. In the late fall, begin basic overall training that includes strengthening exercises with 3 sets of 15–25 reps to build an endurance strength base, and do more climbing-specific aerobic training. The goal is to build a fitness base of aerobic and strength endurance. If you have access to a climbing gym or bouldering area, you can start some light climbing (especially traversing) after 4 weeks of your basic strengthening program. You can also start some basic weight-shifting exercises. It is good to begin some relaxation work early so that you can learn to calm yourself down in tense situations.

After 2 months, increase climbing volume (time on the wall or hanging on fingers) and do some of your strength training (1–2 sets) with reps of 8–12 to build more strength.

After a few more months, build specific climbing strength by working harder on finger and forearm strength, and consider some redpoint training (see Exercise 149).

During this period you may do 1–2 strength training sets with 6–8 reps in a set for maximum strength development. This period before your active climbing season should also be a time to increase the duration of a 1-day-a-week LILD distance if you will be training for climbs that involve an approach of more than a few miles.

During the climbing season have a 2- to 3-day break between a strength training day and a climb. Take a month off from climbing at the end of the season to rest, and continue a base of aerobic and strength training to keep in shape.

BALANCE AND AGILITY

Scramblers and Level 1 climbers should do Exercises 57.4, 59.1, 60.1, and 61.

Level 2 climbers should do the above program, but substitute Exercise 59.3 for 59.1.

GOAL PROGRAMS

Minimum Climbing or Scrambling Program

This is a combination of a scrambling or Level 1 climbing strength training program with traverses (see Exercise 143) and the aerobic program recommended in this chapter for your activity. With this program you can create a base of strength endurance and technique that will enable you to participate in a full day of climbing (i.e., a moderate/novice climb or a strenuous, all-day scramble).

At the end of Week 8 you should be ready for some easy climbs. Do flexibility work with each training session. Weeks 1–8 consist of building the base.

Weeks 1–2: Start very lightly and increase gradually until you can do a set of 15–20 reps before you fatigue. Do 2–3 sets of each strength training exercise for Level 1. Do Exercises 142 and 143.

Weeks 3–4: Strength workout: Two times per week, 2–3 sets each exercise, 12–15 reps of each exercise, gradually increasing the resistance or degree of difficulty of the exercises. Do 30 minutes of climbing 2 times per week. Do Exercises 142 and 143.

Weeks 5–8: Strength workout: Decrease reps to 8–12 per set and do 2–3 sets of each exercise. Do the Week 4 climbing exercises the same, but add Exercises 144, 145, and 148. Gradually increase the difficulty of Exercise 148 (endurance climbing).

Advanced Climbing Goal Periodization Programs

This program trains for techniques and additional strength required in steep, technical climbing. One basic goal is to accomplish a multipitch Grade III or IV rock climb and/or to increase your rock climbing standard by two number grades. Two or 3 months in a goal program should get you ready for all but the most demanding climbing. Remember: Your ability to accomplish a climb successfully is related to many factors besides your conditioning program, including your age, frame size, amount of muscle mass, preexisting injuries, arm and leg lengths, and technique. There is no guarantee that every person completing a goal program will be able to safely complete a climb.

Incorporate a goal program schedule after 8 weeks of the minimum program above, or the equivalent if you are already doing a part of the minimum program. Do flexibility work with each training session. Follow the aerobic guidelines in this chapter.

Weeks 9–15: Do a weight workout 2 times per week. During this time you may want to do 1 set of 15–20 reps for endurance and 2 sets of 8–10 reps for strength. Add the specific forearm and finger exercise in this period as listed in the Level 2 strength program in this chapter. Do climbing-specific exercises 2 times per week. Warm up and divide your workout between Exercises 143–145, 148, and 149.

Weeks 16–24: Sport-specific: Do a weight workout (same as for Weeks 9–15) and consider increasing the finger/forearm strengthening exercises with more emphasis on fingerboards (Exercise 147). Do climbing exercises 2 times a week: Exercises 143–146, 148, and 149.

Weeks 25–41: Climbing season maintenance: Do a weight workout 2 times per week. Leave 2–3 days between a weight workout and a climb. Do 30 minutes of aerobic exercise 3 times per week and 1 hour of climbing twice per week (warm up, and do Exercises 142, 143, 146, and 149).

CLIMBING-SPECIFIC EXERCISES

These exercises are to be used on climbing walls. Do them in conjunction with the strength training program in this chapter.

142 CLIMBING REST POSITION FOR YOUR FINGERS AND BODY

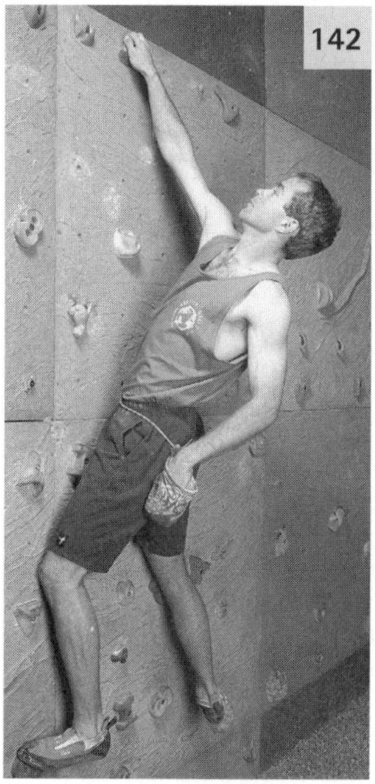

Equipment: Climbing wall (indoor or outdoor) or fingerboard; chalk, tape (to reinforce fingers), rock shoes (slippers are actually best because they help strengthen and train your feet and legs).
Purpose: Warming up your fingers is an essential start to any climbing-specific workout. Initially this exercise is the first step in building fundamental finger strength, weight-shifting skills, and climbing technique. Eventually it becomes a quick prelude to a full workout.

Technique: On a large handhold or the biggest hold on a fingerboard, hang comfortably off a single, straight arm. This is the rest position and is a fundamental technique to any type of climbing. Your feet should also be on good holds (or on the ground). Your legs should be straight and relaxed, hips pressed in, and your back arched. Do 5 seconds on one arm, then switch hands and hang 5 seconds on the other. This position should become second nature. As a warm-up, repeat this process 3 times, resting 20–30 seconds between exercises.

143 TRAVERSING

Equipment: Climbing wall, rock climbing shoes.
Purpose: Do easy climbing sideways back and forth across the wall to practice technique, train your forearms, and begin to develop climbing-specific muscle endurance.

Technique: Traversing can be done solo. You never need to get more than 1 foot off the ground. Begin climbing for 10-minute sessions. Rest 10 minutes, and then climb continuously for another 5 minutes. Build up to 10 minutes climbing, 10 minutes resting, then repeat. With good traversing technique, the climber moves with hips parallel to the wall, shuffling the hands and feet in one direction or the other. Try not to cross hands or feet, and stay on the inside edges of your rock shoes. Imagine Spiderman moving sideways across a wall.

WEIGHT-SHIFTING EXERCISES

The purpose of good weight-shifting is to coordinate the movement of the core of your body to your extremity motions so that you are balanced and move with the least muscular effort. The following exercises will help you to develop skill in moving your center of gravity and extremities while maintaining your balance on a wall.

144 FIVE MOVING PARTS

Equipment: Climbing wall, rock climbing shoes.
Purpose: Develop weight-shifting skills while traversing.

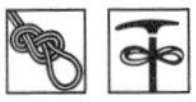

Technique: Imagine that you have five body parts that move when you climb: two hands, two feet, and one torso. Start in a rest position, and then try to climb by moving each part separately and distinctly from the others. Start in the crunch position (144a). Move your left hand to a hold (144b). Then move your right hand to a hold (144c). Then move your left foot up (144d). Then move your right foot up (144e). Then move your core/torso (144f). Have a friend watch you and announce which body part should move, i.e., "hand, hand, foot, body . . . " Never move any two parts at once.
Variations: 144.1. Core move: Try moving your core (back, abdomen, and chest) before you move your legs or your arms. Try to do this smoothly and move a foot or hand when you have first shifted your weight to get yourself in an ideal position for the next move. **144.2.** Next, try moving your core while you initiate an arm or leg motion, to determine the best combination of movements.

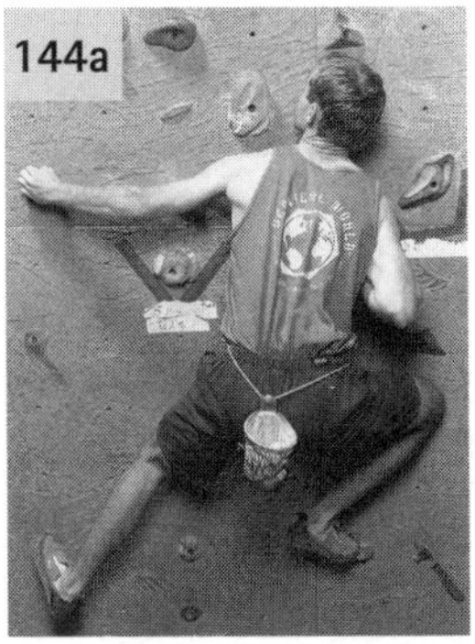

144a

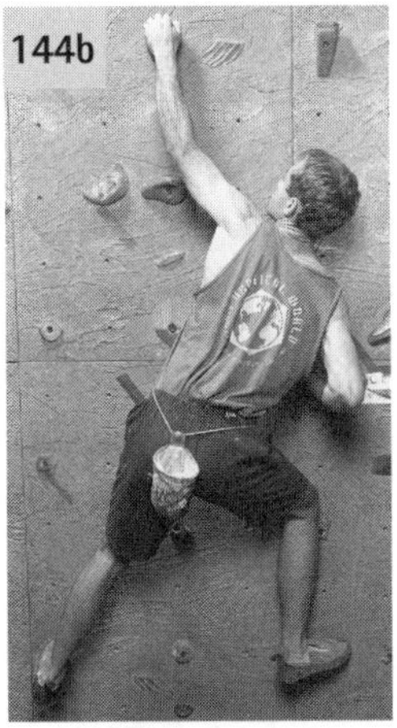

144b

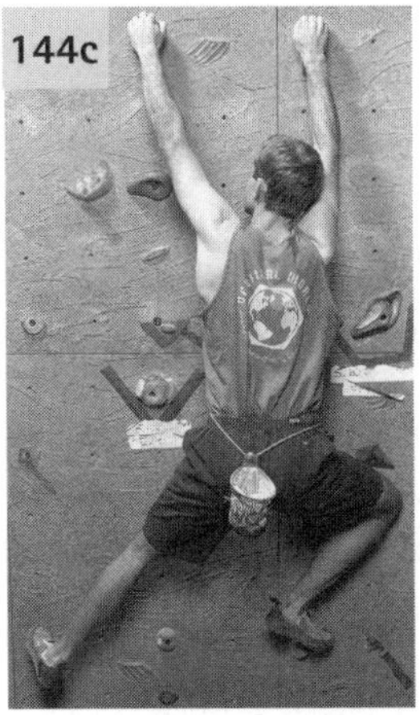

144c

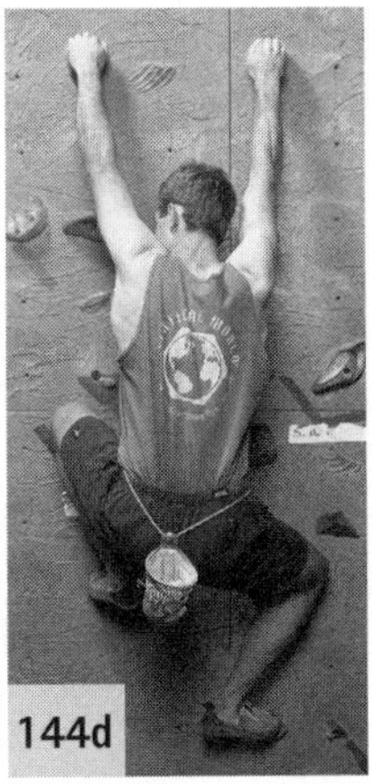

144d

145 ROUND-THE-CLOCK WEIGHT SHIFTING

Equipment: Climbing wall, rock climbing shoes.
Purpose: Improve your balance abilities and efficiency of motion on a climbing wall.

Technique: Locate four suitable holds in a square configuration (two handholds and two footholds). Have both hands and feet on the holds, with hips parallel to the wall. Now move your body around in a circle: shift your weight to the right (145a), then down, then across to the left (145b), up, then back to the middle. Never remove a hand or foot. Feel how shifting your hip and torso positions weights or unweights certain areas. Gradually enlarge your range of motion as you feel more comfortable.

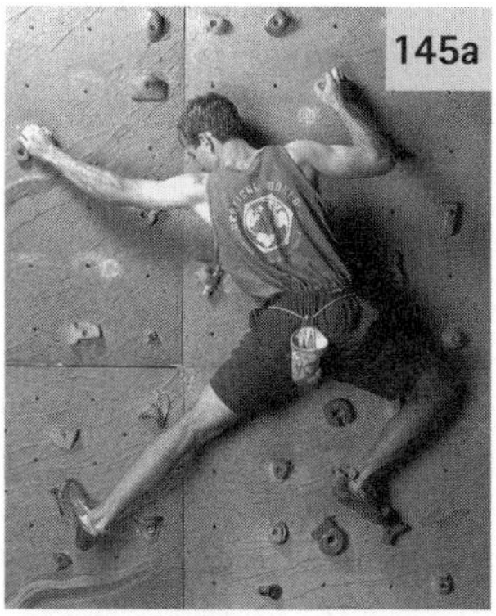
145a

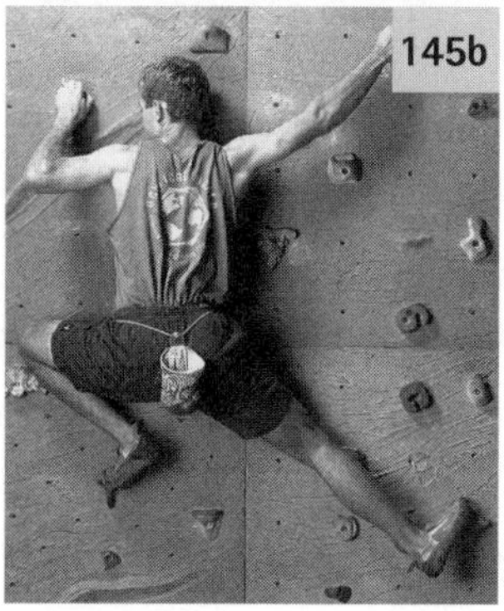
145b

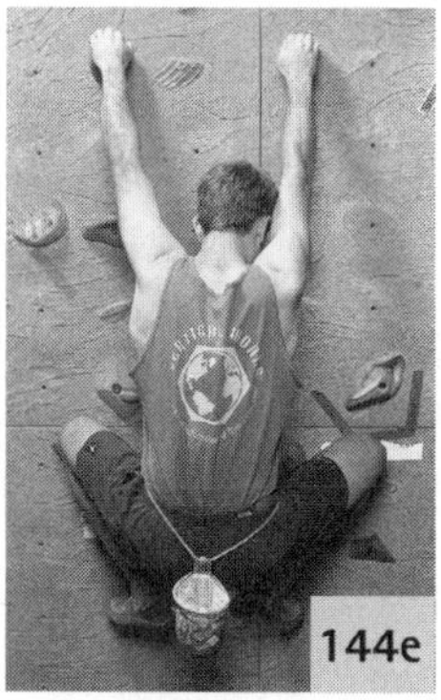
144e

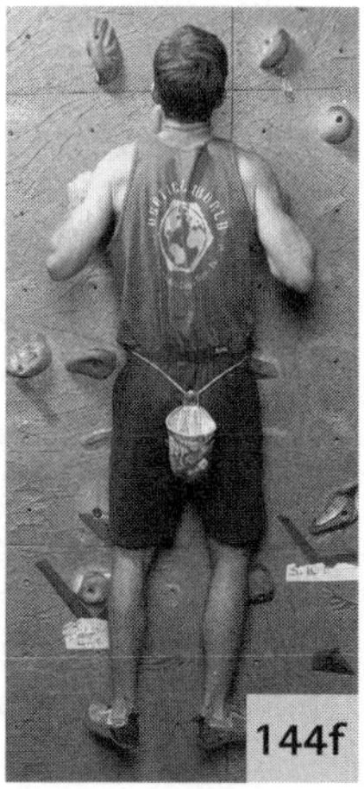
144f

146 FLAGGING

Equipment: Climbing wall, rock climbing shoes.
Purpose: Further improve your balance and weight-shifting on a wall.

Technique: To try flagging out, reach up and to the right with your right hand while lifting your left foot as a counterweight, so you can lean and reach farther to the right. Only your left hand and right foot have weight-bearing contact with the wall (see 146a). Then, to flag in, shift your weight to your left foot and cross your right leg behind your left leg as a counterweight that balances you so you can reach with your right hand up and over your left hand (see 146b). The only two points of contact at this point are your left hand and your left foot. You can try alternating between these positions as you warm up.
Variations: Incorporate other combinations of hand- and footholds.

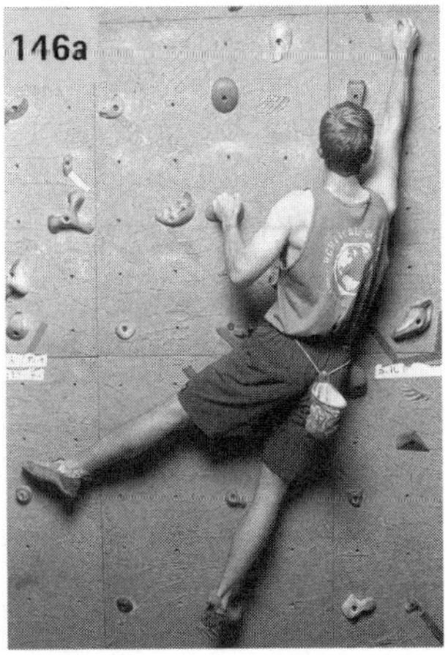
146a

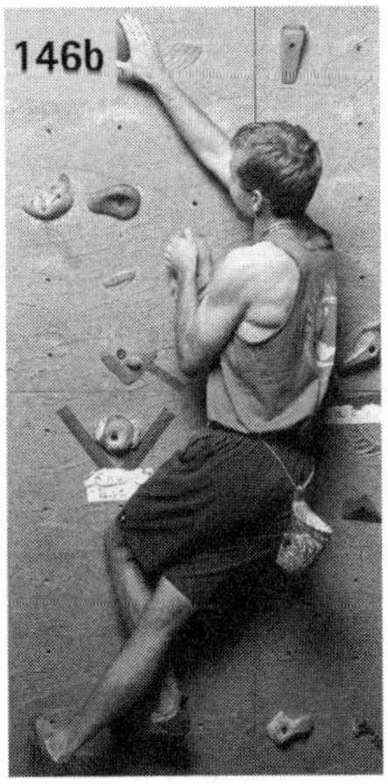
146b

147 FINGERBOARDS

Equipment: Fingerboard.
Purpose: Fingerboards are very effective tools for climbing-specific upper-body strength training. Novice climbers are advised to build a base of strength training before starting fingerboard exercises.

Technique: On a fingerboard, position yourself with an open grip, with your elbows slightly flexed and your lats activated (see 147a). An endurance workout on a fingerboard consists of long, timed hangs off large holds. Try not to hang in a "dead hang" with your weight supported by fully extended shoulders and elbows (see 147b). Note that at this level, appropriate techniques for training will sometimes differ from what is proper technique for climbing. For example, the rest position used while climbing has the climber relaxing all body weight on a straight arm. The "dead hang" is OK while climbing. Also, don't crimp on a fingerboard; use the open grip (see 147c). If you can't hang onto a particular hold without crimping, then don't use that hold. Wait until you have built up sufficient strength to use an open grip.

Variations: 147.1. Time hang: Time yourself for your maximum hang time on a large hold. Rest for at least 2 minutes and repeat your maximum hang. Try to get through the routine 3 times. **147.2.** Try the "20/20": Hang for 20 seconds, then rest for 20 seconds. Repeat 10 times. When you can accomplish the 20/20 on the biggest hold, move to smaller and/or sloping holds. **147.3.** Smaller holds, maximum hang time: Power workouts demand maximum effort of a short duration. Longer rests between sets are necessary. Working on smaller holds is one way to increase power. Time yourself for maximum hang time on progressively smaller holds. Record the number of pull-ups you can do on the smallest hold. If the hang time exceeds 10 seconds, or you can do more than 5 pull-ups, move to smaller holds. Or add resistance (in 2-pound increments) by hanging weight off your chalk bag belt. Adding weight to yourself and then performing pull-ups on a fingerboard is one of the most effective means of increasing finger power for extreme sport climbing. Only attempt this after a very good base of finger strength has been developed.
Tips and Precautions: Always begin a fingerboard workout with a warm-up consisting of 5–10 minutes of easy hanging off big holds. Hang long enough to get your forearms warmed up, but not pumped. Then start the endurance workout on the largest hold.

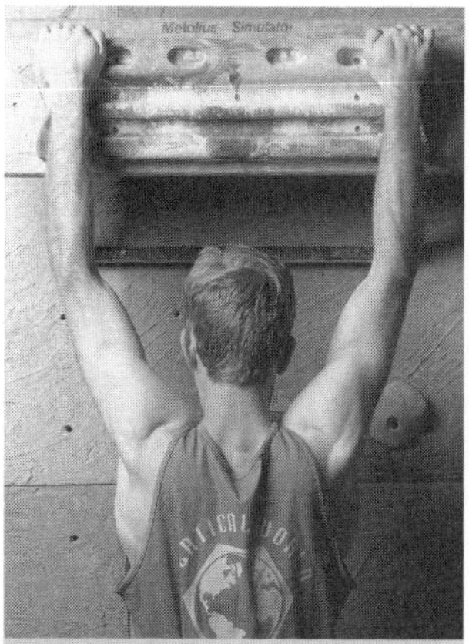

147a. Yes: activate your lats when you hang.

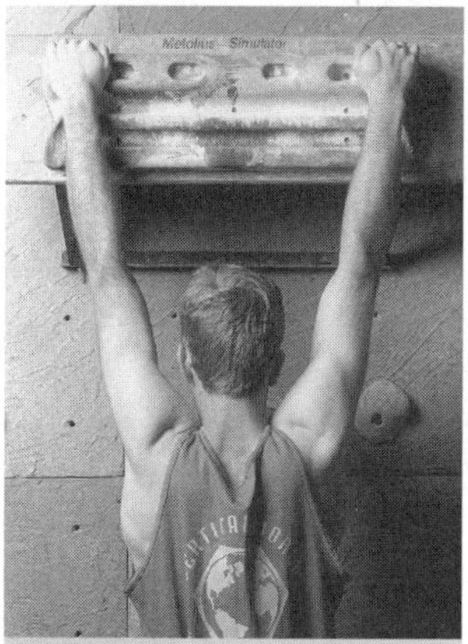

147b. No: don't hang with fully suspended shoulders.

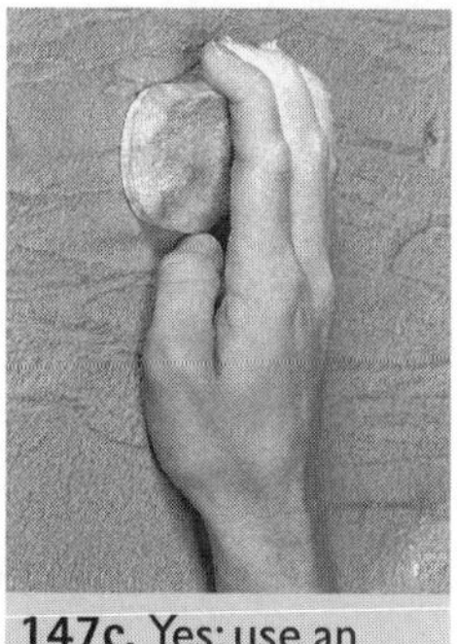

147c. Yes: use an open grip instead of crimping.

148 ENDURANCE CLIMBING

Equipment: Climbing wall, rock climbing shoes.
Purpose: Build climbing-specific endurance by using high repetitions with low resistance.

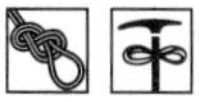

Technique: Choose a relatively easy climb and do "laps" on it. The goal is to climb until you are pumped due to muscle failure. Technical difficulty is not an issue, but the climbing surface must be at least vertical. An excellent goal in a bouldering situation is 30 minutes of continuous climbing, either traversing back and forth, climbing up then down (don't touch the ground), or some creative combination. Try to simulate a long pitch, where you've got to take advantage of rests, move through cruxes, and sometimes downclimb to figure out a problem. If you are top-roping with a partner, take turns climbing several laps in a row on a single climb. Climb to the top, get lowered back to the ground, and then immediately begin climbing again. Build to 5 laps on a typical half-rope-length top-rope climb. In either scenario, the ideal wall is difficult enough that you can just complete the task. If you can't get pumped on a vertical wall, move to progressively steeper and steeper terrain.

149 REDPOINTING

Equipment: Climbing wall, rock climbing shoes.
Purpose: In redpointing, you spend numerous attempts working each section of a specific route. Figure out individual moves by resting on the rope (or "hang dogging") to relax between attempts. The goal is to link each section together without falling on the redpoint attempt. Redpointing generally refers to leading a route without falling, but the concept of working a route to build power can be applied to top-roping or bouldering. It is climbing at, or attempting to push, your limit.

Technique: Pick a hard route, and begin breaking it down into manageable sections. Figuring out each move, and then linking them all, can be a process that takes hours, days, weeks, even months. With each hard move accomplished, you get a little better. Warm up well before a hard session. Use the rating system to keep track of your progress. Breaking through the threshold of each higher grade is one of the more rewarding moments for every climber. The 5.10 level is traditionally a major step for a recreational climber. There are several excellent resources to learn about the complexities of hard redpoint climbing (see Horst, *Flash Training*, and Goddard and Neumann, *Performance Rock Climbing*, in Selected References).

chapter 19 CONDITIONING FOR MOUNTAINEERING

By David Musnick, M.D.

THIS CHAPTER WILL HELP YOU:

- Understand the aerobic and strength demands of mountaineering.
- Plan an exercise program to train to climb a mountain or do significant trekking.

Climbing a mountain with rock, snow, and glacier terrain requires significant aerobic endurance, strength, and balance abilities. Your goal is to get to the top (and get back down), injury free, with the least amount of fatigue. The combination of altitude, heavy loads, difficult and steep terrain, and exposure make it mandatory to modify your conditioning program. Plan a minimum of 12 weeks to train for most mountaineering activities.

MUSCULOSKELETAL DEMANDS

The movement demands of mountaineering are similar to those for climbing (see chapter 18). In addition, there may be more demands on your lower body to take high or long steps without the use of your arms; to do this, it is important to maximize your body positioning.

This can be done by weight-shifting (see chapter 25 for more information on weight-shifting). Practice taking progressively higher steps with Exercises 70 and 98 within 4–6 weeks of your first mountaineering trip. Add a moderately heavy pack to these exercises within 2–3 weeks of your first climb.

MUSCLE IMBALANCES

Muscle imbalances become apparent as physical demands become greater. Muscle weakness or tightness affects your ability to reach or step in a particular range or direction. Characteristic lower-body muscle imbalances of mountaineer athletes include weak gluteals and quadriceps in association with tight hamstrings. This affects your ability to negotiate a steep climb while in a precarious position. This type of muscle imbalance also decreases your ability to decelerate and control your upper body and pack while descending a steep slope.

Upper-body muscle imbalances include weakness of the upper and lower back muscles in comparison to tight and strong chest muscles. Other imbalances may include stronger biceps in comparison to weakened shoulders and latissimus dorsi muscles. The brachioradialis may be weak, making it difficult to do a pull-up in a hand-pronated position (see chapter 16 as well as Exercise 128.2). These muscle imbalances can prohibit you from performing repetitive pulling and climbing tasks associated with mountaineering.

WARM-UP

An appropriate warm-up is important for mountaineers due to the significant demands placed upon all body regions. A minimum warm-up should consist of 5–10 minutes of vigorous walking incorporating repetitive shoulder and arm motions in all directions, simulating climbing motions. Consider performing all or parts of the dynamic warm-up in chapter 4, excluding moves that are unsafe, depending on the terrain and weather conditions. Modify the stretches to use rocks and snow to support your feet.

STRETCHING

Good flexibility of your spine, legs, hips, and ankles as well as chest and shoulders is important. You can do the following exercises during the week or after a warm-up before your climb begins: Exercises 1, 3.1, 3.3, 5, 7–9, 11, 13, 16, 17, and 19.

AEROBIC CONDITIONING

Mountaineering requires a significant amount of aerobic endurance. You will need to improve your maximal aerobic capacity and your ability to work near your lactate threshold, because you will walk on steep slopes at higher altitude. Develop this by doing specific aerobic activities 5 times a week for 30–50 minutes and a longer-duration training activity once every week. Mountaineering-specific training includes:

Inside: Cross-country ski machines, step aerobics, EFX cross trainer, and stair climbing (especially on real stairs or on a revolving stair machine).

Outside: Running, cross-country skiing, snowshoeing, hiking, scrambling, and stair climbing. Stair climbing should be a part of your in-city training within 6 weeks of your first climb. Vary your stair climbing workouts with running single or double stairs and walking double and triple stairs. Do descents of single and double stairs.

Cross training: Cycling and rowing.

STRENGTH TRAINING

Strength training is very important for mountain climbers and should emphasize functional exercises of your whole lower body (buttocks, hips, thighs, etc.), upper body, and lower/upper body combination. Abdominal exercises are important for balance and for back support.

Refer to chapter 18 for more information on strength training if you are going to be doing any significant rock or ice climbing.

Beginning

Lower body: Exercises 28, 29, 35.1, 35.3, 95.1–95.3, 98, 99, 101, and 101.1.

Abdominals: Exercises 72, 78.3, 83–85, 86 (with both feet on the floor), and 92.

Upper body: Exercises 20, 35.1, 35.3, 115, 117.4, 120, 121.1, 122, 123, 127, 128, and 131. Do Exercise 127 and 128 on assisted machines and work up to at least half to three-quarters of your body weight.

Intermediate/Advanced

Lower body: Do the beginning program above for 4 weeks, then omit Exercises 29 and 98, and add Exercises 30, 31, 36, 100.1, 101.2, and 101.3.

Abdominals: Do the beginning program above for 4 weeks, and add Exercises 73, 78.4 or 78.5, 82, 83 (with a pack on), 84 (balancing on one foot), and 93.

Upper body: Do the beginning program above for 4 weeks, then add Exercises 34, 34.1, 114 (decline press), 118, 128.1, 128.2 (as close to unassisted as possible), and 107; substitute Exercise 130 for 115 and 133 for 131.

The Descent

Descending from a climb requires a high degree of strength and control. There are significant forces on your knees and ankles to control the pace of descent and keep you from falling. Often a climber grows fatigued because of awakening early and spending many arduous hours on the ascent. It is important to stay well fueled with food and fluids and to take breaks on the descent.

Training for the descent can be done in town by doing stepping exercises off a step (Exercises 99.1–99.3); by doing walking lunges (Exercises 97.6 or 97.9 on level ground and downhill surfaces); and by descending stairs 2–3 at a time in a controlled manner. Ideally these should be done with a pack and within 4 weeks of your first climb. On weekend hikes, choose steeper terrain and snow as you near your first climb.

BALANCE AND AGILITY

Mountaineering terrain is often unstable (scree, snow, and ice slopes), which challenges your balance while you are under significant loads with a pack. When you are on snow or ice, you must be very stable, balancing on one leg while you are cutting or finding the next step. It is important to be able to balance on one leg with a heavy pack with your legs in variable positions (different amounts of knee bending) and in different planes of motion (front, side, and diagonal).

Start balance exercises within 4–6 weeks of your first climb and do them twice a week. In town, you can do some of these on a hill or a sloped driveway, as well as on a flat surface in your home or in a gym. Practice with a pack once you feel fairly confident without one. You can also practice some of the balance exercises on snow slopes or nonsnow terrain that is not subject to dangerous exposure.

Do Exercises 31.1, 31.2, BST Exercises 49 and 51, Exercises 58.1, 58.2 (especially), 58.3, 59.1, 59.3, 60.1, 61, 61.1, 65, 85.1, and 85.2.

PACK POSITIONING AND LIFTING

Positioning and safe lifting of your pack are described in chapters 14 and 17. Make sure ropes and other gear are packed so your neck and head are not pushed forward. These safe lifting and movement techniques are extremely important on mountaineering trips and should be practiced at all times during the trip to avoid injuries.

GOAL PROGRAM

When setting a mountaineering goal, make sure it is both realistic and that you have enough time to achieve it. For significant aerobic activity goals such as climbing a very high mountain, approximately 5–6 training days a week for 10–12 weeks is usually necessary. Remember that it takes a certain amount of time for physiological adaptation to take place in your cardiovascular, respiratory, and musculoskeletal systems.

Devote approximately 90–120 minutes to strength and balance training per week (with 2 sessions per week).

Break up your available training time by quarters into the aerobic training levels listed below. The percentages listed are related to your in-city aerobic training time. In addition, do a general strength training program 2 days per week. One day a week, do a hike of gradually increasing distance and elevation gain.

Within 10–12 weeks of your first climb, start increasing the duration of 2 of your in-town aerobic sessions from 30 minutes to 50 minutes (by 2 minutes each session).

Within 8–12 weeks of your first mountaineering trip, start your longer, lower-intensity day trips with a hike or, if there is too much snow, a snowshoe or cross-country ski trip. Start with a round trip of 4–6 miles and a 2,000- to 2,500-foot elevation gain. Gradually work your way up each week in length and elevation gain.

Within 4 weeks choose trips with steep and difficult terrain, and with some snow if possible. Gradually increase the weight in your pack as you get closer to your climb. Try to have finished a 1-day trip (and ideally a 2-day trip) of at least 8 hours of difficult hiking with a heavy pack, with some snow and with at least 4,000 feet elevation gain before you attempt your mountaineering climb. Remember that altitude problems can result if you are training above 8,000 feet (see chapter 1 and Cox and Fulsaas, *Freedom of the Hills*).

Within 3–4 weeks of a major climb, try stair climbing with a pack on (on a machine or on stairs). Revolving climbing walls are good for cross training. Your intensity on these activities should be in a range of 60–85% maximum heart rate (max HR). Add interval training to your program if you are healthy (see chapter 3). You can do this with intervals of 15–240 seconds on a stair-climber, on stairs, during running, or while on your training hikes as in Fartlek training.

Below is a sample training program based on a heart-rate training zone approach described in chapter 3. This is just one example of a training program. You can achieve a reasonable level of fitness without doing the interval training outlined below. The main difference may be that you perceive less stamina when brief spurts of high intensity are required on steep or challenging sections of your climb.

Sample Weekly Plan for Heart-Rate Zone Training

Total planned aerobic training time is 5 hours a week in the city and 1 long day of increasing duration (4–8 hours) in an outdoor setting. Spend 45–60 minutes 2 times per week in strength and balance training.

For example, when you are in the increasing endurance level (second month), the amount of time you spend per week is:

20% = 60 minutes in zones 1 and 2
70% = 210 minutes in zone 3
10% = 30 minutes in zone 4

Log your activities to keep on track. An example of a week in the increasing endurance level:

Monday: 8-minute warm-up and 4-minute cooldown (zone 1, 2); 50 minutes (zone 3) preferably on a stair-climber. Strength and balance training 30–45 minutes.

Tuesday: 8-minute warm-up; 30 minutes interval training on the treadmill (50% in zone 4, 50% in zone 3); 4-minute cooldown.

Wednesday: Same as Monday, or substitute another specific aerobic activity.

Thursday: 8-minute warm-up and 30 minutes of intervals (50% in zone 4, 50% in zone 3), 4-minute cooldown.

Friday: 30 minutes cross training (zone 3). Strength training 30–45 minutes.

Saturday: Hike in the mountains (including snow walking as the season and weather permit), carry a pack of gradually increasing weight, and gradually increase the distance, slope, and elevation gain to simulate the climb (zones 1, 2). A few weeks before the climb, you should be up to an 8- to 12-mile hike with 4,000 feet elevation gain if possible. If you don't live in an area where this is possible, spend extended periods of time doing stair running and climbing in a tall building and outside.

Sunday: Same as Monday, except omit strength training.

This schedule can be altered in the third training month by increasing interval training as well as the difficulty of your strength training. At this stage you would add some strength sets of higher resistance, lower reps, and some hops and jumps for power.

Plan a reduced volume of training 1 week before your event so your body can rest and not be overtaxed before your climb. The day before should either be without exercise or no more than light activity.

chapter 20 CONDITIONING FOR SNOWBOARDING AND SKIING

Alpine, Telemark, Cross-Country, and Skate Skiing

By Carl Peterson, P.T., Rich Harrington, and Mark Pierce, A.T.C.

THIS CHAPTER WILL HELP YOU:

- Ski an 8-mile cross-country course with some elevation gain.
- Telemark a course with 3,000-foot elevation gain and loss.
- Ski a full day of advanced alpine skiing.
- Snowboard a moderately difficult slope.

All snowboard and skiing activities are demanding sports that require some form of preseason preparation and training in all areas of fitness. Adequate preactivity preparation not only enhances your enjoyment and performance but minimizes the risk of injury.

MUSCULOSKELETAL DEMANDS

The musculoskeletal demands for skiing and snowboarding are very similar. Your lower body, abdominals, and back muscles are required to initially decelerate your body against gravity and the terrain to prevent falling. The velocities are high in downhill skiing and snowboarding, requiring very rapid and balanced muscular contractions in squatting, lunging, and jumping motions.

Next, these muscles are required to accelerate your body in a chosen direction or pattern of movement. These musculoskeletal demands occur simultaneously in three planes of motion (see chapter 6 for a description of the planes of motion). Alpine, cross-country, and telemark skiing are sagittal plane (forward progression or movement)–dominant sports. When moving in a forward direction, your muscles are required to control joint motion continuously in the other two planes. Skiers may want to pay more attention to the sagittal (forward) and transverse (rotational) planes.

The same applies to snowboarding; however, the dominant plane of motion is the frontal plane (sideways). While progressing in a relative forward direction, the transverse plane (rotation) becomes very important for changes in direction. Snowboarders should emphasize strengthening exercise in the frontal (side-to-side) and transverse (rotational) planes and balance challenges in all three planes.

MUSCLE IMBALANCES

Common muscle imbalances that emerge in skiing and snowboarding are weak gluteals, adductors (including the medial quadriceps), abdominals, hamstrings, and interscapular muscles opposed by the typically stronger and tighter quadriceps, hip flexors, iliotibial band, heel cord, and upper chest muscles. If these imbalances are not corrected, they can contribute to numerous snow-sport injuries.

WARM-UP

A morning warm-up should be done prior to hitting the slopes or trails. In cold conditions it is vital. A proper warm-up prepares your muscles for skiing and snowboarding and also prepares your joints for movement and stability. Start slowly, and progressively increase the intensity of your warm-up. By using ski-specific activities, you will help improve the coordination of your muscles and joints, leading to more efficient movement and performance.

A dynamic warm-up can include an agility drill and is important before performing agility circuits or your snow activity. You could use the dynamic warm-up in chapter 4 as your core dynamic warm-up prior to activity. Modify this routine depending on the safety of the surface available, or include one or two other functional exercises specific to your sport. Other dynamic warm-ups are listed below.

Dynamic Warm-Up 1

This is an easy, quick warm-up before exercise or an activity. It is appropriate for cross-country skiing or any other activity on a cold day. Start with a skipping routine or a light 5-minute jog. Then perform the chapter 4 dynamic warm-up exercises and Exercises 7 and 30.

Dynamic Warm-Up 2

This is appropriate for snowboarders and downhill and telemark skiers.

Do 5 fast hops to your right with your left leg; 5 fast hops to your left with your right leg; 5 vertical jumps; 10 walking lunges; 5 fast hops at 45 degrees to the right with your left leg; 5 fast hops at 45 degrees to the left with your right leg; and 5 continuous jumps—long-high-long-high-long.

STRETCHING

Flexibility is important for technique and minimizing injury potential. You need to be able to bend your knees at least into a half squat and to extend your hips. Ankle flexibility is important for all snow activities.

AEROBIC CONDITIONING

Aerobic and anaerobic conditioning are both important for snowboarding and skiing. Aerobic conditioning is important for telemark, cross-country, and skate skiing. Anaerobic conditioning is important for brief spurts of high-intensity effort such as climbing a hill, skiing a mogul field, or cross-country sprinting.

STRENGTH TRAINING

Strength and power enable you to negotiate turns and terrain. Plan your strength training for each body region 2 times per week. Incorporate your agility and balance training 2 times a week within 6–8 weeks of your activity season.

Skiing and snowboarding require significant abdominal and lower-body strength. Your chest, shoulders, and arms are most used in telemark, skate, and cross-country skiing. They are also used in snowboarding for balance and catching falls. Some exercises should be done on slopes, outdoors on a downhill or traverse pitch, to simulate actual conditions.

Torso (core) strength is very important in skiing and snowboarding. Do the majority of your leg, thigh, and abdominal exercises on your feet so that strength gains will mimic the demands of your activity. Standing positions allow you to perform rotational or side-to-side challenges with your torso and use your abdominal muscles as controllers of motion. Just doing an abdominal crunch will not prepare your abdominal muscles for skiing or snowboarding.

BALANCE AND AGILITY

Moving dynamic balance is critical for snowboarding and all types of skiing, which require a high level of agility, balance, and coordination. Agility is the ability to move quickly and change your body position in a coordinated, controlled fashion. Dynamic balance improves your ability to control rapid changes in direction and adapt to changing snow conditions and terrain. The agility circuits in the exercise section of this chapter are designed to improve your moving dynamic balance.

You can use machines to develop speed and balance. The Fitter (see Exercise 152 in this chapter) is a standing balance machine best for training for snowboarding and downhill skiing with a rapid side-to-side challenge.

See Figure 37 for a brief look at the training components of snowboarding and each type of skiing.

ALPINE (DOWNHILL) SKIING

Dynamic Warm-Up

Do 5 minutes of walking, skipping, or jogging; then do the dynamic warm-up exercises in chapter 4, and add all or part of Dynamic Warm-Up 2, above.

Stretching

Adequate hip, knee, and ankle mobility is required to attain a full squat position. Try Exercises 1–10. For your upper body, do Exercises 21, 34, and 37.

Aerobic Conditioning

Do any continuous standing aerobic activity of 30 minutes or more, including step aerobics and/or "slide" activities. Other aerobic activities are running, using a stair-climber, and using cross-country ski machines.

Anaerobic Conditioning

Do short intervals of a higher intensity. A ski training device (the Fitter) can be used for interval training. Hopping or jumping on a slope can also be an alternative; see Exercises 71, 100, and 101.

Strength Training

Beginning

Upper body: Exercises 22, 114, 127, and 133.

Abdominals: Exercises 80.1, 84, and 85.

Lower body: Exercises 30, 31, 61, 95, 97, and 99.

Intermediate

Upper body: Exercises 21, 22, 33.4, 124, 127, 132, and 133.

Abdominals: Exercises 81, 83–85, and 90.

Lower body: Exercises 30, 31.1, 57.1, 59, 61, 95, 97, 97.3, 97.4, 97.7, 100, 133, and 135.

Advanced

Upper body: Exercises 21–23, 127, 130, 132, and 133.

Abdominals: Exercises 82, 86–88, 91, and 93.

Lower body: Exercises 30 (all variations), 32, 60, 71, 95, 97, 97.3, 97.4, 97.7, 100.3, 101, and 135.

FIGURE 37. TRAINING COMPONENTS

	FLEXIBILITY	ANAEROBIC STAMINA	AEROBIC STAMINA	STRENGTH	AGILITY & BALANCE
Alpine	med	high	low	high	med-high
Telemark	high	med-high	med-high	high	med-high
Cross-Country	med	high	high	med	med-high
Skate Skiing	high	high	high	med	med-high
Snowboarding	high	high	low	high	high

Speed/Power

For alpine skiing, you need to be able to hop repeatedly, side to side, for 30 seconds to 2 minutes.

Beginning: Exercises 100.1, 100.4–100.7.

Intermediate/Advanced: Exercises 100.1, 100.7, 157, 159, 161, 163, 164 or 165, and 166.

Balance and Agility

Beginning: BST Exercises 49, 51, 53, and Exercises 66 and 153.

Intermediate: Exercise 67, 68, 153. Include abdominal challenge stations such as Exercises 80 and 84.

Advanced: Exercises 66.1, 67–69, 153, 165, and 166. Have a downhill component with some traverse sections if available.

At any level, balance can be trained by using a Quadmill (available at some gyms) for 2-minute intervals.

TELEMARK SKIING

Dynamic Warm-Up

Do 5 minutes of walking, skipping, or jogging; then do the dynamic warm-up exercises in chapter 4 and Exercise 29 as a walking lunge.

Stretching

Adequate hip, knee, and ankle mobility are needed to be able to attain a full squat and split squat or lunge position. Do the stretches listed for alpine skiing, above, but spend extra time on the adductor and Achilles stretches.

Aerobic Conditioning

Do any continuous activity for 30–40 minutes. If you are planning to do backcountry touring, train to sustain your activity for a period of up to 2–3 hours at an intensity zone of 50–70% maximum heart rate (max HR). Do a low-intensity, longer-duration (LILD) day and gradually increase the duration and slope to approximately two-thirds to three-fourths of your expected telemark trip. The best activities would be using a cross-country ski machine with a sloped angle, in-line skating, roller skiing, doing an uphill run or treadmill workout, using a stair-climber (especially the revolving stairs), using an EFX elliptical trainer, using the slide board, or using a Fitter machine. Outside, snowshoeing and regular cross-country skiing are also excellent alternatives.

Anaerobic Conditioning

Consider including interval training 2 times per week. Do repeated bursts of activity for 20 seconds–3 minutes. Do intervals in the 85–95% max HR range.

Strength Training

Telemark turns require you to be in a modified lunge position, which exerts a significant amount of internal force on the forward leg. This requires significant strength of the ankle, quad, hamstring, groin, hip, abdominal, and buttock muscles. This force can be simulated with rotational lunges in which a weight is brought toward the front leg and across the midline of your body. Doing these on a hill, in a traverse, or on a downhill pitch is helpful. Start slowly and then increase the speed.

Beginning

Upper body: Exercises 32, 33, and 133.

Abdominals: Exercises 80, 81, and 83.

Lower body: Exercise 30, 31.1, 95, and 97.

Intermediate

Upper body: Exercises 21, 23.2, 38, 124, 128, 132, and 133.

Abdominals: Exercises 80, 81, 83, and 84.

Lower body: Exercise 30, 38, 58.3a, 59, 60, 133, and 135.

Advanced

Upper body: Exercises 21, 33.1, 38, 128–130, 132, and 133.

Abdominals: Exercises 82, 86–88, and 93.

Lower body: Exercises 30, 32, 38, 59, 60, 70, and 135.

Speed/Power

You need to be able to do fast rotational or side-to-side lunges (mimicking telemark turns) for 30 seconds. Do Exercises 159, 162, 164, and 165.

Balance and Agility

You must have adequate balance and coordination to allow total body control with rapid changes of direction over rough terrain.

Beginning/Intermediate: Do Exercises 65, 66.1, and 68. Do the telemark circuit in Exercise 155 with the following modifications: omit Exercises 31, 58.4, and 59.3.

Advanced: Do Exercise 155, the telemark circuit.

At any level, balance can be trained by using a Quadmill (available at some gyms) for 2–4 minutes in the forward- and side-facing positions.

CROSS-COUNTRY SKIING

Dynamic Warm-Up

Do Exercise 170.

Stretching

You need adequate hip, knee, and ankle mobility to be able to attain a stride lunge position. Pay special attention to Exercises 3, 4, and 6–8.

Aerobic Conditioning

You must be able to perform continuous activity for 2–3 hours at 60–80% max HR. Some work on an uphill slope is important if you wish to climb hills. Performing side stepping and V-shaped uphill walking or lunges can help your uphill abilities. Increase your aerobic duration each week. Good activities are running, using an EFX machine, stair climbing, roller skiing, using a cross-country ski machine (especially with some time spent going up a slope), doing a slide routine, or in-line skating. Alternatives are any standing aerobic activity such as hiking, snowshoeing, or running on a hill. Your routines should be 30–50 minutes long with some cross training to prevent overuse injuries. If you intend to race, do some ski interval training (see Fartlek interval training in chapter 3). Your low-intensity, longer-duration (LILD) activities should ideally start on a weekly basis 6–8 weeks before your first full day of skiing.

Anaerobic Conditioning

You must be able to perform occasional bursts of activity for 30–90 seconds. If you wish to enhance your anaerobic abilities, do some interval training.

Strength Training

Do continuous weight-bearing exercises repeated on either both or a single leg for 20–30 reps. Do the skate-skiing strength and balance programs, below.

Beginning

Upper body: Exercises 28, 74, 126, and 127.

Abdominals: Exercises 80 and 84.

Lower body: Exercises 30, 95, and 97.

Intermediate/Advanced

Upper body: Exercises 21, 30, 38, 118, 120, 127, 132, 133, and 136.

Abdominals: Exercises 81, 82, and 84–86.

Lower body: Exercises 24, 29, 30, 31.1, 32, 101, 101.2, and 135.

Speed/Power

You should be able to accelerate on an uphill grade. Interval training and jumping or hopping drills will enhance your speed and power.

Balance and Agility

Beginning/Intermediate: Make a cross-country obstacle course. You can do fast walking or running, and make quick turns (or do Exercise 29) between obstacles that simulate the distance between turns. Incorporate lunge stations as in Exercise 97.5 and step-up stations as in Exercise 98. Use abdominal challenge stations such as in Exercises 80 and 84. Incorporate balance stations such as in Exercises 58.1, 58.2, 59.1, 61, and 63. Link stations with a fast walk, a run, the dynamic warm-up exercises in chapter 4 or do Dynamic Warm-Up 2 earlier in this chapter. You can add a day pack and speed up the pace to make it more challenging.

Advanced: Do Exercise 155, the telemark circuit, with the following modifications: omit Exercises 31, 58.4, 59.3, and 101.

At any level, balance can be trained by using a Quadmill (available at some gyms) for 2 minutes in the forward- and side-facing positions.

SKATE SKIING

Dynamic Warm-Up

Do Exercise 170 along with Exercise 101.2.

Stretching

Do all of the stretches for cross-country skiing, above, especially Exercises 7 and 8.

Anaerobic/Aerobic Conditioning

Using slide boards, EFX machines, stair-climbers, cross-country ski machines, or running or roller skiing are the most sport-specific aerobic activities. Make two of your off-snow (gym) sessions last 40–50 minutes. Consider incorporating 5- to 10-minute intervals of slide-board training at the beginning and end of your aerobic session. Consider doing some anaerobic intervals of 30–90 seconds 2 times per week within 6 weeks of the ski season (see chapter 3). These intervals will help you with hill climbing.

Strength Training

This is similar to the program for cross-country skiing, above, with extra work needed for your groin and hip muscles. Skate skiers should work up to the cross-country advanced program for strength, and add the exercises listed under the advanced program for strength, below.

Beginning

Upper body: Exercise 21, 74, 111, 126, and 127.

Abdominals: Exercises 80 and 84.

Lower body: Exercise 30, 61, 95, and 97.

Intermediate/Advanced

Upper body: Exercises 21, 38, 118.2, 120, 127, 131–133, and 136.

Abdominals: Exercises 81–84.

Lower body: Exercises 30, 32, 95.2, 97.3, 101.2, 101.5 (uphill hopping), 135, 151, 159, and 168.

SNOWBOARDING

Dynamic Warm-Up

Do 5 minutes of walking, skipping, or jogging; then do the dynamic warm-up exercises in chapter 4 and add all or part of the dynamic warm-ups in this chapter.

Stretching

Adequate flexibility and mobility of your legs and hips is necessary for snowboarding in order to assume a prolonged and balanced squat position. To improve your flexibility in these areas try Exercises 5, 6, and 57.

Aerobic Conditioning

Any continuous standing activity of 30 minutes or more that allows you to maintain your target heart rate (see chapter 3) is recommended.

Step aerobics as well as the use of a slide board, stair-climber, or treadmill are all aerobic conditioning activities suitable for snowboarding.

Strength Training

Beginning

Upper body: Exercises 111, 131, and 133.

Abdominals: Exercises 80 or 81, 83, and 85.

Lower body: Exercises 29, 31, 57, 59, 95.1, 109, and 133.2.

Intermediate

Upper body: Exercises 129, 130, 131, 133, and 135.

Abdominals: Exercises 22, 80, 81, 83, 84, and 85.

Lower body: Exercises 29, 31, 34, 58.3, 58.4, 61, 95.2, 95.3, 97, 97.3, 97.4, 97.7, 100, 100.4, 109.2, 133, and 135.

Advanced

Upper body: Exercises 21, 26.2, and 115.

Abdominals: Exercises 22, 82, 86–88, and 93.

Lower body: Exercises 30, 31, 34.1, 68, 71, 95, 97, 97.4, 100.3, 100.4, 109.2, 129, 131, 133, and 135.

Balance and Agility

Beginning: See Exercise 154, the snowboard circuit, and build yourself a 6- to 10-station circuit that includes Exercises 60, 61, 81, 151, and 156. Do each exercise for 20–30 seconds, then jog, skip, or hop to the next station.

Intermediate/Advanced: See Exercise 154, the snowboard circuit, and build an 8- to 12-station circuit that includes Exercises 60, 61, 81, 100.5, 100.6, 101.2, 101.4, 151, 156, and 157. Do each exercise for 20–30 seconds, then jog, skip, or hop to the next station.

SNOWBOARDING AND SKIING EXERCISES

If you are planning to alpine ski, telemark ski, or snowboard, consider adding agility and balance drills to your routine within 6 weeks of your first trip. It is important to have a good aerobic and strength base before adding agility circuits. If you are planning on only cross-country skiing, fine-tune your stamina and strength, and then add balance activities when time permits.

Try to sequence your training and do your agility and coordination drills prior to other types of training, to derive optimum benefit. Also include some agility work as part of your warm-up or during a Fartlek interval aerobic session. In designing balance and agility circuits, make use of natural obstacles for balance and coordination, such as balancing on or jumping back and forth over logs, steps, rocks, or snow slopes.

BALANCE EXERCISES

150 BALANCE BOARDS

Equipment: Balance board, rocker board, or wobble board.
Purpose: Improve your ability to balance in all three planes.

Technique: There are many varieties of ski-applicable balance boards. The basic board is a flat surface with a track that sits in a groove on a roller. The side-to-side rocking motion develops awareness of your body position during motion. The more advanced board has an elevated platform, and the ends of the roller are beveled to allow rocking forward and back, as on a snowboard. As you get comfortable with the balance required, increase the difficulty by holding a tuck position, balancing on one foot, or adding a pack. You can also do this with ski poles to provide added stability.

Rocker boards are rectangular platforms with a thin or thick plank down the center and can be used to challenge your balance in side-to-side or front-to-back directions. Holding a weight in one hand and moving it away from the center of your body will increase the challenge. Other options include performing alternate biceps curls, overhead presses, or rotational punches while balancing on the rocker board.

Wobble boards are either rectangular or circular platforms with a half circle attached to the bottom. These are more challenging in that they create challenges in all three planes simultaneously.

151 SHUFFLE LUNGE WITH REACH

Equipment: None.
Purpose: Improve your ability to balance and recover from a side-to-side and rotational challenge.

Technique: Perform a lateral lunge step to the right, with a left arm reach, as in Exercise 97.8. After reaching in one direction, sidestep to the left for a couple of steps, moving back into a lateral lunge, and reach across your body with the right hand at knee height. For lateral lunge technique, see Exercise 97.3 in chapter 11.

152 THE FITTER

Equipment: Fitter machine, ski poles.
Purpose: Develop your balance and coordination during side-to-side motions used in snowboarding and alpine skiing.

Technique: While holding your ski poles (or two 4-foot lengths of doweling), stand on the Fitter platform. This platform is very wobbly, so allow your knees to slightly bend and find a secure, balanced position. Once you feel balanced, slowly shift your weight to either the right or the left. The stance platform will yield and move sideways in the direction you choose. When you have reached the end point of your initial side, shift your weight and balance while you travel across the Fitter in the opposite direction. This exercise simulates the gliding motion common to alpine skiing. Snowboarders should assume a foot position similar to what you use on your snowboard. The Fitter's resistance can be adjusted by changing the variable-tension cords on the rollers on the undersurface of the machine.

AGILITY EXERCISES AND CIRCUITS

You can practice dynamic moving balance and coordination by creating your own agility obstacle course with cones, poles, trees, balls, and other objects. Place 8–12 obstacles 10–20 feet apart in a Z-shaped pattern to simulate ski or snowboard turns. In an alpine skier or snowboarder course, your stations should be close enough to require you to react quickly from one station to the next. Jog or run between the obstacles. When you reach an obstacle, make a quick change in direction and proceed to the next obstacle. This direction change can proceed from a beginning level of a running cut to more advanced jumps and hops. This will improve your ability to make quick changes in body position.

In ski and snowboard agility and balance circuits, you can work through 8–12 stations (with one station being the obstacle course) 1–2 times. Work hard for 30–45 seconds at each station, then move to the next station. If you are in a gym and are unable to do an obstacle course, do the balance exercises as indicated.

153 ALPINE SKI CIRCUIT

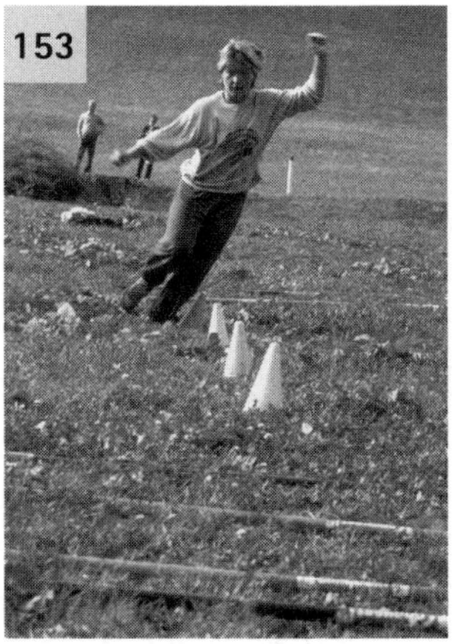

Equipment: Circuit of 8–12 stations, including obstacle course; have a downhill component with some traverse sections if available.
Purpose: Improve your agility and ability to react to changes in direction and various degrees of terrain.

Technique: Include stations such as Exercises 156, 157, 159, and 161. For other stations, use Exercise 151 as well as Exercises 37–61. Use a walking lunge (Exercises 97.9 and 97.11) on a slope if available. See photo 153 for an example of a downhill or snowboard agility course.

154 SNOWBOARD CIRCUIT

Equipment: Circuit with poles, rope, and steps marking areas for jumping drills.
Purpose: Improve your ability to meet the various sudden directional challenges of snowboarding.

Technique: Jump in patterns to simulate snowboarding. Try putting some of the circuit stations on uneven surfaces such as steps, hills, snow piles, and logs if your circuit is outside, and on steps or platforms if indoors. Include stations with lateral shuffles (Exercise 151), lateral hopping (101.2), and rotational jumps of 90–180 degrees (75.4). Consider jumping Exercises 165 and 166.

155 TELEMARK CIRCUIT

Equipment: Telemark agility course with stations and an obstacle course.
Purpose: Improve your ability to change directions and meet the physical demands of telemark skiing.

Technique: You can do fast walking or running and make quick turns between stations. Consider performing Exercise 29 on a downhill obstacle course. When you have reached your obstacle, do the telemark lunge, then quickly jump into an inward quarter turn and proceed to the next obstacle, simulating the distance between telemark turns. Incorporate lunge stations (Exercise 97.5), hop stations (Exercise 101 and 101.1), and step-down stations (Exercise 99). Use abdominal challenge stations such as Exercises 80 and 84. Incorporate balance stations such as Exercises 31, 58.1–58.4, 59.1–59.3, and 61. Link stations with a fast walk, a run, the dynamic warm-up exercises in chapter 4, or Dynamic Warm-Up 2 earlier in this chapter. You can add a day pack and speed up the pace to make it more challenging.

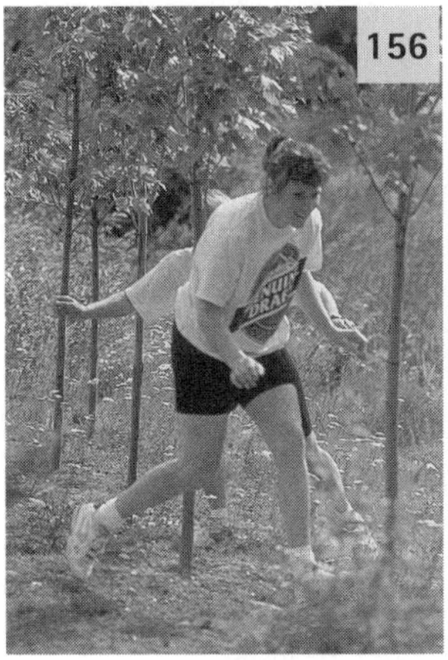
156

156 POLE-RUNNING AGILITY CIRCUIT

Equipment: Ski or garden poles, gentle hill.
Purpose: Develop your lateral agility.

Technique: Set up ski or garden poles along a gentle hill, traverse, or downhill course. Position your poles closely enough so that you have to make quick changes in direction as you run through the course. (Always face forward.)

157 THE "Z" AGILITY COURSE

Equipment: Cones or markers.
Purpose: Improve your ability to decelerate and change directions while improving your anaerobic strength.

Technique: Arrange cones or markers as shown in illustration 157, placing a cone at the end of each arrow. If you have a workout partner, use a stopwatch to time each other. On "Go," sprint from point A to point B and quickly change directions, then proceed on to the

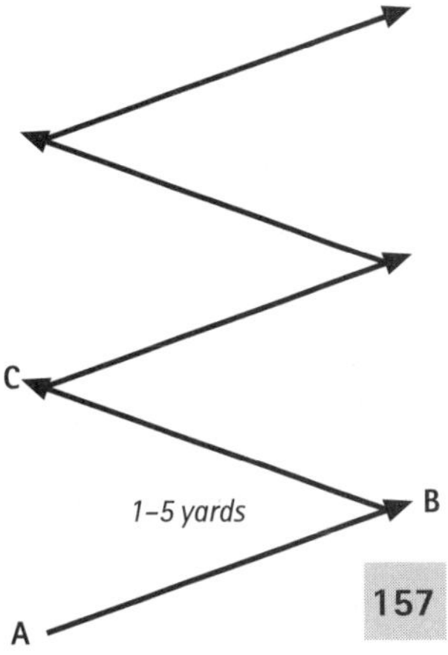

157

next cone. Set as many cones as you like. Complete two trials and record your best time.

Variations: 157.1. Jump turns: When you reach each cone, do a jump turn, then proceed on to the next cone. **157.2.** Cross-body reaches: Reach across your body and touch the base of the cone with your opposite-side hand. Always face front. This simulates a body position similar to skiing.

POWER EXERCISES

These power exercises consist of hopping and jumping plyometrics. Plyometrics train your muscles to reach maximal force in the shortest time possible. Plyometrics are useful for sports that require explosive power, including high-level downhill skiing, snowboarding, and telemark skiing. The U.S. Ski Team uses plyometrics for both preseason training and in-season maintenance.

Beginning

Progression of hops and jumps should follow the rules of easy-to-hard and simple-to-complex. These exercises are most appropriate for downhill skiers, snowboarders, and telemark skiers. Please review the basic technique of jumps and hops in Exercises 100 and 101.

158 DYNAMIC JUMPING WARM-UP

Equipment: None.

Purpose: Warm up before hopping and jumping routines.

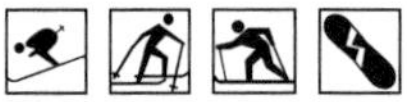

Technique: Do an easy 10-minute running warm-up. Next, stretch your torso (Exercise 21 without dumbbells), shoulders (Exercise 14), and legs, particularly the groin and Achilles tendon (Exercises 1, 3, 6–8, and 10). Next, do some agility drills for 5 minutes at half to three-fourths speed (like the dynamic warm-up exercises in chapter 4).

159 45-DEGREE HOPPING

Equipment: None.

Purpose: Improve your ability to push off and land on one leg.

Technique: Push off from your right foot, moving diagonally forward at a 45-degree angle, land on your left foot, and rapidly contract to push off to land on your right foot. Do 15–20 hops.

160 SIMULATED SKI TURNS

Equipment: None.
Purpose: Practice ski turns during the preseason.

Technique: Do quick jumping on a downhill slope (a park or snowfield) and simulate your ski style in regard to height and frequency of turns. Within 6 weeks of your first downhill trip, start this training with a few jumps and gradually progress to 20 linked jumps. If your knees hurt, perform these exercises on a level surface and take shallower jumps.

161 SLALOM JUMPS

Equipment: Rope.
Purpose: Simulate skiing downhill or snowboarding while connecting multiple turns.

Technique: Lay a rope down a slope that is long enough so that you can do 10–20 jumps. Practice a few jumps, then jump side to side over the rope as if you were connecting multiple turns.

Intermediate/Advanced

162 DYNAMIC JUMPING WARM-UP 2

Equipment: None.
Purpose: Prepare your muscles and joints to accept increasing loads.

Technique: Do the dynamic warm-up exercises in chapter 4. Then do some running drills (forward sprints), and progress to dynamic flexibility exercises such as Exercises 7 and 10; then add some lunge walks (97.9). After this warm-up, add the diagonal hops and progressive power jumps in Exercise 164, or the telemark jumps in Exercise 163.

163

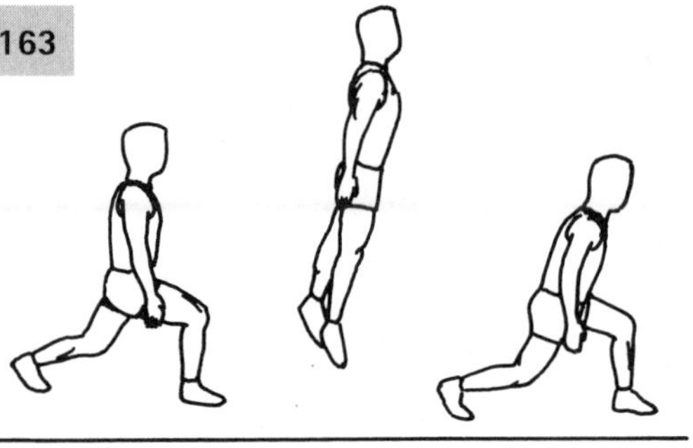

163 TELEMARK JUMP

Equipment: None.
Purpose: Condition your legs and improve your coordination for telemark skiing.

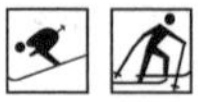

Technique: From the lunge position, jump up and bring the opposite leg forward. This is excellent training for telemark skiing. Work your way up to 10–15 reps.

164 PROGRESSIVE POWER JUMPS

Equipment: Smooth grass or dirt surface or gym floor.
Purpose: Strengthen your legs and gluteals to accelerate out of a turn and increase your vertical leap.

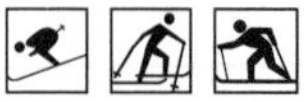

Technique: Do 3 sets of regular, vertical, or rotational jumps (Exercise 75 or 75.1, or 75.4 for snowboarders). First do 3 at 30% maximum height, then do 3 at 60% maximum height, and end with 3 at 90% maximum height. Be careful and progress gradually with these.

165 SINGLE-LEG LATERAL JUMPS

Equipment: Smooth grass or dirt surface or gym floor.
Purpose: Improve strength and agility in snowboarders and alpine skiers.

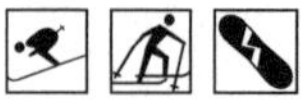

Technique: Jump high and far to your right, recover to ski or snowboarder position, then push off your right foot and jump high and far to your left. Repeat this maneuver for 4–6 times in each direction.

166 CROSSOVER BENCH JUMPS

Equipment: Sturdy bench or wooden box.
Purpose: Closely approximate the side-to-side requirements of skiing or snowboarding.

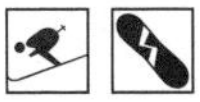

Technique: Position yourself to the left side of a box or platform and place your right foot on the box. Push off with your right foot (assisting with your left foot) and jump up for maximum height, moving sideways. End up with your left foot on the box and your right foot on the ground. Repeat to the opposite direction as soon as your outside foot touches the ground. Do 8–10 jumps to each side.

166

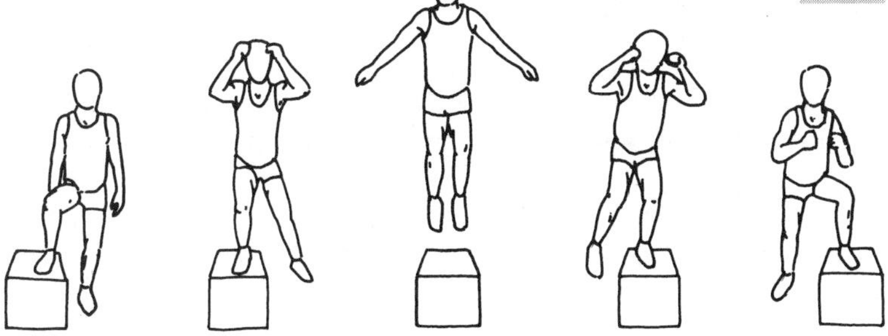

167 THE HEX CIRCUIT

Equipment: 3 hurdles 8 inches high; 1 each of hurdles 10 inches, 12 inches, and 14 inches high.
Purpose: Improve coordination, strength, and agility to make lateral movements with precise foot placement.

Technique: You can make the hurdles from 1 1/2-inch-diameter PVC pipe and elbows available at hardware stores (167a). Hurdles can also be purchased from athletic equipment suppliers. Set up the six hurdles in the pattern shown in illustration 167b. Begin inside the Hex. On "Go," jump to the outside laterally over the first 8-inch hurdle, then immediately back into the center of the Hex. Continue around clockwise, jumping out of the Hex and back in until you have completed all six hurdles. Turn around and return counterclockwise without stopping.

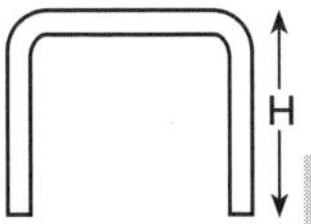

Side View

167a

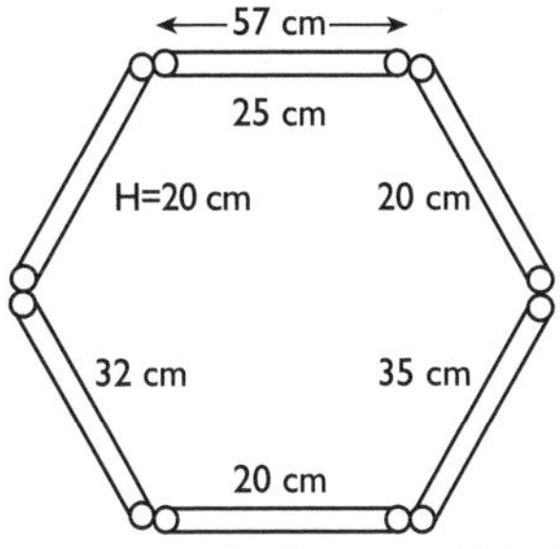

Top View

167b

Variations: 167.1. Spoke pattern: Set up the hurdles in a spoke pattern. Jump over the hurdles, either facing toward or away from the hub. Move clockwise and counterclockwise. **167.2.** Hopping pattern: Hop on one leg and have your training partner call out when to switch legs or directions. **167.3.** Hex in sand: If you have a beach or playground with loose sand available, do the Hex and hurdle variations on sand. This requires more power, and teaches you awareness of your foot and ankle position.

LOWER-BODY ANAEROBIC SPEED/POWER EXERCISES

The following drills can be used separately or in conjunction with the jumping routines above to add interval training and power to your workout.

168 ACCELERATION SPRINTS

Equipment: Field or gymnasium.
Purpose: Prepare your musculoskeletal system and coordination centers for sustained quick movements.

Technique: This is a forward sprint. Start with two 30-meter runs at 65% maximum speed. Then progress to one 30-meter sprint at 80% of your maximum speed by the 30-meter mark. Progress to two 30-meter sprints at 85% of your maximum speed and then three sprints at 90% of your maximum speed.
Precautions: Slow down gradually to avoid excessive strain on your knees. You must be in excellent aerobic shape and meet the interval requirements in chapter 3 to do this.

169 SLIDE BOARDS

Equipment: Smooth surface, fabric shoe covers.
Purpose: Develop both endurance and power in lateral movement patterns. This is very useful in the skating technique of Nordic skiing, giant slalom racing, and any sport requiring lateral agility and power.

Technique: Slide to the right. When you reach a barrier, reach across your body with your left hand at knee height, approximately 1 foot past your body. Repeat this to the left. For strength training, perform this exercise for 45 seconds–1 minute at a higher intensity. For aerobic training, do it for 5–15 minutes at lower intensities.

170 TUCK DRILLS

Equipment: None.
Purpose: Train your muscles and joints to accept quick and constant loads in a tuck position, common to skiing.

Technique: Assume a low tuck position as used in downhill ski racing. Position your back parallel to the floor, arms bent at your elbows, fists forward as if gripping poles, and arms/elbows tucked in at your sides, eyes looking ahead. Hop up and down as fast as possible, with your feet clearing the floor by at least 3 inches. Try to keep your body parallel to the floor, and build up to 2 minutes.
Variation: 170.1. Step and jump: From the low tuck position, step to the right, bring your left leg in next to your right leg, and immediately spring straight up for maximum height as in rebounding a basketball; then drop back to the low tuck and step to the left. Repeat for 10 reps on each side.

chapter 21 CONDITIONING FOR CANOEING, KAYAKING, AND ROWING

By Sherri Cassuto, Certified Rolfer™, and Dan Nelson, D.C.

THIS CHAPTER WILL HELP YOU:

- Become aware of the basic muscle groups used in propelling boats.
- Understand the musculoskeletal demands of these boating activities.
- Identify areas of the body that commonly exhibit muscle imbalances.
- Be aware of areas of the body that are susceptible to injury.
- Be able to implement appropriate water- and land-based training methods for each sport.

Human-propelled oar and paddle craft rely on an unstable and constantly shifting surface (the hull) from which to exert a driving force through the face of the paddle/oar blade to the water. To improve your strength and endurance in boating sports, there is no real substitute for time on the water in variable conditions. This book assumes that you either have the necessary skill base and are preparing for your season, or you are enrolled in a skill development course. This is especially important for whitewater boating and sea kayaking. This chapter includes suggestions for both water-based and land-based training to help improve your performance and reduce the likelihood of injury. Training information is designed for the recreational boater, although the stretching, agility, and strength training programs are also applicable to racers.

MUSCULOSKELETAL DEMANDS

Canoeing, kayaking, and rowing are total body exercises. All involve translation of power from your feet/knees through your body and hands to the paddle/oar. All involve significant load to the muscles of your back, torso, shoulders, and arms.

In canoeing and kayaking, your legs provide a stable connection to the boat and are used to initiate the stroke and rotation of your pelvis and torso. Side bending of the spine is a necessary and integral part of paddle sports, because hull placement in the water is variable. Your torso is used as a lever in both the front-to-back and side-to-side planes, with all intermediate positions possible.

In rowing, the use of your legs is more propulsive and your torso undergoes very little side bending. Your torso is primarily used as a lever in the front-to-back plane of motion. The rowing shell is designed to ride on a stable hull surface. Sweep rowing involves some rotation.

Back Position

A proper neutral low-back position can be achieved by putting your low back through a range of motion from full extension to full flexion, as outlined in Exercise 180 in chapter 25. This neutral position is just slightly off full extension. You can practice it by pushing upon the boat slightly to unweight your spine. Finding your neutral position intermittently throughout the day is important to protect your low back from excessive strain.

If you have very tight hamstrings, stretching them is necessary to enable you to sit in the boat with your spine in good position, avoiding the compensation of excessively flexing (or forward slumping) your low back. You need to be able to tolerate sitting in this position for at least 3–4 hours consecutively to be able to tolerate a full day of boating. For rowing, the same flexibility requirements are necessary for less time on the water.

Rounding of your mid back or excessive forward head and neck positions can lead to shoulder fatigue and injury as well as neck pain. Accomplishing the stroke by excessive use of your upper trapezius instead of allowing your shoulder to drop, relax, and reach forward also leads to neck pain.

MUSCLE IMBALANCES

The following recommendations are for the average recreational boater. If you have been very active in your sport over a number of years, it is likely that your body has changed to accommodate it. The major muscle groups used repetitively will become hypertrophied compared to the rest of your body. For this reason, strength training should be used to produce a general and balanced effect: as your body becomes adapted to your sport, the goal of strength training shifts to create more balance in the underdeveloped body regions. Boaters involved in asymmetrical sports (whitewater canoeing and sweep rowing) will find themselves more developed on one side than the other. More important is the effect of overdevelopment and repetitive motion on flexibility. As time goes by, continue to evaluate your flexibility.

Shoulder, Chest, and Upper Back (Upper Torso)

In many individuals the shoulder and upper back muscles are less developed and less coordinated than the muscles of the chest and lower extremity, due to less awareness of the need for a balanced strengthening program. Any or all of these may be poorly conditioned, but a very common pattern is for the chest muscles to be significantly stronger than the upper back. Most shoulder injuries in water sports are the result of relative weakness in the upper back and in the rotator cuff muscles. The prevalence of rib injuries is largely due to muscle imbalances as well as the significant repetitive load experienced in this region. To prepare for these activities, spend time strengthening this region, especially emphasizing the rotator cuff, middle and lower trapezius, serratus anterior, latissimus, teres, and rhomboids (see chapter 15 and the strength recommendations in this chapter for further details on these muscles).

Hip, Abdominal, Low Back, and Buttock (Lower Torso)

Another common problem is weakness in the torso stabilizing muscles. These include the abdominal muscles; muscles associated with extension, lateral flexion, and rotation of the back; hip flexors; and muscles associated with the ribs and chest. All boating activities rely heavily on the torso/buttocks/hips region for stability of the boat and placement of the hull. The torso region is used as a lever for transferring force from the powerful lower extremity to the upper extremity and ultimately to the paddle/oar.

Wrist, Forearm, and Elbow

This region is a relatively weak link in the musculoskeletal system because most of us don't significantly use these muscles in our daily lives. All water sports use the forearm for strength, endurance, and agility. Keeping this area stretched and limber is extremely important. When it is poorly prepared to absorb the large forces and repetitive motion of paddling or rowing, this region may become susceptible to a variety of forearm/elbow tendon inflammation syndromes and/or carpal-tunnel (nerve) problems.

WARM-UP

You can do all or part of the following warm-up before boating or working out: Do a short aerobic period (5–10 minutes) of fast walking or jogging. Before your on-land training, perform 5–10 minutes on a rowing ergometer. After that, stretch (you can do Exercise 14 with your paddle). Before beginning your paddle do Exercise 18 in the boat in calm water. Include Exercises 19 and 130.1 (push-ups against a bench or boulder). Once on the water, begin with 10–15 minutes of paddling at low intensity. Concentrate on form and gradually build intensity, as you feel ready.

STRETCHING

Flexibility of your hamstrings is vital to maintain a safe and effective body position in all three types of boating. In whitewater boating especially, your quadriceps and hip flexors need to be very limber. Other muscles in your lower body benefit from stretching in order to meet the inherent balance challenges in these sports. This can be accomplished by doing stretching Exercises 1–3, 5, 6, 8, and 9.

Flexibility in the upper/lower back, chest, and shoulders is important in all of these activities. It becomes especially important for boaters who have been very active in their sport over a number of years. This can be accomplished by doing Exercises 11, 12, and 14–18.

AEROBIC CONDITIONING

In this chapter, the aerobic training intensities are defined as follows:

Low intensity: Any level of effort below medium intensity.

Medium intensity: 70–85% maximum heart rate (max HR) for the duration of the training interval. This type of training is not an all-out sprint, but is a fast enough pace to make you feel like you are working harder than normal.

High intensity: Above 85% max HR for the duration of the training interval.

STRENGTH TRAINING

See the strength training programs for the various types of boating, later in this chapter.

BALANCE AND AGILITY

On the Water

Try these training drills for canoe and kayak. For whitewater boating, do drills 1–3 with more sudden, higher-amplitude motions.

1. In a tandem canoe/kayak, have one person make sudden side-to-side movements requiring a bracing response from the other paddler.
2. If the water is warm enough (or you have a wet suit on), have a friend suddenly grab at the sides of the canoe/kayak, requiring a bracing response. If you are a whitewater kayaker, challenge yourself further by having someone straddle your bow or stern while making sudden movements.
3. Using obstacle courses (abrupt turns, etc.) helps develop coordination and balance for sudden changes in attitude of the boat due to outside forces. Set up a course by throwing oranges (or tennis balls, buoys, or life preservers) into the water, creating the obstacles to turn around. Alternatively, make abrupt turns randomly. Random turns can be done in response to a countdown timer or to a friend yelling out, "Turn to the right," etc.
4. Consider canoeing/kayaking a safe distance from motorboat wakes, but paddling through them or riding them at various angles.

On Land

It is important to utilize exercises to enhance sitting balance. These are best done within 4–6 weeks of starting your sea kayak or whitewater training. You can expect to spend 5–10 minutes per session twice a week on balance training. Do the following: Exercises 62 and 94. Secondarily, choose from Exercises 38 and 39.

TOURING OR FLAT-WATER CANOEING

Flat-water canoeing is a repetitive motion that involves rotation and flexion of your torso (initiated with your legs) in concert with pulling of your paddle-side arm and shoulder (and to a much lesser degree, pushing of the opposite side). It is symmetrical in that the paddler switches sides regularly.

The primary propulsive muscles are those of your hips, thighs, torso, and large muscles of your shoulder girdle. The paddler's feet or knees are linked to the boat and provide a base to utilize the power of the lower body. The drive phase of the stroke involves a rotation of your torso, followed by a slight flexion of your elbow, resulting in the draw of the blade against the water. In performance flat-water paddling, the leg on the same side of the paddle extends, initiating the drive. All of these muscles must function as a linked system to yield efficient power. Your scapular stabilizer (upper back) and serratus anterior muscles are extremely important in providing a base to transfer the forces from your large torso muscles through your shoulder and arm to the paddle. Significant weakness or imbalance in these chains of muscles may compromise performance and lead to injury. Areas that are particularly susceptible to injury include your back, shoulder, forearm, and wrist.

Aerobic Conditioning

Flat-water canoeing depends on muscular and aerobic endurance. There are occasional periods when high-intensity activity prevails (inclement weather, exposed open-water conditions). Most training should focus on longer sustained efforts at lower to moderate intensities.

On-the-water training should involve variety, with time devoted to both technique training and progressively longer cardiovascular exercise. Most training days on the water should be 45–90 minutes. If you are preparing for an extended trip on exposed water, spend 1 longer water training day per week, gradually building up to a full day of paddling. Occasionally load your boat up with weight to approximate the gear you will be carrying. Try to do some paddling in challenging water conditions. On land, aerobic training could consist of the use of a rowing ergometer (including Exercise 37), cross-country ski machine, aerodyne bike, or swimming.

Interval training can be helpful to improve your general aerobic endurance, as well as to prepare for unexpected high-intensity paddling efforts. Consider starting your interval training after you have established an aerobic base (about 4 weeks into your paddling training). Once a week, work toward moderate-intensity intervals of 10–20 minutes. Return to low-intensity paddling for 1–2 times the duration of the interval. Alternatively, rest only as long as you need to and start the next interval when you feel ready. Try to do 2–3 intervals per interval training session. As your conditioning level improves, the duration of each work interval is increased and the time for rest is decreased. The duration of training should not increase more than 15–25% per week. If a long trip is planned during the season, adjust training to prepare for it by gradually increasing the duration of low- to moderate-intensity paddling until 4 hours of Fartlek-type paddling is comfortable. When this level is reached, you are ready for a full day of paddling. This can usually be achieved within 8 weeks of beginning training.

Strength Training

In addition to aerobic training, your time on land should be a time to work on stretching and strengthening any musculoskeletal deficiencies as regards canoeing. Common areas of strength deficiency include the torso, upper back (scapular stabilizers), and forearm muscles. Appropriate exercises are rows, lat pulls, biceps curls, triceps extensions, pull-ups, dips, and sitting balance exercises on a gym ball. Several of these exercises should include a trunk rotational component. A basic strength training program can be done twice a week and would include:

Upper body: Exercise 24.1, 39, 115, 117.4, 118 (parallel grip), 120, 120.3, 121.1, 124, 125 (parallel grip), 127, 131, and 134. If you will be on a multiday trip doing portages, add Exercises 20 and 122.

Abdominals: Do Exercises 78.1, 78.2, 84, and 92. Add a rotary torso machine exercise if you have access to one in your gym. Alternatively, do Exercise 80.

Lower body: If you will be on a trip involving portages, add squats and lunges to your program: Exercises 30, 95, and 97.

WHITEWATER CANOEING

Whitewater canoeing in anything above Class II water is classically done with your body positioned differently than for flat water. The boater assumes a kneeling position with both knees apart and braced into the bottom of the boat. This keeps the center of mass lower and adds to hull stability. The sitting balance challenges in whitewater boating are among the most significant of any sitting activity, and the speed demands of intermediate and above levels of whitewater canoeing require that the paddler not switch paddle grip while in a drop. Because of this, more load (often in unexpected and awkward positions) is placed on rotational muscles of your torso as well as shoulder stabilizers. In addition, aggressive use of your hip flexors, quadriceps, gluteus, and hamstrings in concert with rotation of your trunk provides the base to paddle from. Therefore, trunk strength, flexibility, and shoulder stability are primary requirements. Due to the potential for asymmetry in whitewater canoeing as opposed to flat water, pay particular attention to equal development and flexibility on both sides of your body.

If you are an advanced whitewater canoeist, the strength demands increase, especially due to the addition of rolling and extreme bracing.

Aerobic Conditioning

Whitewater boating is not as demanding aerobically, but is very skill dependent. Spend at least 30 minutes 2 times per week paddling on flat water. On land, aerobic training uses the same equipment suggested for flat-water boating for 30-minute sessions. After 3–4 weeks of base-level aerobic training, add high-intensity intervals (15- to 90-second bursts) once or twice a week. Have some of your aerobic training be interval-free.

Strength Training

Strength training is similar to that for flat water, but should include some advanced strengthening exercises for your upper body to improve bracing strength and to protect against dislocations.

Upper body: Do Exercises 111, 115, 116, 117.4, 118 (parallel grip), 119, 120, 120.2. 120.3, 121, 121.1, 123, 124, 125 (parallel grip), 126, 127, 130, 131, 133, 134, 139, and 140. To help simplify this program, choose two from the rowing exercises (118, 119, 131, 133, and 134); choose one from each of the following groups: 123 or 124, 126 or 127, and 111, 115, or 130; and do Exercises 139 and 140. After 6 weeks of gradually increasing the resistance, add 1 set of higher resistance, with lower reps per set (4–6 reps per set), except for Exercises 88, 120, 120.2, 121, 133, and 134.

Abdominals: For whitewater boating, abdominal development is especially necessary. Do Exercises 78.5, 79.2 or 92, 82, 84, 88, and 93. Add a rotary torso machine exercise if you have access to one. Alternatively, do Exercise 80.

Lower body: Do Exercises 29, 95, and 97.

Balance and Agility

Spend at least 30 minutes 2 times per week on agility and balance practice. Gradually intensify these sessions to quick and higher-amplitude balance and agility challenges. Particularly focus on doing on-the-water agility drill 3, earlier in this chapter, at high-speed intervals. Work toward doing a 2-minute obstacle course 8–10 times. Once this fitness base has been established (about 4–6 weeks), start on easy rivers. Continue the agility training and roll practice throughout the season (see the Rolling section in Sea or Lake Kayaking, below). For additional balance training, see the general dry-land balance exercises listed earlier in this chapter.

SEA OR LAKE KAYAKING

Kayakers should read Touring or Flat-Water Canoeing, above, which contains basic information for both canoeing and kayaking.

Kayaking, like canoeing, uses symmetrical, repetitive, linked motion that involves same-side leg and paddle drive. Your hips are flexed and your knees are nearly extended, which places a continuous load on your low back. The drive phase is accomplished through leg extension and rotation of your torso, followed by elbow bending. The kayaking stroke involves a significant degree of torso rotation and side bending, which requires a high level of torso strength and endurance. Your hip flexors are used for control of hull position as well as for maintaining slight forward flexion of your torso during the stroke. This makes flexibility in your hamstrings, hip flexors, and low back very important. In kayaking, your chest and back need to be equally well developed. The major muscles of the upper body listed for flat-water canoeing also apply to kayaking.

Rolling

Rolling is considered an advanced skill for sea kayakers and a necessary skill for whitewater kayakers. Rolling the kayak requires a very rapid, powerful combination of hip, back, abdominal, shoulder, chest, and arm muscles. The movement is primarily initiated from your hips, then progressively with your back, abdomen, and shoulders. It is best to practice this in a class or pool with other people around who can assist before trying it in cold water or with a loaded kayak. You should have good flexibility and torso strength before trying your first roll. Don't practice rolling if you have active shoulder or back problems, as they might be significantly exacerbated by it.

Stretching

When doing the stretching exercises outlined in the Stretching section earlier in this chapter, pay particular attention to the hamstrings (Exercises 1 and 2).

Aerobic Conditioning

Your aerobic training is best done on the water in a kayak with a program similar to the one suggested for flat-water canoeing earlier in this chapter. Start in calm waters with 30–60 minutes of low-intensity kayaking. Once weekly, do a long paddle, increasing the duration by 20 minutes per week up to 1 half day. By week 3–4, include 1–2 sessions of moderate-intensity intervals of 10 minutes (initially) and gradually work up to 60 minutes (see the on-water moderate-intensity interval suggestions for flat-water canoeing). After increasing the duration of your moderate-intensity training to 30 minutes, take your kayak out during windy conditions on a lake to practice your higher-intensity kayaking under rougher conditions. After 4–6 weeks, consider adding some high-intensity interval training.

Off-the-water training emphasizes aerobic base training with rowing ergometers (or use Exercise 37), cross-country ski machines, or other equipment that combines upper- and lower-body training. Use the same principles outlined for on-the-water training.

Interval Training for Rough or Windy Conditions

Sea or rough-water lake kayaking demands the stamina and skill level to do long-term, high-intensity paddling in order to get through windy conditions or rough water. Training for this should include higher-intensity intervals and should incorporate training time in challenging sea conditions. Start this type of interval training after you have been able to do approximately 45 minutes of on-water medium-intensity training (as outlined above).

Get comfortable with 1–2 hours of moderate- to high-intensity paddling if you would like to handle rough, windy conditions in sea kayaking, common during full-day or multiday sea kayaking trips. For high-intensity training, start with intervals of 1–2 minutes. Alternate this with periods of low-intensity paddling of double the duration of the high-intensity interval, to have some relative rest. Start with a few intervals mixed in with your regular paddling practice, and work up to 4–6 intervals. Gradually add some longer intervals. Intervals can also be done as Fartlek training (see chapter 3).

Strength Training

Upper body: Do the flat-water canoeing program earlier in this chapter, with the following modifications: Exercises 120.2 and 121.

Abdominals: Do the exercises outlined for whitewater canoeing earlier in this chapter.

Lower body: Do Exercises 29 and 95.

Balance and Agility

Dynamic sitting balance and agility are particularly important for rough, exposed water conditions. If you are training for difficult conditions, do the strength training outlined for whitewater kayaking, below.

Goal Program for a Full-Day or a Multiday Sea Kayak Trip

Begin approximately 8–10 weeks before your expected first day trip. You can feel reasonably prepared to embark on a 1-day or multiday sea kayak trip when you are able to sit comfortably for 4 hours and kayak at low intensity, do 30–45 minutes of moderate-intensity kayaking on smooth and rough water, do 6 intervals of 2- to 4-minute very high-intensity paddling, and handle capsizes.

Within 4–6 weeks of your sea kayak trip, practice some rolling or wet exits/reentries in a swimming pool with a partner or preferably in a class, especially if you don't have any active injuries in your back and shoulder. Make sure you feel comfortable tipping and exiting the kayak in open water and getting back in with or without the assistance of another boater. If you will be boating in cold water, make sure you have tried your roll/wet exit in cold water before going on your trip.

WHITEWATER KAYAKING

The paddle stroke is much the same in whitewater kayaking as in sea kayaking; however, the boat is normally fit snugly to the paddler in order to make immediate use of hip movements for boat placement. Hamstring stretching is even more important for proper spine position, as the kayaker's lower body position varies little over the course of the day.

The sitting balance challenges in whitewater boating are among the most significant of any sitting activity. The speed demands of intermediate and above levels of white water require that the paddler often perform in highly loaded, awkward positions. This places tremendous demands on the muscles of your torso as well as shoulder stabilizers. Shoulder injuries are not uncommon. In addition, aggressive use of your hip flexors, quadriceps, gluteus, and hamstrings in concert with rotation of your trunk and pelvis provides the base to paddle from. Therefore, trunk strength, flexibility, and shoulder stability are primary requirements.

Aerobic Conditioning

Follow the whitewater canoeing program discussed earlier in this chapter.

Strength Training

Your time on land should be a time not only to train aerobically, but also to work on stretching and strengthening any musculoskeletal deficiencies as regards kayaking. Common areas of strength deficiency include the torso, upper back (scapular stabilizers), and forearm muscles. Appropriate exercises are rows, lat pulls, biceps curls, triceps extensions, pull-ups, and sitting balance exercises on a gym ball. Several of these exercises should include a trunk rotational component.

See the Whitewater Canoeing section earlier in this chapter for a good basic strength training program.

Balance and Agility

Follow the whitewater canoeing program described earlier in this chapter.

Goal Program for a Full Day of Whitewater Kayaking

You should be ready for your full-day trip when you can spend 3–4 hours in your kayak, do 8–12 intervals on an obstacle course, roll, and feel comfortable bracing and turning in rough water. You should have mastered the strength and balance training program. This includes doing some sets of the upper-body exercises at higher speed and some sets at higher resistance.

ROWING (SCULLING AND SWEEP)

Sport rowing involves mechanics that are in many ways very different from canoeing and kayaking. Rowing shells have extremely little side-to-side stability and are generally designed to run on a stable hull surface on calm waters; therefore, the rowing motion involves very little side bending of your trunk. The plane of travel of the oar handle remains fairly constant, and your body is required to adjust to it around your shoulder joint. When rowing, your feet are secured to the bottom of the boat, and you move forward and back on a rolling seat positioned just slightly higher than your feet. This allows your legs to become the primary propulsive element in the stroke. Rather than the alternating right/left cycles of canoe or kayak paddling, rowing involves simultaneous extension of both knees with contraction of both arms.

The propulsive phase of the stroke is initiated with a powerful contraction of the gluteal and quadriceps muscles. This power is transferred through a neutral spine through your shoulders and arms to the face of the blade. This is accomplished by rolling on your sit bones (ischial tuberosities of the pelvis), rather than dramatically flexing and extending the low back. The power generated by your lower body is sudden and considerable. The support structure of your shoulders and arms must be strong enough to absorb the load, and to transfer those forces to the oars.

Sculling, in which you grasp two oars, is a symmetrical activity. Unless you are in rough, open conditions in an appropriate open-water boat, there is negligible torso side bending or torso rotation. Your spine has a high requirement for flexibility in flexion and extension and, as mentioned above, hamstring flexibility is quite necessary to attain proper positioning. Scullers may race or tour on flat or open water.

Sweep rowers (crew) grasp a single oar. It is unlikely that sweep rowers will be touring. Generally, sweep is a specifically competitive activity. It involves a rotational component to your torso, and, most important, your torso is rotated and slightly side-bent when your legs impose their greatest load. Sweep rowers row on one side only, at least during any given workout, so their potential for asymmetrical body development is quite high. It is therefore important to understand the high level of flexibility necessary in this activity.

Aerobic Conditioning

It is beyond the scope of this book to design appropriate training programs for sprint and distance rowing races. The rower with those intentions has adequate other published materials to draw upon and is likely involved in a coached competitive program. The stretching, resistance, and balance training aspects of this book, however, are certainly applicable to the competitive rower. The focus here is to enable the recreational touring rower to be adequately prepared. Because rowing shells are particularly unstable, it is also assumed that the rower attempting to follow this program has the necessary skills to handle the boat during periods of hard work.

On the water: Rowing is very aerobically demanding, as it engages an enormous number of muscles and is done in an explosive manner. It is also highly skill-dependent. Although some of each training time should be used to focus particularly on skill development, it is important to maintain good body mechanics by remaining aware of them with every stroke. Otherwise, the potential for injury increases greatly.

Begin with sessions of 30–60 minutes of low-intensity training while focusing on balance and technical skills. Once a week, take a longer row, increasing the duration by 15–30 minutes. Your regular training sessions should build to 45–90 minutes, and your longer row to 2 hours. If you are training for a long rowing trip, adjust the maximums accordingly. Remember that the load on the extensor muscles of your spine is great in rowing, and that the increases in time should be made only if they can be done comfortably.

By week 3–4, include 10-minute intervals of moderate intensity, working toward 2–3 in a session. Gradually increase the proportion of medium-intensity work until you are able to spend your whole row (excepting warm-up) at medium intensity.

After increasing your medium-intensity interval to 30 minutes and doing so with good, relaxed control, begin adding high-intensity bursts of anywhere from 30 seconds to 2 minutes at a higher stroke rate. This is necessary to develop the boat-handling skills needed when encountering foul weather, boat wakes, or even other boats. Do this in a Fartlek-type format (see chapter 3).

On land: A rowing ergometer is a good tool for aerobic training. It is widely available in health clubs and closely mimics the actual rowing motion. If being on the water is not an option, use an erg to do the aerobic training outlined above. Consider varying your stroke rate to music as you keep at a moderate intensity. The different beat of different tunes will vary the workout and the aerobic demand. Try to make it fun.

If an ergometer is unavailable, a cross-country ski machine is the next best option. If you choose running for your aerobic cross training, use hills and/or stair running (not stair-climbers) as part of your training, but remember that running does little for the upper body.

Strength Training

Your time on land should be used not only to train aerobically, but also to work on stretching and strengthening any musculoskeletal deficiencies as regards rowing. Common areas of strength deficiency include the legs, back, abdomen, and upper back (scapular stabilizers). In sweep rowing, trunk rotation is also necessary to prepare for load. Flexibility deficiencies are common in the hamstrings and muscles of the forearm.

Upper body: Exercises 116, 117.4, 118, 120 or 128.1, 121, 124, 125, 127, 131, and 134 (sweep only).

Abdominals: Exercises 78.4, 79 (or better, 92), 80 (sweep only), 87 (sweep only). Sweep rowers add a rotary torso machine if you have access to one in your gym.

Lower body: Exercises 31, 32, 95, 95.2, 95.4, and 97 (with weights).

chapter 22 CONDITIONING FOR ROAD AND MOUNTAIN BICYCLING

By Erik Moen, P.T.

THIS CHAPTER WILL HELP YOU:

- Appreciate the physiological demands on the cyclist.
- Create a basic mileage plan for a known ride.
- Establish a functional strengthening program specific for bicycling.
- Successfully perform coordination drills to enhance cycling confidence.

The first objective of anyone who is interested in bicycling should be proper equipment fit and then development of an aerobic base. Following this you can add interval, strength, balance, and agility training depending on the demands of your activity. Mountain cyclists should spend extra time on strength and agility training.

MUSCULOSKELETAL DEMANDS

Quadriceps, hamstrings, and gluteals play a big role in the propulsion of a cyclist. Your hamstrings should be strengthened to approximately four-fifths the strength of your quadriceps. Your shoulders and arms are used for pulling but are primarily used in the maintenance of torso posture and the absorption of shock from the terrain. More upper-body, balance, and agility training is required for mountain bikers.

MUSCLE IMBALANCES

Muscle imbalances commonly associated with cycling are mid- and upper-back weakness contrasted with tight pectorals (chest). This can lead to other upper-body imbalances, which can affect the neck and front of the shoulders. In the lower body, inadequate hamstring-to-quadriceps strength can lead to early leg fatigue during a cycling trip.

WARM-UP

Warm up for cycling by doing 5–10 minutes of low-resistance pedaling.

STRETCHING

Follow the warm-up with stretching Exercises 1–3, 6, 9, 11–13, 17, and 19.

AEROBIC CONDITIONING

Effective training for a selected bicycling event requires answers to two questions:

1. What is the goal riding volume (as defined by distance or time)?
2. How much time prior to the event do you have to achieve your goals?

Phasic training and preparation time for different bicycling events are suggested in Figure 38. Each event is listed by distance or time and has a minimum preparation time suggested in weeks prior to that event. Your total preparation time is broken into three phases of training: Phase 1, base mileage; Phase 2, strength and aerobic capacity; and Phase 3, specific preparation for the event. Each typical event has a suggested weekly training plan, outlined in Figure 38, to help create weekly training specific for your goals (weekly training specifics are shown in Figure 39). There is room for individual variation of basic training.

Please be aware that rushing preparation time may lead to an overuse injury. The following training programs assume that your bicycle is properly fit and that you are not adjusting to new equipment.

Calculating Weekly Goal Mileage

The next step of planning is to define weekly mileage goals as a function of how many weeks you need to prepare for an event. Always count backward from the event date in determining mileage goals. A reasonable peak mileage goal (PMG) for whatever event you pick is the distance of the event. In the example of a 2-day event, a reasonable PMG would be the most miles expected in 1 day. Each phase of training has a reasonable percentage of volume change (VC) per week to ensure progression of mileage. Net VC per week is discussed in each phase below. Weekly mileage goals (WMG) are calculated as a function of PMG, and calculations are given for each phase.

Phase 3, or the specific preparation phase, allows a rider to adapt to the basic mileage/time volumes required for successful completion of a goal. The VC for Phase 3 is 10% of PMG, so the generic formula is: WMG = PMG–(0.10 × PMGx4).

Example: Lance chooses to train 12 weeks for a 150-mile 1-day ride. Phase 3 of a 12-week plan has 3 weeks. Lance's PMG should equal 150 miles, thus WMG for weeks 10–12 are as follows:

Week 12 150 miles – (0.10 × 150 × 1) = 135 miles
Week 11 150 miles – (0.10 × 150 × 2) = 120 miles
Week 10 150 miles – (0.10 × 150 × 3) = 105 miles

Phase 2 is designed to increase a rider's bicycle-specific strength and aerobic capacity. Peak mileage goals will be no more than 70% of PMG. The VC for Phase 2 is 5% of PMG and the generic formula is: WMG = PMG × 0.7 – (0.05 × PMG × 4). Continuing with the example:

Week 9 150 miles × 0.7 – (0.05 × 150 × 1) = 98 miles
Week 8 150 miles × 0.7 – (0.05 × 150 × 2) = 90 miles

FIGURE 38. PHASIC TRAINING FOR BICYCLE EVENTS

WEEKS PRIOR TO EVENT	TYPICAL EVENT	PHASE 1 (WEEKS)	PHASE 2 (WEEKS)	PHASE 3 (WEEKS)	SUGGESTED WEEKLY TRAINING PLAN
14	2 days of 100 miles each on road	6 weeks	5 weeks	3 weeks	2D
13		5	5	3	
12	150 miles on road in 1 day	5	4	3	2D
11		5	4	2	
10		4	4	2	
9	100 miles on road or 5 hours on MTB	3	4	2	1D or MTB
8		3	3	2	
7		3	2	2	
6	50 miles on road or 3 hours on MTB	2	2	2	1D or MTB

D = day, MTB = mountain bike, 2D or 1D = mileage covered in 1 or 2 days

Week 7 150 miles × 0.7 – (0.05 × 150 × 3) = 83 miles

Week 6 150 miles × 0.7 – (0.05 × 150 × 4) = 75 miles

Phase 1 is designed for your body's adaptation to basic miles on the bicycle. Peak mileage goals for this phase will be no more than 60% of total PMG. The VC for Phase 1 is 8% of PMG and the generic formula is: WMG = PMG × 0.6 – (0.08 × PMG × 4). Continuing with the example:

Week 5 150 miles × 0.6 – (0.08 × 150 × 1) = 78 miles

Week 4 150 miles × 0.6 – (0.08 × 150 × 2) = 66 miles

Week 3 150 miles × 0.6 – (0.08 × 150 × 3) = 54 miles

Week 2 150 miles × 0.6 – (0.08 × 150 × 4) = 42 miles

Week 1 150 miles × 0.6 – (0.08 × 150 × 5) = 30 miles

Thus, 12 weeks prior to the event, the highlight of Lance's first week of training will be a 30-mile ride. Mileage overlap between Phases 1 and 2 is designed to allow your body to compensate for Phase 2's added intensity as described in Weekly Training Plans, below.

Weekly Training Plans

Figure 39 shows suggested weekly training plans for ride distances given in Figure 38. These are suggested weekly plans as a function of phase and WMG to create a sufficient aerobic base to achieve your goals. Please note the inclusion of physiological intervals and skill drills. These are described later in this chapter.

Five to 7 days prior to your goal event should be a period of relative rest. Relative rest includes activities of minimal intensity and significantly reduced mileage. Volumes are not to exceed 30% of your most recent WMG.

Pedaling Cadence

Basic pedaling mechanics are of high priority for efficiency, aerobic conditioning, and avoiding overuse injury. These pedaling drills don't have to be performed exactly as described here. They may be altered to suit your level.

Optimal pedaling cadence for the cyclist is largely individual and dependent on terrain, but generally should be 80–90 revolutions per minute (rpm). Maintenance of this relatively quick pace allows you to ride more efficiently and thus decreases the possibility of injury or fatigue. The use of a bicycling computer that measures cadence is suggested. But even without one, monitoring cadence is as simple as taking your heart rate.

This self-test should be done on a quiet stretch of road. Simply monitor your watch as you pedal. Count the number of pedal strokes in a 15-second period and then multiply that number by 4. This will give you an rpm value. Now that you have an appreciation for rpm, practice maintaining your goal.

Work your way through the progression of pedal cadences found in Figure 40. Practice your ability to determine approximate levels of cadence. This is easiest when using an indoor trainer or exercise bike. This may and should also be done outdoors. Pay attention to your path of travel to avoid obstacles. *Note:* Although the word interval is used, these drills should be done in an aerobic level below 75% maximum heart rate (max HR).

When the more difficult interval becomes easy, maintain your 90 rpm value for the duration.

High-cadence intervals are performed to overload your body's ability to perform pedaling at levels greater than 90 rpm. The ability to pedal greater than 90 rpm for short periods of time is important in both road and mountain bicycling. It may be difficult for an individual to perform this task efficiently. You frequently see inefficient cyclists bounce on their saddles when attempting high-cadence efforts. Bouncing compromises your ability to control the bicycle's, steering, braking, shifting, and traction.

FIGURE 39. WEEKLY TRAINING PLANS

2D: 2 DAYS OF LONG ROAD RIDING

	PHASE 1	PHASE 2	PHASE 3
M	off	off	off
Tu	30% WGM	35% WGM	30% WGM
W	off	off	off
Th	40% WGM	30% WGM, Lactate threshold interval*	35% WGM
F	off	off	off
Sat	100% WGM	100% WGM	100% WGM
Sun	55% WGM	65% WGM	85% WGM

1D: 1 DAY OF LONG ROAD RIDING

	PHASE 1	PHASE 2	PHASE 3
M	off	off	off
Tu	45% WGM	30% WGM	30% WGM
W	off	off	off
Th	20% WGM	30% WGM, Lactate threshold interval*	30% WGM
F	off	off	off
Sat	100% WGM	100% WGM	100% WGM
Sun	20% WGM	25% WGM	25% WGM

MTB: MOUNTAIN BIKE RIDING

	PHASE 1	PHASE 2	PHASE 3
M	off	off	off
Tu	30% WGM	40% WGM	45% WGM
W	off	off	off
Th	50% WGM on road	Lactate threshold interval*	Anaerobic power interval
F	off	off	off
Sat	0.5 hour of skill and agility	0.5 hour of skill and agility	0.5 hour of skill and agility
Sun	100% WGM	100% WGM	100% WGM

*Lactate threshold interval should be performed and included as part of the daily volume.

FIGURE 40. BASIC PEDAL CADENCE DRILLS

	BEGINNER	INTERMEDIATE	ADVANCED
Total number of efforts	3	4	8
Sets	1	2	2
Repetitions in a set	3	2	4
Duration	3 minutes	5 minutes	2 minutes
Rest between reps	5 minutes	3 minutes	1 minutes
Rest between sets	—	10 minutes	3 minutes
Cadence for efforts	70–90 rpm	70–90 rpm	70–90 rpm

FIGURE 41. HIGH-CADENCE INTERVALS

	BEGINNER	INTERMEDIATE	ADVANCED
Total number of efforts	6	4	8
Sets	2	2	2
Repetitions in a set	3	2	4
Duration	30 seconds	3 minutes	45 seconds
Rest between reps	1 minute	2 minutes	1 minute
Rest between sets	5 minutes	5 minutes	5 minutes
Cadence for efforts	100 rpm	110 rpm	120 rpm
Cadence during rest	70 rpm	70 rpm	70 rpm

The intervals shown in Figure 41 should be performed so you don't bounce on the seat or create excessive motion in your upper body. Using an indoor trainer or stationary bike in front of a mirror is an excellent way to monitor your progress.

Interval Training

The following intervals are included to enhance your efficiency in pedaling. See chapter 3 regarding precautions and other information on interval training.

Intervals can be done on level surfaces and hills. The mountain bicyclist should do some intervals on trails and off-road terrain. All interval training requires a warm-up that includes 10–15 minutes of low-intensity, easy riding, stretching, and surveying the interval course for possible hazards. All intervals should be ended with a 10- to 15-minute cooldown period of easy, low-intensity riding and stretching.

Anaerobic Power Intervals

These are short, all-out intervals of 20 seconds or less.

Terrain: Section of uninterrupted hill approximately 2–3 blocks long. May be either dirt or pavement. Dirt better simulates real mountain biking terrain and requires attention to proper weight-shifting in order to maintain traction. Pavement allows you to focus clearly on the pure physiological effort.

Required time: Approximately 30–45 minutes.

High-intensity effort: Should last 10–20 seconds.

Cadence: 60–70 rpm.

Recovery: 3–5 minutes of easy, low-intensity pedaling to regain normal breathing.

Total number: Start with 4 intervals and work up to 8.

Moderate-Duration Intervals

Terrain: Long, straight roads, hills, or trails with long straight sections

Required time: 40–60 minutes.

High-intensity effort: 20 seconds–4 minutes, with the majority at 3 minutes.

Cadence: 70–90 rpm.

Recovery: 5 minutes of easy, low-intensity pedaling to regain normal breathing.

Total number: 4–8 intervals.

Lactate Threshold Longer Intervals

These build fitness for sustained efforts such as long hill climbs. These efforts are aerobic in nature, less intense than the above intervals, and sustained for 5–10 minutes. You should be in a heart rate zone of 75–85% max HR.

Terrain: 2–4 miles of flat or rolling uninterrupted terrain, or a 1- to 3-mile section of gradual climbing.

Required time: 40–60 minutes.

Interval: 5–10 minutes of sustained heavy breathing while maintaining your pedal cadence.

Cadence: 70–90 rpm.

Recovery: 5 minutes of easy, low-intensity pedaling to regain normal breathing.

Total number: Start with 2 intervals and work up to 4.

STRENGTH TRAINING

The following exercise recommendations can help the cyclist improve performance and balance. Exercise each body region 2 times per week.

Road Cycling

Lower body: Exercises 57.5, 95, 95.2, 96 (hamstring curls done with a single leg, sitting if possible as in exercise 96.2), and 97 (basic lunge).

Abdominals: The road cyclist should do these if riding hills, doing fast cornering, and so on. Do Exercises 81, 83, 84, and 94.

Upper body: Exercises 111, 113 or 115, 117, 118, 120.1, 121, 127, and 131.

Mountain Biking

Lower body: Do the road cyclist program above, adding the following: Exercises 97.10, 100, 100.1, 100.3 (advanced cyclists can try 100.4), 101, and 101.1.

Abdominals: Mountain cyclists have a significant demand on their arms, legs, torso, and abdominal muscles to maintain balance. Do the road cyclist program above, adding Exercise 62. See the agility exercises below.

Upper body: Do the road cyclist program above, adding Exercise 128, and substituting Exercise 130 for 115 and 104 for 131.

FUNCTIONAL BIKING AGILITY EXERCISES

The development of agility takes practice. The following exercises are considered dynamic and functional exercises. They challenge your moving balance in simulated environments. Effective practice means calculated risk. Please be aware that bicycling in general, and possibly these exercises, can be dangerous. The successful practice of the following exercises will help to decrease the potential danger of bicycling. Please use common sense and a properly fitted helmet when on your bike.

ROAD AND MOUNTAIN BIKING SKILLS

171 BALANCE-READY POSITION

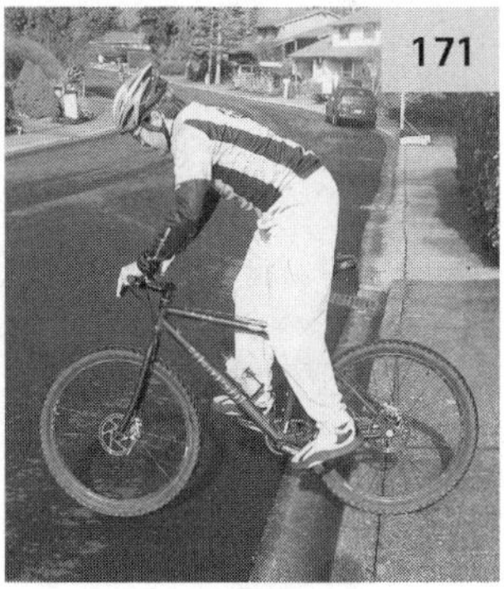

Equipment: Bicycle, curb.
Purpose: The balance-ready position is your most effective posture on the bike for meeting challenging situations. This position should be learned and readily accessible for both road and mountain biking.

Technique: The balance-ready position maintains your center of mass over the bottom bracket of the bicycle. This exercise takes the rider down off the curb. You should be off the saddle with your cranks horizontal, knees and elbows slightly bent, head upright, vision forward, with a firm grasp on the handlebars. Approach the curb in an easy gear while on the saddle. As you approach the curb perpendicularly, control your speed with your rear brake as you attain the balance-ready position. Roll off the edge of the curb, landing the front wheel as softly as possible; continue to control your speed as you slowly roll the back wheel off the curb. Repeat until you are able to roll your bike off the curb as smoothly and quietly as possible.

172 MAINTAINING A STRAIGHT LINE

Equipment: Bicycle, quiet road.
Purpose: The maintenance of a straight line while riding your bicycle is important for injury prevention. It requires balance and concentration.

Technique: Find a line on a quiet road that you can ride along for 30–120 seconds. Concentrate on your pedal speed and rhythm. Try not to pedal off the line.

173 LEVEL SLALOM

Equipment: Uninterrupted level surface approximately 30–100 feet long; objects such as cones, water bottles, hats, and so on, set up in a slalom course.

Purpose: Steering through challenging surfaces such as hills takes concentration, coordination, balance, steering, speed control, and vision (picking a line) to put together a clean ride. It is important that you be able to avoid consecutive objects.

Technique: Place the objects 4–6 feet apart, with an exit gate 2 feet wide. Start with a short course with objects at 6-foot distances and gradually progress to shorter object-to-object distances and more challenging courses. Enter the course traveling slalom-style around the objects. Control your speed as you travel through the challenge so that you exit through the gate without knocking over any obstacles.

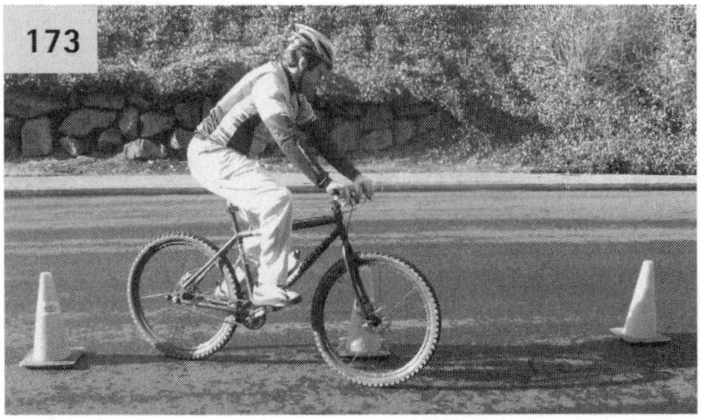
173

Variation: 173.1. Decreased slalom distances: You may include shorter distances between objects, or see how quickly or slowly you can do the course. Mountain bikers should set up obstacle courses on hills (uphill and downhill sections).

MOUNTAIN BIKING–SPECIFIC DRILLS

174 DOWNHILL SLALOM

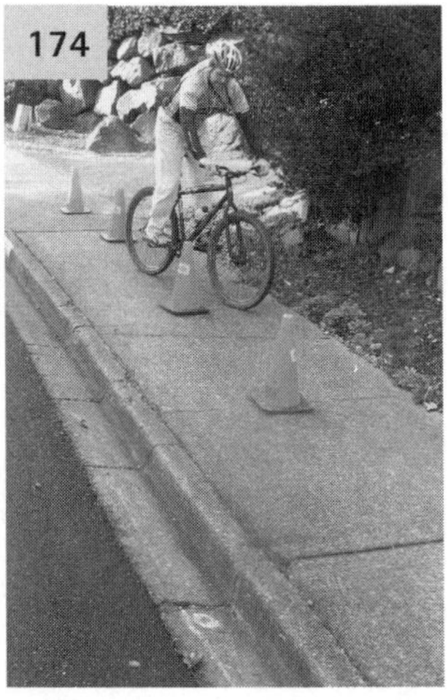
174

Equipment: Slalom course setup for Exercise 173, on a downhill grade 100–300 feet.

Purpose: Control your speed and maintain your balance on downhill trails.

Technique: Start at the top of a downhill grade. You don't have to pedal much for this exercise, but an appropriate (easy-to-pedal) gear should be predetermined in the event that you have to regain balance. Enter the course with your weight slightly behind the saddle in a balance-ready position. Control your speed with the rear brake as you navigate the slalom course. Remember to keep your weight over the bike rather than leaning out to the side.

Variation: 174.1. Increased downhill grade: You can make this exercise more difficult by increasing the pitch of the slope.

175 RIDE THE 2X4 LINE

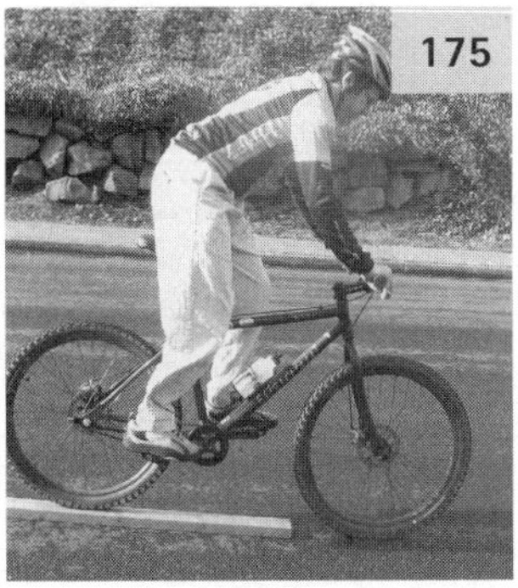

Equipment: 3- to 10-foot-long 2×4.
Purpose: Challenge your ability to maintain a narrow path and refine ability to balance on the bike in tricky off-road areas.

Technique: Set the 2×4 down flat, 4-inch side down, on a quiet lot. Approach the 2×4 with enough speed to carry yourself along its length. As you near the board, assume the balance-ready position. Control your speed with your rear brake. Lightly lift, or unweight, the front wheel by leaning slightly back on the bike. Move back to the balance-ready position as you traverse the wood. Pay attention to keeping your head up and forward. Focus on where you are going rather than your immediate front wheel; you should have already seen that territory.

BUNNY HOP

Mastering the bunny hop and its components takes skill, agility, and coordination. This is an important survival skill for both the off-road and road cyclist. It allows you to avoid objects such as potholes without swerving into traffic or other riders, and to avoid objects that would otherwise cause a flat tire.

176 LIFTING THE FRONT WHEEL

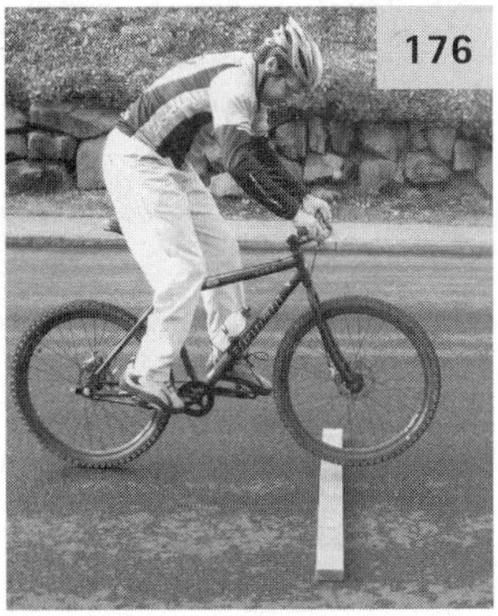

Equipment: 3- to 5-foot-long 2×4.
Purpose: The first component of the bunny hop is helpful in activities such as going up a curb.

Technique: Pick a gear that can be easily pedaled. Make a slow, perpendicular approach to the board. Attain the balance-ready position. Just before you get to the wood: (a) crouch down, loading your weight over the pedals; (b) spring up and back, unloading the pedals (feet continue their contact with the pedals), and lift up on the handlebars; (c) let your rear wheel roll over the 2×4. Use caution to not make the lifting up and back too ballistic, as you may fall over backward. The 2×4 is an excellent object to work with, as you can easily roll over it if you do not adequately lift your front wheel. Try many times until you have a sense of control and are able to quietly clear the 2×4 with your front wheel.
Variation: 176.1. Curb lift: You can increase the difficulty by using a curb or larger piece of wood.

177 LIFTING THE BACK WHEEL

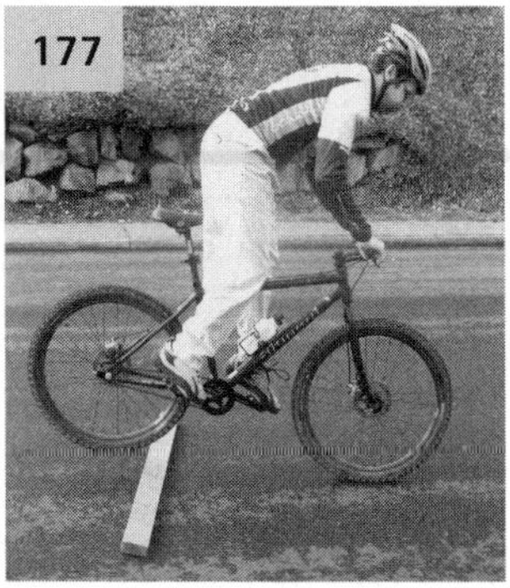

Equipment: 3- to 5-foot-long 2×4.
Purpose: The second component of the bunny hop is a handy skill to master for off-road proficiency.

Technique: Make a perpendicular approach to the 2×4 with controlled speed. Hop the front wheel over the board and then: (a) shift your weight forward so your center of mass is in front of the bottom bracket of the bicycle; (b) simultaneously push down on the handlebars and lift up on the pedals. You will notice a hop of the rear wheel. Again, use caution to not make too large a leap when trying to hop the rear wheel, as there is potential to go over the handlebars onto your head. Lifting up on the pedals can be done without toe straps. This is achieved by pointing your toes slightly down prior to lifting up. The combination of this with leaning slightly forward creates the lift. Try this exercise repeatedly, with a goal of control and ease.
Variation: 177.1. Curb lift: You can increase the difficulty by using a curb or larger piece of wood.

178 BUNNY HOP

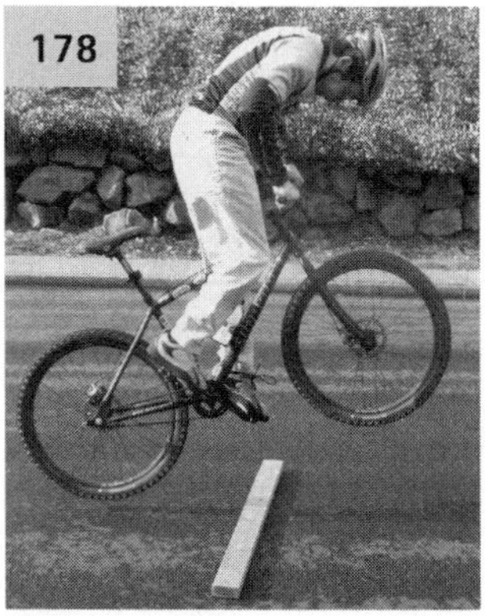

Equipment: 3- to 5-foot-long 2×4.
Purpose: The intentional full clearance of bike and rider off the ground incorporates the skills of front and rear wheel hops.

Technique: The 2×4 is an excellent practice piece, as you will know if you don't clear it, but 99% of the time it will not cause you to crash. Make the usual perpendicular approach to the board. Making a faster approach will not necessarily ensure that you will clear the board with greater success; therefore, maintain a controlled speed. Attain the balance-ready position as you approach the 2×4: (a) crouch down, loading your weight over the pedals; (b) spring up, lifting the front wheel up via the handlebars; (c) quickly shift your weight forward, pushing the handlebars forward to help lift the rear wheel up and over the object. It helps to use the same foot lift in the last part of the hop as you used to lift the back wheel in Exercise 177. As you can see, the bunny hop is a combination of the two single-wheel hops.
Variation: 178.1. Line hop: If you are a little tentative about using a 2×4 to start with, establish a line in the dirt as your first practice setup. You can work on becoming proficient at hopping a line in the dirt prior to moving to a 2×4.

chapter 23 CONDITIONING FOR RUNNING

By Lisa Fox, P.T., and David Musnick, M.D.

THIS CHAPTER WILL HELP YOU:

- Put together a comprehensive conditioning program to meet distance goals from a 5K run through a marathon.
- Use running as a part of your outdoor fitness program.

Running can be used for general fitness, to train for other activities, or as a goal in itself. From the information in this chapter, you can develop a conditioning program to improve your running. In this chapter, most distances are listed in miles, except for some shorter distances and marathon distances, which are in meters or kilometers (abbreviated as K). The Appendix at the back of this book gives conversions for standard and metric units of measurement.

MUSCULOSKELETAL DEMANDS

Running is primarily a forward-motion activity that also involves side-to-side and rotational forces. It generates an impact of two to four times your own body weight and is thus considered a high-impact and repetitive activity. Running involves alternating deceleration forces by pronation (foot flattening, internal rotation of your leg, and flexing and side bending of your hip and spine), followed by propulsion or supination (foot arching, external rotation of your leg, and extending of your hip and spine). Because of the forces involved, it makes sense to follow an aerobic and strength training program to avoid foot, knee, and hip injuries.

Muscles Used in Running

All of the muscles from your buttock to your feet are used in running. They work to push you off the ground and to decelerate you. Leg, thigh, and buttock muscles are stressed the most when they slow down your knee, hip, and ankle from bending excessively and your foot from pronating. They are functionally strengthened during squats, lunges, and hops. Step-ups and step-downs are important if you are planning to run on hilly terrain. You may improve your running speed and endurance by doing functional strength training.

Risk Factors That May Lead to an Injury

Overuse injuries can occur in running as a result of foot problems, muscle imbalances, and low-back problems as well as from common training errors, including:

- Excessive mileage (especially when easy days are not incorporated into the program)
- Excessive interval or hill training
- Running on improper terrain (including running on canted or very uneven surfaces and excessive downhill running)

Build your weekly mileage slowly, and vary the routes and the terrain. For example, don't always run the same route that requires you to face traffic on the left side of a canted road. Also, don't run the same hilly route each time you go out for a run.

MUSCLE IMBALANCES

The most common areas of imbalance in runners are tighter heel cords in comparison to the weaker tibialis anterior; tighter iliotibial bands compared to their counterparts, the adductors and medial quadriceps; and gluteal weakness and tight quadriceps in relation to the hamstrings and hip flexors. These common areas of imbalance can be addressed with exercises to enhance flexibility (such as Exercises 1, 3, and 5–10) and strength (Exercises 23 and 98).

WARM-UP

You can warm up for running with a fast walk for 5 minutes followed by 1–3 minutes of skipping, or a jog of increasing intensity until you get up to your running pace.

STRETCHING

Running predominantly strengthens the calves, hamstrings, lower back, and front hip muscles. Over time, as these muscles become stronger, they will also become tighter. Do the following stretches after a warm-up or after your run: Exercises 1, 3.1, 3.2, 5, and 7–9.

AEROBIC TRAINING

Aerobic training for running is best done by running, with occasional cross-training sessions. Running is a high-impact activity, so be careful to increase your duration of each run by no more than 10–15% per week. Training for races can be done by following the training tables (Figures 42–45) later in this chapter.

Interval Training

You can do interval training with running to enhance your general aerobic endurance and your ability to do sprints. See chapter 3, as well as the sections on the second and third pyramid levels later in this chapter, for details on interval training.

Cross Training

If running is your major activity, you can use cross-training options to use your leg muscles and decrease the impact of running. These include hiking, cross-country skiing or using cross-country ski machines, snowshoeing, using a stair-climber, using an EFX cross trainer, using a slide board or a step, or doing regular aerobics workouts. Cycling can also be used, but it uses the muscles in a different way.

You can also use running as a cross-training tool for other activities. Running is an excellent form of aerobic conditioning. It is good preparation for participation in hiking, mountaineering, snowshoeing, and cross-country skiing.

STRENGTH TRAINING

Strength training should focus on higher-rep sets rather than bulking exercises (high resistance, low repetitions) for the lower body. You can do these strengthening exercises 2–3 times per week. For the lower-body exercises, do 2–3 sets of 15–20 reps. *Note:* An abdominal and upper-body strength training program can enhance your running, but doesn't yield as much of a return in performance as do lower-body exercises. (For definitions of *beginning* and *intermediate/advanced*, see Developing a Training Program section below.)

Beginning

Lower body: Exercises 28, 28.3, 29, 95, 95.2, 96, and 98.

Abdominals: Exercises 23, 78.3, 79.1, and 80.

Upper body: Exercises 111, 126, and 127.

Intermediate/Advanced

Lower body: Do the beginning program, adding Exercises 31, 101, and 101.3. Consider adding Exercise 30 and omitting Exercises 28 and 29.

Abdominals: Exercises 23, 78.4, 79.2, 81, and 86.

Upper body: Add Exercise 133 to the beginning program.

BALANCE AND AGILITY

Balance and agility are crucial components of function for runners. Poor balance and poor reaction to unpredictable surfaces are primary factors contributing to injury. To improve your balance and agility for running, do BST Exercises 44 and 46, and Exercises 58, 59, 66.1, 80.1, and 101.2 twice a week.

DEVELOPING A TRAINING PROGRAM

You can train for distance running or races in many different ways. The tables at the end of this chapter (Figures 42–45) will help you gradually build up your mileage. You can also progress your training in a pyramid method (described below) that adds mileage, long runs, and then hill and speed work.

The program should look like a stack of building blocks, with each level providing the foundation for the next one. This program may take 4–6 months to safely reach the goal of a specific marathon. Training for 5K, 10K, and half-marathon runs will take less time, depending on your fitness level and running experience.

Beginning runners are those with 0–1 year of experience. *Intermediate/advanced runners* have more than 1 year of experience, have run races, and have been in training programs for increasing mileage or speed in the past 1–2 years. Beginning runners should start with the first pyramid level and refer to the beginning training schedule later in this chapter (see Figure 42).

The beginning runner may need at least 4 weeks to slowly introduce a running program that is injury free. At the fourth week, you will be running with alternate cross-training days. You should initially walk briskly for 30 minutes, 3 times per week, for 2 weeks. Then progress into jogging by inserting short jogging distances during the walk. An example would be to insert 400-meter (440-yard) jogs (the distance once around a standard track) repeatedly throughout the session. Initially insert 1 jog per mile, then 2 jogs, and so on, until you are jogging a mile, and then gradually increase the jog until you are jogging 30–40 minutes 3 times per week.

At this point you can begin a pyramid training schedule, especially if you have goals for running races. The first pyramid level, called base training, develops greater endurance and aerobic capacity for distance or race running. It accounts for 50% of the training program. During the second level, add strengthening drills (with strength training and hill running), speed interval workouts, and longer runs. The third level also incorporates interval training. (See chapter 3 for information and guidelines on various types of interval training.) The beginning runner can follow the guidelines under base training and the second pyramid level, or simply follow the training tables in Figures 42–45 to achieve various race distances.

A reasonable first running goal would be a 5–10K. See Figures 42 and 43. Beginning runners should start with the walking program described in the Warm-Up section earlier in this chapter. Weekly runs should include a long run in addition to 2–3 additional easier days. Intermediate runners with 4 months of a consistent base can insert speed work once a week if they are able to tolerate 20–30 miles a week. The distance of your long run depends upon what your experience level is at the time that you begin the program. An intermediate runner can enter a training schedule in line with your present weekly mileage. Strength training can be done on your cross-training or off days.

Do long runs every 1–2 weeks to prepare your body to tolerate longer distances and prepare you for races or longer-duration outdoor activities. Advanced runners may tolerate long runs every week. Beginning runners should initially do them every other week.

The pace for a long run is 1½–2 minutes

per mile slower than your current 10K race pace, or 2 minutes per mile slower than your expected marathon pace. Long runs are developed by taking the longest run in the past 2 weeks and increasing it by 1–2 miles. If you are running for fitness alone, do your long run based on time and add a 10–15% increase in time or distance.

> **PRACTICAL POINT**
> Plan an easy activity for 1–2 days after a long run to assist in recovery.

Rules for Training

There are a few simple rules that apply whether you are training for that first 5K run, have set a goal to break the 3-hour barrier for the marathon, or are conditioning for a weekend hike.

Rule 1: Start slow and with short distances.

Rule 2: Always incorporate a warm-up and cooldown phase into the daily program.

Rule 3: Don't increase the total exercise time or mileage by more than 10% per week.

Rule 4: Beginning and intermediate runners should take a rest week of fewer miles each third or fourth week.

Rule 5: Beginning runners should run at an intensity in which they are able to carry on a conversation while running.

Rule 6: Beginning runners should target distance before speed. The beginner will notice consistent improvements simply by adding distance.

Rule 7: Don't rigidly follow someone else's training schedule. Be flexible. If you feel tired, run easy for 1–2 days. If after 2 days of rest you are still tired, think about reducing the entire week of training and reevaluating the schedule.

Rule 8: Always follow a hard training day with an easy day of running or cross training.

Rule 9: Provide an adequate tapering-down period prior to a race.

Rule 10: Allow sufficient time to recover from a race. The recovery of muscle strength and endurance capacity are attained sooner if you rest for 6–7 days after a marathon vs. continuing to run.

Rule 11: Limit the number of races you participate in. Most runners can't tolerate more than 2 short-distance (10k or less) races a month and 3 marathons a year.

The First Pyramid Level: Base Training

Base training consists of daily runs, long runs on alternate weeks, and occasional participation in races. The goals are to develop endurance and aerobic capacity, which will lead to improved speed and ability to run longer distances.

Pace should be a comfortable speed, and you should be able to easily talk while running (70–80% maximum heart rate). The pace should be 1 1/2–2 minutes per mile slower than your current 10K race pace (if known). These runs should be relatively easy and enjoyable.

Races should be of moderate pace and done no more than every other week.

Mileage: Do up to 40 miles a week if training for a half or full marathon.

Long runs: If you are a beginning runner, take long runs on alternate weeks at a relaxed pace. Intermediate and advanced runners can do long runs every week.

The Second Pyramid Level: Hill Repeats

Once a week, run hill repeats on a 5–15% grade only. The distance can be from 150 yards to 1/2 mile. Proper form includes looking at the top of the hill and bringing your hips forward rather than slumping and leaning into the hill.

Improved form on a hill allows you to propel yourself up with less effort. You should feel your hamstrings and gluteals working while your legs move behind your body. Emphasize pushing off your feet and pumping your arms.

Pace: Run uphill at an intensity of 80–90% maximum heart rate (max HR) and jog easily back down to recover.

Frequency: Start with two hills, and increase by one to two hills per week to build up to 6–8 repeats for the longer hills and 8–10 repeats for the shorter hills. Perform this session once or twice per week.

Duration should be once or twice a week for 4–6 weeks, and should not be performed during the third pyramid level, the speed-training phase.

Mileage remains the same as the for first pyramid level, except for adding 1–2 days of hills.

The Second Pyramid Level: Fartlek Training

Fartlek training consists of interval training runs of varying speeds designed to build stamina. It allows you to control the pace in different environments, on cross-country trails or on roads, with the goal of feeling challenged but not exhausted when you are done (see chapter 3 for more details on Fartlek training). Examples:

1. Run 1,200 meters moderately hard, then run at an easy pace for equal or double the time.
2. Do speed bursts (80–90% max HR) of 100–400 meters with short, easy jogs between each sprint.
3. Run with a moderately hard effort up hills you encounter, followed with an easy pace between each hill.
4. Run for 1-, 2-, and 3-minute intervals (at approximately 85% max HR), with equal or double rest times of easy jogging between efforts.

Pace: During a jog, randomly mix in intervals of higher intensities (80–85% max HR) and distances when you feel like it. These can be done as timed segments of 30 seconds–4 minutes or as distances. Go back to a jog pace in between the interval.

Frequency is 1–2 times per week.

Duration is 20–50 minutes after a warm-up of easy jogging.

The Third Pyramid Level: Speed Training

The speed-training phase is the building block preceding the targeted goal. A runner who has more than a year of experience may need to target speed work in order to reach a new plateau in performance. Speed training results in markedly improved efficiency in your cardiovascular system within the initial 7 weeks. After 7 weeks the gains are slower. This phase is shorter because of the increased risk of injury due to the greater stress placed upon the body.

The best speed work for marathon distances is long intervals of 1/2 mile or more. Typically, 800 meters–3 miles are utilized for 10K and half-marathon training. Shorter distances of 400 meters–1 1/2 miles are utilized for 10K or 5K goals. Discontinue hill repeats and begin speed or interval workouts 1–2 times per week using one of several variations listed in the Third Pyramid Level: Interval Training, below.

Frequency: The intermediate runner should start speed work after 4–6 months of base training, then only once a week until the following season. During the second season, increase this to twice a week.

Duration is 4 to a maximum of 7 weeks.

Mileage: Cut total mileage by 10%.

Long runs can be continued, gradually increasing them to your goal distance.

PRACTICAL POINT

Speed training cannot be performed year-round except by experienced runners. The average runner should develop a speed program of 7 weeks to avoid injury and to take advantage of the best peaking time.

The Third Pyramid Level: Tempo Running

This is fast distance training that can be performed on a road or track. The goal is to maintain a consistent pace.

Pace is slightly slower than race pace for the same distance. For example, if your 5K pace is 7:45 minutes per mile, then practice a 5K course at an 8:15-minutes-per-mile pace.

Mileage is 2 miles or more.

The Third Pyramid Level: Interval Training

Anaerobic intervals are intervals of less than 4 minutes' duration done at anaerobic intensities of 85–95% max HR, with rest periods of lower-intensity running or fast walking (at 60–70% max HR) for 1–2 times the interval duration. Work up to 3–8 shorter anaerobic intervals of 30 seconds, 1 minute, 2 minutes, 3 minutes, and 4 minutes, or do them as distances of 200, 400, and 800 meters.

Aerobic intervals of longer duration (greater than 4 minutes) should be done at 80–85% max HR. Other interval examples:

- 2 at 5 minutes
- 400 meters, 800 meters, 1,200 meters, 800 meters, 400 meters
- 4 at 400 meters
- 3 at 1,200 meters
- 3 at 1 mile

Duration is 5 to 30 minutes.

Mileage is 800 meters–3 miles for longer race distance goals (half or full marathon).

At the Top of the Pyramid: The Goal Event/Tapering

This is the 2–4 weeks before the big race or the planned climbing trip, for example. Start about 14 days prior to a shorter event, reducing total mileage by 30–50%; at 7 days, reduce by 70–80%, with the final 2–3 days consisting of only 1–3 miles daily. You can continue the same speed with each run since the fewer miles will allow ample rest. Begin tapering 3–4 weeks prior to a marathon, tapering to 50% by week 3, and at 7 days reduce by 70–80%, again with the final 2–3 days consisting of only 1–3 miles daily.

With a running training program it is easy to see that one distance goal can be the base of the next. For example, a 5K schedule in May will provide the strength and skill for a half marathon in the fall. A half marathon in February will provide a base for a weekend glacier climb in the late spring.

FIGURE 42. EXAMPLE TRAINING PROGRAM FOR A 5K (BEGINNING)

WK	MON	TUE	WED	TH	FRI	SAT	SUN	TOTAL MILEAGE
1	off	3	CT	3	off	CT	4	10
2	off	3	CT	3	off	CT	3	9
3	off	3	CT	3	off	CT	5	11
4	off	3	CT	3	off	CT	3	9
5	off	3½	CT	3½	off	CT	5	12
6	off	3½	CT	3½	off	CT	4	10
7	off	3½	CT	3½	off	CT	4	11
8	off	3	CT	3	off	CT	3	10
9	off	3	CT	3	off	CT	2	9 tapering
10	off	3	CT	2	off	CT	1	5
11	off	2	CT	1	off	CT	race	5K

CT = cross training
Distances are in miles.
Races of 10K or shorter should be followed by 1 easy week.

FIGURE 43. EXAMPLE TRAINING PROGRAM FOR A 10K (WITH A 5K AS A BUILDING BLOCK)

WK	MON	TUE	WED	TH	FRI	SAT	SUN	TOTAL MILEAGE
1	off	3	CT	3	CT	3	5	14
2	off	4	CT	4	CT	3	4	15
3	off	4	CT	3½	CT	3	6	16½
4	off	4	CT	4	CT	3	4	15
5	off	4	H + CT; 1 x ¼ mile	4	CT	3	7	18
6	off	4	H + CT; 1 x ¼ mile	5	CT	3	5	17
7	off	2	H + CT; 1 x ¼ mile	3	CT	2	3	10
8	off	3	H + CT; 1 x ¼ mile	2	CT	1	race 5K	
9	off	rest	CT	rest	CT	rest	rest	0
10	off	4	CT	5	CT	3	7	20
11	off	4	CT	5	CT	3	5	17
12	off	5	CT	6	CT	3	8	22
13	off	5	CT	6	CT	3	5	19 tapering
14	off	5	CT	6	CT	3	8	22
15	off	3	CT	3	CT	2	3	11
16	off	2	CT	2	CT	1	race 10K	
rest	rest	rest	rest	rest	rest	rest	rest	rest

CT = cross training

H = hill training

Distances are in miles. Total mileage at the beginning should be no greater than 20–30 miles per week.

Note: Hill training can be added to any of the running days at the end of a workout.

Races of 10K or shorter should be followed by 1 easy week.

FIGURE 44. EXAMPLE TRAINING PROGRAM FOR A HALF-MARATHON

WK	MON	TUE	WED	TH	FRI	SAT	SUN	TOTAL MILEAGE
1	off	4	CT	4	CT	3	6	17
2	off	4	CT	4	CT	3	7½	18½
3	off	5	CT	4	CT	3	4	16
4	off	5	CT	5	CT	3	7½	20½
5	off	6	CT	5	CT	3	4	18
6	off	6	CT	5	CT	3	8½	22½
7	off	6	CT	6	CT	3	5	20
8	off	6	H + CT; 1 x ¼ mile	6	CT	3	10	25
9	off	6	H + CT; 1 x ¼ mile	6	CT	3	5	20
10	off	6	H + CT; 2 x ¼ mile	6	CT	3	10	25
11	off	6	H + CT; 2 x ¼ mile	6	CT	3	5	20
12	off	2	H + CT; 3 x ¼ mile	4	CT	3	4	13
13	off	2	H + CT; 3 x ¼ mile	2	CT	1	3	8
14 tapering	off	3	H + CT; 3 x ¼ mile	2	CT	1	race 10K	
15	off	rest	CT	rest	CT	rest	rest	0
16	off	6	CT	6	CT	3	10	25
17	off	6	CT	6	CT	3	6	21
18	off	6	CT	6	CT	3	12½	27½
19	off	6	CT	6	CT	3	8	23
20	off	7	CT	6	CT	3	14	30
21	off	7	CT	7	CT	3	7	24
22	off	8	CT	8	CT	3	14	33
23 tapering	off	4	CT	5	CT	3	5	17
24	off	2	CT	3	CT	1	4	10
25	off	2	CT	2	CT	1	race ½ marathon	

CT = cross training

H = hill training

Distances are in miles. Total mileage at the beginning should be no greater than 20–30 miles per week.

Note: Hill training can be added to any of the running days at the end of a workout.

FIGURE 45. EXAMPLE TRAINING PROGRAM FOR A MARATHON

WK	MON	TUE	WED	TH	FRI	SAT	SUN	TOTAL MILEAGE
1	off	6	CT	6	CT	3	10	25
2	off	6	CT	6	CT	3	5	20
3	off	6	CT	6	CT	3	10	25
4	off	6	CT	6	CT	3	5	20
5	off	6	CT	6	CT	3	12½	27½
6	off	6	CT	6	CT	3	8	23
7	off	7	CT	6	CT	3	14	30
8	off	7	H + CT; 1 x ¼ mile	7	CT	3	7	24
9	off	7	H + CT; 1 x ¼ mile	7	CT	3	6	33
10	off	7	H + CT; 2 x ¼ mile	7	CT	3	16	27
11	off	8	H + CT; 2 x ¼ mile	7	CT	3	10	36
12	off	8	H + CT; 3 x ¼ mile	7	CT	3	18	28
13 tapering	off	4	CT	4	CT	3	10	14
14	off	3	CT	2	CT	1	race ½ marathon	
15	off	rest	CT	rest	CT	rest	rest	0
16	off	8	CT	7	CT		10	28
17	off	8	CT	7½	CT	3	21	39½
18	off	8	CT	7½	CT	3	10	28½
19	off	8	CT	7½	CT	3	22	41½
20 tapering	off	8	CT	7½	CT	3	10	28½
21	off	4	CT	6	CT	3	7	20
22	off	2	CT	3	CT	1	4	10
23	off	2	CT	2	CT	1	race marathon	
rest week								
rest week								

CT = cross training
H = hill training
Distances are in miles. Total mileage at the beginning should be no greater than 20–30 miles per week.
Note: Hill training can be added to any of the running days at the end of a workout.
Completely rest the first week following a marathon and allow at least 3 easy months for a full recovery, especially if you are prone to injuries.

chapter 24 CONDITIONING FOR WINDSURFING

By Mark Pierce, A.T.C., and David Musnick, M.D.

THIS CHAPTER WILL HELP YOU:

- Develop an exercise program that will increase your balance and musculoskeletal ability to meet the rigorous demands of windsurfing.

Typically, a windsurfing run lasts between 10 and 30 minutes before a rest or fall, followed by about 2 minutes of recovery and repositioning. This requires a moderate amount of sustained and intermittent strength.

MUSCULOSKELETAL DEMANDS

Windsurfing requires significant balance and agility along with sustained whole-body strength. The typical body posture while windsurfing is hands grasping the boom; hips, knees, and ankles bent with your shoulders forward; and upper back in a flexed position. Most of your body weight is supported by a belt harness around your hips or chest and hooked to the boom. Assuming this posture allows you to change the position of your center of gravity and direct the sail for maneuverability while reacting to the constant movement of your board. Windsurfing requires significant quad, back extensor, and shoulder girdle strength in order to decelerate and respond to quick forces. Throughout this chapter, exercises preceded by an asterisk (*) are considered to be the most important for windsurfers.

MUSCLE IMBALANCES

Considering the sustained posture required to maneuver your board and boom, muscle imbalances can become apparent. Imbalances common to the sport of windsurfing are weaker hand and wrist extensors in comparison to their counterparts, the flexors; a weaker upper back as compared to the chest; and weaker gluteals and hamstrings as compared to the quadriceps. When physically preparing yourself for the challenges of windsurfing, consider training these usually weaker areas more intensely than their stronger counterparts. The functional exercises listed in this chapter will challenge your musculoskeletal system to respond with improved functional muscular balance.

WARM-UP

Before windsurfing, consider doing all or parts of the following warm-up to prepare yourself for the agility and flexibility demands: Do the dynamic warm-up in chapter 4. Before your in-city workouts, consider doing a modified warm-up consisting of 5 minutes of aerobic activity; the dynamic warm-up drills Carioca, Crazy Legs, and Shuffle Run (chapter 4); followed by stretching Exercises 7, 10, 11, 13, 15, and 16.

STRETCHING

Adequate flexibility of your ankles, knees, and hips along with spinal and shoulder mobility is essential for windsurfing. Do Exercises 1, 3, 5.1, 5.2, and 7–18, 3–4 times per week.

AEROBIC CONDITIONING

A good windsurfing run may last up to 30 minutes. This duration places a great deal of aerobic demands on your body. Do the minimum aerobic program in chapter 3. Make sure that 2 sessions per week are 40 minutes long. Aerobic training options are running, using a stair-climber, using an EFX cross trainer, using cross-country ski machines, or using rowing ergometers.

STRENGTH TRAINING

The exercises listed below are designed to enhance your ability to meet the key physical components of windsurfing. Make sure to do the warm-up and stretching exercises described above before starting your strengthening program.

For best results, select 3–4 exercises from each category and construct a 12-station circuit. Perform each exercise for 45–60 seconds. This is a very effective way of challenging and enhancing your response to the physical demands of windsurfing. If you choose to exercise each body region individually, choose 3–4 exercises and follow the recommended number of sets and reps found in the exercise technique descriptions.

Beginning

Upper body: Exercises 39; 111 or 115; *118, 119, or 131; 120.1; 120.2; 121; *127; and 129.

Abdominals: Exercises 78.3, 80, 80.1, *82, *83, *84, 86, and 92.

Lower body: Exercises *32, 32.1, 57.6, 95, 95.2, 97, and 97.3.

Upper/lower body: Exercises *32, *34, *133, 133.2, and 135.

Intermediate/Advanced

Upper body: Do the beginning program above.

Abdominals: Do the beginning program above.

Lower body: Do the beginning program above, adding Exercises 30, 31, *100.1, 100.4, and 100.5, and omitting Exercise 97.

Upper/lower body: Do the beginning program above.

BALANCE AND AGILITY

Because your board is continually moving, good balance and agility in all directions are crucial to coordinate your board and boom. Do Exercises 58, 58.1, 58.3, 58.4, *59.1, 59.2, 59.3, 61, 63, 65, 67, 100.5, 100.6, and 150–152. For advanced agility training do Exercise 154.

PART IV

Optimal Wellness

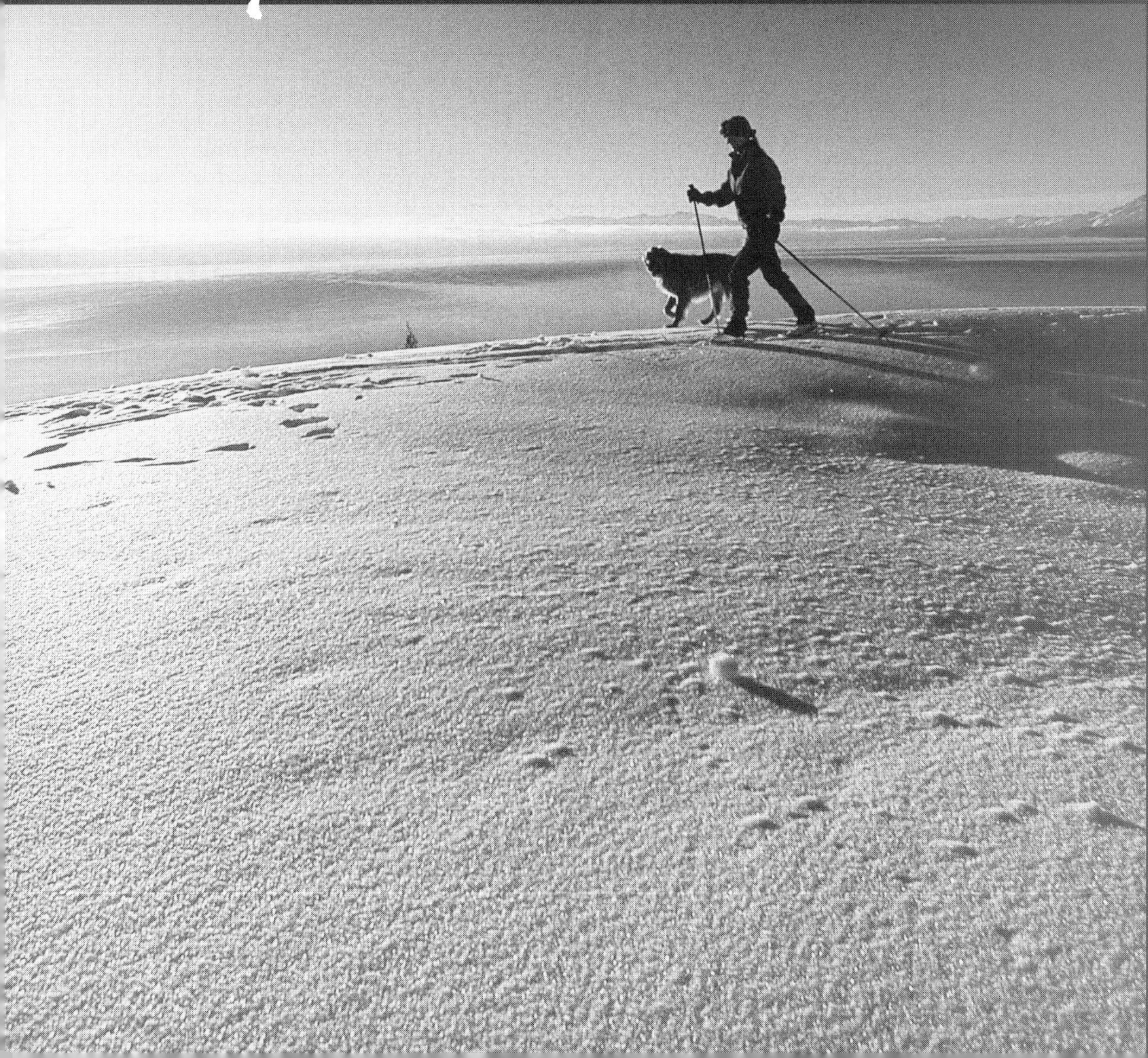

chapter 25 BODY POSTURE AND MOVEMENT PATTERNS

An Aston-Patterning™ Approach

By Judith Aston, M.F.A., and Joani Gelinas, P.T., Certified Aston-Patterner

THIS CHAPTER WILL HELP YOU:

- Increase your awareness of posture and your options in movement.
- Understand neutral spine posture in sitting and standing positions.
- Enhance your performance by using ground reaction forces and weight-shifting.
- Prevent injuries.

Finding our potential begins with the discovery that we all have posture and movement options. The choices we make affect the functioning of our muscles and joints, make us more or less efficient, and make us more or less prone to injury. This chapter presents basic principles that can help you move in a more balanced and efficient manner, along with movement exercises to let you discover how to use these principles and feel the benefits. You may find that by applying these principles to your activities, you decrease symptoms of musculoskeletal distress or improve efficiency.

There are many schools of movement. Some such as yoga or Tai Chi have definite exercise forms that each person practices. Others such as the Aston approach (as well as Feldenkrais, Alexander technique, etc.) are individually tailored to each person's body. To get the most out of a movement awareness technique, try some of the exercises in this chapter.

MOVEMENT PATTERNS

We all have unique movement patterns that we have developed throughout our lives. There's usually a good reason why they occur and stay with us, without our even knowing it, long after they have served their initial purpose. They have become habitual and unconscious. Often they restrict the way we move, causing injuries or pain. Your usual movement patterns during the day are probably similar in everything you do.

A movement pattern requires many repetitions to change, which is why you need to do any movement exercise often. Gradually you will begin to sit, stand, and move differently as you choose movement options that are easier and more efficient. Here are four basic concepts and applications for various activities:

1. You can modify how gravity affects your body and how you use ground reaction force to move.
2. You can become aware of your neutral posture and how to find and maintain it.
3. You can change your base of support in standing or sitting positions to provide better central body stability for motion.
4. You can shift your center of gravity (weight-shifting) to move your whole body and extremities more efficiently.

Gravity and Ground Reaction Force

Gravity is the force we all live with, and it takes work to move against it. Its influence on a particular movement or exercise is variable, depending on the plane of the movement in relation to gravitational forces. Gravity has a counterforce that most people don't know about: ground reaction force (GRF). This is the force that you can create by pushing down onto any surface that you are contacting, such as the ground, the floor, a kayak, and so on. It acts to support you against the downward force of gravity. Together, these two forces create a dynamic synergy that can work for you.

The downward pull of gravity acts as a stabilizer. It can lock you into any posture you are holding, good or bad. That is why we want to find a neutral position, as described below. Often, people are locked into a slouched posture and think about getting into good posture by pulling themselves up from there (i.e., a military posture). This might look good, but it feels stiff because it requires that you continue to use your muscles to hold yourself up. If you find a neutral posture before you settle into gravity and get locked in, you can use gravity to your advantage. It will mechanically stabilize your spine into its place of balance, and your muscles can be at rest.

Neutral alignment, using gravity and GRF, and weight-shifting all contribute to continuous movement through your body. This creates a fluidity to movement that massages your tissue rather than creating tension. This fluidity brings motion to your body's soft tissue and enhances flexibility. Remember what it feels like to jump on a trampoline or off a diving board? There is a springing effect and you are elongated gently upward. As you come down again, you give in to gravity as you absorb the shock of impact and then push up again.

Often, we forget to come down and let go into gravity, or "give." Think about hiking down a long, steep grade and putting a great amount of effort into controlling the impact abruptly rather than letting go slightly into the motion. The force is driven back up into a system that is rigid, creating jarring. Problems such as shin splints can result, or if the jarring moves up to a joint that is not well aligned (knees or hips), it may cause pain there. Think instead of receiving the impact, giving in to gravity slightly, and then distributing the motion throughout.

The secret is that the body is always in motion. Absorbing impact and distributing the different movements through the whole body make for movement with less effort and make it more powerful, with injury less likely. Try Exercise 179 to experience the effect of ground reaction force.

Neutral Postures

A neutral posture is one in which your body, including your spinal joints and discs, is the least stressed and in the best possible position. Most people have learned to think of posture as something static and rigid. But your neutral posture is dynamic, fluid, and flexible. There is a "zone" of neutral posture alignment.

Neutral is a position that your body can maintain with minimal effort or resistance to gravity. Neutral is your own unique position of a dynamically balanced alignment. Think of each of your body parts as being symbolized by a ball: your head, neck, chest, pelvis, knees, and feet all taking that round form. Think of neutral posture as the position of maximum balance, with each ball being balanced directly over the ball below it. These balls progressively lean just slightly forward, which centralizes your weight over your feet.

When any given part or segment of your body moves away from its balance point, increased effort or stress is required. This can take a variety of forms: a tensing, holding, tightening, or shortening in some areas, which causes excessive compression or stretching and compensatory motion in other areas. Injury can result. This puts stress and strain on the affected soft tissue and joints. Balanced posture has the effect of distributing support in all the dimensions of your body. This more evenly distributes your effort as well, so any activity occurs throughout your whole body. Neutral posture may increase the efficiency of your muscles, because you are alleviating stress and strain, and your muscles are able to contract better.

Many of us don't know how to sit or stand in an easy or efficient way. This is amplified when we walk, move, or perform recreational activities. The posture you have when you sit, stand, and walk makes a tremendous difference in the effort required and the amount of discomfort you feel. The posture you have when you ride your bike, carry a backpack, in-line skate, or lift weights can make the activity enjoyable or tedious and injury-prone. The more time you spend in any activity, the more important it is to find an optimal neutral position. It is important to establish balanced posture before trying to increase repetitions or power in your activities.

Neutral Sitting Posture

Exercise 180 can assist you in finding your own neutral sitting posture, which will feel balanced, relaxed, and easy to maintain. Once you have practiced this, you can perform it on a bicycle, in a kayak, or while doing any sitting activity. Exercise 181 will help you experience gravity's effect on your sitting posture. Together, these exercises will help you to develop an awareness of your efficient sitting posture.

Note: The two bony prominences on the bottom of your pelvis (the ischial tuberosities) that you feel when you are sitting upright are called your sit bones in this chapter.

Neutral Standing Posture

Exercise 182 will help you to find your neutral standing posture, in which your body parts are more easily balanced on each other. When this happens, activities in upright positions become easier, as your body is not spending as much energy on merely supporting structures that are out of alignment. This may result in an improved position; a body in neutral balance allows your muscles to work more evenly, which allows for greater efficiency.

Finding your neutral standing posture will also allow you to feel your upright base of support: your feet. People often align themselves over only the posterior third of the foot. Or maybe we stand with more weight on the balls of our feet, or with most of our weight on only one foot. We may be unaware that we are using only a portion of the surface available to us for support (though such unbalanced support can definitely be important in activities such as rock climbing).

According to Aston-Patterning, the dynamic plumb line in relation to standing has a slightly forward inclination similar to the line used in relation to sitting. This takes into consideration the front part of your foot as part of your base of support. This helps distribute your body's weight over your whole foot rather than only your heel, which is a common base of support for a more perpendicular plumb line. Using your whole foot—feeling the ball, heel, and arch simultaneously—gives a broader base of support for your whole body, reducing unnecessary strain and tension and allowing easier movement.

Base of Support

Your body receives support in many ways: from your skeleton, from GRF, as well as from the tone and resiliency of your soft tissues. Another important way in which your body receives support has to do with its base of support (BOS). The base of support for any particular part of your body is the part directly underneath it, and the base of support for the whole body comes from whichever segment contacts the ground. In sitting, it is your pelvis and your feet. In standing, as noted above, it is your feet. Base of support also takes into account the total effect of all of these parts supporting each other. If any part of your body does not have adequate support underneath it, it will have to tense or compensate to perform any action.

Base of support has to do with how your body parts rest one on the other, or line up underneath one another. Therefore, if you are standing, your feet have to be in a good position to support your knees, and your knees to support your hips. Whenever you perform an activity, it is important to understand in which direction you will be moving and to try to make your foot placement match the body motion above it. When you are reaching for a ball in tennis or racquetball, if you step and then reach for the ball, you have given your arm the BOS it needs for the reach. Because of the support gained for your arm by stepping under the action, you are less likely to strain another part of your body. The same could be said for aerobics, climbing, and so on. When you are lifting your arms, remember to modify your foot position to support the various arm and trunk positions you are performing.

Exercise 183 will help you find your base of support while standing.

Weight-Shifting

And now it's time to move! Movement is most easily initiated by shifting your weight. This allows your center of gravity and spine to move to allow more stability for movements of your arms and legs. Weight-shifting involves maintaining a neutral but not rigid center.

In Exercises 179–184, you'll experience the importance of GRF in helping to counteract gravity. You'll have a balanced neutral position, and a good base of support. Now you need to add movement, so first find neutral, and then find your BOS. Third, identify the joints bearing the greatest weight. If you are sitting, these will be your pelvis and hips. If you are standing, these will be your feet, ankles, knees, and hips. Finally, rock and shift your weight across these joints to begin the movement with your aligned body. Exercise 184 describes weight-shifting in detail.

Weight-shifting can assist you in many standing activities in which you reach with an arm or a leg or simply step. This shifting of your center of gravity can be very helpful in hiking or mountaineering when you are taking a long or high step up a steep section. It is also very important in rock and indoor gym climbing.

APPLICATIONS OF ASTON-PATTERNING TO ACTIVITIES

Below are Aston-Patterning applications to a few activities, but the basic principles can be applied to many outdoor activities.

Cycling

Practice sitting arcing (Exercise 180) on a bicycle seat to find a comfortable neutral position. This will also help you determine how to adjust the seat, pedals, and handlebars to your body. It can also be helpful as a range-of-motion exercise during a long ride to keep from getting too stiff in your low back.

Backpacking and Mountaineering

Always try to practice safe spine postures and movements when putting on your pack. (See chapter 17 for more details on lifting and positioning your pack.)

You can try doing modified standing arcing (Exercise 182) with your pack on and during your hike to find the most comfortable low-back position. Most people end up in an excessively flexed position. Try unweighting your pack slightly by pushing up on the top tube of an external frame pack or on the straps of an internal frame pack. You can also have someone lift up on the bottom of the pack. Do the standing arcing with less flexing and extending to avoid a back injury. Try to arrive at a posture that is away from full flexion and closer to neutral.

Kayaking

Many people find themselves sitting slouched in the seat of a kayak because of the design of the seat. This takes the support away from your shoulders and you lose good leverage for paddling. A slouch in flexion also compresses your low back because your spine is not in neutral and therefore your discs and spinal joints are at risk.

If you find yourself slouched, with your arms doing all the work and your low back becoming sore, try pushing your hands down onto the kayak so you can lift and unweight yourself and elongate your trunk. Then move your sit bones back so they rest snugly against the back of the seat. Find neutral and then settle into this position. Next, weight-shift by leaning forward through your hip hinge for the initiation of the paddling—right hip hinge, left hip hinge, right, left—while using your feet to push on the footholds. This will increase your ground reaction force (GRF) and the feeling of power coming through your whole body. If you reach forward with only your arms and shoulders when you start to paddle, most of the effort is in your arms and your back, and you will move out of neutral and undo the good that has been achieved by finding your neutral position.

Weight Training

Begin by lifting free weights in a familiar exercise such as a biceps curl. Identify the effort, specifically in your arms and generally in your whole body. Now perform the standing arcing exercise (Exercise 182) so that your weight is centered over your whole foot. From neutral, shift your weight slightly forward through your ankles and push slightly through your feet on the same side as you lift the weight. If you do one arm at a time, you can put one foot slightly in front of the other with a weight shift on the forward foot (the same side as the curling arm). Note that whichever foot is forward should be directly under your center of gravity.

Stretching

There is much that could be said about how to maximize the benefits of stretching, but here's one important point to remember so you do actually stretch rather than simultaneously compress other body areas. Many stretching techniques involve bending forward or sideways to stretch your spine, legs, or arms. Sometimes, in performing this bending, you actually shorten and compress the joints and deeper structures of your body while trying to stretch. Try lengthening your spine by pushing down through your feet while standing, or into your pelvis while sitting, to lengthen your spine before you lean and stretch. You can maintain the length of your deep and superficial muscles by using GRF and hinging at the greatest weight-bearing joint.

POSTURE AND MOVEMENT-PATTERN EXERCISES

179 GROUND REACTION FORCE

Equipment: None.
Purpose: Experience the effect of ground reaction force on your body.

Technique: While standing with your feet about shoulder-width apart, place your right foot a few inches in front of your left foot. Then raise your right arm in front of you parallel to the floor. Hold it there for a moment and feel how the weight of your arm seems to increase. You have now felt the effect of gravity. As you hold it there, your arm feels heavier and more difficult to hold up. Feel which muscles have to work and how hard they have to work. Can you also feel the muscles in your shoulder and neck tensing?

Now try it another way. First slightly shift most of your weight from your left onto your right foot. Next push off your right foot and move more off the ball of your left foot while elevating your arm in front of you. Progressively increase the length and tone up your right side, as you lift your right arm parallel to the floor. This utilizes ground reaction force, lengthening your body and increasing support for your arm. Do you feel that your arm is lighter and easier to lift? Can you feel that the elevation of your arm is being assisted with the GRF and push-off from your feet, legs, and buttock?

Tips: In any standing activity, if you remember not only to concentrate on the action of the activity but also to support your activity and spine by initiating effortful moves with GRF first, you may feel that the movement is easier.

180 SITTING ARCING EXERCISE: FINDING NEUTRAL IN SITTING

Equipment: Chair.
Purpose: Learn to find a neutral low-back position in sitting.

Technique: Sit on the edge of a chair that is tall enough that your hips are slightly higher than your knees. Place your knees a comfortable distance apart, with the front of your ankles under your knees. Let all your movements be smooth, without strain. Starting at the hip joint, roll your pelvis backward and down toward your tailbone.

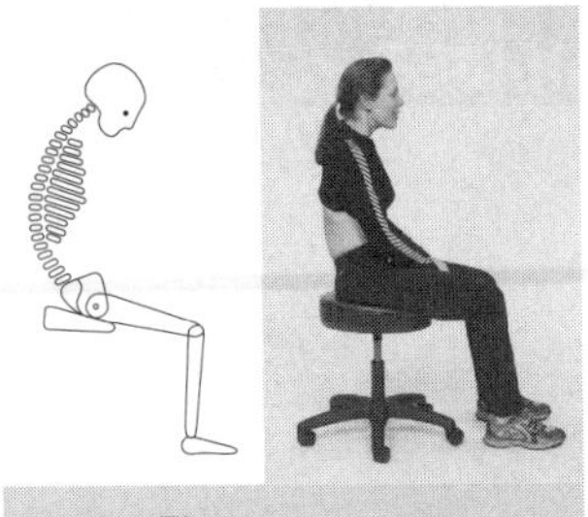
180a. Flexion

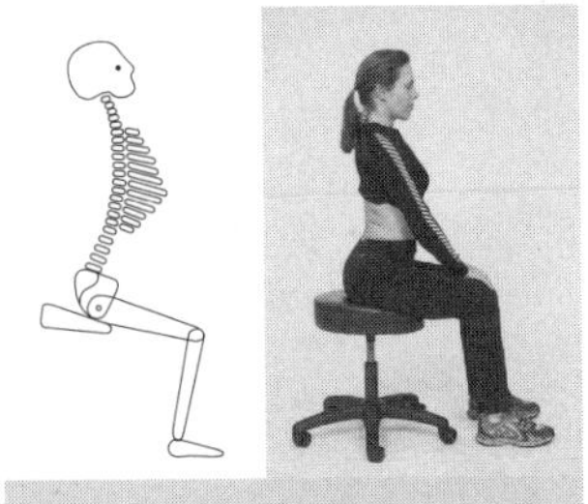
180b. Extension

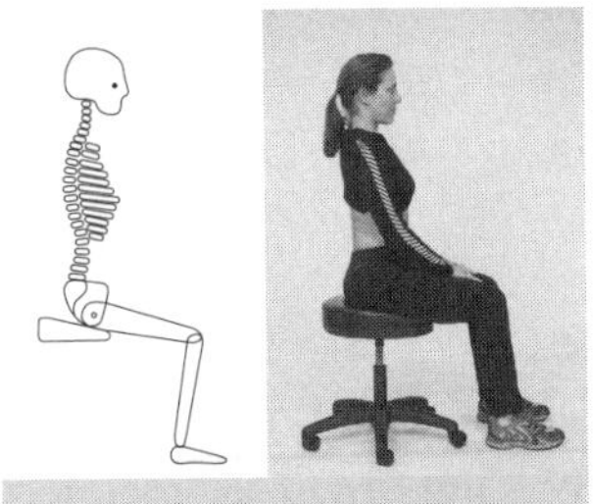
180c. Neutral

Your belly button will go in a posterior direction. Let your spine fall evenly into a C shape, your chest falling forward, letting all the segments of your spine bend about the same amount. Let your head nod slightly to match the bend through the rest of your spine. Exhale as you roll down. This is a "letting go" motion, called flexion (180a).

Next, start arching your back. Shift your weight slightly forward so you are rocking your pelvis through your chest forward, and feel your weight shift toward the front of your hips. Push down and back into the seat with your sit bones, which brings your tailbone up and away from the seat. Push down into the floor with your feet, creating a slight but even arch throughout your whole spine. Your spine will be pushed gently into extension, and the front of you will be lengthened. Your belly button should move in a forward direction. Inhale as you finish the movement. Allow your head and eyes to match the movement in the rest of your spine (180b).

Settle back into a midpoint between flexion and extension, where the length of your front approximately equals the length of your back. You will feel that you are sitting directly on your sit bones. Let your body find its place of rest. This will likely be closer to extension than flexion. This is neutral (180c).

Variations: 180.1. Relaxed neutral: Once you find your neutral position, you can find relaxed neutral by letting go into gravity just a little, sliding down into a slightly flexed pattern. **180.2.** Toned neutral: Toned neutral is found by adding GRF to your neutral position by pushing down into the seat with your sit bones and by pushing down into the floor with your feet. This toned position readies you for any movement action so you have the tone to support yourself in neutral while you move. This is important when you are lifting objects and during certain exercises.

Tips: Sitting arcing should be performed daily. You can use it whenever you first sit down or after a long duration of sitting. It can help you become more comfortable in sitting activities, from sitting in your car to lifting weights, kayaking, or bicycling. Sitting on a small wedge to tip your pelvis slightly forward may make neutral sitting easier.

Note that in the Aston method of sitting arcing you don't lift against gravity, but rather you push and use ground reaction force. Your inhalation will naturally lift your rib cage, which also assists in tractioning your spine. Once your spine is released from the locking mechanism of gravity, it is easy to find your balanced posture, in which the segments of your body rest one on top of the other without much effort.

181 GRAVITY'S EFFECT ON SITTING

Equipment: Chair.
Purpose: Feel a decrease in muscle tension during sitting posture.

Technique: Sit on a seat in a slouch and let yourself settle down into gravity, letting it lock your spine in this position. Then attempt to sit up tall by pulling up against gravity with your back muscles. Feel the tension in your back and shoulder blades; feel the rigidity in your muscles. Realize that if you don't continue to tighten your muscles, you will fall back down into a slouch.

Now try to do it differently. Practice Exercise 180 again, this time noticing that as you use ground reaction force and breathe in, you unlock your spine. Find your neutral, and then settle in, letting gravity stabilize your spine into neutral. Feel that your hips, pelvis, ribs, neck, and head are balanced on top of each other. Feel the absence of muscle tension and the overall stability and ease in your body. Because your muscles are not tensing to hold you up, there is more resilience and fluidity in your position. You should feel less tense and tired, since your muscles are not overworking just to sustain your posture.

182 STANDING ARCING EXERCISE: FINDING NEUTRAL IN STANDING

Equipment: None.
Purpose: Experience neutral spine position in standing.

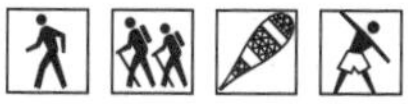

Technique: Stand in a comfortable position with your feet directly under your hip joints (about shoulder-width apart). Let your toes turn out slightly. Rock forward through your ankle hinge (or joint), which allows you to shift your body weight toward the balls of your feet, and then rock backward, moving your weight slightly toward your heels. You have found the neutral position when you feel the whole length of your foot supporting you. Transfer your weight back slightly, rocking through your ankle hinge, so you feel your weight on the heels of your feet. Bend slightly forward at your hip hinge. Let your spine flex slightly and curve forward gently, remembering to distribute the shape of the curve evenly throughout your spine. Your back will be lengthened. Then let your knees bend. Exhale as you flex (182a).

Rock forward by transferring the weight to the balls of your feet. Push into the ground, letting your whole body lengthen upward and

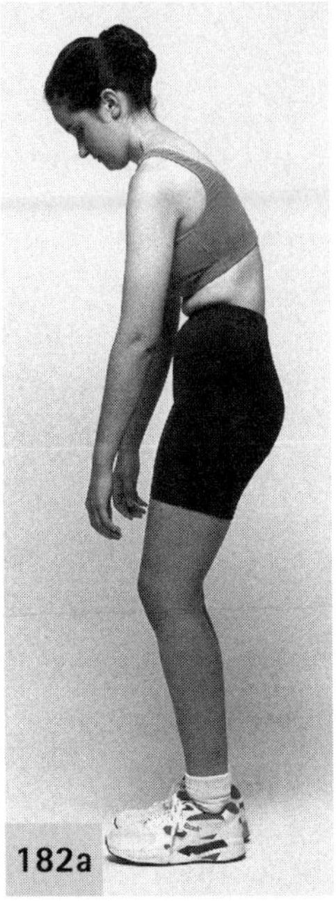

182a

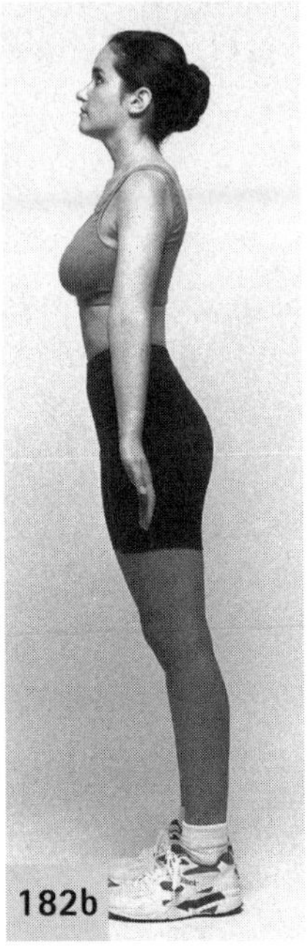

182b

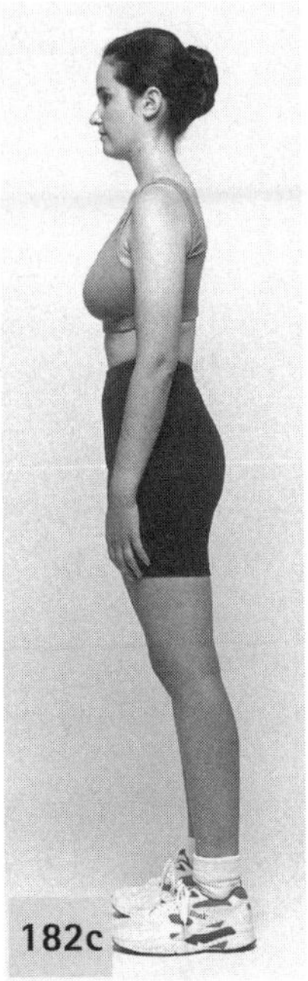

182c

arch slightly (extend) as you inhale. Gradually progress the movement along your spine toward your neck, and the front of you will be lengthened. Your whole body will be inclined slightly forward. Inhale as you go up. Let your arms respond with your palms facing forward (182b).

From your feet, move slightly back to a place that feels balanced, where the length of your front equals the length of your back (neutral). All of your body parts can balance over each other (182c). Move your whole body by rocking through your ankles to distribute your weight over your whole foot, front to back and side to side.

183 BASE OF SUPPORT

Equipment: None.
Purpose: Become aware of your base of support.

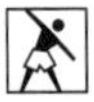

Technique: Stand with your feet very close together and find how far you can reach with one arm—in front of you, beside you, or behind you—before you lose your balance or feel yourself tense up. Feel how the placement of your feet—base of support (BOS)—is too narrow for your body to feel stable during your reaching action. Now move your feet to a wide stance so your feet are placed wider than your shoulders. Notice that this makes it very easy if you want to reach your arm to the right or left side of you, but how far does a wide stance's BOS support you for leaning forward? Not very far. You now have a base of support that supports side-to-side movements well, but lacks support for backward and forward movements. This makes it easy for you to face forward or for someone to push you over from behind. Finding the right base of support for your movements in hiking, climbing, weight training, and other activities can be helpful.

184 WEIGHT-SHIFTING IN STANDING

Equipment: None.
Purpose: Experience weight-shifting to improve your movement patterns.

Technique: Position your right foot about 18 inches to the side of your left foot, with your knees slightly bent. Now reach to the right side with your right hand as if you were reaching for an object, a rock, or a wall hold. Notice that it feels a bit off balance. Now initiate the movement from your base of support by transferring your weight over your right foot, knee, and hip before you reach or while you are reaching. Notice a feeling of more control and balance.
Variations: 184.1. Staggered stance weight shift: Also try this exercise with your right foot in front of your left. Reach in front of you for an imaginary rock hold first without weight-shifting, and then with weight-shifting. You can do this in a diagonal pattern with your right foot at about a 2:00 position to your left. **184.2.** Step-up weight shift: Try this exercise while stepping onto a step, stool, rock, or log. Place your right foot onto a high step or other surface and feel the effort when you try to push off with your right foot. Now place your foot onto a high step and, before you push off, shift your whole body more over the right foot until you feel yourself just moving forward. At this point, push off with your right and left foot.
Tips: If you step onto a higher surface without weight-shifting, you will likely use more effort and possibly tilt backward, especially if you have a pack on. Weight-shifting can make the step-up more balanced and decrease your risk of injury.

chapter 26 EXERCISE, NUTRITION, AND LIFESTYLE FOR OPTIMAL WELLNESS

By David Musnick, M.D., and Mark Pierce, A.T.C.

THIS CHAPTER WILL HELP YOU:

- Develop an exercise program with aerobic and functional strength and balance components for optimal health at any age.
- Use nutrition to optimize your energy and support your cells and organs.
- Slow your aging process and help prevent major diseases.
- Learn lifestyle changes to stay optimally well.
- Develop a total program for wellness.

Optimal wellness and excellent health are worthy goals for people of every age. In this chapter we give you guidelines for exercise, nutrition, and lifestyle that can help you prevent diseases, slow down the aging process, and feel more vitality. Feeling good is a product of many interrelated systems working well together and at full function. These include your cellular energy systems and your cardiovascular, endocrine (hormonal), immune, detoxification, and gastrointestinal systems.

Today, serious health problems are costing countries a tremendous amount of money and are impairing peoples' well-being. Obesity is a problem in all developed countries and is on the rise in both adults and teenagers. One out of three people get cancer. Cardiovascular disease is still a national killer. Inflammation has now been linked to heart disease, cancer, and Alzheimer's disease. Many people are suffering from pain, fatigue, and depression. New infectious diseases are arising and viruses are becoming more potent each year. In addition, our world is now quite challenged by pollution and environmental issues that adversely affect our health.

Conventional medical approaches don't seem to be working well to address these challenges. Focusing instead on prevention through exercise, nutrition, and lifestyle changes is key to helping us solve our health problems and to reducing health-care costs.

Exercise is essential for preventing diseases, decreasing stress, and maintaining strength and muscle. Optimal nutrition can fuel every cell and organ in your body, can give you enough amino acids for your muscles, and can help to detoxify chemicals and slow the formation of free radicals. Furthermore, making wise choices to limit your exposure to toxicity and eating to improve your detoxification systems can decrease your risk for many health problems.

The new field of *functional medicine* has evolved in the last ten years, taking this integrated approach. Functional medicine looks at the interrelationship of internal systems and aims to improve function and to treat and prevent diseases and symptoms. Similarly, *environmental health and medicine* has developed over the last twenty years and has increased awareness and understanding of how toxins and changes in the environment affect our health.

In this chapter we combine the perspectives from functional medicine, environmental medicine, and exercise science to outline the Musnick-Pierce (MP) Optimal Health Program: a total program for exercise, nutrition, supplements, and lifestyle habits that will enhance your health, your mood, and will help you to prevent diseases.

EXERCISE

The MP Optimal Health Program combines warm-up and flexibility, aerobic exercise, strength training, balance, and bone-density components.

Warm-Up

A warm-up is always recommended prior to any activity that stresses your muscles, joints, or cardiovascular system. Warming up helps prepare your body for strenuous activities and decreases your chances of injury. Do the aerobic warm-up (with or without the weight-lifting warm-up) described in chapter 4 before starting your general conditioning program.

Flexibility

General flexibility is important for joints, muscles, and tendons to function optimally. It also aids the functioning of your musculoskeletal system during any home, work, or athletic endeavor.

Recommended flexibility exercises are in chapter 4: 1, 3, 5, 8, 9, 17, and 19.

Aerobic Exercise

Aerobic exercise is your most powerful wellness tool. Done regularly, it can give you many health benefits, including prevention of strokes and heart disease. Chapter 3 discusses the minimal aerobic program, the concept of the heart-rate training zone, and interval training, as well as detailing the many benefits of aerobic exercise.

Before starting, consult with your health-care provider to make sure you are healthy enough to do moderate-intensity aerobic exercise. Start slowly in your aerobic program if you are just beginning. You can start with as little as 10 minutes, 3 days a week of low-intensity walking, cycling, or using an aerobic machine. Gradually increase the duration until you are up to 30 minutes in your heart rate zone. Then you can increase the number of days that you work out to 5–6 days per week. This is equivalent to the minimal aerobic program as outlined in chapter 3, which is designed to give you significant health benefits.

For optimal wellness, modify the minimal aerobic program as follows. Aim for 2 days a week in which you do activity in your target heart-rate range for 40–45 minutes. Use two aerobic machines or activities instead of one to give yourself some variety and to decrease exercise boredom. If you are injury-free and have a low risk for heart disease, consider adding one or two short interval workouts. Consider a long walk or a leisurely bike ride to keep your joints limber and to burn more calories. Take short walking breaks at work even if they are only 10 minutes long. If you are not at your ideal body weight, consult chapter 29 for suggestions concerning exercise for weight loss.

Strength Training

Maintaining your muscle mass and basic strength is very important throughout your life. Doing strength training helps to build strength, prevent injuries, and prepare you for activities. It also helps you to maintain the shape and tone that you want. As we age we loose muscle tissue, so one goal of strength training is to slow this loss and to maintain muscle mass. Strength training can also stimulate growth hormone, which can help decrease muscle loss, sagging tissue, and wrinkles. To achieve these benefits, you must use your large muscles (chest, upper back, thighs, buttocks). Select your exercises from the strength training workouts listed in this chapter with these body regions in mind (and see chapter 5 for a full discussion of strength training). You may wish to see a health professional trained in biomechanics, physical therapy, or athletic training to determine if you have any strength imbalances that need addressing.

At the start of a strength training program it is important to train safely for the first 3 weeks and to develop a base strength level before increasing resistance or adding exercises. This is true for anyone beginning a strength training program for the first time or for those who have not exercised for more than 3 months and are starting back.

Consider the first 1–3 weeks of a new strength training program as a learning curve for both your mind and your body. Not a lot of muscular gains happen during this initial time frame. Almost all gains are due to your neuromuscular system adapting to the coordination and resistance challenges. Along with this neuromuscular learning curve, your joints and deep connective tissues adapt to the added stress and gain the tensile strength required for harder, more intense loads.

Strength training can be done in a number of ways. You can add a few strength training exercises to your current exercise program 2–3 times a week; you can do them before or after an aerobic workout; you can do them in a circuit for possible additional aerobic benefit.

In this chapter we outline basic, intermediate, and advanced strength training programs (see Strength Training Workouts for Optimal Wellness). If you are a beginner, start with the basic program, doing the first three exercises for each body region for 2–3 sets of 8–12 reps. Train each body region 2–3 times a week for 3–4 consecutive weeks before adding any additional exercises. For optimal results, diversify your training routine every fifth or sixth workout. Try changing the order of your workout by training your lower body first, then your abdominals and upper body, or change the order of the exercises within the body regions.

Once you have developed a base, consider blending your body regions into a circuit training workout once every week. To do this, choose 2–3 exercises from each body region and perform 8–12 reps of each exercise, moving from one exercise to the other with a 30-second rest between stations. Do this for 2–3 consecutive circuits of 6–9 stations.

After 4 weeks of consecutive training, progress to the intermediate level for at least 3 more weeks before moving on to the advanced level. Train each body region 2–3 times a week for best results.

STRENGTH TRAINING WORKOUTS FOR OPTIMAL WELLNESS

BASIC

Lower body: Exercises 95, 96, 97.3, and 97.6.

Abdominals: Exercises 78.1–78.3.

Upper body: Exercises 114.1, 117, 118, 120, and 127 (unloaded on an assist machine).

INTERMEDIATE

Lower body: Exercises 31.1, 95, 96, 97.2, and 97.6.

Abdominals: Exercises 78.3, 80, 83, 84, and 92.

Upper body: Exercises 114.1, 117, 118, 120, 121.1, 121.2, 125.1, 126.1, and 127 (unloaded on an assist machine).

ADVANCED

Lower body: Exercises 30.1 and 30.2, 31.1 or 31.2, 95, 96.1, 109.1, and 135.

Abdominals: Exercises 23.1, 80, 88 or 90, 92, and 92.2.

Upper body: Exercises 20, 21, 114 or 115, 118, 120, 125, 126, 127 (on an assist machine), and 131.

Balance

Balance is the most fundamental component of biomechanical function. Good balance enables you to move, change direction, reach, push or pull objects, and to control your body (core) on unstable or unpredictable surfaces. Before you start incorporating balance challenges into your workout program, take a few moments and test your balance strengths and weaknesses.

See chapter 6 and perform balance self-test Exercises 40, 41, 43, 45, and 47 to assess your individual static balance proficiencies. You may find that you have good balance in one or two planes, but less than desirable balance in another. Find the plane of balance that challenges you the most and concentrate your balance exercises in that plane. Adding any balance challenge to an exercise increases the muscular activity and accelerates strength gains.

As your balance improves, routine activities will become easier and more efficient. To continue developing your balance, try to do BST Exercises 43, 45, 47, and Exercises 59, 59.1, 60, and 61 at least twice a week as part of your workout, or do them separately sometime during your day.

Bone Density Program

To maintain and/or build bone density you need to load the bones in your legs, hips, and arms regularly. This means impact loading your legs and your arms at least 3 days a week, more if you don't have a back, hip, or knee problem.

For your legs, try aerobic activities such as walking, hiking, jogging, using treadmill and EFX machines, and doing aerobics classes (done in standing positions).

For your arms, try biceps curls and dips (see exercises in chapter 15). Try each exercise for 2 sets of 10 reps 3 times a week.

Your bone density program should also consist of adequate bone maintenance minerals, including about 1,000 milligrams of calcium per day (if you are a woman, see chapter 28) and 500 milligrams of magnesium per day. These can be from a combination of food and supplements. Recent studies have found that Vitamin D has a potential role in cancer prevention. For this reason, consider supplementing vitamin D with 400–1,000 IUs a day. In the winter months, limited sunlight inhibits our skin's ability to make adequate vitamin D, so supplementation is critical.

NUTRITION

In chapter 2 we discuss basic nutritional concepts in detail, and reading that chapter will give you essential background information. Here, we build on that base to outline an optimal nutrition program designed to provide and achieve the following:

- Optimal and safe protein to help you maintain or build muscle and support your body's needs for amino acids
- Low- to moderate-glycemic and high-quality carbohydrates for energy
- Healthy fats, while limiting unhealthy fats
- Decreased inflammation
- Decreased toxins
- A reasonable blood-sugar level
- Decreased risk for cardiovascular disease, type 2 diabetes, and cancer

The quality of the food you consume can influence all of the above variables. We urge you to keep up with developments regarding the quality and safety of foods in regard to nutrient content, toxins, and infectious disease issues in your city, state, and country.

Food Quality, Toxins, and Purity

It has become apparent since this book's first edition that there are significant factors that influence the purity and quality of the food supply in the United States and likely in most other countries. Soils have become depleted of essential minerals because of excessive use without replenishment, so it is more difficult to meet mineral needs by eating nonorganic foods alone.

Produce, grains, legumes, and meat products may have varying amounts of pesticides and toxic metals due to agricultural practices that allow industrial waste to be converted into fertilizer, which allows heavy and toxic metals to be in the fertilizers used on many farms. Vegetables, grains, and animals fed from these crops may contain significant amounts of these heavy metals, which in turn can accumulate in human tissues if such contaminated food products are eaten regularly. This can potentially cause a number of physiological problems in your mitochondria, cell membranes, and nerves. Pesticides on and within produce appear to be stored within fat tissues when ingested and may influence human health and contribute to free-radical production and inflammation.

Because of these health concerns, we recommend that you make food choices as wisely as possible and choose organically grown and produced foods whenever possible. It is also important to choose whole foods, which are the least processed and contain the fewest additives.

Food Additives

Food additives are used to enhance flavor, sweeten, give color, and to preserve. Certain additives may produce side effects and some individuals are more susceptible than others. If you have food sensitivities, consider getting a blood test for food allergies, as you might be reacting to a food that you eat regularly.

A comprehensive list of additives to avoid is beyond the scope of this book; refer to Selected References for book- and Internet-based information on food additives. It is important to limit and avoid your intake of aspartame, MSG (monosodium glutamate), and partially hydrogenated oils, as these may affect your health as well as cause possible symptoms. MSG, for example, is a form of free glutamic acid used to enhance flavor, and it can lead to muscle aching, headaches, and mood disorders, among other symptoms. It also goes by names other than MSG. Keep up with the literature and the media on food additives to inform yourself about what may not be safe for you and your family. Whole, unprocessed foods are always preferable to processed foods.

> **HEALTH TIP**
>
> Food sensitivities are fairly common and can lead to a range of symptoms. These can include, but are not limited to, achy muscles and joints, headaches, fatigue, sleepiness, and abdominal bloating and pain. If you experience any of these symptoms and think they could be related to foods, it may be helpful to get a blood test for food allergies. Ask your health-care provider to consider ordering a food-allergy panel.

Carbohydrates

Carbohydrates are your primary source of calories for energy, as well as containing B vitamins, phytochemicals, and fiber (see discussions below). Choose carbohydrates that are low to moderate on the glycemic index in order to keep your blood sugar level. (See chapters 2 and 29 for a discussion of the glycemic index). If you are a high-level athlete, you will need more carbohydrate calories than the average person in order to supply your body with energy.

Limit simple sugars and highly processed starches and carbs (including bread, potatoes, rice, crackers, cookies, muffins, and other sweets). Try to consume vegetables, fruits, whole grains, and legumes (beans, lentils, etc.) as your primary sources of carbohydrates. Such whole-food sources (with very little or no processing) are beneficial in part because they contain fiber, which modulates the conversion of carbohydrates into sugar. Try to eat organic fruits and vegetables whenever possible, and try to have a minimum of five servings of fruits and vegetables per day.

Protein

The amino acids in protein are essential building blocks of your muscular tissues as well as of your vital organs. Amino acids are also necessary for many processes in your body. The average person needs 0.8–1 gram of protein per day for every kilogram of lean body weight (which is your approximate ideal weight). Take your weight in pounds and divide it by 2.2 to get your weight in kilograms. Then multiply this by 1–1.2 and this will be about the amount of protein you need unless you are vigorously doing aerobic exercise or significant hours of strength training. For protein needs for particular endurance or strength training goals, see chapter 2.

Try to consume organic sources of protein. Protein in meat, poultry, fish, and dairy concentrates toxins. Seek out grass-fed beef and other meat sources that are fed with organic feed. For lunch meats, use only those that are nitrite-free to limit your colon cancer risk. Avoid large fish such as tuna, swordfish, and mackerel to limit your mercury exposure. Avoid farm-raised salmon because of potential toxins. If you eat fish for protein, choose ocean salmon and other smaller fish and use them sparingly because of mercury and other toxin content. Pregnant or lactating women should strongly consider staying away from fish entirely for this reason, and should instead seek out vegetarian sources of the beneficial nutrients found in fish (see Healthy Fats below).

If you are a vegetarian, you can combine foods to get adequate amino acids. For example, eat grains (corn, rice, rye, quinoa, wheat) in breads, crackers, cereals, or cooked, in combination with organic dairy products. Or eat grains with legumes (beans, lentils, soy) or legumes with seeds (pumpkin, sesame, sunflower).

FOOD TIP

Try to start your day with 20–30 grams of protein in a healthy protein smoothie. In a blender, combine 8–10 ounces of liquid (e.g., organic milk, soy, oat, rice, or almond milk) with protein powder. Choose a protein that is pure and that you are not allergic to (rice, soy, or whey). Read the protein powder's label to determine how many scoops will give you enough protein; it is usually 1 1/2–2 scoops. If you use a whey protein powder, try to find one that is from organically fed, hormone-free cows. For flavor, add organic berries or a banana.

To improve your nutritional intake, consider eating a snack with protein and healthy carbohydrates in between meals. This could be some nuts and sunflower or pumpkin seeds. You could also try an apple or celery with almond butter.

If these snacks are difficult to make or you miss a meal, you can try a protein bar. Choose a protein bar without partially hydrogenated oils, food colorings, or MSG. Also make sure that you are not allergic to the bar's protein source and that it is good-tasting. Some people have difficulty digesting certain protein bars, and bars very high in protein are often unpalatable. Some of the higher-quality protein bars have added vitamins and minerals. Also look at the total calories and carbohydrates to see if the bar fits your needs. Many bars in grocery and health-food stores are not good choices based on these criteria. See Selected References for suggested sources of healthy protein bars.

Healthy Fats

Fats come in many forms and they are classified according to their biochemical structure. *All* fats have been given a bad rap because *some* fats do increase the risk of heart disease. These latter fats are cholesterol, saturated fat, and partially hydrogenated oils. Become a label reader and be on the lookout for partially hydrogenated fats in cookies, crackers, and other processed foods. These fats are harmful and increase inflammation and risk of heart disease. Limit your intake of saturated fats. Minimize or eliminate deep-fried foods. Minimize or try to avoid cottonseed and safflower oils.

Healthy fat, on the other hand, is essential for the health of your brain, heart, skin, and every cell membrane. Even some cholesterol is healthy, as it is used to make hormones. Healthy fats are essential fatty acids and include monounsaturated fats (such as olives and olive oil) and some healthy omega-6 and omega-3 fats.

Try to consume these healthy fats every day. Good sources are avocados, macadamia nuts, walnuts, and other nuts (as long as they are not cooked in cottonseed or partially hydrogenated oils), olives and extra-virgin olive oil, seeds (sunflower, sesame, and pumpkin), and the oils found in small cold-water fish.

Consider using vegetable sources of omega-3s (e.g., flaxseed oil) mixed with monounsaturated oils to make a salad or vegetable dressing. A tasty combination is 2–4 parts extra-virgin olive oil and 4 parts flaxseed oil, mixed with 1–2 parts walnut oil and some sesame oil to taste. You can also add a tablespoon of flaxseed oil into a morning smoothie.

EPA/DHA oil is an omega-3 fish oil that has been studied extensively. It has been shown to be anti-inflammatory and useful in the treatment and prevention of coronary artery disease, gastrointestinal problems, and some arthritis conditions. EPA/DHA oil can also improve mood and prevent or limit depression. Consider taking a fish oil supplement to get a gram of fish oil and at least 650 mg of EPA/DHA per day. Make sure your fish oil is tested for PCBs, pesticides, and mercury. The DHA component of fish oil appears to be essential for proper brain development in children and teenagers. It is also essential for pregnant and nursing women to get some DHA oil each day. Purified fish oil is a good source, or it can be found in flaxseed oil or in other vegetarian sources available in health food stores. It is probably a good idea to take a mixed antioxidant or multivitamin supplement with your fish oil to prevent oxidation of the oil.

Phytochemicals

Phytochemicals are compounds that have antioxidant or anticancerous properties, and they are found primarily in fruits and vegetables. Phytochemicals in the cruciferous family (broccoli, cabbage, kale) are especially known for their cancer prevention activity. Eat from the onion family (onions, leeks, garlic, chives, shallots) as well as from the cruciferous family to improve detoxification and the elimination of toxins.

Berries, especially blueberries, are a good fruit choice, as they have fiber and phytochemicals that are helpful for brain function and for protection from oxidation (free radicals). Apples provide excellent fiber, and citrus fruits also contain valuable phytochemicals. If you eat a colorful variety of fruits and vegetables you will maximize your phytochemical intake (again, organic fruits and vegetables are best). Try to eat fruits and vegetables of the following colors every day: dark green, red, purple, yellow, and orange. Eat a minimum of five servings of these colorful fruits and vegetables each day.

Fiber

Fiber is a polysaccharide (a complex carbohydrate) and occurs exclusively in plants. Fiber does not directly provide energy, but it confers many health benefits.

Fiber is important for keeping your colon healthy and for helping to prevent colon cancer. It helps bulk stool and decreases constipation and other gastrointestinal problems. It helps your body to bind and eliminate toxins. It can help lower cholesterol and thereby decrease the risk of coronary artery disease. It is important for people who would like to lose weight; by improving the health of your gastrointestinal system, fiber may indirectly contribute to improved metabolic function. Fiber also plays an important role in reducing insulin secretion and improving insulin sensitivity (see discussion of insulin sensitivity in chapters 2 and 3). Increasing fiber is important for people who have type 2 diabetes and the metabolic syndrome (which includes hypertension, hyperlipidemia, and insulin resistance with or without type 2 diabetes).

There are basically two types of fiber, insoluble and soluble. Insoluble forms are in wheat bran and vegetable fibers. This type of fiber is the most important for stool bulking and for preventing constipation and colon cancer. Soluble fiber comes from foods like beans, oats, brown rice, and psyllium. This type of fiber is helpful in reducing levels of the "bad," low-density cholesterol (LDL) as well as in providing fuel to keep colon cells healthy.

The average person should eat 20–35 grams of fiber per day. The best way to get your fiber is through your diet, by eating a variety of whole-grain products as well as at least five servings of vegetables and fruit per day. If you cannot eat enough fiber-containing foods, you can consider taking a fiber supplement. Remember to mix adequate water with fiber supplements.

Water

All of our cells need water to carry out primary metabolic function, so drinking enough water is a cornerstone of good health. Try to drink 6–8 glasses of water or other healthy, noncaffeinated fluids per day. Choose water that is filtered through a high-quality filter with multiple layers. Avoid drinking out of soft plastic containers, as the plastic residues may leach out into the water (this effect is worse in warm weather). Instead, drink out of ceramic mugs or glass containers whenever possible.

Supplements

We live in a time when soils are depleted of vitamins and minerals, and we face health challenges from the foods we eat, the products we use, and the air we breathe. Adding supplements to your diet can be valuable. In chapter 2—in the section Vitamins, Minerals, and Free Radicals—we discuss several vitamins and minerals and their recommended dosages. At the very least, a multivitamin mineral supplement is now recommended by medical associations and numerous health-care providers to meet your minimum daily needs for vitamins, minerals, and antioxidants. Choose a multivitamin wisely; a good one will usually require 3–6 capsules per day to provide you with what you need. It should have at least 100% of the daily value for the vitamins included, 400–800 micrograms of folic acid, 400 IUs of vitamins E and D, 20–30 milligrams of zinc, 400–500 milligrams of magnesium, 500–1,000 milligrams of calcium (depending on your dietary intake), and 100–200 micrograms of selenium.

LIFESTYLE HABITS

Toxins

Practice a low-toxin lifestyle by minimizing your exposures to products that emit a smell. Learn about "green" household products that have a minimal effect on your health and the environment. Minimize your exposure to products that off-gas volatile organic compounds (VOCs), such as formaldehyde. Try to improve the quality of the air that you breathe and minimize indoor air pollution (by using an air filter, for example). Avoid spraying pesticides and

FIGURE 46. FIBER CONTENT OF COMMON FOODS

Food	Serving Size	Total Fiber (gm)	Soluble Fiber (gm)	Insoluble Fiber (gm)
100% Bran cereal	½ cup	10	.3	9.7
Peas	½ cup	5.2	2	3.2
Kidney beans	½ cup	4.5	.5	4.0
Apple	1 small	3.9	2.3	1.6
Potato	1 small	3.8	2.2	1.6
Broccoli	½ cup	2.5	1.1	1.4
Oats	½ cup	1.6	.5	1.1
Strawberries	¾ cup	2.4	.9	1.5

Note: See *www.nal.usda.gov/fnic/foodcomp* for the fiber content of other food.

herbicides, and avoid your exposure to these chemicals. Investigate the ingredients of skin products such as deodorants, makeup, and lotions, and make safe choices. Practicing a low-toxin lifestyle can decrease your body's chemical burden and can improve your health.

Stress Management

Minimizing and managing stress well is a key to being healthy. There are many types of stress: financial, interpersonal conflicts, health-related, work-related, environmental, political, and so on. It is important to learn to decrease your exposure to stress and to learn to manage that which you are exposed to. Excessive stress has been associated with many health problems, including ulcers and heart attacks. Excessive stress can even contribute to weight gain and to difficulty in losing weight.

There are several methods for unloading and managing stress. Daily exercise can be very helpful. Time management and organizational skills can also decrease stress. Try to listen and communicate as well as possible to decrease interpersonal stress. Consider learning more about listening and conflict resolution skills.

Prolonged stress can decrease your body's ability to respond to stress with adequate energy, and your adrenal glands can become quite compromised. It is appropriate to get your adrenal hormones tested with lab tests if you feel you are under constant stress and don't feel like you are managing it well.

Preventative Health Tests

Keep up with your preventative health testing regarding cancer, bone density, and cardiovascular screening. Books, lectures, and the Internet abound with new and developing information on such testing. You may want to insist that your doctor run some preventative tests that you have investigated. In addition to the usual tests (such as a lipid panel), there are numerous tests available for more complete cardiovascular screening (homocysteine, lipoprotein(a), lipid subfractions, cardio-CRP, etc.). There are also tests available that measure the competency of your immune function.

Connections

Having close friends and connections can help to decrease stress and improve your health. Studies have shown that married people live longer than single people and that people in support groups have lower overall mortality. Talk and listen to your close connections regularly to stay more healthy. Consider joining a group that meets once a month, as support groups can break isolation and lead to improved health.

These suggestions of the MP Optimal Health Program will help you on your road to improved health. Most important for wellness are regular aerobic, strength, and balance exercise; good dietary habits; a low-toxin, low-stress lifestyle; and a good set of connections and friendships. These are all things that make our lives enjoyable.

chapter 27 CONDITIONING FOR SENIORS, DECONDITIONED INDIVIDUALS, AND PEOPLE WITH NEURODEGENERATIVE CONDITIONS

By David Musnick, M.D., and Mark Pierce, A.T.C.

THIS CHAPTER WILL HELP YOU TO:

- Improve your balance and prevent falling.
- Maintain and improve your muscle mass.
- Gain flexibility.
- Improve your energy.
- Improve your nutritional status.

In this chapter we outline the Musnick-Pierce (MP) Program for Seniors. Though the program is addressed to seniors, its recommendations apply to a broader group of people. Most of this chapter's suggestions will work equally for you if you have become deconditioned through illness or lack of activity, or if you have a neurological condition that alters your balance and strength. If you fall into any of these categories, this is the perfect place to start working your way toward health and wellness. As always, and especially if you are just getting into better shape, it is best to consult your health-care provider prior to beginning any exercise program.

As we age, and especially as we pass 60, we experience several aging-related processes that can be counteracted to achieve better health: balance abilities and flexibility decline; endurance and energy levels decline; muscle mass and strength decline; bone density declines, which can be critical in a fall; and risk for cardiovascular and other diseases increases.

Participating in the MP Program for Seniors can help to address all of the above challenges. The program lays out guidelines for flexibility and stretching; aerobic conditioning for disease prevention and better energy; strength training for increased muscle mass and strength for daily tasks and activities; balance exercises for increased steadiness and to prevent falling; and tips for maintaining bone density and preventing fractures.

Either before you start or as you fine-tune your program based on the recommendations in this chapter, consider seeking help in assessing your balance and strength. It is quite reasonable by the age of 60–65 to get evaluated by a physical therapist, even if there is nothing hurting or bothering you. A good evaluation and plan can help you determine your specific balance and strength challenges and can help you to plan exercises more specifically.

FLEXIBILITY

It is good to have reasonable flexibility of your Achilles, quads, hamstrings, and back. To do a stretch, you should get into position carefully and hold the stretch for about 20 seconds. You should feel a stretch, but otherwise it should be pain-free.

Chapter 4 discusses warming up and stretching in detail. Do the following chapter 4 stretches in this order: 9 (Achilles), 4 (quadriceps), 2 and 2.1 (hamstrings), and 19 (spine rotations).

AEROBIC CONDITIONING

Aerobic exercise is basically any form of exercise that will elevate your heart rate by using your arms and legs. Plan on wearing supportive shoes that lace up and are designed for walking or running.

If you have not been doing an aerobic program, we suggest that you start by walking 10 minutes 3 times a week. Walking will load your bones and will help to improve your bone density. Your walking should be at a pace that allows you to feel like you are working moderately. If you work, you can add walking to your breaks. If you are able to get to a health club, you may want to try an EFX machine, as it also loads your bones but is low impact. If you are quite overweight, walking might cause knee or hip pain, in which case a stationary bike or water aerobics might be more appropriate.

You can gradually increase the duration of your chosen activity by 1 minute each session until you are up to 30 minutes 5–6 days per week. Studies have shown that this amount of aerobic activity results in significant health benefits, such as decreasing your risk of heart attack and stroke.

You can create variety by mixing what you do. Some days you can walk and other days you could use an EFX machine or stationary cycle. It is important to do an activity that loads your legs at least 3 times a week in order to maintain your bone density. If you start getting any pain in your chest, feet, knees, or hips, consult a health professional.

STRENGTH TRAINING

Your strength training should build and maintain the major muscles of your body including your legs/thighs, abdominals, chest/upper back, and arms. By doing the following program 2–3 days a week, you will experience less sagging, more strength, and better tone, and you may be able to stimulate anti-aging growth hormone. You will find these exercises described in other chapters in this book, complete with pictures. Please read the exercises carefully. You can do these at home, with light weights available at sporting goods stores, or in a gym.

Legs and Thighs

Chapter 11 contains written explanations for how to do the following exercises. Use those descriptions and the associated pictures to learn the proper technique. Some of the exercises are pictured below, demonstrated by one of our patients who is an active senior.

Start with a basic squat, Exercise 95. Do a set of 5 squats initially and take a minute break, then try another 5. Eventually work your way up to 10 squats in a set. Remember to do this with your back in good alignment. It is OK to stick out your buttocks. You can also do this squat by holding onto 2 chair backs to assist your balance.

After this is easy, try a squat with a biceps curl as described in Exercise 95.2 (see Figures 47a and 47b). You could try this with a 3- or 5-pound weight.

After you can do a squat with a curl, try a basic lunge, Exercise 97. Try doing it between 2 chairs initially and use the chair backs for balance. You can have a tight grip if your balance is poor or a slight finger-touching grip if your balance is reasonable (see Figure 48). Try doing 5 lunges with only a slight knee bend and make sure that you are not wobbling too much in your thighs and knees. You can gradually increase the number of your lunges to 10 in a set, and try to get up to 2 sets of 10 reps.

Once you can do these smoothly and without pain or wobbling, try a lunge without hold-

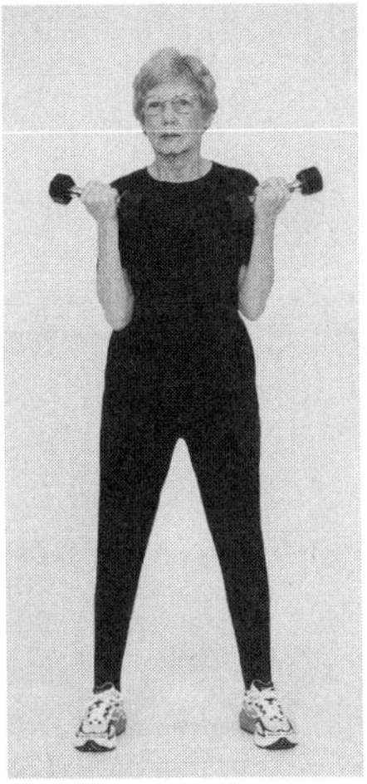

FIGURE 47a. Squat with biceps curl start.

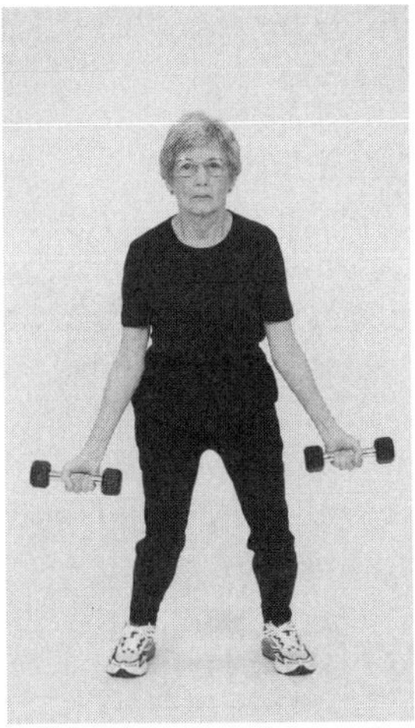

FIGURE 47b. Squat with biceps curl end.

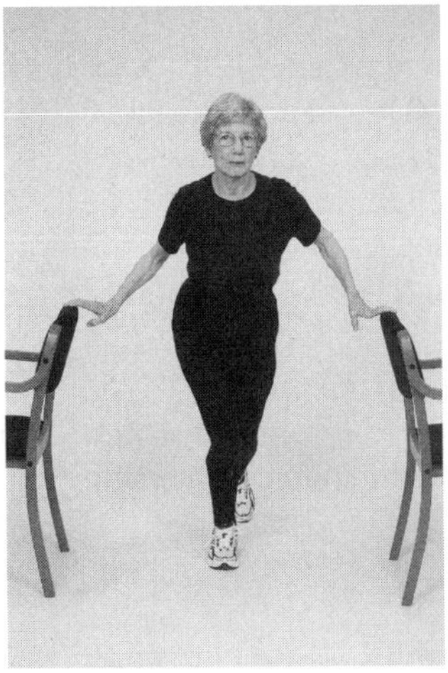

FIGURE 48. Lunge with light finger-touching grip.

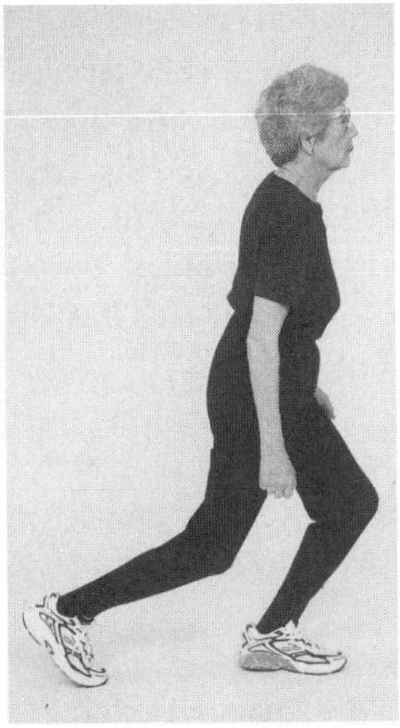

FIGURE 49. Lunge end position, without chair.

ing onto a chair (see Figure 49, which shows the end position).

Once you can do 10 of these easily, you are ready to try the lunge with a biceps curl, Exercise 97.6 (see Figures 50a and 50b).

For your routine, do a squat and a lunge exercise in each of your 2–3 weekly strength training sessions. Your lunge should be done in functional motions to simulate your needs for movement in your kitchen, yard, and in your normal activities.

Abdominals

These recommended exercises can be found in chapter 10, with descriptions and pictures.

Try Exercise 78 and then attempt the progression described. Add Exercise 79. Then add Exercise 84, initially with one foot toe-touching to support your balance.

Chest and Upper Back

These exercises can be found in chapter 15, with detailed descriptions and pictures.

Start with an assisted dip, Exercise 127. Instead of using a machine to unload some of your body weight, you can do a basic squat between 2 chairs but use your arms to push up from the squat. Use a stable chair with sturdy armrests. Hold onto the armrests and straighten your elbows while you assist by pushing with your legs. Do 2 sets of 8–10 reps.

Next, try a single-arm dumbbell row with 5 pounds, Exercise 131.

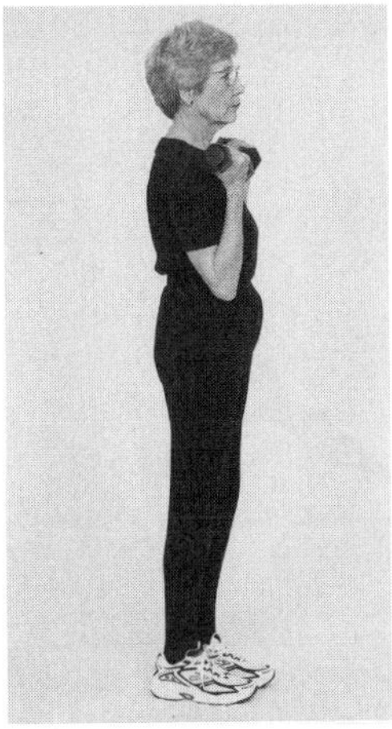

FIGURE 50a. Lunge with biceps curl start.

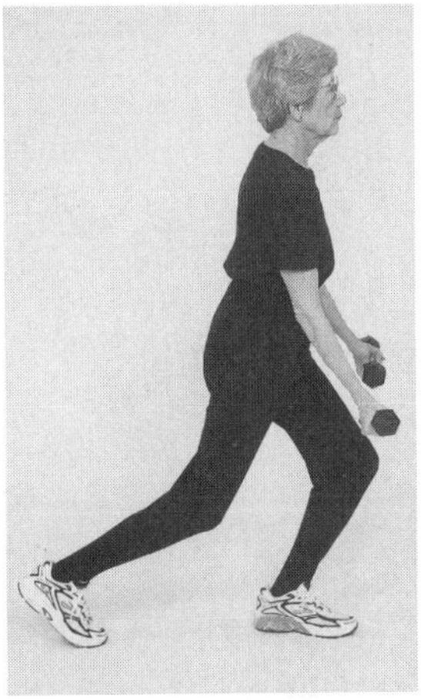

FIGURE 50b. Lunge with biceps curl end.

Arms

These exercises will strengthen your biceps and triceps, and they are pictured and described in chapter 15. Choose a weight that enables you to do 10–12 reps in a set pain-free and with fatigue for the last few reps.

Start with a basic biceps curl with 5 pounds, Exercise 125.

For your triceps, do Exercise 126.1 if you have access to a high pulley at a gym. You can also exercise your triceps with Exercise 98, using two chairs or an assisted dip machine.

BALANCE

These balance exercises can be found in chapter 6, with written descriptions and pictures. Below, we include some demonstration pictures of our active senior patient.

First, try balance self-test (BST) Exercise 44 to assess your front-to-back (sagittal plane) balance (Figures 51a and 51b).

Then try BST Exercise 46, which will test your balance in the frontal (side-to-side) plane (Figures 52a and 52b).

When these balances are comfortable, add Exercise 59, in which you balance on one leg and reach your opposite leg around an imaginary clock.

BONE DENSITY

By following the aerobic and strength training recommendations above, you will be loading the bones in your arms, back, and hips, thus helping to maintain bone density and slow osteoporosis. You should do this along with taking about 1,500 milligrams of calcium citrate, 400–500 milligrams of magnesium, and 400–800 IUs of vitamin D per day.

NUTRITIONAL RECOMMENDATIONS

The nutritional recommendations for optimal wellness in chapter 26 are important for health maintenance. Additional background on nutrition can be found in chapter 2.

After about age 60, levels of stomach acid may decline. As this occurs, digestion can be impaired and digestive enzymes may not be secreted in reasonable quantities. If you experience digestive problems you may benefit from digestive enzymes.

Vitamin B_{12} absorption from dietary sources

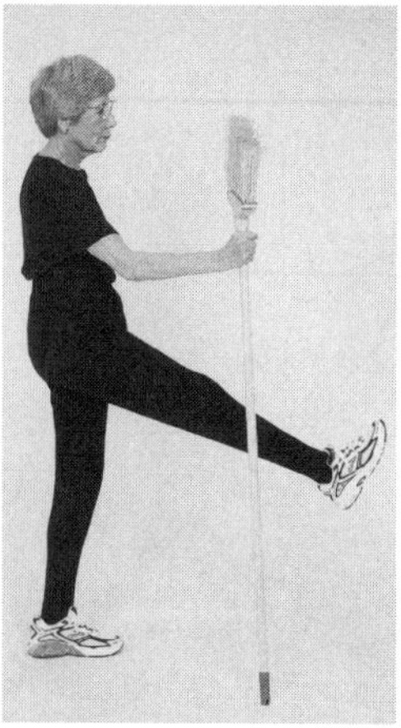

FIGURE 51a. Balance self-test Exercise 44, forward swing.

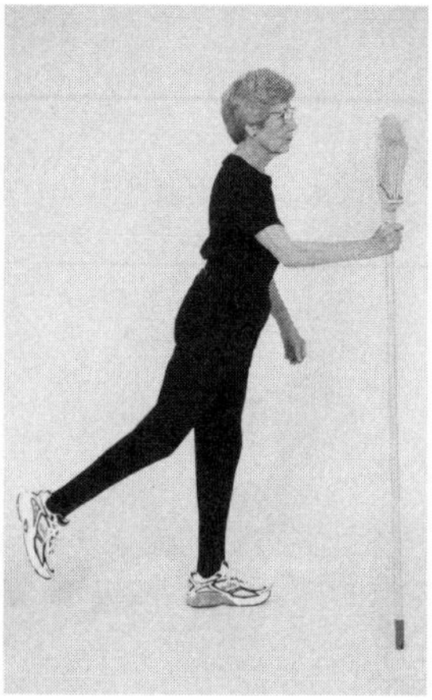

FIGURE 51b. Balance self-test Exercise 44, backward swing.

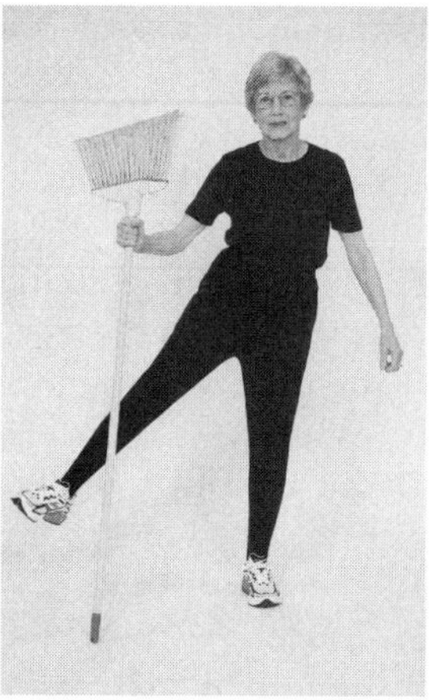

FIGURE 52a. Balance self-test Exercise 46, outward swing.

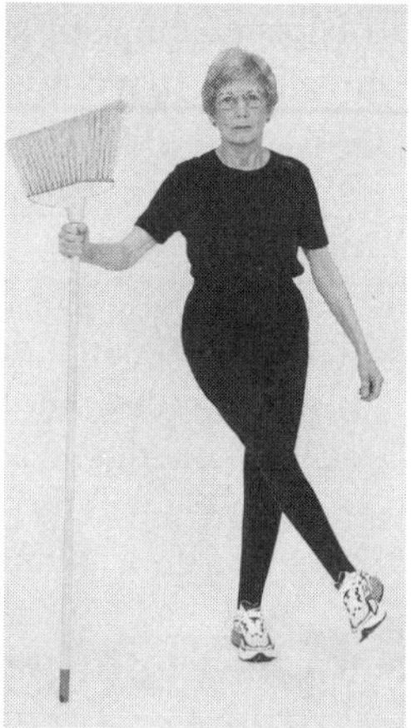

FIGURE 52b. Balance self-test Exercise 46, inward swing.

can also become limited because of stomach changes associated with aging. If your B_{12} level gets too low, you can develop problems with balance. You might need to turn the light on in order to feel steady on your feet in the middle of the night, and your balance may be impaired during the day. It is important to get blood work for vitamin B_{12} levels every year. Consider supplementing your diet with the form of vitamin B_{12} that you simply put under your tongue, as this ensures adequate absorption and bypasses the age-related low-stomach-acid issue.

Another common nutritional deficiency that comes with aging is low vitamin D levels, especially in the winter in more northern latitudes, when there is less sunlight. Vitamin D relates to bone density and may be related to other important health issues. It is good to get a blood-level test for vitamin D and supplement your diet, at least during the winter, with 400–800 IUs per day.

Overall, it is important to take at least a few supplements to ensure that you are getting an adequate base of vitamins and minerals. This is good advice for everyone, not just for seniors. Choose a multivitamin wisely; a good one will usually require 3–6 capsules per day to provide you with what you need. It should have at least 100% of the daily value for the vitamins included, 400–800 micrograms of folic acid, 400 IUs of vitamins E and D, 20–30 milligrams of zinc, 400–500 milligrams of magnesium, 500–1,000 milligrams of calcium (depending on your dietary intake), and 100–200 micrograms of selenium. Most one-a-day multivitamins are quite inadequate. Remember to take your multivitamins two or three times a day with food and liquid to avoid an upset stomach. A physician or nutritionist may recommend additional supplements depending on your health concerns, conditions, and health risks.

One of the most important nutritional considerations is to remember to get enough quality protein at every meal. You will need a minimum of 0.8 gram of protein per kilogram of your ideal lean body weight. If you consider yourself to not be overweight, divide your weight in pounds by 2.2, then multiply that number by 0.8 to arrive at your total number of protein grams needed per day.

Try to divide this protein requirement between three meals. It is good to have about one-third of your protein at breakfast. This could be in the form of a protein smoothie, a two- to three-egg omelet, and so on.

It is also important for you to get high-quality fruits and vegetables at each meal, as these help to keep your gastrointestinal tract working well and they help to prevent cancer. Remember to try to eat three meals a day and consider eating two snacks to keep your blood-sugar level and energy up. Please read chapter 26 for more specific information on how to choose foods with protein as well as fruits and vegetables. Fresh and organic foods are always preferable.

Following this MP Program for Seniors, whether you are over 60, are getting back into shape, or are living with a challenging neurodegenerative condition, will set you on your way toward improved health. Follow these recommendations for at least 6 weeks to improve your vitality, decrease your risk of injuries, improve your strength, and help to slow down the aging process.

chapter 28 SPECIAL ISSUES FOR THE CONDITIONING WOMAN

By Jane A. Moore, M.D., and David Musnick, M.D.

THIS CHAPTER WILL HELP YOU:

- Learn about eating disorders and how they can lead to health problems in women.
- Understand menstrual disorders and their relationship to osteoporosis and injuries.
- Understand the special nutritional needs of women.
- Learn about osteoporosis in younger and older women.
- Become aware of a functional approach to menopause.

We are gaining information on problems specific to women athletes, including unique medical and nutritional problems and the effects of training on the menstrual cycle. Can women be as good as men in outdoor activities such as kayaking, hiking, rock climbing, and glacial mountaineering? Absolutely! In these activities, there are no significant limiting factors based on male vs. female physiology and structure.

WEIGHT CONTROL AND DISORDERED EATING

Attempts to control weight in order to improve performance are very common in women athletes. One study found that 32% of collegiate women athletes used vomiting, laxatives, diuretics, or diet pills on a regular basis. Such behavior is more common in women involved in endurance sports, sports with weight classes, and sports where judging can be influenced by appearance, but may be seen in athletes in any sport.

Eating disorders that lead to decreased calorie intake are more common in women than men because of cultural patterns in regard to appearance and self-esteem, and expected norms for female athletes. The spectrum of disordered eating behaviors ranges from mild to severe. Behavior may progress from mild disturbances to the severe, clinically defined disorders of anorexia or bulimia.

Anorexia nervosa is a medical syndrome in which the individual consumes an inadequate number of food calories compared to the amount needed to maintain body weight at a reasonable level for that person's age, height, build, and so on. Characteristics of anorexia nervosa include:

- Refusal to maintain body weight at or above 85% of that expected for age and height.
- Intense fear of gaining weight or becoming fat, even when very thin.
- Disturbance in the way one's body weight or shape is perceived, or seeing oneself as fat even when one is very thin.
- Undue influence of body weight or

shape on self-evaluation.

- Denial of the seriousness of a low body weight.
- *Amenorrhea,* or the absence of at least three consecutive menstrual cycles after periods have become established.

Bulimia is a medical problem in which a person may take in adequate calories but will try to decrease the amount their body retains by vomiting or using laxatives. Characteristics include:

- Recurrent episodes of binge eating (at least twice a week for 3 months).
- Recurrent inappropriate compensatory .behavior or purging (at least twice a week for 3 months).
- Self-evaluation unduly influenced by body shape and weight.

Personality traits such as compulsiveness, perfectionism, and high achievement expectations may help a high-level athlete but may also be associated with the development of disturbed eating patterns. Low self-esteem is common in those with disordered eating, and there may be a history of previous sexual or physical abuse. A woman may also lack a sense of identity other than being an athlete.

An athlete suspected of disordered eating should be approached thoughtfully about the problem. It is appropriate to see a medical professional when this problem is recognized.

DISORDERS OF MENSTRUAL FUNCTION

Disorders of menstrual function can occur in women as a result of an intense conditioning program in relation to inadequate calories consumed. These include changes in the cycle length, lack of ovulation, and lack of periods (amenorrhea). Secondary amenorrhea is the absence of 3–6 consecutive menstrual cycles in a woman who has already been menstruating. Exercise-associated amenorrhea may be related to vigorous/high-volume exercise and to inadequate calorie intake to meet energy balance. Athletic women with amenorrhea or infrequent periods are at risk for early osteoporosis because of low female hormone (especially estrogen) levels. A very low level of estrogen can lead to calcium and bone density losses.

PRACTICAL POINT

If you have stopped menstruating for more than 2 cycles, seek a medical evaluation. It could help prevent serious medical problems.

OSTEOPOROSIS AND CALCIUM AND OTHER NUTRIENT SUPPLEMENTATION

Osteoporosis is a disease associated with extensive bone density loss. This results in low bone mass and changes in bony architecture that can lead to fragile bones and an increased risk of stress and regular fractures. It is most common in women after menopause. It may occur at any age when bone mass falls below a critical threshold. Women with absent or infrequent periods might have hormonal levels similar to those of postmenopausal women and so may develop premature osteoporosis.

Exercise, calcium intake, and reproductive hormone status are major factors in controlling bone density. Bone mass declines with age because the remodeling (rebuilding) process is inefficient and results in a small deficit at the end of each cycle of remodeling. These deficits gradually accumulate, resulting in the decline in bone mass. Peak bone mass is a factor in protection from osteoporotic fractures. Peak bone mass is reached in the early to mid 20s in women. After this, women lose up to 1% per year until menopause. They may lose 4–6% per year for the first 4–5 years after menopause. Men maintain bone mass until about age 50, after which they lose about 0.4–0.5% per year.

PRACTICAL POINT

To decrease your risk of osteoporosis, consider combining the following:

- Strength training, especially of your arms
- Low- to moderate-impact aerobic exercise of your legs
- Calcium supplementation
- Vitamin D supplementation with 400–800 IUs per day, especially in winter months
- Minimal soft drink consumption
- Other minerals, including magnesium, zinc, copper, manganese, boron, and silicon
- Treatment for menstrual disorders if you are a premenopausal female
- A bone density study to determine bone density in your hips, back, and wrists

Calcium is stored in the skeleton. Adequate amounts of calcium and other minerals in the diet are required to maintain healthy bones. Dietary calcium is most critical during the adolescent growth spurt and into the 30s, so that peak bone mass can reach its full potential. Large amounts of caffeine, phosphorous, and protein in the diet may increase calcium loss.

Recommended Daily Amounts of Calcium

Adolescence and up to age 24: 1,200 milligrams per day

Postadolescence and premenopause: 800–1,200 milligrams per day

Pregnancy and menopause: 1,500 milligrams per day

Sources of calcium include milk products (about 300 mg per 8 ounces), broccoli, canned salmon, soy products (many are enriched with calcium), and calcium supplements. In general, calcium bound to amino acids (calcium citrate, etc.) is more absorbable than the calcium carbonate form. Calcium in the form of hydroxyapatite is also a highly beneficial form.

Osteoporosis Prevention and Treatment Exercise Program

Exercise is an important component in maintaining bone mass. Physical activity provides mechanical stress to bone, which stimulates bone formation. It is important to do strength training such as biceps curls and modified dips so as to put forces through your forearm to help prevent significant declines in arm bone density. Do Exercises 28 or 125 for your curls. For your dips, do Exercise 127 with 2 chairs and with your feet firmly on the ground. For both the curls and dips, do 2 sets of 12 reps 3 times per week.

Aerobic exercise that involves moderate-impact loading through your feet and legs (see chapter 3) can help slow bone loss in your hips and spine. Women should do impact-loaded aerobic exercise 3–5 times per week as part of their conditioning program. This could be walking, using a treadmill, doing aerobic classes, hiking, or jogging.

THE FEMALE ATHLETE TRIAD

The *female athlete triad* refers to the combination of amenorrhea, osteoporosis, and disordered eating. If a female athlete has disordered eating and a high training volume, she is more likely to develop amenorrhea. If she develops both of these conditions, she is more likely to develop early osteoporosis and possibly stress fractures. If a woman with the triad doesn't receive early medical attention, she can have serious medical problems.

HORMONES AND BIRTH CONTROL PILLS

Birth control pills can have numerous side effects, including a risk of thrombosis (excessive clotting) in the deep veins of the legs, pelvis, and so on. This may manifest with calf swelling or pain in the leg, thigh, or chest. Chest pain and shortness of breath at rest, or markedly decreased stamina, are more serious symptoms. Women on climbing expeditions or other prolonged outdoor trips should be aware of this risk. Consider going off the medication approximately 2–4 weeks before the trip and using another form of birth control. If you experience any of the above symptoms while on or off birth control pills, seek medical attention promptly.

MENOPAUSE

Exercise is extremely important for the postmenopausal woman because it can help decrease risks of cardiovascular disease, maintain a good body image, slow down osteoporosis, and maintain good strength and balance. Low- to moderate-impact aerobic exercise and strength training can have a role in decreasing the decline of bone density. Balance training and functional strength training exercises, such as lunges and mini squats, can be helpful to prevent falls that could lead to hip, spine, and wrist fractures.

Since the publication of the first edition, studies have indicated that hormone replacement therapy may contribute to a significant risk of uterine and breast cancer. For this reason, peri- and postmenopausal women are urged to consult a physician who is knowledgeable about nonhormone approaches to menopause.

The basic strategy for moving through menopause without hormone therapy is as follows:

1. Determine whether you are in perimenopause (very irregular periods after the age of 45) or menopause (the complete absence of a menstrual period).
2. If you are in perimenopause, consider getting your hormone levels tested with standard blood tests as well as a saliva profile, which can monitor hormones throughout an entire cycle.
3. Support the clearing and detoxification of estrogen so that it does not build up to harmful levels in your body. You can do this by eating from the cruciferous family of veggies, eating 20–35 grams of fiber, and by taking certain supplements recommended by your health-care provider.
4. Seek the care of a health-care provider who can work on symptoms and functional endocrinology with herbs, diet, and supplements.
5. Do the recommended exercises for osteoporosis prevention listed earlier in the chapter.

chapter 29 WEIGHT LOSS: A FUNCTIONAL AND HOLISTIC APPROACH

By David Musnick, M.D., and Teri Johnson, N.D.

THIS CHAPTER WILL HELP YOU:

- Choose your foods for weight loss.
- Control cravings.
- Understand the role of supplements in weight loss.
- Plan your exercise program to burn calories more efficiently and lose fat while gaining muscle.
- Decide which types of aerobic exercise are good for you.
- Understand the role of metabolic testing in weight loss.

Integrating functional medicine with a well-thought-out exercise program is an excellent approach to unloading unwanted pounds. In the United States and in many other developed countries, there is an epidemic of weight problems and obesity in adults and teenagers. *Overweight* is defined as a body mass index (BMI) of 25 to 29.9. *Obese* is defined as a BMI greater than 30. Note that if you are muscular, you could fall into the lower end of the overweight category.

BMI can be calculated using two methods. The first is to divide your weight in kilograms (pounds divided by 2.2) by your height in meters squared (height in meters × height in meters). The second method is to divide your weight in pounds by your height in inches squared (height in inches × height in inches). The Centers for Disease Control and Prevention's website has a BMI calculator, making the calculation simple (*www.cdc.gov/nccdphp/dnpa/bmi/calc-bmi.htm*).

There are many reasons for this explosion in weight gain, including genetic predisposition, dietary habits, inadequate physical activity, and exercise and environmental factors. Being overweight may have once conferred an advantage to people during famines, when survival depended on having enough fat on one's body to outlast times of food scarcity. But it no longer confers a survival advantage. In fact, being at a BMI of greater than 25 is associated with increased risks of type 2 diabetes, coronary artery disease, stroke, arthritis, and sleep apnea, among other disorders. So it is best to understand why weight gain occurs and how to approach attaining a healthy body weight from both metabolic and exercise angles.

WHY PEOPLE GAIN WEIGHT

People gain weight when they take in more calories than they use. A pound equals 3,500 calories; eat that in a day, and use fewer calories, and you gain weight.

We expend calories through our resting metabolic rate (RMR: the amount of energy it takes in calories to keep us alive each day in all of our organs and cells), through the amount of energy used to break down the food we eat (this takes very little energy), and through the amount of energy we expend in light activity or in directed exercise.

Most people have gained weight by consistently eating high-calorie, nutrient-depleted foods (e.g., starches, sugars, and high-fat foods) without adequate exercise and energy expenditure to balance it out. Many people have problems controlling appetite. Extra calories are consumed to satisfy cravings and to deal with uncomfortable emotions. Even worse, in many weight-loss diets, pounds are lost only to be regained, and then some, within 6 months to a year.

ATTAINING A HEALTHY WEIGHT

Try using the following guidelines for a complete approach to maintaining or achieving a healthy weight:

- Control cravings and limit your appetite by applying environmental and behavioral controls to habit-induced eating. Eat smaller portions and consider supplements to control cravings.
- Gain greater awareness of emotional patterns that are linked to eating.
- Choose your food wisely to end up with lower-calorie, nutrient-dense foods and level blood sugar. Minimize or eliminate beverages and snacks that are nutrient depleted.
- Choose low- to moderate-glycemic index foods.
- Limit incoming toxicity and support detoxification because toxins are released as you lose weight.
- Do regular aerobic exercise and try to burn at least 300, preferably 500, calories per session 6 days a week.
- Do strength training to build more muscle and increase your metabolic rate.
- Get your RMR tested. Realize that as you lose weight, your RMR will likely decrease, meaning you will have to tune up your eating and exercise.
- Get an analysis of your most efficient exercise fat-burning zone by getting a cardiorespiratory test.
- Try some safe supplements that might help you to use fat for fuel.

CONTROL CRAVINGS AND YOUR APPETITE

The regulation of a person's appetite is a complex issue. There are many biochemical, environmental, emotional, and social issues at play. Aim to feel satisfied, having had enough to eat without stuffing yourself. Colorful, tasty, and appealing food helps with this. Using your brain and self-control mechanisms rather than only relying on instincts is also helpful. This is a big factor in controlling cravings. Exercise can also help control appetite, partially because it can decrease stress-related eating by unloading stress.

NUTRITION TIP

Load up your salad with fiber-filled veggies, including broccoli, cauliflower, spinach, chard, celery, and so on. Make them more appealing by lightly steaming them the night before and putting some olive oil or toasted sesame oil, garlic powder, ground rosemary, or other herb flavoring on them. The fiber in the veggies helps prolong your blood glucose levels. Beans or cooked grains can also supply fiber and prolong your blood sugar level.

Cravings occur for many reasons. The primary reason is that your blood sugar may drop too low, signaling an urge to eat. This can be prevented by eating snacks and meals that will prolong your blood sugar. The guidelines below for carbohydrate, protein, and fat intake will help you choose foods that do this. The usual quick breakfast (coffee and a bagel or a scone) and the usual lunch (a salad) are culprits in quick declines in blood sugar. Skipping a meal will also cause your blood sugar to dip, making you prone to unhealthy snacking. Plan on a snack between lunch and dinner to avoid such pitfalls.

NUTRITION TIP

Healthy snack ideas: If you crave sweets, your blood sugar may be a bit low, or you may be feeling fatigued, sleepy, or down in the dumps. Sweets don't treat these symptoms for very long. Instead, try one-third to half of a protein bar, or some apple or celery with nuts or almond butter. If the craving is occurring before bedtime, you could try some fruit (like an apple or an orange), but avoid the juices. Melons in season are good snacks because they are filling, but note that they will not prolong your blood sugar.

ENVIRONMENTAL AND BEHAVIORAL CONTROLS

Many cravings are stimulus-response based: you pass by a fast-food place and all of a sudden want something that you know is not healthy. Try to avoid stimuli that you know will trigger this type of response.

Make a list of foods that you don't want to buy or eat and keep it in your car, wallet, purse, and/or on your refrigerator. Give the list a negative title (e.g., Fat Foods)—something you will associate with an unpleasant feeling so that you won't be so tempted to buy or eat the listed foods, even if others in your family do. A good rule is not to walk the grocery store aisles where your tempting foods are shelved.

Other tips are to only serve yourself portions that are reasonable or that have been determined for you by a certified nutritionist. Also, never sit down at the computer or TV with a pint of ice cream and expect to eat only a few spoonfuls. In fact, avoid buying high-calorie foods such as ice cream or cookies that will draw you into mindless eating if they are in your kitchen. Most of us cannot limit ourselves to small portions of tasty, high-calorie snacks.

Avoiding such simple, snack-type carbohydrates (carbs), which are not good for weight control, can be a big help. Similarly, avoid grocery shopping when you are hungry, because those simple carbs and unhealthy snacks will be tempting.

Some things will reliably inhibit cravings. Eating protein seems to inhibit the urge for quick carbs. This could be in the form of one-third to half of a low-carb protein bar or a few slices of turkey. Chromium is a mineral that may work in some people to decrease carb cravings. The dose would be 200 micrograms 1–2 times per day. The herb *Gymnema sylvestre* taken orally as capsules 3 times a day seems to decrease cravings. You can also use it as a liquid and put 3–5 drops on your tongue. This herb will make carbs taste bland and so will limit snacking. It is good to use before a party or if you are home alone and have carb cravings. It is best to use before the cravings start if you have predictable times of cravings.

Emotional cravings require both an awareness of the uncomfortable emotion and a food substitute. Become aware of the emotions by catching yourself reaching for food and asking, "Is this healthy? Is this a regular meal time? Am I covering up an emotion? What is the emotion that I am trying to cover up with food?" Usually it is a feeling of depression, fear, grief, loneliness, shame, and/or anger—in other words, any of the uncomfortable emotions. Become your own expert at identifying these food craving emotions. Develop other ways to deal with them, such as exercise, journal writing, and/or counseling (see Selected References for some websites that have suggestions).

If you are clinically depressed, you may eat less or crave carbs. Get help with your depression by seeing a health-care provider. If it is mild, you may be able to treat it with regular exercise, fish oils (1–2 grams per day), and some amino acids (see both Ross titles in Selected References). An amino acid precursor to serotonin, 5 HTP, can also improve mood and in some cases can help with cravings. For nighttime cravings, start with one 50 milligram capsule 1–2 hours before your cravings begin. You may increase it to two to three 50 mg capsules. Don't use 5 HTP if you will be driving, as it can make you sleepy. Also avoid it if you are already taking a serotonin-type medication for depression.

FOOD ALLERGIES AND CRAVINGS

Food allergies and sensitivities can lead to craving the food that you are sensitive to. It is not unreasonable to get a physician to order a food allergy panel and to eliminate foods that you are sensitive to for at least a month. You can then consider reintroducing one such food at a time, watching for any severe allergic reaction (e.g., shock, hives, asthma).

CHOOSE YOUR FOOD WISELY

Chapter 26 discusses healthy food choices for optimal wellness, and chapter 2 provides detailed background information on nutrition in general and for conditioning. Read those chapters as well as the specific guidelines for weight loss below for a good understanding of nutrition and weight loss.

Carbohydrates

The goal for weight loss is to minimize simple sugars and nonnutritive carbs. Chapter 2 describes the glycemic index, and understanding where foods fall on the index is important for weight loss. Avoid high glycemic-index carbs like white rice, potatoes, donuts, scones, cookies, and crackers. Minimize carbs such as pasta, as their calories add up quickly. This is especially true when you consider that such dishes are usually loaded with high-calorie and high-fat dairy

FIGURE 53. Glycemic Index of Common Foods

	Low (<55)	**Moderate (56–69)**	**High (>70)**
Cereals	Oatmeal 48 All bran 38		Grapenuts 71
Breads		Wholewheat 65 Rye (wholemeal) 58 Spelt (wholegrain) 58	
Grains	Brown rice 50 Corn on the cob 48 Wholegrain rye <40 Pasta 35		
Crackers		Rye Crisp 63	
Beans/legumes	Soy beans 20		
Dairy and milk substitutes	Soy milk 40–45 Yogurt 35 Skim milk 32		
Fruits	Banana 51 Orange 50 Strawberries 45 Apple 30–40		
Juices	Carrot (fresh) 43 Apple (unsweetened) 40 Tomato 38		

products (butter, cream, and cheeses). Limit bread and don't eat it with meals. Try to limit your carbs to mostly low glycemic index choices (less than 55). Figure 53 lists several food choices that are low to moderate on the glycemic index. Extensive lists can be found on the websites listed in Selected References.

Avoid carbs mixed with saturated fats, such as such as chips, nachos, and pizza; these have a high calorie count for a small amount eaten. Especially limit french fries and chips, as they contain a lot of deep-fried high-calorie oils.

Instead, eat most of your carbs as organic fruits, vegetables, beans, and legumes. Vegetables are especially useful for weight loss. They are low-calorie, and certain types aid in detoxification, which is important because toxins are released from fat as you burn it (see Toxicity and Detoxification below). Eat a variety of vegetables and try to have two kinds at each meal. Include at least a half cup of cruciferous veggies (broccoli, cauliflower, cabbage, kale, brussels sprouts) at lunch and dinner. These veggies help your body clear toxins. Eat salad at least once a day (don't heap on the dressing, and add some protein to it as noted below). A good strategy at lunch or dinner is to fill up on vegetables and salad to create a feeling of fullness and to minimize the amounts of breads and starches you eat.

Protein

First, calculate your daily protein needs based on your ideal body weight: Divide your ideal weight in pounds by 2.2 to get your weight in kilograms. Then multiply this by 1–1.2 to get your protein needs.

Use organic protein sources when possible, depending on availability and your finances. This includes dairy products; free-range, organic, grass-fed meats; free-range, hormone-free, organically fed turkey and poultry; and eggs. The protein sections in chapters 2 and 26 discuss vegetarian protein sources. Those such as legumes (beans, lentils, soy, etc.) can be good for weight loss because they have some fiber and can be more filling than meat or dairy sources. The important thing is knowing how to prepare them in a tasty fashion. Avoid protein options high in saturated fat, such as pizza, sausage, and most red meat (unless lean).

NUTRITION TIP

Start your day with about one-third of your protein needs or a maximum of 30 grams. You can do this with a protein smoothie. Use two scoops of a protein powder (organic whey, rice, or soy) with 12 ounces of liquid (soy, oat, almond, or rice milk). Use organic berries instead of bananas. Bananas are high on the glycemic index, unlike berries, which are also low-calorie and contain healthy phytochemicals and fiber. Add a scoop of a powdered fiber supplement and blend.

Starting your day with protein and fiber will help your blood sugar to stay level through the morning and should curtail any before-lunch cravings, especially those quick-carb cravings. You can take some in a to-go container and have it as a midmorning snack if you do get a craving.

Include high-quality, low-fat protein at every meal, including lunch. Too often lunches are salads with little or no protein, and this leads to midafternoon hunger and cravings. If you do eat a lunch salad, try adding some nitrate-free turkey to it. If you are vegetarian, or even a meat eater, you can load up on different beans as well as on different veggies (fiber-filled veggies are the best). Avoid the usual dressings and use olive oil and vinegar instead.

Consider a low-carb protein bar to curb your cravings for sweets. Some of these bars come in flavors that will satisfy your sweet cravings. (See Selected References for chapter 26 for some suggestions.)

NUTRITION TIP

If you eat sandwiches, try the following: avoid mayonnaise and butter on the bread; eliminate one of the two slices of bread; ask for extra lettuce, tomato, and other veggies to fill you up; and ask for extra protein.

Fats

Chapter 26 discusses healthy fats for optimal wellness, and that information also applies to weight loss. Healthy fats are extremely important for your skin, heart, mood, and your general health, so please use them daily, even when trying to lose weight.

Make your own salad dressing, because most store-bought varieties are high in calories and lacking in good oils. Use extra virgin olive oil with flaxseed and walnut oil, and add sesame oil to taste. Seasonings will add flavor. You can use this oil mix on salads and veggies to increase your intake of healthy oils and to inhibit your appetite.

Healthy fats such as fish oil can help in improving insulin sensitivity if you are overweight and have insulin resistance. Nuts have healthy fats, and you can use them as fat/protein snacks for a prolonged boost of your blood sugar. Make sure they are not cooked in cottonseed oil.

Fats have 9 calories per gram, so it is important to limit unhealthy fat calories. Do this by eliminating all deep-fried foods. Avoid fast-food restaurants. Avoid all products with partially hydrogenated oils. Limit saturated fats in snacks, ice cream, and so on. Avoid cream-based gravies and toppings on biscuits. Limit foods with cooked cheese in them, such as pizza and lasagna. These foods usually have a lot of calories and saturated fats.

TOXICITY AND DETOXIFICATION

Toxins are at high levels in industrialized society. We are exposed to them in the food we eat and in the products we use on our skin, hair, and in and around our home. It is important to limit toxin exposure so that we don't overwhelm our organs of elimination. Therefore, eat organic foods as much as possible. Stay away from pesticide and herbicide sprayings. Limit your exposure to chemicals in fumes, sprays, perfumes, and so on.

Studies have sampled the fat of the average person not occupationally exposed to pesticides. Surprising results show that people living in the United States routinely have very high levels of more than five pesticides as well as PCBs and other toxic chemicals. The toxins that cannot be removed by your liver, kidney, and skin are stored in different compartments in your body, mostly in your fat stores because the toxins are fat soluble.

A goal of weight loss is to break down your fat stores and to use them for energy. If toxins released in the process are not eliminated, they will be mobilized and restored in your body. If toxins are not processed well, they can lead to symptoms such as achiness, headache, and stiffness.

You can support your body's ability to biotransform toxins as your fat stores are broken down. Veggies from the cruciferous and the onion families (respectively: broccoli, cabbage, kale; onions, garlic, leeks, chives, shallots) provide your liver's enzyme systems with materials to aid your body in detoxification. Other things that can be helpful in biotransforming toxins and in protecting your liver are milk thistle, N-acetyl cysteine, mixed antioxidants, and other liver-supportive nutrients.

MODIFIED CARBOHYDRATE-TO-PROTEIN RATIO DIETS

There is evidence that certain ratios of macronutrients (carbohydrates, protein, and fat) can be more beneficial for an individual trying to lose weight. Higher-carb diets are definitely essential for athletes to supply daily energy needs. Lower-carb and higher-protein diets (e.g., the Atkins Diet), however, have been popularized and appear to be helpful for many people trying to lose weight. For instance, these diets appear to have favorable effects on blood cholesterol levels. If you choose such a diet, remember that the quality of the protein and fat is quite important. Healthy fats and protein sources should be emphasized.

Some people lose weight better on a metabolic typing diet. This diet follows a specific ratio of macronutrients depending on your metabolism, and certain foods and supplements are more emphasized. There have been no randomized control trials on this approach, but clinical experience has shown it to be helpful for some overweight individuals.

RESTING METABOLIC RATE AND CARDIORESPIRATORY TESTING

Your resting metabolic rate (RMR) is an important number to know if you are trying to lose weight. It can be estimated by the formula in chapter 3, but for a more accurate measure seek out a clinic that has specialized equipment. Once your RMR is measured, a nutritionist or trained physician can calculate the total number of calories that your body uses each day. You can then decide how many calories short of this you will eat per day. Remember that 3,500 calories equals 1 pound, so 500 calories less than you need per day will lead to a safe weight loss of 1 pound per week.

You can vary the calorie deficit to change the amount of weight you would like to lose. A nutritionist can help you with these decisions. As you lose weight, your RMR can decrease, so it is a good idea to get it remeasured periodically in order to keep losing weight.

Cardiorespiratory exercise testing is a specialized type of exercise test that can give you information about your aerobic and anaerobic exercise heart rate zones. This test can give you a more specific heart-rate training zone for burning more fat (chapter 3 tells you how to derive general heart-rate training zones).

Some clinics have computer programs and the equipment to give you a very refined exercise prescription based on the above tests. Call around or do an Internet search to find a clinic in your area.

EXERCISE FOR WEIGHT LOSS

Exercise is essential for weight loss in order to burn calories, increase your lean muscle mass, increase your RMR, and to replace fat with muscle. Aerobic exercise will burn the most calories. Chapter 3 explains aerobic exercise in detail, chapter 5 provides strength training guidelines, and chapter 26 contains some aerobic exercise guidelines and specific strength training exercises for optimal wellness. Your aerobic exercise goals are to:

- Work out 6–7 days per week, working up to at least 30 minutes of aerobic exercise each day.
- Make 2 of your aerobic workouts be of longer duration (40–50 minutes).
- Achieve at least 2,000 kilocalories burned through exercise per week.

The issues for weight loss are how to start (or increase) what you are doing as well as what aerobic and strength training exercises to do.

Starting is basically a matter of making a commitment and scheduling your exercise for when you have the most energy. If you work, start taking 10- to 15-minute walks on your breaks. If the weather is really bad, you could climb stairs during your break. Try getting in some short exercise sessions every day; avoiding elevators and using the stairs for brief bouts is a good way to do this. Try to go to a facility to exercise, such as a gym or a YMCA, as the environment is suitable for exercising, and there are many equipment options. Use footwear such as a running shoe with a heel counter and medial arch stability. This type of shoe can also be used for walking.

Choose aerobic options that will not hurt your knees, feet, or back. At a health club, ask a trainer to show you around initially and explain how to use the aerobic equipment. The best equipment choices for overweight people are the stationary cycles and the EFX and treadmill machines. The best classes are water aerobics and low-impact aerobics.

On equipment, start with 10 minutes of low- to moderate-intensity exercise and gradually increase by 1 minute the duration of each workout. You may want to use two different pieces of equipment when your sessions get to be 30 minutes or longer, to avoid overuse injuries. Try to increase the duration of your average workout to a minimum of 30 minutes. To start, aim for aerobic sessions 2 days a week that last 45–60 minutes. This can be very helpful in increasing weekly calorie burning. Consider 1 day a week of a low-intensity activity that lasts a few hours, such as walking, hiking, and so on. In the city, you can try walking in malls and parks.

At some point you may be ready for some interval training on a bike or an EFX machine. See chapter 3 for details, but this will basically involve doing 3–6 1-minute spurts of increased aerobic activity during your aerobic workouts 2 times per week. Follow the guidelines and precautions in chapter 3 for these intervals and avoid them if you have a cardiac or an orthopedic condition. Doing intervals can increase the levels and efficiency of some of the enzymes in your muscles that can help to make weight loss easier.

Strength training should be done 2–3 times per week. It will help to build muscle and to increase your RMR, which can make it easier to lose weight and keep it off. You can get all of your strength training done in about 15–20 minutes after or before your aerobic workout. Start with the exercise suggestions in chapter 26, doing 2 sets of 10–12 reps. Add any other exercises from the Part II body region chapters that you can enjoy and do safely.

NUTRITIONAL AIDS TO FAT BURNING WHILE EXERCISING

A number of supplements might help with fat burning and energy expenditure. L-carnitine helps to shuttle fatty acids to mitochondria (your cells' energy-producing organelles), where they can be burned for energy. It may help you to use more fat for fuel as you exercise. It may also limit appetite. Try a dose of 1,000 milligrams in the morning and again in mid-afternoon. Drinking green tea may also increase thermogenesis and calorie burning. Try drinking two to three cups per day (note that green tea does contain caffeine). Green tea may also aid in cancer prevention.

WHAT ABOUT DIETS, SUPPLEMENTS, AND NUTRITIONISTS?

There are many diets that you can read about, including the Atkins and the South Beach diets. We have used concepts from these diets in this chapter, but have gone beyond them with weight-loss strategies that have worked over time. No one diet has the answer for everyone, and there is no replacing the basic nutritional and exercise concepts in this chapter.

A good multivitamin and mineral that requires 3–6 capsules per day can supply B vitamins, minerals, and antioxidants helpful for your basic metabolism. An additional mixed antioxidant may be helpful if you are quite overweight and experience metabolic syndrome (hypertension, hyperlipidemia, and insulin resistance with or without type 2 diabetes); such antioxidants can combat the excess of free radicals generated by weight loss.

It is not unreasonable to consult a certified

nutritionist, especially if that person is familiar with the basic weight-loss concepts in this chapter. A certified nutritionist can help you with meal plans, food portions, calorie counts per day, and rotation diets for allergenic foods, among other weight-loss strategies.

Taking a functional and more holistic approach to food choices, supplements, and exercise can make a big difference in losing weight and keeping it off. Diets for weight loss change continually, so we urge you to keep up with the literature on such diets as well as that on supplements.

chapter 30 ENERGY, FATIGUE, OVERTRAINING, AND EXERCISING WITH FIBROMYALGIA

By David Musnick, M.D.

THIS CHAPTER WILL HELP YOU:

- Understand what to consider if you have low energy.
- Identify the signs of overtraining syndrome.
- Learn how to exercise with fibromyalgia or chronic fatigue.
- Learn about a few supplements to improve energy.

How much energy you have depends on many variables. Reading chapter 1 can give you a good idea about how cells work to produce ATP, your energy storage units. Toxins, free radicals, and viruses, among other things, can damage your mitochondria. If this occurs to a significant level, you may feel like you don't have enough energy to exercise aerobically at a high level. If there is enough mitochondrial damage, it may be difficult to exercise at all except for strength training and balance. Some people have even more significant energy problems and have fatigue all day long, as in fibromyalgia and chronic fatigue syndrome.

Other health conditions that can lead to fatigue include overtraining syndrome; iron deficiency anemia; hormonal problems including thyroid and adrenal dysfunction; mood disorders such as depression; and cardiac, kidney, and lung disorders. If you have fatigue, it is important to see a health-care provider who can rule out serious and treatable medical problems that can lead to fatigue.

OVERTRAINING SYNDROME

If you are athletic and doing a lot of training, it is important to be aware of what can cause fatigue and plan on doing things to prevent it. Have blood work done periodically to check your complete blood count (CBC) and ferritin levels to screen for iron deficiency anemia. Have a TSH thyroid test done every few years. Have a general chemistry panel with a magnesium level every 1–2 years. Make sure that you are eating enough carbohydrates to supply your muscles with glycogen and to load or rebuild the glycogen stores pre- and postevent (see chapter 2).

Also learn to recognize the symptoms of overtraining syndrome, a dysfunction in adrenal and sex hormone systems as well as other metabolic abnormalities. Check your morning pulse when you first awaken and record the number on a calendar. Be on the lookout for a rise of 5 or more points. This, along with a recurrent sore throat and exercise-related fatigue, might be a sign of overtraining. If you suspect overtraining syndrome, immediately decrease your exercise volume in regard to duration and intensity. Also make sure you are not losing weight, and consult a physician familiar with the intricacies of managing this syndrome.

FIBROMYALGIA SYNDROME

Fibromyalgia syndrome (FMS) is characterized by tenderness in certain areas of the body above and below the waist and on the right and left side of the body. There are a number of possible reasons why a person might develop this. In conventional medicine, there is no known cause, and treatments include antidepressants and muscle relaxers. A more integrative and functional medicine approach uses certain lab tests, diet changes, supplements, and lifestyle changes to try to achieve less pain and improved sleep.

If you have FMS, it is important to modify aerobic exercise and weight lifting. Start with a shorter duration of the exercise period, say 10–15 minutes, and only very gradually increase it. Low-impact aerobic activities like walking, using EFX machines, and stationary cycling should be tried before more aggressive activities such as running, aerobic step classes, Tae Bo, and so on. Increase the duration of the exercise by increments of 1 minute per every two aerobic sessions and make sure there is no pain or exhaustion after the exercise or the next day.

With strength training, always start with lower resistance (weight) and fewer reps even if the exercise seems too easy. Try biceps curls with 5 pounds, or even 3 pounds, and do a set of 5 reps initially, eventually working up to a set of 10–12 reps. For your upper body, try basic exercises like a biceps and triceps curl before doing lat pulls or dips. Try the strength training program as outlined in chapter 27, as it is easier and less likely to cause injury. As you improve in your symptoms, you can gradually increase the weight that you use in your exercises.

CHRONIC FATIGUE SYNDROME

People with chronic fatigue syndrome (CFIDS) have mitochondrial dysfunction and can get too exhausted from aerobic activity other than light walking. If you have CFIDS, it is best to focus on balance exercises and strength training until your energy levels are much improved. Follow the strength training and balance program in chapter 27, as it is easier and less likely to lead to injury.

A functional medicine approach to this condition involves more in-depth lab testing than most conventional labs will do. Once these labs are obtained, a functional medicine physician can determine more specifically what is wrong and can work on specific issues to support your immune system and energy production.

You should not do aerobic exercise until you have no significant fatigue during a day. When you do start, make sure it is low impact and for a brief duration, for example, light walking for 10 minutes. This will allow you to gain aerobic benefit without using up all of your available energy supply for exercise.

ENERGY, MOOD, AND SLEEP

Depression can lead to low energy. If you are depressed and have some of the associated symptoms (critical thoughts, early awakening, lack of ability to experience pleasure, low mood, etc.), seek evaluation by your physician. Did you know that regular exercise as well as 1 gram of fish oil per day has been found to partially alleviate or prevent depression? The exercise needs to be about a half-hour long and be almost daily. Mild depression may also be treated by amino acids in some cases. For this, you would see a physician familiar with using amino-acid support for depression.

Sleep is also extremely important for energy. Most people need 8 hours of sleep to feel well rested. There are many reasons for insomnia, which can be evaluated and often treated with sleep hygiene suggestions.

ADRENAL AND THYROID ISSUES

Dysfunction of either the adrenal or thyroid gland can lower an individual's energy level. Fatigue is a well-known symptom of hypothyroidism. Get a TSH test and perhaps a free T3 and T4 test to screen out more subtle causes of a low thyroid condition. If your thyroid is hypofunctioning, this can be supported with thyroid medication.

Adrenal dysfunction is much more subtle for a physician to diagnose because the conventional ACTH stimulation test may only pick up the most severe cases. There can be varying levels of adrenal dysfunction and a salivary adrenal test done 4 times during the day may be able to detect more subtle cases. If results are positive, your adrenals can be supported by supplements to improve function. Stress management is also very important in supporting the adrenal system.

FOOD ALLERGIES AND FATIGUE

Food allergies can be severe and life threatening, as when a person with an allergy to peanuts eats the nut and has difficulty breathing. There can also be milder forms of allergic reaction or sensitivity to foods that can cause joint or muscle aching, fatigue, headaches, and other symptoms. If you find that you are feeling low energy after eating certain foods, it might be that you are actually sensitive to them. It can be helpful to have a blood test with a panel for food allergies, along with measures of antigliadin and antiendomysial antibodies to determine gluten sensitivity. If the test returns with high values for particular foods, it is wise to eliminate the food for a month and to monitor your energy level.

GAINING MORE ENERGY

If you are experiencing decreased energy, it is important to thoroughly look for causes before using supplements to support cell energy production. Review the major causes of low energy discussed above and have a minimum of the following tests done: TSH thyroid testing; adrenal testing including salivary hormone testing; and complete blood count chemistry panel. If nothing shows up on these tests, many others can be done, including a test for free T3 and T4, one for urinary organic acids, screening for food allergies, and various other metabolic tests. A functional or environmental medicine physician or a naturopathic physician can run all these tests. If specific abnormalities are found, they can be treated.

Also look at your diet. It is best to eat in a way similar to that outlined for optimal wellness in chapter 26. If you have done all of the above tests and your diet is sound, it is not unreasonable to try a few supplements and then to monitor your response in regard to your energy level. Try an energy supplement for at least 1 week before judging its effectiveness.

Coenzyme Q10 can be taken in doses of 100 milligrams 2–3 times a day. Take it with nuts or some other oil (olive oil with a salad) so that the CoQ10 will be better absorbed. A second supplement to try is L-carnitine, at a dose of 500–1,000 milligrams twice a day. This can help shuttle fat to your cells' mitochondria and help to burn it.

Be alert for fatigue; it is an important symptom. As prevention, exercise regularly but not excessively, get adequate rest, and eat a healthy diet. A close look at your exercise program and a functional medicine approach can usually get to the root of the problem and lead to supportive measures.

chapter 31 ARTHRITIS AND NUTRIENT SUPPORT FOR JOINT HEALTH

By David Musnick, M.D.

THIS CHAPTER WILL HELP YOU:

- Choose exercise options if you have arthritis.
- Understand which supplements may help your joints.

The most common form of arthritis is degenerative osteoarthritis (DJD). This involves a thinning of cartilage, narrowing of joints, and extra bone formation. DJD occurs most commonly in the feet, ankles, knees, hips, low back, and neck. It is more common a few years after a serious sprain injury or after a person reaches their mid 40s. There are many other forms of arthritis that are beyond the scope of this book, but similar principles of exercise will apply.

If you have arthritis that is significant enough to narrow a joint or to cause limited motion or pain in a joint, get evaluated, try to avoid exercises that cause the condition to flare up, and consider nutritional support for your joints. Remember that stable, proper-fitting shoes that have laces and rear foot support are important in order to minimize mechanical overload of any arthritic problem of the knee, hip, or back.

JOINT EVALUATION

If you are having pain, swelling or limitation of movement, consider getting evaluated by a medical practitioner. Imaging studies (such as X-rays) may be helpful in evaluating the health of your joints. A combined exercise and nutritional supplement program, along with proper shoe wear, can be very helpful in maintaining and improving the health of your joints.

KNEE AND HIP ARTHRITIS

If you have arthritis in your knee or hip, your best choices for aerobic workouts are the stationary cycle, the EFX machine, and water aerobics. Your aerobic and strength training choices should not put you into joint ranges of motion that will be uncomfortable, but the exercises should still move the arthritic joints. Try not to put your joints at the end of their range of motion, as this can injure them or cause pain. Use hiking poles if you walk to unload your knees, especially when you are walking downhill or on snow.

Knee and hip DJD responds fairly well to supplements after 6–8 weeks of supplementation (see Supplements for Your Joints). But if a knee or hip continues to hurt or if such pain restricts your activities, see a physician or physical therapist.

LOW-BACK ARTHRITIS

Low-back DJD can cause leg or foot weakness, or pain in your back or down one of your legs. If you have these symptoms, see your chiropractic or medical physician. Read chapter 14, which discusses anatomy and function of the neck, mid back, and low back/core, as well as safe lifting techniques. Learn how to activate your core muscles and use good body mechanics to avoid further injury.

Most DJD of the low back will limit running

or treadmill use. Swimming and cycling are usually very well tolerated. Also consider cycling, EFX machines, water aerobics, and outdoor activities that you enjoy and tolerate well.

NECK ARTHRITIS

Neck arthritis can cause pain in your neck, shoulders, arms, and hands. It can also cause weakness of your arms, wrists, or fingers. To alleviate symptoms, it is very important to maintain good posture in all of the chairs that you use. You might consider an ergonomic chair. Please read chapter 25 to learn neutral spine sitting.

Choose lower impact aerobic activities such as EFX machines, water aerobics, and stair-climbers if they do not aggravate your symptoms. When strength training, use less weight than you can maximally lift if your neck is irritable; your neck is involved in many weight-lifting exercises. If you hike, find a pack that fits you well and that does not sway much side to side, as such movement will put excessive pressure on your neck and low back.

FOOT ARTHRITIS

DJD of the big toe can make it difficult to run and walk. Your big toe should be able to move 45–60 degrees when extended from a flat-on-the-floor position to an extended-toward-the-ceiling position, but arthritis can limit movement. When this is significant, it may affect the way that you walk. It is important to use stable and supportive shoes for work and recreation if you have this problem. You might consider a shoe with a slight rocker bottom (forefoot arched upward) to help decrease the amount of motion that walking puts your foot through.

There are many other foot conditions, such as plantar fasciitis, that can also cause pain. Plantar fasciitis is not an arthritic problem, but is rather an inflammation and mechanical problem leading to pain in your arch and heel area. Consider a generic orthotic and seek medical attention if such a condition does not improve after 4 weeks.

SUPPLEMENTS FOR YOUR JOINTS

There have been numerous studies to determine which supplements may be helpful for DJD. Most studies have looked at the effect of supplements on DJD of the knee. Glucosamine sulfate is a biochemical that is in your joints, and it is a rate-limiting nutrient in the repair and making of cartilage. Studies have shown that taking a minimum of 1,500 milligrams of glucosamine sulfate per day for a minimum of 6–8 weeks can decrease pain and other symptoms of knee arthritis. This appears to also be true for DJD of the foot, hip, and spine. It is important to take pure glucosamine sulfate for at least 8 weeks, as cartilage is very slow to build and heal. If you have a shellfish allergy, avoid the shellfish-origin glucosamine and use the vegetarian-origin glucosamine. For arthritis in any of your joints, as well as after joint sprains, you might consider taking 2,000 milligrams of glucosamine sulfate every day divided in two doses. Also consider using it if you have a kneecap pain problem with exercise or activities.

Other important nutrients for joint healing are vitamin C and zinc. Chondroitin sulfate has been studied for arthritis of the knee and has been shown to be beneficial. It is found in most products that also contain glucosamine. The majority of chondroitin comes from cow trachea, which may not be a safe and pure source. Chondroitin is less well absorbed than glucosamine because of its large molecular weight. If you have bad arthritis consider using a special type of chondroitin sulfate—"low molecular weight chondroitin sulfate" (at least 1,200 mg per day)—along with glucosamine sulfate.

Finally, MSM may be helpful for cartilage support. The minimal dose for MSM is 3–4 grams per day in divided doses.

Because information on supplements changes as research occurs, use additional resources such as those in Selected References to help keep yourself informed.

Appendix

U.S.–METRIC CONVERSIONS

U.S. Weight	Metric Weight
1 ounce (oz)	28.35 grams (gm)
1 pound (lb)	453.59 grams (gm)
1 pound (lb)	0.454 kilograms (kg)

U.S. Length	Metric Length
1 inch (in)	2.54 centimeters (cm)
1 foot (ft)	30.48 centimeters (cm)
1 yard (yd)	9.1 meters (m)
1 mile	1600 meters (m)
1 mile	1.6 kilometers (K)

METRIC–U.S. CONVERSIONS

Metric Weight	U.S. Weight
1 gram (gm)	0.035274 ounces (oz)
1 kilogram (kg)	35.274 ounces (oz)
1 kilogram (kg)	2.2046 pounds (oz)

Metric Length	U.S. Length
1 centimeter (cm)	0.3937 inches (in)
1 meter (m)	39.37 inches (in)
1 meter (m)	3.281 feet (ft)
1 meter (m)	1.0936 yards (yd)
1 kilometer (K)	0.6 mile

Selected References

CHAPTER 1

Adams, J. Crawford. *Outline of Orthopedics*. 10th ed. New York: Longman Group, 1986.

Ainsworth, B. E., et al. "The Compendium of Physical Activities; Classification of Energy Costs of Human Physical Activities." *Medicine and Science in Sports and Exercise* 25, no. 1 (January 1993).

Cox, Steven, and Kris Fulsaas, eds. *Mountaineering: The Freedom of the Hills*. 7th ed. Seattle: The Mountaineers Books, 2003.

McArdle, W. D., F. I. Katch, and V. L. Katch. *Exercise Physiology: Energy, Nutrition, and Human Performance*. Philadelphia: Lippincott Williams and Wilkins, 2001.

CHAPTER 2

Ainsworth et al. "Compendium" (see chapter 1 references).

American Dietetics and American Diabetes Associations. *The Exchange Lists for Meal Planning*. Alexandria, Va.: American Dietetics and American Diabetes Associations, 2003.

Berning, S., and S. N. Steen. *Nutrition for Sport and Exercise*. Gaithersburg, Md.: Aspen Publishing, 1998.

Broun, Fred. *Nutritional Needs of Athletes*. New York: John Wiley and Sons, 1995.

Burke, Louise, and V. Deakin. *Clinical Sports Nutrition*. 2nd ed. New York: McGraw-Hill Professional, 2000.

Clark, Nancy. *Sports Nutrition Guidebook*. 3rd ed. Champaign, Ill.: Human Kinetics Publishing, 2003.

Gaby, Allan R. *Preventing and Reversing Osteoporosis*. Rocklin, Calif.: Prima Publishing, 1994.

Gretebeck, R., et al. "Glycemic Index of Popular Sports Drinks and Energy Foods." *Journal of the American Dietetic Association* 102, no. 3 (2002): 415–416.

Lukaczer, Dan. *Functional Medicine: Adjunctive Nutritional Support for Syndrome X*. Gig Harbor, Wash.: HealthComm International, Inc., 1998.

McArdle, Katch, and Katch. *Exercise Physiology* (see chapter 1 references).

Powell, K. Foster, S. Holt, and J. Brand Miller. "International Table of Glycemic Index and Glycemic Load Values." *American Journal of Clinical Nutrition* 76 (2002): 5–56.

Sears, Barry. *Enter the Zone*. New York: Regan Books, 1995.

Wilson, Duff. *Fateful Harvest*. New York: Harper Collins, 2001.

Wolinksy, Ira, ed. *Nutrition in Exercise and Sport*. Boca Raton, Fla.: CRC Press LLC, 1998.

Websites

Food composition of carbs, fats, and proteins: *www.nal.usda.gov/fnic/foodcomp/Data/index.html*

Glycemic index: *www.glycemicindex.com; www.glycemicdietsw.com*

Natural medicine: *www.naturaldatabase.com*

Omega-3 fats: *www.nal.usda.gov/fnic/foodcomp/Data/index.html; www.annecollins.com/dietary-fat/omega-3-efa-6-chart.htm*

Protein: *www.caloriecountercharts.com; http://teaching.ucdavis.edu/nut10/handouts/content.pdf*

Sports drinks: *www.ais.org.au/nutrition/SuppFS01.htm*

CHAPTER 3

Bakoulisbloch, Gordon. *Cross Training*. New York: Simon and Schuster, 1992.

Blair, S. N., M. J. LaMonte, and M. Z. Nichaman. "The Evolution of Physical Activity Recommendations: How Much Is Enough?" *American Journal of Clinical Nutrition* 79, no. 5 (May 2004): 9135–9205.

Edwards, Sally. *The Heart Rate Monitor Book*. Sacramento, Calif.: Heart Zones Co., 1993.

———. *Sally Edwards' Heart Zone Training: Exercise Smart, Stay Fit and Live Longer*. Holbrook, Mass.: Adams Publishing, 1996.

McArdle, Katch, and Katch. *Exercise Physiology* (see chapter 1 references).

Paffenbarger, Ralph F. Jr., and Eric Olson. *Life Fit*. Champaign, Ill.: Human Kinetics Publishing, 1996.

Shephard, Roy. *Aerobic Fitness and Health*. Champaign, Ill.: Human Kinetics Publishing, 1994.

CHAPTER 4

Anderson, B., and E. R. Burke. "Scientific, Medical and Practical Aspects of Stretching." *Sports Medicine* 10, no. 1 (1991).

Anderson, R. A. *Stretching*. Bolinas, Calif.: Shelter Publications, 1980.

Janda, Vladimir, and Gwendolen A. Jull. "Muscles and Motor Control in Low Back Pain: Assessment and Management," in *Physical Therapy of the Low Back*, ed. Lance T. Twomey and James R. Taylor. New York: Churchill Livingstone, 1987.

McAtee, R. *Facilitated Stretching*. Champaign, Ill.: Human Kinetics Publishing, 1993.

Powers, S. K., and E. T. Howley. *Exercise Physiology*. Madison, Wis.: Brown and Benchmark, 1994.

Smith, C. A. "The Warm Up Procedure: To Stretch or Not to Stretch." Review, *Journal of Orthopedic and Sports Physical Therapy* 19, no. 1 (1994): 12–17.

CHAPTER 5

Anderson, Bob. *Getting in Shape*. Bolinas, Calif.: Shelter Publications, 1994.

Baechle, Thomas R., ed. *Essentials of Strength Training and Conditioning*. Champaign, Ill.: National Strength and Conditioning Association and Human Kinetics Publishing, 2000.

Colgan, M. *The New Power Program*. Richmond, Canada: Apple Publishing Company, 2001.

Fleck, Steven J., and W. J. Kraemer. *Designing Resistance Training Programs*. Champaign, Ill.: Human Kinetics Publishing, 1997.

Gray, Gary. *Chain Reaction Festival*. Adrian, Mich.: Wynn Marketing, 1996.

———. *Lower Extremity Functional Profile*. Adrian, Mich.: Wynn Marketing, 1995.

Hakkinen, K., et al. "Neuromuscular Adaptation during Prolonged Strength Training, Detraining and Re-Strength-Training in Middle-Aged and Elderly People." *European Journal of Applied Physiology* (Germany) 83, no.1 (September 2000): 51–62.

Izquierdo, M., et al. "Effects of Strength Training on Submaximal and Maximal Endurance Performance Capacity in Middle-Aged and Older Men." *Journal of Strength and Conditioning Resources* 17, no.1 (February 2003): 129–139.

Kostka, T. "Resistance (Strength) Training in Health Promotion and Rehabilitation." *Pol. Merkuriusz. Lek.* (Poland) 13, no. 78 (December 2002): 520–523.

Kramer, W. J. "Endocrine Responses to Resistance Exercise." *Medical Science and Sports and Exercise*, suppl. 29 (1988): 152.

McArdle, Katch, and Katch. *Exercise Physiology* (see chapter 1 references).

McCarthy, J. P., M. A. Pozniak, and J. C. Agre. "Neuromuscular Adaptations to Concurrent Strength and Endurance Training." *Medical Science and Sports Exercise* 34, no. 3 (March 2002): 511–519.

Paliquin, Charles. *Modern Trends in Strength Training, Volume 1, Reps and Sets*. 3rd ed. Richmond, Canada: Apple Publishing Company, 2001.

Slade, J. M., et al. "Anaerobic power and physical function in strength-trained and non-strength-trained older adults." *Journal of Gerontology* 57, no. 3 (March 2002): 168–172.

Smith, Mark J. *A Comparison: Moderate-Intensity Continuous Activity and High-Intensity Intermittent Activity*. Philadelphia: Mark J. Smith, 2002.

VanHelder, W. "Growth Hormone Responses During Intermittent Weight Lifting Exercise in Men." *European Journal of Applied Physiology* (Germany) 53 (1984): 31–34.

White, Thomas P. *The Wellness Guide to Lifelong Fitness*. New York: Rebus, 1993.

Websites

Exercise equipment: *www.performbetter.com; http://xiser.com*

CHAPTER 6

Aydin, T., et al. "Proprioception of the Ankle: A Comparison Between Female Teenaged Gymnasts and Controls." *Foot/Ankle International* 23, no. 2 (February 2002): 123–129.

Chong, R. K., et al. "Source of Improvement in Balance Control after a Training Program for Ankle Proprioception." *Perception and Motor Skills* 92, no. 1 (February 2001): 265–272.

Dean, C., R. Shepherd, and R. Adams. "Sitting Balance I: Trunk-Arm Coordination and the Contribution of the Lowe Limbs during Self-Paced Reaching in Sitting." *Gait Posture* (Netherlands) 10, no. 2 (October 1999): 135–146.

Gauchard, G. C., et al. "Beneficial Effect of Proprioceptive Physical Activities on Balance Control in Elderly Human Subjects." *Neuroscience Letters* (Ireland) 273, no. 2 (October 1999): 81–84.

Hirsch, M. A., et al. "The Effects of Balance Training and High-Intensity Resistance Training on Persons with Idiopathic Parkinson's Disease." *Physical Medicine and Rehabilitation* 84, no. 8 (August 2003): 1109–1117.

Kavounoudias, A., et al. "From Balance Regulation to Body Orientation: Two Goals for Muscle Proprioceptive Information Processing?" *Experimental Brain Research* (Germany) 124, no. 1 (January 1999): 80–88.

Lin, S. I., and R. M. Lin. "Sensorimotor and Balance Function in Older Adults with Lumbar Nerve Root Compression." *Clinical Orthopedics* 394 (January 2002): 146–153.

Lord, S. R., et al. "Sit-to-Stand Performance Depends on Sensation, Speed, Balance, and Psychological Status in Addition to Strength in Older People." *Journal of Gerontology* 57, no. 8 (August 2002): M539–M543.

Ringsberg, K., et al. "Is There a Relationship Between Balance, Gait Performance and Muscular Strength in 75-Year-Old Women?" *Age Ageing* (England) 28, no. 3 (May 1999): 289–293.

Robinovitch, S. N., et al. "Effect of Strength and Speed of Torque Development on Balance Recovery with the Ankle Strategy." *Journal of Neurophysiology* 88, no. 2 (August 2002): 613–620.

Schlicht, J., D. N. Camaione, and S. V. Owen. "Effect of Intense Strength Training on Standing Balance, Walking Speed, and Sit-to-Stand Performance in Older Adults." *Journal of Gerontology* 56, no. 5 (May 2001): M281–M286.

Shimada, H., et al. "Relationship with Dynamic

Balance Function During Standing and Walking." *American Journal of Physical Medicine and Rehabilitation* 82, no. 7 (July 2003): 511–516.

Spring, H., A. Pirlet, and T. Tritschler. "How Much Strength is Needed for Fitness?" *Ther. Umsch.* (Switzerland) 58, no. 4 (April 2001): 213–219.

Timonen, L., et al. "A Randomized Controlled Trial of Rehabilitation after Hospitalization in Frail Older Women: Effects on Strength, Balance and Mobility." *Scandinavian Journal of Medical Science and Sports* (Denmark) 12, no. 3 (June 2002): 186–192.

Toole, T., et al. "The Effects of a Balance and Strength Training Program on Equilibrium in Parkinsonism: A Preliminary Study." *NeuroRehabilitation* 14, no. 3 (2000): 165–174.

Wang, W. Y., and S. M. Chen. "Balance and Muscular Strength in Normal Children Aged 9-12 Years." *Kaohsiung Journal of Medical Science* (China) 15, no. 4 (April 1999): 226–233.

Wernick-Robinson, M., D. E. Krebs, and M. M. Giorgetti. "Functional Reach: Does it Really Measure Dynamic Balance?" *Physical Medicine and Rehabilitation* 80, no. 3 (March 1999): 262–269.

Websites

Balance and agility equipment: *http://bodyblade.com; www.fitness1st.com; www.fitter1.com; www.optp.com; www.performbetter.com; www.powersystems.com*

CHAPTER 7

Bompa, Tudor. *Periodization: Theory and Methodology of Training.* 4th ed. Champaign, Ill.: Human Kinetics Publishing, 1999.

Galloway, Jeff. *Galloway's Book of Running.* Bolinas, Calif.: Shelter Publications, 1984.

Gambetta, Vern. "Building the Complete Athlete," in *Optimum Sports Training.* 4th ed. Sarasota, Fla.: Performance Conditioning, Inc., 1997.

———. *The Gambetta Method: Common Sense Training for Athletic Performance.* 2nd ed. Sarasota, Fla.: Gambetta Sports Training Systems, 2002.

Gray. *Chain Reaction Festival* (see chapter 5 references).

Sleamaker, Ross. *Serious Training for Serious Athletes.* Champaign, Ill.: Leisure Press, 1989.

Website

Training: *www.truestarhealth.com*

CHAPTER 9

Hall, Carrie F., and Lori Theim-Brody, eds. *Therapeutic Exercise: Moving Toward Function.* Philadelphia: Lippincott Williams and Wilkins, 1999.

Kendall, Florence. *Muscles: Testing and Function.* 4th ed. Philadelphia: Lippincott Williams and Wilkins, 1993.

Maffetone, Philip. *Complementary Sports Medicine.* Champaign, Ill.: Human Kinetics Publishing, 1999.

Renstrom, P. *Sports Injuries, Basic Principles of Prevention and Care.* London: Blackwell Scientific Publications, 1993.

Schamberger, Wolf. *The Malalignment Syndrome.* New York: Churchill Livingstone, 2002.

Zachazewski, James E., David J. McGee, and William F. Quill. *Athletic Injuries and Rehabilitation.* Philadelphia: W. B. Saunders Co., 1996.

CHAPTER 10

Gray. *Lower Extremity Functional Profile* (see chapter 5 references).

Hall and Theim-Brody. *Therapeutic Exercise* (see chapter 9 references).

Hall, Carrie M. *Fitness in Balance*. Unpublished handbook. St. Louis, Mo.: Professional Physical Therapy, 1989.

Kendall. *Muscles: Testing and Function* (see chapter 9 references).

Sahrmann, Shirley A. *Diagnosis and Treatment of Movement Improvement Syndromes*. St. Louis: Mosby, 2002.

Sahrmann, Shirley A., et al. "Diagnosis and Treatment of Muscle Imbalances and Musculoskeletal Pain Syndromes." Course notes presented at a seminar in Seattle, 1995.

CHAPTER 11

Gray. *Lower Extremity Functional Profile* (see chapter 5 references).

Hall and Theim-Brody. *Therapeutic Exercise* (see chapter 9 references).

Kendall. *Muscles: Testing and Function* (see chapter 9 references).

Krivickas, L. S. "Anatomical Factors Associated with Overuse Sports Injuries." *Journal of Sports Medicine* 24, no 2 (August 1997): 132–146.

Mangine, R. E., ed. *Physical Therapy of the Knee: Anatomy and Biomechanics*. New York: Churchill Livingstone, 1988.

Marshall, J. L., F. G. Girgis, and R. R. Zelko. "The Biceps Femoris Tendon and Its Functional Significance." *Journal of Bone and Joint Surgery* 54, No. 1444 (1972).

Seebacher, J. R., A. E. Inglis, and R. F. Warren. "The Structure of the Posterolateral Aspect of the Knee." *Journal of Bone and Joint Surgery* 64A no. 536 (1982).

Siemoens, W. A., "Iliotibial Band Friction Syndrome." *JBR-BTR* 85(3): 152–153.

Warren, L. F., and J. L. Marshall. "The Supporting Structures and Layers on the Medial Side of the Knee." *Journal of Bone and Joint Surgery* 61A, no. 56 (1979).

Williams, P. L., et al. *Gray's Anatomy*. 37th British ed. London: Longman, 1989.

CHAPTER 12

Gray. *Lower Extremity Functional Profile* (see chapter 5 references).

Hall and Theim-Brody. *Therapeutic Exercise* (see chapter 9 references).

CHAPTER 13

Hall and Theim-Brody. *Therapeutic Exercise* (see chapter 9 references).

Nawoczenski, Deborah, et al. *Orthotics in Functional Rehabilitation of the Lower Limb*. Philadelphia: W. B. Saunders Co., 1997.

CHAPTER 14

Janda and Jull. "Muscles and Motor Control" (see chapter 4 references).

Lee, Diane. *The Thorax: An Integrated Approach*. White Rock, Canada: Diane G. Lee Physiotherapist Corporation, 2003.

Lee, Diane, and Andry Vleeming. *The Pelvic Girdle: An Approach to the Examination and Treatment of the Lumbo-Pelvic-Hip Region*. 2nd ed. Edinburgh: Churchill Livingston, 1999.

Preuss, Grenier, and S. McGill. "The Effect of Spine Position on Lumbar Spine Position Sense." *Journal of Orthopedic Sports and Physical Therapy* 33 (2003): 73–78.

Richardson, C., et al. *Therapeutic Exercise for Spinal Segmented Stabilization in Low Back Pain*. Edinburgh: Churchill Livingston, 1999.

Sahrmann. *Diagnosis and Treatment* (see chapter 10 references).

Vleeming, Andry, ed. *Movement, Stability, and Low Back Pain*. New York: Churchill Livingstone, 1997.

Website

American Association of Orthopedic Medicine (AAOM): *www.aaomed.org*. 1-800-992-2063. This is an association of physicians who specialize in prolotherapy ligament injections and techniques other than surgical ones to decrease pain to stabilize the SI and other joint areas.

CHAPTER 15

American Association of Orthopedic Medicine (see chapter 14 website reference).
Baechle. *Essentials of Strength Training* (see chapter 5 references).
Gray, Gary. *Chain Reaction Plus*. Adrian, Mich.: Wynn Marketing, 1994.
Hall. *Fitness in Balance* (see chapter 10 references).
Hall and Theim-Brody. *Therapeutic Exercise* (see chapter 9 references).
Kendall. *Muscles: Testing and Function* (see chapter 9 references).
Keshner, E. A. "Controlling Stability of a Complex System." *Physical Therapy* 70 (1990): 854–884.
Norkin, C., et al. *Joint: Structure and Function*. Philadelphia: F. A. Davis Co., 1983.
Pearl, B., et al. *Getting Stronger*. Bolinas, Calif.: Shelter Publications, 1986.
Sahrmann. *Diagnosis and Treatment* (see chapter 10 references).
Sahrmann et al. "Diagnosis and Treatment of Muscle Imbalances" (see chapter 10 references).

CHAPTER 16

Hall and Theim-Brody. *Therapeutic Exercise* (see chapter 9 references).

CHAPTER 17

Cox and Fulsaas. *Freedom of the Hills* (see chapter 1 references).
Edwards, Sally. *Snowshoeing*. Champaign, Ill.: Human Kinetics Publishing, 1995.
Griffin, S. *Snowshoeing*. Mechanicsburg, Pa.: Stackpole Books, 1998.
Seeborg, E. *Hiking and Backpacking*. Champagne, Ill.: Human Kinetics Publishing, 1994.

CHAPTER 18

Cox and Fulsaas. *Freedom of the Hills* (see chapter 1 references).
Goddard, Dale, and Uno Neumann. *Performance Rock Climbing*. Mechanicsburg, Pa.: Stackpole Books, 1993.
Holtzhausen, Lucy-May, and T. Noakes. "Elbow, Forearm, and Hand Injuries Among Sport Rock Climbers." *Clinical Journal of Sport Medicine* 6, no. 3 (1996): 196–203.
Horst, Eric. *How to Rock Climb Series: Flash Training*. Evergreen, Colo.: Chockstone Press, 1994.
Long, John. *How to Rock Climb Series: Gym Climb!* Evergreen, Colo.: Chockstone Press, 1994.

CHAPTER 19

Cox and Fulsaas. *Freedom of the Hills* (see chapter 1 references).

CHAPTER 20

Gullion, Lori. *Nordic Skiing: Steps to Success*. Champaign, Ill.: Human Kinetics Publishing, 1993.
Hart, L. *The Snowboard Book*. New York: W. W. Norton Co., 1997.
Witherell, W. *The Athletic Skier*. Boulder, Colo.: Johnson Books, 1993.

CHAPTER 21

Borne, Gilbert C. *A Textbook of Oarsmanship: A Classic of Rowing Technical Literature*. Toronto: Sports Book Publishers, 1987.
Cunningham, F. *The Sculler at Ease*. Boulder, Colo.: Avery Press, 1992.
Gullion, L. *Canoeing and Kayak Instruction Manual*. Birmingham, Ala.: American Canoe Association and Menasha Ridge Press, 1987.
Heed, P., and Dick Mansfield. *Canoe Racing*. Syracuse, N.Y.: Acorn Publishing, 1992.

CHAPTER 22

Bompa. *Periodization* (see chapter 7 references).

Broker, Jeff, Ph.D. Paper presented at the Elite Coaching Symposium/International Symposium USA Cycling, Colorado Springs, Colo., 1997.

Davis, D. *Mountain Biking*. Champaign, Ill.: Human Kinetics Publishing, 1994.

LeMond, Greg, and Kent Gordis. *Greg LeMond's Complete Book of Bicycling*. New York: Putnam Publishing Group, 1990.

Lombardi, Blair. *Bicycling in Balance Instruction*. Paper presented at the Elite Coaching Symposium/International Symposium USA Cycling, Colorado Springs, Colo., 1997.

USA Cycling, Inc. *Training Manuals*. Colorado Springs, Colo.: USA Cycling, 1996.

CHAPTER 23

Brown, R. *Fitness Running*. Champaign, Ill.: Human Kinetics Publishing, 1994.

Burfoot, A. *Runner's World Complete Book of Running*. Emmaus, Pa.: Rodale Press, 1997.

Galloway. *Galloway's Book of Running* (see chapter 7 references).

Triathlete Magazine. September 1994.

CHAPTER 24

Winner, K. *Windsurfing*. Champaign, Ill.: Human Kinetics Publishing, 1995.

CHAPTER 25

Aston, Judith. *Aston Postural Assessment Workbook: Skills for Observing and Evaluating Body Patterns*. San Antonio, Tex.: Psychological Corp., 1999.

Physical Therapy Today. Summer 1991.

Physical Therapy Today. Fall 1993.

CHAPTER 26

Baechle. *Essentials of Strength Training* (see chapter 5 references).

Bland, Jeffrey. *20-Day Rejuvenation Diet Program*. New Canaan, Conn.: Keats Publishing, 1997.

Challem, Jack. *The Inflammation Syndrome: The Complete Nutritional Program to Prevent and Reverse Heart Disease, Arthritis, Diabetes, Allergies, and Asthma*. Hoboken, N.J.: John Wiley and Sons, 2003.

Farlow, Christine H. *Food Additives: A Shopper's Guide to What's Safe and What's Not*. Rev. ed. Escondido, Calif.: Kiss for Health Publishing, 2001.

Fletcher, Robert. "Vitamins for Chronic Disease Prevention." *Journal of the American Medical Association* 287, no. 23 (June 19, 2002): 3127–3129.

Gray, Gary. *Chain Reaction*. Adrian, Mich.: Wynn Marketing, 1998.

Mahler, Donald A. *ACSM Guidelines for Exercise Testing and Prescription*. Philadelphia: Lippincott Williams and Wilkins, 1995.

Roitman, Jeffrey. *ACSM Resource Manual for Guidelines for Exercise Testing and Prescription*. 3rd ed. Philadelphia: Lippincott Williams and Wilkins, 1998.

Stoll, Andrew L. *The Omega-3 Connection: The Groundbreaking Antidepression Diet and Brain Program*. New York: Simon and Schuster, 2002.

Weil, Andrew. *Eating Well for Optimum Health*. New York: Quill, 2001.

White. *The Wellness Guide* (see chapter 5 references).

Wilson. *Fateful Harvest* (see chapter 2 references).

Winter, Ruth. *A Consumer's Dictionary of Food Additives*. 5th ed. New York: Three Rivers Press, 1999.

Wolcott, William Linz, and Trish Fahey. *The Metabolic Typing Diet*. New York: Broadway Books, 2002.

Websites

Fiber content: *www.nal.usda.gov/fnic/foodcomp*

Food additives: *www.truthinlabeling.org;*

www.allergy-network.co.uk/index.html
Food composition of carbs, fats, and proteins: *www.nal.usda.gov/fnic/foodcomp/Data/index.html*
Glycemic index: *www.glycemicindex.com; www.glycemicdietsw.com*
Healthy protein bars: *www.bio-genesis.com*
Natural medicine: *www.naturaldatabase.com*
Nutrition and supplements: *www.truestarhealth.com*
Omega-3 fats: *www.nal.usda.gov/fnic/foodcomp/Data/index.html; www.annecollins.com/dietary-fat/omega-3-efa-6-chart.htm*
Protein: *www.caloriecountercharts.com; http://teaching.ucdavis.edu/nut10/handouts/content.pdf*

CHAPTER 27

Brill, Patricia A., and Carol A. Macera. "Clinical Feasibility of a Free-Weight Strength-Training Program for Older Adults." *Journal of the American Board of Family Practice* 11, no. 6 (1998): 445–451.
Dalsky, G. P., et al. Weight-Bearing Exercise Training and Lumbar Bone Mineral Content in Postmenopausal Women. *Annals of Internal Medicine* 108 (1988): 824–828.
Grossman, Melanie D., and Anita L. Stewart. "'You Aren't Going to Get Better by Just Sitting Around': Physical Activity Perceptions, Motivations, and Barriers in Adults 75 Years of Age or Older." *American Journal of Geriatric Cardiology* 12, no. 1 (2003): 33–37.
Gutin, B., and M. J. Kasper. "Can Vigorous Exercise Play a Role in Osteoporosis Prevention? A Review." *Osteoporosis International* 2 (1992): 55–69.
Kannus, P. "Preventing Osteoporosis, Falls and Fractures Among Elderly People." *British Medical Journal* 318 (1999): 205–206.
Karlsson, M. K., et al. "Exercise During Growth and Bone Mineral Density and Fractures in Old Age." *Lancet* 355 (2000): 469–470.
Peedo, F. J. "Physical Activity Interventions in the Elderly: Cancer and Comorbidity." *Cancer Investigation* 22, no. 1 (2004): 51–67.
Vincent, K. R., et al. "Strength Training and Hemodynamic Responses to Exercise." *American Journal of Geriatric Cardiology* 12, no. 2 (2003): 97–106.

CHAPTER 28

Agostini, Rosemary. *Medical and Orthopedic Issues of Active and Athletic Women.* Philadelphia: Hanley and Belfus, 1994.
American College of Sports Medicine. "The Female Athlete Triad." Unpublished slide set. Indianapolis: American College of Sports Medicine, n.d.
Bradley, Michael. *The Female Athlete: Train for Success.* Terre Haute, Ind.: Wish Publishing, 2004.
Dalsky et al. "Weight-Bearing Exercise Training." (see chapter 27 references).
Gaby. *Preventing and Reversing Osteoporosis* (see chapter 2 references).
Haycock, Christine, ed. *Sports Medicine for the Athletic Female.* Oradell, N.J.: Medical Economics Books, 1980.
Kai, M. C. "Exercise Intervention: Defusing the World's Osteoporosis Time Bomb." *Bulletin of the World Health Organization* 81, no. 11 (2003): 827–830.
O'Connor, Bob. *Complete Conditioning for the Female Athlete.* Terre Haute, Ind.: Wish Publishing, 2001.
Shangold, M., and G. Mirkin. *Women and Exercise: Physiology and Medicine.* Philadelphia: F. A. Davis Co., 1988.

CHAPTER 29

Agatston, Arthur. *The South Beach Diet.* Emmaus, Pa.: Rodale Press, 2003.
Atkins, Robert. *Atkins for Life: The Complete Controlled Carb Program for Permanent Weight Loss.* New York: St. Martins Press, 2003.

Eckel, Robert. *Obesity: Mechanisms and Clinical Management*. Philadelphia: Lippincott Williams and Wilkins, 2003.

Foster, Gary. "A Randomized Trial of a Low Carbohydrate Diet for Obesity." *New England Journal of Medicine* 348 (2003): 282–290.

Layman, Donald. "A Reduced Ratio of Dietary Carbohydrate to Protein Improves Body Composition and Blood Lipid Profiles During Weight Loss in Adult Women." *Journal of Nutrition* 117 (2003): 411–417.

Muller, D. M. "Effects of Oral L Carnitine Supplementation on In Vivo Long Chain Fatty Acid Oxidation in Healthy Adults." *Metabolism* 51, no. 11 (2002): 1389–1391.

Murase, T., et al. "Beneficial Effects of Tea Catechins on Diet-Induced Obesity: Stimulation of Lipid Catabolism in the Liver." *Journal of Nutrition* 132, no. 6 (2002): 1282–1288.

Rosenblatt, Steven, and Cameron Stauth. *The Starch Blocker Diet*. New York: HarperResource, 2003.

Ross, Julia. *The Diet Cure*. New York: Penguin, 2000.

———. *The Mood Cure*. New York: Viking Press, 2002.

Websites

Dealing with uncomfortable emotions: *www.emofree.com; www.rc.org*

Glycemic index: *www.glycemicindex.com; www.glycemicdietsw.com*

Resting metabolic rate (RMR) and cardio respiratory metabolic testing: *www.newleaf-online.com*

CHAPTER 30

Fennell, Patricia A., Leonard A. Jason, and Renee R. Taylor, eds. *Handbook of Chronic Fatigue Syndrome*. Hoboken, N.J.: John Wiley and Sons, 2003.

Fitzgerald, Matt. *Triathlete Magazine's Complete Triathlon Book: The Training, Diet, Health, Equipment, and Safety Tips You Need to Do Your Best*. New York: Warner Books, 2003.

Starlanyl, Devin J., and Mary Ellen Copeland. *Fibromyalgia and Chronic Myofascial Pain: A Survival Manual*. 2nd ed. Oakland, Calif.: New Harbinger Publications, 2001.

Teitelbaum, Jacob. *From Fatigued to Fantastic!: A Proven Program to Regain Vibrant Health, Based on a New Scientific Study Showing Effective Treatment for Chronic Fatigue and Fibromyalgia*. Rev. ed. New York: Avery Penguin Putnam, 2001.

Wilson, James L. *Adrenal Fatigue: The 21st-Century Stress Syndrome*. Petaluma, Calif.: Smart Publications, 2002.

Websites

Environmental medicine: *www.aaem.com*

Fibromyalgia and chronic fatigue: *www.afsafund.org/resource.htm; www.fmnetnews.com; www.haworthpress.com*

Functional medicine: *www.functionalmedicine.org*

Natural medicine: *www.naturaldatabase.com*

CHAPTER 31

Jacob, S. *The Miracle of MSM: The Natural Solution for Pain*. New York: Penguin Putnam, 1999.

Leeb, B. F. "A Meta-Analysis of Chondroitin Sulfate in the Treatment of Osteoarthritis." *Journal of Osteoarthritis* 27 (2000): 205–211.

Mathewson, A. J. "Glucosamine: A Review of Its Use in Osteoarthritis." *Drugs and Aging* 20, no. 14 (2003): 1041–1060.

Ruane, R. "Glucosamine Therapy Compared to Ibuprofen for Joint Pain." *British Journal of Community Nursing* 7, no. 3 (March 2002): 146–152.

Website

Natural medicine: *www.naturaldatabase.com*

Index

A
abdominal muscles
  anatomy of, 185–86
  exercises for
    balance, 188–92
    functional, 192–205
    in seniors, 371
    strengthening, 187
  function of, 185–86
  imbalances of, 186
  injury prevention, 187
  lower, 186
  spine protection from, 186
  strength of, 186
  upper, 186
abduction, 176
acclimatization, 28
Achilles tendon
  anatomy of, 180
  stretch of, 77, 227
acromioclavicular joint, 179
active stretching, 69–70
additives, 364
adduction, 176
adductors (hip)
  anatomy of, 180
  stretch of, 76–77
adenosine triphosphate, 24–25
adrenal dysfunction, 388–89
aerobic conditioning log, 61, 64, 160
aerobic conditioning/exercise
  aerobics classes, 58–59
  anaerobic exercise vs., 25
  for backpacking, 281
  calendar for tracking, 62–63
  for canoeing, 320–23
  cardiovascular benefits of, 27
  characteristics of, 25
  circuit training for, 59
  cooldown period after, 55, 157
  cross training, 52–53
  cross-country skiing machine for, 57
  for cycling, 327–32
  definition of, 44
  description of, 24, 361
  diabetes mellitus considerations before, 32
  duration of, 46
  EFX elliptical trainer for, 57
  equipment for, 52
  evaluations of, 61
  fat burning during, 26
  free radical production during, 45
  frequency of, 46
  glycogen depletion by, 26
  goals for, 60–62, 153–55
  health benefits of, 44–45, 361
  heart-rate zone training approach to, 55–56
  for hiking, 281
  impact from, 59–60
  improvement stage of, 55
  initial stage of, 55
  in-line skating for, 59
  insulin resistance decreased by, 44–45
  intensity of
    calories expended per unit of time, 47
    description of, 46–47
    factors that affect, 47
    heart rate and, 48–49
    lactate threshold and, 49–50
    methods of expressing, 47
    rating of perceived exertion and, 47–48
  interval training. *See* interval training
  maintenance stage of, 55
  maximal oxygen uptake during, 27
  minimum amount of, 46
  modes of, 56–59
  muscle benefits from, 27
  for outdoor activities, 46
  program for, 61–62
  progression of, 52–55
  respiratory benefits of, 26–27
  risks of, 45
  rowing machine for, 58
  scrambling, 287
  for seniors, 370
  session of, 55–56
  skiing, 302–06
  snowboarding, 302, 306–07
  for snowshoeing, 281
  specificity of, 52
  spinning class, 58
  stair-climbers for, 56–57
  stationary cycle for, 58
  stress test before initiating, 48
  treadmill for, 57
  treadwall for, 58
  variables associated with, 45–55
  walking, 59
  warm-up for, 65–66
  weight loss benefits of, 45, 385
  for windsurfing, 347–48
aerobic stamina, 157
agility
  definition of, 126–27, 162
  sports that require, 126–27
  training for, 127, 156–57, 162
  warm-up for, 66
agility circuit, 127, 163, 309–12
agility exercises
  for canoeing, 320–23
  for cycling, 333–36
  description of, 126
  for kayaking, 320–21
  for mountaineering, 299
  in outdoor settings, 162–63
  for rowing, 320–21
  for running, 127, 339
  for skiing, 302–06, 309–12
  for snowboarding, 302–03, 307, 309–12
  for windsurfing, 348
agonists, 177
alpha-lipoic acid, 40
alpine skiing, 303–04
altitude
  caloric requirements, 42–43
  description of, 28
amenorrhea, 375
amino acids, 26, 35, 364
anaerobic exercise
  aerobic exercise vs., 25
  circuit training, 173–74
  description of, 24–25
  in outdoor settings, 163
  for skiing, 303–06
anaerobic reactions, 24–25
anemia, 41
ankle, 226–27
anorexia nervosa, 374–75
antagonists, 177
antioxidants, 40–41
arm exercises
  functional exercises, 264–72
  in seniors, 372
  strength training, 120–21
arthritis, 390–91
Aston-Patterning, 352–54

B
B_{12}. *See* Vitamin B_{12}
back
  low. *See* low back
  mid, 234, 252–56
  rock climbing demands, 286
backpacking
  aerobic conditioning for, 281

Aston–Patterning applications, 353
balance exercises for, 282
boots for, 284
conditioning programs for, 284
muscle imbalances for, 280–81
musculoskeletal demands of, 280
pack posture during, 282–83
strength training for, 281–82
warm-up for, 281
balance
definition of, 125
importance of, 125–26
training for, 126, 156–57
warm-up for, 66
balance beams, 130
balance board, 308
balance equipment, 129–32, 150–53
balance exercises
for abdominal muscles, 188–92
for backpacking, 282
for canoeing, 320–23
equipment for, 129–32, 150–53
for hiking, 282
for kayaking, 320–21, 324
for mountaineering, 299
in outdoor settings, 162
for rock climbing, 289
for rowing, 320–21
for running, 339
for scrambling, 289
for seniors, 372
for skiing, 145–46, 302–06, 308–09
for snowboarding, 302–03, 307–09
for snowshoeing, 282
types of, 145–53
for windsurfing, 348
balance pads, 131
balance self-tests, 99, 133–44
balance steps, 131
base of support, 352–53, 358–59
biceps
anatomy of, 180, 245
strengthening exercises for, 259–60
bicycling. *See* cycling
birth control pills, 376–77
BMI. *See* body mass index
boating
agility exercises for, 127
balance exercises for, 134
Body Blade, 130, 153
body mass index, 378
body movements, 176–77
body posture. *See* posture
bone density, 100, 363, 372
bone mass, 375
boots, 284
Bosu balance trainer, 131, 152, 199–200
brachioradialis, 180
breaks, 284
bulimia, 375
bunny hop, 335–36
bursitis, 177
buttocks. *See also* gluteal muscles
anatomy of, 206–07
muscle imbalances of, 207–08
strengthening exercises for, 223–25

C

calcaneus, 178
calcium, 367, 375–76
canoeing
aerobic conditioning for, 320–23
agility exercises for, 320–23
back position during, 318–19
balance exercises for, 320–23
flat-water, 321–22
interval training for, 321
muscle imbalances, 319
musculoskeletal demands of, 318–19
strength training for, 321–22
stretching before, 320
warm-up for, 320
whitewater, 322–23
carbohydrates
calories from, 31–32
classification of, 30–31
complex, 30–32
composition of, 25–26
description of, 364, 381–82
energy from, 25–26, 30–35
glucose production from, 26, 31
glycemic index of, 32–34
loading of, 34–35
low-carbohydrate diets, 35
meal timing suggestions for, 34–35
simple, 30–31, 364
in sports drinks, 42
training-related intake of, 31
weight control and, 381–82
cardiac output, 27
cardiorespiratory exercise testing, 384
carioca, 66
L-carnitine, 385, 389
carpal bones, 273
carpal tunnel, 273
cartilage, 177
cervical spine, 178–79, 234
chest exercises
functional exercises, 106
in seniors, 371
strength training, 248–51
stretching, 78
chin-ups, 264
chondroitin sulfate, 391
chromium, 380
chronic fatigue syndrome, 388
circuit training
agility, 127, 163
description of, 59
outdoor, 172–74
weight training, 88
circumduction, 177
clavicle, 179, 245
climbing. *See* rock climbing
climbing stairs, 56–57
closed-chain activity, 98
coenzyme Q10, 389
cold weather, 43
complex carbohydrates, 30–32
conditioning
aerobic. *See* aerobic conditioning
goals for, 154–56
for mountaineering, 299–300
in outdoor settings, 161–63
conditioning program
components of, 156–57
intensity period for, 158
periodizing of, 157–60
phases of, 157–59
cooldown, 55, 157
coordination, 126
copper, 40–41
core, 234–36, 286
core muscles, 93–94
cravings, 379–80
crazy legs, 66
creatine monohydrate, 41
creatine phosphate, 25
cross training, 52–53, 338
cross-country skiing, 305–06
cross-country skiing machine, 57
cycling
aerobic conditioning for, 327–32
Aston-Patterning applications, 353
exercises for
agility, 127, 333–36
balance, 134, 137
Fartlek interval training for, 51
interval training for, 331–32
mileage goals for, 328–29
muscle imbalances, 327
musculoskeletal demands for, 327
pedaling cadence, 329–31
spinning class for, 58
strength training for, 332
warm-up for, 327

D

deceleration, 182–83
degenerative joint disease, 390–91
deltoid, 180–81, 245
depression, 380, 388
descent, 298–99
detoxification, 383
DHA, 366
diabetes mellitus
aerobic exercise considerations, 32, 44
hypoglycemia associated with, 32
diet. *See also* nutrition
high-protein, 37
low-carbohydrate, 35

metabolic-type, 35
modified carb-to-protein-ratio, 38, 383–84
vegetarian, 37–38
dips, 169–70
disc pillow, 131, 152
DJD. *See* degenerative joint disease
dorsiflexion, 226
downhill skiing, 303–04
dynamic balance
definition of, 126, 133
self-tests of, 143–44
dynamic constant-resistance equipment, 96
dynamic variable-resistance equipment, 96
dynamic warm-up, 67
dynamic warm-up drills, 66–67

E
eating disorders, 374–75
EFX elliptical trainer, 57
elastic resistance equipment, 97
elbow flexors, 245
endurance climbing, 295
endurance training
for lower body, 173
strength training repetitions and sets for, 91
energy
from carbohydrates, 25–26, 30–35
from fats, 26, 38
fuel sources for, 25–26
gaining of, 389
from protein, 26, 35
requirements for, 29–30
environmental health and medicine, 360
EPA, 366
ergogenic aids, 41
Essential fatty acids, 38–39
exercise
aerobic. *See* aerobic conditioning/exercise
anaerobic. *See* anaerobic exercise
benefits of, 360
calorie calculations during, 30
in cold weather, 43
glycogen reserves during, 34
at high altitudes, 28
lactic acid produced during, 25
protein requirements based on, 36
warm-up before, 361. *See also* warm-up
weight loss benefits of, 384–85
extension
definition of, 176
spine, 240–41
external oblique, 180, 185
external rotation, 176

F
Fartlek interval training, 51–52, 287, 341
fascia, 177
fast-twitch fibers, 85
fat(s)
burning of, 26
characteristics of, 26
daily requirements of, 39, 383
energy from, 26, 38
essential fatty acids, 38–39
functions of, 38
healthy types of, 365–66
intake guidelines for, 39
weight control and, 383
fatigue
food allergies and, 389
glycogen depletion and, 31
overtraining-related, 156
strength training sets and, 91
fatty acids
omega-3, 38–39
omega-6, 38–39
female athlete triad, 376
femur, 178, 207
fertilizers, 313
fiber, 31, 366–67
fibromyalgia syndrome, 387–88
fibula, 178–79, 227
finger taping, 275
fish oils, 39
Fitter, The, 130
5 HTP, 313
flat-water canoeing, 321–22
flexibility
conditioning program for, 156
in deconditioned individuals, 369–70
description of, 67
importance of, 361
performance and, 67
in seniors, 369–70
flexion, 176
flexor tendon, 273
fluids
daily intake of, 41–42
sweating-related loss of, 42
foam cylinders, 130
food
as fuel, 30–39
carbohydrate sources, 30–31
fiber content of, 367
glycemic index of, 33–34, 381
food additives, 364
food allergies, 381, 389
food quality, 30, 363–64
foot, 228–31, 391
footwear, 228–30
force closure, 233
forearm
anatomy of, 273–74
injury prevention in, 275
muscle imbalances in, 274–75
strengthening exercises for, 276–78
stretching exercises for, 80
forward-tilted pelvis, 186
free radicals
aerobic exercise and, 45
description of, 40
free weights, 96
FreeMotion integrated core stability program, 106–11
frontal plane
definition of, 128, 130, 135
dynamic balance self-tests in, 144
motion in, 177
peripheral balance self-tests in, 141–42
static balance self-tests in, 138–39
functional exercises
for abdominal muscles, 192–205
for arms, 264–72
characteristics of, 98–100
definition of, 83
designing of, 123–24
frequency of, 100
guidelines for, 99–100
repetitions for, 91
for shoulder, 264–72
for triceps, 272
types of, 104–23
for upper body, 264–72
warm-up using, 66
functional medicine, 360
functional self-tests, 99

G
gastrocnemius, 180–81
general preparation period, 138
glucosamine sulfate, 391
glucose. *See also* hypoglycemia
from carbohydrates, 26, 31
steady blood levels of, 33
gluteus maximus
anatomy of, 180–81, 206
strengthening exercises for, 223–24
gluteus medius
anatomy of, 180
strengthening exercises for, 223–24
glycemic index, 32–34, 381
glycemic response, 33
glycogen
fatigue caused by depletion of, 31
pre-exercise levels of, 34
production of, 26
replacement of, 34–35
reserves of, 34
gravity, 350–51, 357
ground reaction force, 350–51, 355
growth hormone, 28, 84, 91, 101

H
hamstrings
  anatomy of, 180–81
  stretching exercises for, 72–73, 210–11, 318–19
hand
  anatomy of, 273–74
  injury prevention in, 275
  muscle imbalances in, 274–75
  strengthening exercises for, 276–78
healing, 183–84
health tests, 368
heart rate
  aerobic conditioning intensity based on, 48–49
  calculation of, 48–49
  intensity zones, 49
  stress testing of, 48
heart rate monitor, 49
heart–rate zone training, 55–56, 300
heavy metals, 40–41
heel cord stretch, 77
hiking
  aerobic conditioning for, 281
  balance exercises for, 282
  boots for, 284
  conditioning programs for, 284
  Fartlek interval training for, 51–52
  muscle imbalances for, 280–81
  musculoskeletal demands of, 280
  pack posture during, 282–83
  strength training for, 281–82
  warm–up for, 281
hill repeats, 340–41
hill running, 163
hip
  abductors of, 206
  adductors of, 206
  anatomy of, 206
  arthritis of, 390
  function of, 206, 207
  muscle imbalances, 207
  strengthening exercises for, 208–25
  stretching exercises for, 76
hip flexor stretch, 75
hops, 164, 219, 222–23, 312
hormone(s)
  adrenal, 388–89
  description of, 376–77
  estrogen, 377
  growth, 28, 84, 91, 101
  testosterone, 101
hormone replacement therapy, 377
horse gallop side shuffle, 67
humerus, 179, 244
hypoglycemia, 32–33

I
iliotibial band
  anatomy of, 180, 206
  stretch of, 74–75
infraspinatus, 245
injuries
  description of, 177
  healing of, 183–84
  phases of, 183–84
  predisposing factors, 177–83
  running–related, 337
  shoulder, 246–47
  stretching after, 70–71
in–line skating, 59
insoluble fiber, 366–67
insulin resistance, 44–45
insulin sensitivity, 44
intensity
  of aerobic conditioning. *See* aerobic conditioning/ exercise, intensity of
  of conditioning program, 158
  neuromuscular adaptations to, 90
  repetition maximum, 90
internal oblique, 185
internal rotation, 176–77
interval training
  for canoeing, 321
  for cycling, 51, 331–32
  definition of, 50
  endurance, 51
  Fartlek, 51–52, 287
  goal of, 50
  intermediate, 51
  for kayaking, 323–24
  risks associated with, 50
  for running, 338, 341–42
  sample workout for, 50–51
iron, 38, 41
isometric exercise, 87–88

J
joint(s)
  definition of, 177
  dysfunction of, 69
  evaluation of, 390
  hypermobility of, 69
  hypomobility of, 69
  loose, 182
  supplements for, 391
  tight muscle effects on, 68–69
jumps, 164, 219–22, 312–14

K
kayaking
  aerobic conditioning for, 320, 323
  agility exercises for, 320–21, 324
  Aston–Patterning applications, 353–54
  back position during, 318–19
  balance exercises for, 320–21, 324
  interval training for, 323–24
  kilocalories burned during, 47
  muscle imbalances, 319
  musculoskeletal demands of, 318–19
  sea, 323–24
  strength training for, 324–25
  stretching before, 320
  warm–up for, 320
  whitewater, 324–25
Kegel exercises, 235
kilocalories
  calculation of, 29–30
  food sources of, 30
knee
  anatomy of, 206–07
  arthritis of, 390
  function of, 207
  strengthening exercises for, 208–25
krebs cycle, 25

L
lactate threshold
  aerobic conditioning intensity based on, 49–50
  definition of, 25
lactic acid, 25
lateral movement, 176
latissimus dorsi
  anatomy of, 181
  strength training exercises for, 115–20
legs, 226–27, 370–71
lifting, 238–39
ligament
  definition of, 177
  laxity of, 182
  sprains of, 177
low back
  anatomy of, 232–33
  arthritis of, 390–91
  muscle imbalances in, 237
  postural considerations, 238
  stretching precautions for, 70
low–carbohydrate diets, 35
lower body
  endurance training for, 173
  outdoor training exercises for, 165–67
  plyometrics for, 88
  rock climbing demands, 285–86
  scrambling demands, 285–86, 286
  stretches for, 72–77
lumbar spine, 178–79
lumbopelvic complex, 234
lunges, 111–15, 144, 211–16, 225
lungs, 26–27

M
malalignment, 178
manganese, 40–41
maximal oxygen uptake, 27
maximum lifts, 94
medial movement, 176

medicine ball
  abdominal exercises using, 197, 204
  description of, 97
menopause, 377
menstrual disorders, 375
mercury, 37, 314–15
metabolic function, 93
metabolic syndrome, 44–45
metabolic-type diet, 35
metacarpals, 273
metric conversions, 392
mid back
  anatomy of, 234, 238
  strengthening exercises for, 252–56
monosaccharides, 30
motor units, 27
mountain biking. *See* cycling
mountaineering, 297–300, 353
movement
  patterns of, 350–53
  planes of, 127–29, 177
  rock climbing demands for, 286–87
  scrambling demands for, 286–87
MSG, 313–14
MSM, 391
multifidi, 235–36
multipitch climbing, 288
multivitamins, 385
muscle(s). *See also specific muscle*
  actions of, 87
  aerobic training effects on, 27
  anatomy of, 27
  closed-chain activity of, 98
  concentric action of, 87
  eccentric action of, 87
  ecocentric action of, 87
  fast-twitch, 85
  functions of, 98
  hypertrophy of, 102
  inhibited, 178, 181
  interrelationships among, 98–99
  isometric action of, 87
  isotonic action of, 87
  length tension relationship of, 84–85
  neural control of, 85
  open-chain activity of, 98
  overloading of, 92
  phasic, 85
  shaping of, 102
  skeletal, 85–86
  slow-twitch, 85
  soreness of, 95
  strength training effects on, 27–28
  symmetry of, 94–95
  tight, 68–69, 178
  tonic, 85
  toning of, 102
  weak, 178
muscle fibers, 85–86
muscle imbalances
  abdominals, 186
  ankle, 227
  from backpacking, 280–81
  buttocks, 207–08
  from canoeing, 319
  from cycling, 327
  foot, 228
  forearm, 274–75
  hand, 274–75
  from hiking, 280–81
  hip, 207
  from kayaking, 319
  leg, 227
  low back, 237
  from mountaineering, 297
  from rock climbing, 287
  from rowing, 319
  from running, 337–38
  from scrambling, 287
  shoulder, 246
  from skiing, 301
  from snowboarding, 301
  from snowshoeing, 280–81
  spine, 237–38
  stretching to improve, 67–68
  from windsurfing, 347
muscle strains, 177
musculoskeletal system
  anatomy of, 177–81
  description of, 176
  injuries of, 177–84

N

neck arthritis, 391
neuromuscular adaptations, 90
neutral posture, 351–52
neutral sitting posture, 352
neutral spine, 70, 176, 236–37
neutral standing posture, 352
noncontractile tissue, 61, 155
nonfunctional exercise, 89–92
nutrition. *See also* diet
  antioxidants, 40–41
  carbohydrates. *See* carbohydrates
  description of, 363–67
  ergogenic aids, 41
  fats. *See* fats
  fluids, 41–42
  free radicals, 40
  protein. *See* protein
  for seniors, 372–73
  water, 41–42

O

obese, 378
oligosaccharides, 30
omega-3 fatty acids, 38–39, 366
omega-6 fatty acids, 38–39
one repetition maximum, 83, 90
open-chain activity, 98
optimal wellness, 360–68
oral contraceptives, 376–77
organic, 382
orthotics, 231
osteoporosis, 375–76
outdoor training
  agility exercises, 162–63
  anaerobic exercises, 163
  balance exercises, 162
  circuit training, 172–74
  conditioning in, 161–63
  lower-body, 165–67
  program for, 164
  strength exercises, 161–62
  tips for, 163–64
  torso, 168–69
  types of, 161
  upper-body, 169–71
  warm-up for, 66
overloading, 92
overstretching, 70
overtraining, 156, 387
overuse injuries, 52
overweight, 378
oxygen
  altitude effects on, 28
  metabolism of, 40

P

pack posture, 282–83, 299
paired muscle active stretch, 70
passive stretching, 69
patella, 178, 180
patellar tendon, 180
patellofemoral joint, 207
pectoralis major, 68, 180
pectoralis minor, 68, 180
pedaling cadence, 329–31
pelvic floor muscles, 235
pelvis
  anatomy of, 178
  forward-tilted, 186
periodization
  conditioning program, 157–60
  plan for, 159–60
  strength training, 95–96, 158, 289
peripheral balance
  definition of, 126, 133
  self-tests of, 140–43
peroneus longus, 180
pesticides, 37, 313, 315, 317, 333
phalanges, 273
phasic muscles, 85
physioball
  abdominal exercises using, 202–03, 205
  description of, 97, 132
  spine exercises using, 241–42
phytochemicals, 366

planes of motion, 127–29, 177
plantar flexors, 227
plyometrics
  description of, 88
  equipment for, 88–89
  lower body exercises, 88
  precautions regarding, 89
  push-ups, 171
  upper body exercises, 88
polysaccharides, 30
postural muscles, 86
posture
  description of, 350
  exercises for, 355–59
  during lifting, 238–39
  low back, 238
  mid back, 238
  neck, 239
  neutral, 351–52
  pack, 282–83
  poor habits, 182
  during strength training, 94
  tight muscle effects on, 68
power, 83–84
pronation, 129, 177, 207
protein
  amino acids, 26, 35, 364
  composition of, 26, 35
  daily requirements of, 35–36, 382
  description of, 364–65
  energy from, 26
  excessive amounts of, 37
  exercise-based requirements for, 36
  food sources of, 35–36, 365
  modified carb-to-protein-ratio diet, 38, 383–84
  organic sources of, 382
  on outdoor excursions, 37
  quality of, 35
  supplementation of, 36–37
  in vegetarian diets, 37–38
  weight control and, 382–83
protein bars, 36
psoas muscle, 206
pull-downs, 255–56
pulleys
  description of, 96–97
  strength training exercises using, 106–11, 122–23
pull-ups, 170
push-ups, 170–71, 250–51, 266

Q

quadriceps
  anatomy of, 180, 207
  stretching exercises for, 73–74

R

radius, 179
rating of perceived exertion, 47–48
reactive hypoglycemia, 32
recovery period, 159
rectus abdominis, 180, 185
remodeling phase of injury repair, 184
repetitions, 90–92
resistance, 89–90
resistive exercise. *See also* strength training
  benefits of, 84
  isotonic, 87
  resistance amounts, 89–90
respiratory system, 26–27
rest period, 159
resting metabolic rate, 29, 378, 384
rhomboid
  anatomy of, 181
  stretch of, 78
rib cage, 178
road bicycling. *See* cycling
rock climbing
  balance exercises for, 289
  isometric exercises for, 88
  jumping exercises for, 219–22
  lower body demands for, 285–86
  movement demands for, 286–87
  multipitch, 288
  muscle imbalances, 287
  musculoskeletal demands of, 285–87
  strength training and exercises for, 288–96
  upper body demands for, 286
  warm-up for, 287
rocker boards, 130, 150–51
rolling, 323
rotator cuff
  muscles of, 244
  strengthening exercises for, 256–57
  stretch of, 79
rowing
  aerobic conditioning for, 320, 325–26
  agility exercises for, 320–21
  back position during, 318–19
  balance exercises for, 320–21
  description of, 325
  muscle imbalances, 319
  musculoskeletal demands of, 318–19
  strength training for, 326
  stretching before, 320
  warm-up for, 320
rowing machine, 58
running
  aerobic training for, 338
  exercises for
    agility, 127, 339
    balance, 339
    stretching, 338
  Fartlek interval training for, 341
  injuries during, 337
  interval training for, 338, 341–42
  muscle imbalances, 337–38
  musculoskeletal demands for, 337
  speed training for, 341
  strength training for, 338
  training program for, 339–46
  warm-up for, 338

S

sacroiliac joints, 70, 179, 233–34
sacrum, 178
sagittal plane
  definition of, 127–28, 130
  dynamic balance self-tests in, 143–44
  motion in, 177
  peripheral balance self-tests in, 140–41
  static balance self-tests in, 137–38
sarcopenia, 100
sartorius, 180
scapula
  anatomy of, 178–79, 244
  strengthening exercises for, 252–56
scrambling
  aerobic conditioning for, 287
  balance exercises for, 289
  Fartlek-type interval training for, 287
  lower body demands for, 285–86
  movement demands for, 286–87
  muscle imbalances, 287
  musculoskeletal demands of, 285–87
  strength training and exercises for, 288
  upper body demands for, 286
  warm-up for, 287
sculling, 325–26
sea kayaking, 323–24
selenium, 40
seniors
  aerobic conditioning for, 370
  arm exercises for, 372
  balance exercises for, 372
  bone density considerations, 372
  chest exercises for, 371
  description of, 369
  flexibility concerns, 369–70
  nutritional considerations for, 372–73
  strength training for, 370–71
serratus anterior, 180
serratus posterior inferior, 181
sets, 90–92
shoes, 228–30
shoulder
  anatomy of, 244–46
  exercises for
    functional, 264–72
    strength training, 115–21, 247, 256–59

stretching, 78–79
functions of, 245–46
injuries of, 246–47
muscle imbalances, 246
muscles of, 244–46
shoulder capsule stretch, 79
shuffle run, 66–67
simple carbohydrates, 30–31, 364
sitting balance
exercises for, 122–23
training for, 162
sitting ball, 168
skate skiing, 306
skeletal muscle, 85–86
skiing
aerobic conditioning for, 302
alpine, 303–04
cross-country, 305–06
exercises for
agility, 127, 302–03, 309–12
balance, 145–46, 302–03, 308–09
lower-body anaerobic speed, 316–17
power, 312–16
muscle imbalances, 301
musculoskeletal demands, 301
skate, 306
strength training for, 302–06
stretching before, 302
telemark, 304–05
warm-up for, 302
sleep, 388
slide board, 130
slow-twitch muscle, 85
snacks, 365
snowboarding
aerobic conditioning for, 302, 306–07
exercises for
agility, 127, 302–03, 307, 309–12
balance, 302–03, 307–09
lower-body anaerobic speed, 316–17
power, 312–16
muscle imbalances, 301
musculoskeletal demands, 301
strength training for, 302, 307
stretching before, 302, 306
warm-up for, 302
snowshoeing
aerobic conditioning for, 281
balance exercises for, 282
conditioning programs for, 284
muscle imbalances for, 280–81
musculoskeletal demands of, 280
strength training for, 281–82
warm-up for, 281
soluble fiber, 366–67
speed training, 341
spine. *See also* low back
abdominal muscles' protection of, 186
active rotation of, 82
anatomy of, 178
cervical, 178–79, 234
core muscles training, 93–94, 234–36
exercises for, 239–43
flexion of, 176
function of, 232–34
injury prevention in, 238
lumbar, 178–79
mid back region of, 234
muscle imbalances in, 237–38
neutral, 70, 176, 236–37
sacroiliac region of, 233–34
stability of, 235
static loading of, 237
stretching exercises for, 81–82
thoracic, 178–79, 238
tight muscle effects on, 68
spinning class, 58
sport climbing, 288
sports drinks, 42
sprinting, 163
squat, 110–11, 118, 166–67, 209–10, 370
stability ball, 97
stabilization, 129
stair running, 163–64
stair-climbers, 56–57
static balance
definition of, 126, 133
exercises for, 137–40
self-tests of, 134–40
stationary cycle, 58
step-downs, 217–18
steps, 97
step-ups, 165–66, 216–17
sternocleidomastoid, 180
strength
definition of, 83
determinants of, 84–85
strength endurance, 83
strength training
for backpacking, 281–82
benefits of, 84
bone density benefits of, 100
for canoeing, 321–22
circuit weight training, 88
conventional, 83
for cycling, 332
definition of, 83
for endurance athletes, 91
equipment for, 96–97
exercises for, 104–23
fibromyalgia syndrome and, 388
form during, 89
frequency of, 93
goals of, 100–102, 156
guidelines for, 92–96
health benefits of, 361–63
for hiking, 281–82
imbalances in, 69
injury prevention by, 102
isometric, 87–88
isotonic, 87
for kayaking, 324–25
log for, 102–03
maximum lifts, 94
metabolic function benefits of, 100
for mountaineering, 298–99
muscle benefits of, 27–28
muscle soreness during, 95
muscle symmetry goals of, 94–95
in outdoor settings, 161–62
overloading, 92
periodization in, 95–96, 158, 289
plateaus in, 95
plyometrics, 88–89
programs for, 362
range of motion during, 93
repetitions, 90–92
resistance during, 89–90
for rock climbing, 288–96
for rowing, 326
for running, 338
for scrambling, 288
for seniors, 370–71
sets, 90–92
for skiing, 302–06
for snowboarding, 302, 307
for snowshoeing, 281–82
spine postures and movements during, 94
timing of, 289
uses of, 83
warm-up for, 92–93
for weight loss, 385
weight management benefits of, 100–101
for windsurfing, 348
for women, 91
stress management, 368
stretches
Achilles tendon, 77
adductors (hip), 76–77
chest, 78
forearm, 80
hamstring, 72–73
heel cord, 77
hip, 76
hip flexor, 75
iliotibial band, 74–75
lower-body, 72–77
quadriceps, 73–74
rhomboid, 78
rotator cuff, 79
shoulder, 78–79
shoulder capsule, 79
spine, 81–82

triceps, 80
upper-body, 78–80
stretching
active, 69–70
after injury, 70–71
Aston-Patterning applications, 354
goal of, 67
low-back protections during, 70
methods of, 69–70
for mountaineering, 298
muscle imbalances improved by, 67–68
passive, 69
precautions regarding, 70–71
for running, 338
for skiing, 302
for snowboarding, 302
subscapularis, 245
supination, 129, 177, 207
supplements, 367, 373, 385–86
supraspinatus, 245
sweating, 42
sweep rowing, 325–26
swimming, 47
Syndrome X, 44–45

T
talus, 178, 227
tapering, 342
taping, 275
telemark skiing, 304–05
tendon, 177
tendonitis, 177
tensor fasciae latae, 180
teres minor, 245
testosterone, 101
thoracic spine, 178–79, 238
thyroid dysfunction, 388–89
tibia, 178–79, 227
tibialis anterior, 180
tone, 86
tonic muscles, 85
torso. *See* trunk
toxic chemicals, 333
toxic metals, 313
toxicity, 333
toxins, 363–64, 367–68, 383
trace minerals, 40–41
transverse plane
definition of, 128–29, 135
dynamic balance self-tests in, 144
motion in, 177
peripheral balance self-tests in, 142–43
static balance self-tests in, 139–40
transversus abdominis, 180, 185, 235
trapezius, 180, 181
treadmill, 57
treadwall, 58
triceps
anatomy of, 181, 245
functional exercises for, 272
strengthening exercises for, 261–64
stretching exercises for, 80
triplanar function, 129
trunk
muscle imbalances, 319
outdoor exercises for, 168–69
strength training of, 302

U
ulna, 179
upper body
functional exercises for, 264–72
outdoor exercises for, 169–71
plyometrics for, 88
scrambling demands, 286
stretches for, 78–80
urea, 37

V
vastus medialis oblique, 180
vegetarian diet, 37–38, 365
vitamin B_{12}
deficiency of, 37
description of, 372–73
vitamin C, 40
vitamin D, 367, 373
vitamin E, 40, 367
VO_2 max, 27
volatile organic compounds (VOCs), 317

W
walking
aerobic benefits of, 59
downhill, 284
kilocalories burned during, 47
uphill, 284
warm-up
aerobic, 65–66
agility, 66
for backpacking, 281
balance, 66
description of, 65
dynamic, 67
dynamic drills for, 66–67
exercises for, 72–82. *See also* stretches
functional exercise, 66
for hiking, 281
for kayaking, 320
for mountaineering, 297
for outdoor activity, 66
for rock climbing, 287
for rowing, 320
for running, 338
for scrambling, 287
for skiing, 302
for snowboarding, 302
for snowshoeing, 281
strength training, 92–93
weight-lifting, 66
for windsurfing, 347
water
during altitude exercise, 42–43
daily intake of, 41–42, 367
weight control
behavioral controls for, 380–81
cravings and, 379–80
description of, 374–75
environmental controls for, 380–81
fats and, 383
food choices and, 381–83
modified carb-to-protein-ratio diet, 38, 383–84
protein intake and, 382–83
tips for, 379
weight gain
cravings and, 379–80
description of, 378
reasons for, 378–79
weight loss
dietary supplements and, 385–86
exercise for, 384–85
weight-lifting
Aston-Patterning applications, 354
circuit-based, 88
warm-up for, 66
weight-shifting
description of, 353
exercises
for backpacking, 282
for rock climbing, 292–96
for scrambling, 292–96
for snowshoeing, 282
in standing position, 359
whitewater canoeing, 322–23
whitewater kayaking, 324–25
windsurfing, 347–48
wobble boards, 130, 151
women
birth control pill use by, 376–77
calcium supplementation for, 375–76
eating disorders in, 374–75
female athlete triad, 376
hormonal considerations, 376–77
menopause in, 377
menstrual disorders in, 375
osteoporosis in, 375–76
strength training for
benefits of, 100
repetitions and sets, 91
weight control in, 374–75
wrist
anatomy of, 273–74
taping of, 275

Z
zinc, 40–41, 367

Acknowledgments

I would like to thank the following people: my family, for their encouragement; Gary Gray, P.T., for his excellent exercise seminars and insights into closed kinetic chain exercise; Jock Bradley for his kind donation of his photography services for many of the exercise photos in the book; Sandy Elliott, P.T., for helping out in the photography and organizational efforts; Jeffrey Bland for his superb contributions to the field of functional medicine; the doctors and staff at the Comprehensive Medical Center; and Mark Pierce, A.T.C., for his encouragement, friendship, many hours of work, and creativity in exercise design.

David Musnick, M.D.

My devoted thanks go to the following people for making my work on this project possible: my parents, James and Janet Pierce, for your balance of knowledge, wisdom, and understanding, from which I and my four brothers find our sense of self; my daughter Tara, your brilliance has shown me incredible joy; David Musnick, M.D., for your friendship, encouragement, and successful completion of the second edition; Gary Gray, P.T., for your insightful seminars on biomechanics and functional exercise; my business partner, Neil Chasan, P.T., M.M.T., for your inspired creativity and constant support; and to Kerri Kanegae—thank you for reappearing in my life with your radiance, charm, and love. Thank you all.

Mark Pierce, A.T.C.

About the Contributors

Judith Aston, M.F.A., is the originator of Aston-Patterning™. She teaches internationally and maintains a practice in Incline, Nevada.

Kimberly B. Bennett, Ph.D., P.T., is an orthopedic manual physical therapist at Olympic Physical Therapy in Seattle, with many years in practice, and is a clinical assistant professor in the physical therapy department at the University of Washington. Bennett has a Ph.D. in anatomy. Her practice emphasizes care of multisystem orthopedic problems, including acute and chronic spine and peripheral joint dysfunction, and various rheumatological problems, including fibromyalgia.

Sherri Cassuto is a Certified Rolfer™ with a private practice in Seattle. She was on the 1984 U.S. Olympic Sweep Rowing Team and the 1988 U.S. Olympic Sculling Team. In the 1988 World Masters Games she won silver medals in single and double marathon canoeing. She is an avid sea kayaker and a reasonable whitewater kayaker.

Dan Cauthorn is co-founder and director of instruction at Vertical World, America's first indoor rock climbing gym, located in Seattle. A graduate of Western Washington University, he has taught, trained, and guided climbers since 1978. He is a Seattle native who began climbing in the Cascades at an early age. He has completed numerous difficult ascents of mountains from Alaska to Patagonia, including Cerro Torre and Burkett Needle.

Dorothy Sager Dolan, B.A., L.M.P., works for Technogym, an exercise equipment company in Seattle.

Sandy Elliott, P.T., is a physical therapist in Seattle. She assisted with photography sessions and initial organizational work on the first edition of the book, especially for Part II, Body Regions.

Lisa Fox, P.T., is a physical therapist in private practice in Seattle. She is an avid runner.

Joani Gelinas, P.T., is a physical therapist and certified Aston-Patterning™ practitioner in Seattle. She incorporates the Aston-Patterning™ movement principles in her treatment of patients.

Carrie Hall, M.H.S., P.T., is a physical therapist at and owner of Movement Systems Physical Therapy in Seattle. She is on the clinical faculty in physical therapy at the University of Washington and is a national instructor on the topic of muscle imbalances based on the Shirley Sahrmann physical therapy approach. Hall is the author of *Therapeutic Exercise: Moving Toward Function*.

Michael Hansen, P.T., is a physical therapist and owns Biosports in Wenatchee, Washington.

Rich Harrington is a co-owner of Sound Mind and Body Gyms in Seattle. He teaches ski conditioning classes at Sound Mind and Body and is an avid skier.

Teri Johnson, N.D., is a naturopathic physician in Seattle.

Craig London, P.T., is a physical therapist and the owner of Olympic Physical Therapy in Everett, Washington.

Mark Looper, M.S., P.T., C.O.M.T., holds a master's degree in physical therapy from the University of Southern California. He is a nationally recognized speaker, instructing for the McConnell Institute, and provides therapeutic care for the Seattle Sea Dogs, a professional indoor soccer team. Mark received his certification in manual therapy (C.O.M.T.) from the North American Institute of Manual Therapy, and is the owner of Olympic Physical Therapy in Kirkland, Washington.

Bobbi Lutack, N.D., is a naturopathic physician at Evergreen Natural Health Clinic in Seattle. Her specialty is nutrition and sports medicine.

Sarah Meeker, P.T., M.S., A.T.C., is a physical therapist and certified athletic trainer in private practice in Seattle. She specializes in manual therapy and movement re-education.

Erik Moen, P.T., is a physical therapist. He is the clinic director of PRO Sports Club Physical Therapy–Seattle. He specializes in bicycling biomechanics and bicycling-related injury rehabilitation. He holds an Elite coaching license with the U.S. Cycling Federation, is a Certified Strength and Conditioning Specialist with the National Strength and Conditioning Association, and is an active member of the American Physical Therapy Association.

Jane A. Moore, M.D., F.A.A.F.P., F.A.C.S.M., has had a private practice in family and sports medicine since 1984, currently located in Tacoma, Washington. She has much experience with women's health, U.S. swimming, and U.S. Masters swimming sports medicine.

Leslie Moskowitz, M.S., R.D., is a registered dietician living in New Jersey. She does consulting and clinical work with sports medicine and family practice patients.

David Musnick, M.D., M.P.H., is a sports and internal medicine physician at the Center for Comprehensive Medicine in Bellevue, Washington. In his private practice he specializes in disease prevention, exercise planning, functional medicine, internal medicine, nutrition, weight loss, and nonsurgical approaches to musculoskeletal injuries and pain problems. He approaches medicine from a holistic perspective. He is an instructor in the Department of Orthopaedics at the University of Washington; a lecturer and seminar instructor for physical therapists and physicians at a national level; and is on the adjunct faculty of Bastyr University. He is a physician examiner for the North American Institute of Orthopedic Manual Therapy and has studied numerous physical therapy techniques and theories. He has contributed chapters to four other books. He is a frequent lecturer for The Mountaineers Club and REI on conditioning for various outdoor activities. He has taught hiking, backpacking, cross-country skiing, rock climbing, canoeing, and mountaineering. He works out regularly and is an avid hiker, backpacker, scrambler, snowshoer, and cross-country skier. More information about David Musnick can be found at *www.comprehensivemedicalcenter.com* and *www.drm.meta-ehealth.com.*

Dan Nelson, M.S., D.C., D.A.B.C.O., is clinical director and founder of Olympic Rehabilitation Specialties. He has a master's of science in exercise physiology from the University of Washington and 13 years of experience in competitive rowing. His training in biomechanics and orthopedics has resulted in a diagnostic protocol based on identifying functional deficits. He does research with Group Health Cooperative and teaches postgraduate exercise physiology and rehabilitation at three chiropractic colleges. He emphasizes the use of osseous manipulation to enhance normal joint function coupled with exercise prescription. He is currently implementing a back fitness testing program to identify patients at risk for back problems and to help direct specific conditioning exercise programs to meet their lifestyles.

Darcy Norman, P.T., A.T.C., C.S.C.S., is a physical therapist and athletic trainer. He currently is working in Phoenix, Arizona. He has competed internationally in all four disciplines of alpine skiing.

Carl Peterson, P.T., has worked for 12 years as a physiotherapist/fitness coordinator for the Canadian Alpine Ski Team and has recently been appointed the director of sport science for Alpine Canada. He has coached and designed recovery programs for Olympic, World Champion, and World Cup medalists as well as for recreational-level athletes. Petersen, who resides in Vancouver, British Columbia, lectures nationally and internationally and has published more than 50 articles.

Mark Pierce, A.T.C., is co-owner of the Sports Reaction–Physical Therapy, Body Balance for Performance and Smart Metabolism Centers in Bellevue and Redmond, Washington. He has been a sports medicine practitioner certified by the National Athletic Trainers Association for over 20 years. He is a two-time NCAA All-American in track and field, and winner of top regional bodybuilding competitions. He is also a clinical instructor at Bastyr University and the Washington State Criminal Justice Training Association.

John Rumpeltes, P.T., is a physical therapist and owner of Olympic Physical Therapy in Seattle. He specializes in manual therapy.

Peter Shmock, C.S.C.S., is a two-time Olympian in track and field who is nationally known for his nontraditional approach to athletic performance training. He worked as the director of strength and conditioning for the Seattle Mariners for 11 years. He is a private fitness trainer for executives, youth, recreational athletes, and fitness professionals. Shmock specializes in outdoor and functional strength training; he was one of three top finalists for the Nike Fitness Innovation Award. He is the owner of ZUM, a personal training studio in Seattle.

Katrina Sullivan, D.P.M., is a podiatrist at the Joslin Clinic in Seattle.

Anne Marie Trumbold, P.T., and **Mark Trumbold**, P.T., are physical therapists at Proformance Physical Therapy in Seattle. They specialize in spine care and muscle activation techniques.

Maria Zanoni, P.T., is a physical therapist in Elm Grove, Wisconsin. She specializes in manual therapy and functional exercise.

Photo and Illustration Credits

Jock Bradley: Figures 4, 8a–c, 9, 30, 31, 33, 34, 36 and Exercises 2.1, 3, 4, 9a–b, 33.1, 33.4, 38, 39, 58.3a–b, 60a–b, 78, 78.1a–b, 78.2a–b, 78.3a–b, 78.4, 78.5a–b, 79a–b, 79.1, 79.2, 99, 99.3, 115.1, 117, 117.1, 117.2, 117.3, 120, 120.1a–b, 122a–b, 142, 144a–f, 145a–b, 146a–b, 147a–c

Scott Gaudette: Exercises 100.2, 100.3a–b, 163, 166

Michelle Lewis and Gail Smith: Figures 17, 18, 19, 35a–b and Exercises 1a–b, 2, 3.1, 5, 5.2, 7a–b, 10, 14a–b, 14.1, 15.1, 16, 17a–b, 19, 20a, 29, 31.2a–b, 32.1a–b, 34.1a–b, 35.1, 36a–b, 57, 57.3, 57.4, 58.4, 59.1, 61a–c, 62a–c, 68, 70.3a–b, 71.1a–c, 71.2a–c, 72, 73a–b, 74.1, 74.3, 75.1, 77.2a–c, 82a–b, 83a–b, 84, 85.1, 85.2, 86a–b, 92.1, 93a–b, 94.1, 97.3, 98a–b, 100a–c, 101a–b, 117.5a–b, 117.6a–b, 118.1a–b, 119a–b, 121a–b, 121.1a–b, 121.2a–b, 122a–b, 129a–b, 130a–d, 130.1a–b, 131a–b, 133, 133.2, 138, 139a–b, 141a–b

Erik Moen: Exercises 171, 173–178

Carl Peterson: Exercises 71.2d, 153, 156

Ani Rucki: Figures 2, 3, 5, 6, 11, 14, 15, 16

Cheri Ryan: Figures 24a–c, 25a–c, 26, 29, 32

Jennifer Shontz: Figure 7 and Exercises 157, 167a–b

Gavin Sisk: Exercises 6, 8.1, 20b–c, 20.1a–b, 22a–d, 23a–c, 23.1a–b, 24a–b, 24.1a–b, 25a–b, 26a–c, 27a–b, 28, 28.3a–b, 28.4, 30a–d, 30.1, 30.2, 31a–b, 31.1a–b, 40, 40.1, 41, 42a–b, 43a–d, 44a–b, 45a–b, 46a–b, 47a–b, 48a–b, 49a–b, 51, 54, 56, 63, 64, 66.1a–b, 67, 80a–c, 81a–d, 87a–b, 87.1, 87.3a–b, 88a–b, 88.1a–b, 89a–b, 90, 90.1, 91a–b, 97, 97.1, 97.2a–b, 97.5a, 97.5b–c, 97.6a–c, 102a–b, 103, 104, 104.1, 105, 106a–b, 107a–c, 108, 108.1a–b, 108.2, 108.3, 108.4a–b, 109a–b, 109.1, 109.2, 110a–b, 125.1a–b, 125.2a–b, 125.3a–b, 125.9a–b, 126.1a–b, 126.3a–b, 126.5, 127, 128, 134a–c, 134.1, 135a–c, 135.2, 135.3a–c, 180a–c, 180b, 180b

Kristy Thompson: Figures 10, 13, 20, 21, 180a–c

PhotoDisc, Inc.: Part openers, pages 23, 175, 279, and 349 © EyeWire *Outdoor Adventures* CD.

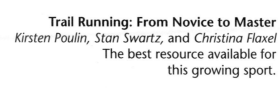

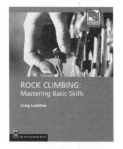

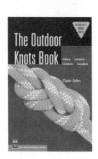

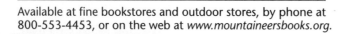